**IF YOU ARE LIVING WITH DIABETES,
YOU ARE NOT ALONE.**

In the United States, 24 million people—8% of the population—have diabetes, and 1.9 million new cases are diagnosed every year. More than 79 million people, and counting, are considered prediabetic.

**IF YOU ARE LIVING WITH DIABETES,
WHAT YOU EAT IS THE KEY
TO GOOD HEALTH.**

***THE DIABETES COUNTER*, 5th Edition**

is your one-stop guide for managing diabetes and reducing complications. This one-of-a-kind book provides carbohydrate, calorie, sugar, fiber, and fat counts for thousands of foods—all the information you need to count carbs and set up a healthy eating plan. Use this reliable meal-planning guide to customize your diet to your likes and dislikes, your culture, and your life's demands.

***Managing diabetes has never been easier!
It's up to you.***

Books by Karen J. Nolan and Jo-Ann Heslin

The Calorie Counter (Sixth Edition)

The Fat and Cholesterol Counter

The Complete Food Counter (Fourth Edition)

The Ultimate Carbohydrate Counter (Third Edition)

The Protein Counter (Third Edition)

The Diabetes Counter (Fifth Edition)

The Most Complete Food Counter (Third Edition)

Books by Annette B. Natow, Jo-Ann Heslin and Karen J. Nolan

The Cholesterol Counter (Seventh Edition)

The Fat Counter (Seventh Edition)

The Healthy Wholefoods Counter

Books by Annette B. Natow and Jo-Ann Heslin

Eating Out Food Counter

The Healthy Heart Food Counter

The Vitamin and Mineral Food Counter

Ebooks by Karen J. Nolan, Jo-Ann Heslin and Annette B. Natow

The Most Complete Food Counter (Second Edition)

The DIABETES COUNTER

Fifth Edition

Karen J. Nolan, Ph.D.
and Jo-Ann Heslin, M.A., R.D.

GALLERY BOOKS
New York London Toronto Sydney New Delhi

Gallery Books
An Imprint of Simon & Schuster, LLC
1230 Avenue of the Americas
New York, NY 10020

This Gallery Books trade paperback edition November 2024

GALLERY BOOKS and colophon are registered trademarks of Simon & Schuster, LLC

Simon & Schuster: Celebrating 100 Years of Publishing in 2024

For information about special discounts for bulk purchases, please contact Simon & Schuster Special Sales at 1-866-506-1949 or business@simonandschuster.com.

The Simon & Schuster Speakers Bureau can bring authors to your live event. For more information or to book an event, contact the Simon & Schuster Speakers Bureau at 1-866-248-3049 or visit our website at www.simonspeakers.com.

Manufactured in the United States of America

10 9 8 7 6 5 4 3 2 1

ISBN 978-1-6680-8500-4

The authors and publisher of this book are not physicians and are not licensed to give medical advice. The information in this book has been collected for the convenience of the reader. The nutrient values for prepared foods are subject to change and may now differ from listings herein, which are based on research conducted prior to Summer 2013. Such information does not constitute a recommendation or endorsement of any individual, institution, or product, nor is it intended as a substitute for personalized consultation with your physician. The authors and publisher disclaim any liability arising directly or indirectly from the use of this book.

For
Our families,
who support us through every project.

ACKNOWLEDGMENTS

For all her continuous support and help, our agent, Nancy Trichter.

For her suggestions and editing skills, Sara Clemence.

For all her patience, comments, and questions—our favorite reviewer, Jean Schwarsin.

Without the tireless cooperation of Stephen Llano and the production department at Pocket Books, *The Diabetes Counter*, 5th edition, would never have been completed.

A special thank-you to our editor, Emilia Pisani.

And we would like to thank all of our readers for their suggestions and questions. Your input helps us provide you with the most useful information.

The regulation of the diet is the most important consideration in the treatment of diabetes mellitus. . . . While certain general principles in regard to diet for diabetes can be laid down, each patient presents an individual problem. . . .

Mary Swartz Rose, Ph.D.
Feeding the Family
The Macmillan Company, 1919

CONTENTS

INTRODUCTION

You've just been told that you have diabetes.

OR

Someone close to you has diabetes.

OR

Your doctor said you have risk factors that increase your chance of getting diabetes in the near future.

Every day, 5200 new cases of diabetes are diagnosed in the U.S. At first, most newly diagnosed people feel devastated. Having to change the way they eat, and being told to lose weight, to exercise, and to take medication is overwhelming. But there is good news. Diabetes is a condition over which you have a great deal of control. And the more control you exercise, the healthier and more complication-free your life will be. Most importantly, you can look forward to a very long life.

There is no question that being diagnosed with diabetes is a jolt—emotionally, physically, and even socially. It is a condition that requires constant attention and modifications in how you lead your life. It isn't unusual to feel down. If you do, discuss your feelings with your doctor. Depression can be caused by feeling that you can no longer control your body and your life. But you can.

With some adjustments, life will be normal again—and sooner than you think. Initially, it is going to take work on your part and a commitment to follow your doctor's orders. The payoff is that your body will respond—in ways that may amaze you—to your new diet, exercise, and medication plan.

The two major goals of *The Diabetes Counter,* 5th Edition are:

- To give you the tools needed to understand and manage diabetes, whether you are newly diagnosed or trying to fine-tune your management plan.
- To sort through the research and provide you with accurate, current information on meal planning, carbohydrate counting, using sugar, understanding fiber, and the value of the glycemic index.

You Should Know—

Knowledge Is Power

The more you know about diabetes,
the better you can take care of yourself
and the healthier you will be.

Let's get started putting you in control.

UNDERSTANDING DIABETES

What is diabetes?

Diabetes is a group of conditions that results in too much sugar in your blood. After you eat cereal and juice at breakfast, the food is broken down into a sugar called *glucose,* which floods into your bloodstream. Your blood carries glucose to cells throughout your body. *Insulin,* a hormone made by the pancreas, is spilled into the bloodstream to help glucose move from the bloodstream into muscles, where it is burned for energy to keep your body functioning. Glucose may also be moved into fat cells to be stored for future use. With diabetes, either your body no longer makes insulin (type 1) or your body can't use the insulin it makes (type 2).

Insulin resistance happens when your body's cells don't recognize insulin and glucose can't get out of the bloodstream into the cells. This creates a buildup of sugar in the blood. To compensate, the pancreas pumps out more insulin. Now the blood has both too much sugar and too much insulin because the route into the cells is not working. Having too much insulin or too much sugar in your blood will cause damage to important body cells over time.

> **Preventing Insulin Resistance**
>
> ***Lose weight***—*Losing weight makes fat and muscle cells more sensitive to insulin.*
>
> ***Eat right***—*Eat lots of fruits and vegetables, choose whole grains, use more avocado, nut, olive, and canola oils, which make cells more responsive to insulin.*
>
> ***Move it and lift it***—*Exercise of all kinds improves insulin resistance.*
>
> ***Get enough sleep***—*Aim for at least 7 to 8 hours each night. Research shows 1 night of poor sleep can decrease insulin sensitivity in cells by 25%.*

For more information on insulin resistance, see pages 13 to 16.

What causes diabetes?

In most cases, it's your genes. But some very new research shows that changes in the way your cells work could trigger diabetes, too. In the U.S., over 8% of the population has diabetes—that's close to 26 million people. It's estimated that a person born in 2000 has a 1 in 3 chance of developing diabetes in their lifetime.

But the good news—are you getting the picture, that there is always good news?—is that lifestyle choices can alter the action of your genes and prevent changes in the way your cells function.

Just because you carry the risk for diabetes doesn't mean you will get diabetes. People who lead the healthiest lives are 80% less likely to develop diabetes. Those who stay slim, exercise regularly, don't smoke, and eat generally healthy diets decrease their odds of developing diabetes no matter what their genetic profiles say. People with diabetes can control the condition, and in some cases even reverse it, with lifestyle changes.

You Should Know—

- *1.9 million new cases of diabetes are diagnosed every year.*
- *7 million people have diabetes and don't know it.*
- *79 million Americans have prediabetes, putting them at risk for type 2 diabetes in the future.*

It is important to be tested.

What puts a person at risk for diabetes?

The risk of developing diabetes increases with each of the following that apply to you.

- Being 45 or older
- Being overweight
- Having a parent or close relative with diabetes

- Being African-American, American Indian, Asian-American, Pacific Islander, or Hispanic/Latino American
- Having had diabetes during pregnancy
- Giving birth to a baby weighing more than 9 pounds
- Having high blood pressure
- Having high cholesterol
- Having high triglycerides
- Exercising very little or not at all
- Having polycystic ovary syndrome (a disorder affecting the female reproductive system)
- Having dark, thickened skin around the neck or armpits (acanthosis nigricans)
- Having a history of blood vessel disease
- Having higher than normal blood glucose levels at previous screenings

What are the symptoms of diabetes?

Diabetes often goes undetected for a long time because many people have no symptoms—or they ignore symptoms because they seem harmless. See your doctor if you experience any of the following problems.

- Being very thirsty
- Needing to urinate frequently
- Being very hungry
- Unexplained weight loss

- Feeling tired and weak
- Blurry vision
- Cuts and bruises that heal very slowly, or do not heal at all
- Tingling or numbness in your hands or feet
- Recurring or hard-to-heal infections
- Annoying itching

Asian-Americans at Higher Risk

- *Often doctors do not routinely screen Asian-Americans for diabetes because they are slim.*
- *If you are of Asian descent (and 13 million Americans now identify themselves as at least part Asian), you have a 60% higher risk for diabetes than non-Hispanic whites.*
- *Your risk of developing type 2 diabetes increases for each generation that your family has lived in the U.S.*

How is diabetes diagnosed?

Your doctor can screen for diabetes when you have blood tests. Everyone over the age of 45 should be screened. If everything is normal, screenings should be repeated every 3 years. Younger individuals need to be tested earlier if they have a number of the risk factors noted above. Children who are overweight should be tested periodically, too.

Screening Tests for Diabetes

Random Blood Glucose—*Your doctor checks your blood glucose without regard to when you last ate. A normal result is less than 200. If your results are normal, you will be retested at some time in the future based on your risk.*

Fasting Blood Glucose—*Your doctor tests your blood after you have not eaten for at least 8 hours. Results below 100 are normal. Between 100 and 125 indicates you may have prediabetes, which signals your risk of developing diabetes in the future. If the results are 126 or higher, the test is usually repeated on another day. If the numbers stay high, this confirms a diagnosis of diabetes.*

Oral Glucose Tolerance Test—*Your blood is tested in the morning after you have not eaten for at least 10 hours, then it is tested a second time 2 hours after you drink a sweetened beverage. Results of 139 or below are normal. Between 140 and 199 indicates you have prediabetes. Results over 200 indicate diabetes. Some doctors repeat the results on another day just to confirm the diagnosis.*

A1C—*A nonfasting blood sample is taken to get a snapshot of your blood sugar levels over the last 3 months. Values between 5.7 to 6.4 indicate a risk for prediabetes. Values over 6.5 indicate a risk for diabetes. Those at very high risk may be screened annually; those at moderate to high risk can be screened every 3 to 5 years.*

How do I manage my diabetes?

Diet, exercise, and medication all play roles in managing diabetes. Once you're diagnosed, your primary care doctor will help you organize your health care team, a group of health professionals who will help manage all aspects of your condition. The most important member of the team is YOU.

Every person with type 2 diabetes is different. A one-size-fits-all treatment plan simply won't work. It is all about YOU—what you can do and what you are willing to do. Personalization has to be the cornerstone of an effective treatment plan. The American Diabetes Association (ADA) and the European Association for the Study of Diabetes (EASD) are both advocating an individualized patient-centered approach to diabetes care.

Patient-centered care is responsive to what the person wants, their values, and to some degree what medications they are willing to use. This approach may seem like you are receiving less-than-effective treatment, but even the best instructions are useless if they are not followed. Treatment options that you agree to and are willing to follow, even when not optimum, will provide better results.

Only you know how you feel. You will be the first to notice any problems. And you will set the pace for what you are willing and able to do. The rest of the team depends on you to be honest and to thoroughly report on your home care.

YOUR HEALTH CARE TEAM

Health Professional	Seen How Often	To Help You With
Primary Care Doctor	Every 3 months	Providing general care Monitoring blood sugar Referring you to other specialists
Certified Diabetes Educator (CDE) May be a nurse or dietitian with special training in diabetes management	As needed	Putting your drug, diet, exercise, and daily care plan in place Managing problems such as sick days Answering all questions about your self-care routine
Registered Dietitian (RD) May also be a CDE	As needed	Setting up a meal plan tailored to your treatment goals and personal choices
Eye doctor	Yearly	Monitoring the health of your eyes Preventing and treating complications from diabetes

(continued)

Health Professional	Seen How Often	To Help You With
Podiatrist	As needed	Caring for your feet and lower legs To treat corns, calluses, sores
Dentist	Twice yearly	Monitoring the health of your mouth Preventing or treating gum disease and infections

You Should Know—

The evidence shows that those who get counseling from a certified diabetes educator (CDE) or a registered dietitian (RD) are more capable of managing their diabetes. These services are often covered by insurance and always covered by Medicare. You will benefit from this help.

TYPES OF DIABETES

Diabetes—or, more correctly, *diabetes mellitus*—is a group of similar conditions all resulting in the same outcome: too much sugar in the blood.

Why one person develops diabetes and another does not is the result of a complicated interaction between genes and environment. Researchers classify diabetes into four main groups—type 1, type 2, pregnancy diabetes, and "from other causes." This last group accounts for a very small percentage of cases in which the development of diabetes is usually secondary to another condition like Down syndrome.

Type 2

This is by far the most common form, accounting for a whopping 90% to 95% of people with diabetes.

You Should Know—

Approximately 50% of men and 70% of women who develop type 2 diabetes are overweight. Weighing less could delay the onset of the disease—and in some cases prevent diabetes entirely.

The number of people with this condition is increasing daily, and experts believe that as time goes on more and more people, even children, will develop type 2 diabetes because so many people are overweight and inactive. Couple this with the fact that our population is aging (type 2 is most common in those over 30), and the number of new cases could be overwhelming.

You Should Know—

Type 2 and Kids

- *One in three children diagnosed with diabetes has type 2, largely due to the dramatic increase in childhood obesity that has taken place over the last 3 decades.*
- *In 2013 the American Academy of Pediatrics published the first guidelines to help doctors manage type 2 diabetes in children.*

Maintaining a normal weight could prevent many of these cases.

With type 2 diabetes, your body is unable to effectively use the hormone insulin, which is produced by the pancreas. The cells don't recognize insulin, so the hormone can't attach to cells to help deliver glucose (blood sugar) into cells to be used for energy. This is referred to as insulin resistance—cells become resistant to recognizing and using insulin.

To better understand insulin resistance, it might be helpful to understand how insulin works. After you eat, your digestive tract breaks down the carbohydrate (starches and sugars) you eat into simple sugars that pass into your bloodstream. When the sugar in the blood reaches a certain level, the pancreas is signaled to release insulin to move the sugar out of the blood and into the cells, where it is either burned as energy or stored for future use. If the cells are insulin resistant, insulin builds up in the blood, along with excess sugar.

To try to get around this problem, the pancreas makes more insulin in the early stages of insulin resistance. At first this works, but after a while the pancreas gets exhausted from all the extra work, and it loses its ability to make enough insulin.

The reasons why insulin resistance develops are not completely understood, but several factors do increase your risk.

- Does anyone else in the family have insulin resistance or diabetes?
- Are you overweight?
- Are you inactive?
- Are you dealing with other health issues?
- Are you taking medication that may contribute to insulin resistance?
- Are you older?

You Should Know—

Why Insulin Overload Is Unhealthy

Insulin resistance happens when the body's cells don't recognize and use insulin.

Too much insulin in the bloodstream:

- *Increases the risk for type 2 diabetes*
- *Impairs kidney function, increasing the risk for high blood pressure and gout*
- *Increases the risk for polycystic ovary syndrome (PCOS)*
- *Lowers good HDL cholesterol and raises bad LDL cholesterol*
- *Raises triglycerides*
- *Increases the risk for liver disease*
- *Increases the risk for dementia*
- *Increases the risk for certain cancers*

The good news about type 2 diabetes is that it can be managed very effectively by lifestyle changes—diet, weight loss, exercise, and, when needed, medication and possibly insulin. Don't be discouraged; much of the control is in your hands. In some cases type 2 diabetes can actually be reversed.

You Should Know—

Research Has Shown

Eating less meat and fatty food and more salads and cooked vegetables reduces the risk of developing type 2 diabetes.

Alzheimer's Disease and Diabetes

New research shows that the memory loss in Alzheimer's disease could be caused by insulin resistance in the brain. When this happens, brain cells don't recognize insulin, which prevents glucose from entering the cells to be used for energy. Insulin not only helps brain cells use glucose but also promotes their growth, survival, repair, and normal functioning. Over time, high insulin levels in the brain increase the risk for memory loss. Preventing insulin resistance and controlling diabetes may lower the risk for Alzheimer's.

Type 1

In the past, this form of diabetes was called *juvenile diabetes* because most people developed it in childhood or early adulthood, but it can occur at any age. Only 5% to 10% of people with diabetes have type 1. It develops when something happens to destroy the cells in the pancreas that produce insulin. A person with type 1 cannot make any insulin and must supply it daily by injection, through an insulin pump, or in a recently approved inhalable form. The amount of insulin taken daily must be balanced with diet and exercise. There is no known way to prevent type 1, and it cannot be reversed.

Pregnancy Diabetes

Gestational diabetes mellitus occurs only during pregnancy and usually disappears after the baby is born. Over 230,000 women who have babies each year have gestational diabetes. Being overweight or having a family history of diabetes can increase a woman's risk. To prevent problems, all pregnant women are tested. If their blood sugar levels are too high, they are taught to adjust their food intake and may be given insulin until their baby is delivered. Having pregnancy diabetes increases a woman's risk of developing type 2 diabetes in the next 5 to 10 years.

You Should Know—

Treating pregnancy diabetes is not only important to the health of the mother but it also reduces the baby's risk for childhood obesity. A pregnant woman with untreated diabetes has an 82% higher risk of her child being overweight by age 5 to 7.

Complications

The key to being healthy and avoiding complications from diabetes is working with your health team to keep your blood sugar down, your blood pressure down, your blood fats low, and taking your medication or insulin as prescribed.

You Should Know—

Diabetes Is Serious

Terms such as "a touch of diabetes," "mild diabetes," or "my sugar is a little high" shouldn't be used, because they minimize a serious health problem.

Regardless of the type, when diabetes is not well controlled you are at risk for complications—heart disease, stroke, eye disease, kidney disease, nerve damage, gum disease, tooth loss, and even amputations. It's a pretty scary list. But as we said before, with the bad news comes some really good news. *Serious complications are not inevitable.*

- Keeping blood sugar levels within the normal range can reduce the risk of eye, kidney, and nerve problems by as much as 40%.
- Reducing your systolic blood pressure (the top number) by 10 reduces the risk for all complications by 12%.
- Lowering blood fats (triglycerides and cholesterol) can reduce the risk of heart disease and stroke by 20% to 50%.
- Visiting your eye doctor regularly can reduce the risk of vision problems by 50% to 60%.

- Visiting your podiatrist regularly can reduce amputation rate by 45% to 85%.

The most important thing you need to know about diabetes is that you are in control. By keeping your condition under control, you reduce your risk for complications and serious health problems.

You Should Know—

Diabetes and Infections Are Linked

High blood sugar levels smother or block systems in your body that detect and fight infections. High blood sugar can put you at greater risk for viral infections, the flu, or even heart disease, which has its roots in inflammation in the body.

A Word About Prediabetes

Prediabetes is not a disease but a condition that doubles your risk for heart disease and quadruples your risk for diabetes. With prediabetes your blood sugar levels are higher than normal but not high enough for a diagnosis of diabetes. It is estimated that 79 million adults in the U.S. have prediabetes. Over age 65, 50% have prediabetes. If we don't reduce the incidence of prediabetes soon, there could be a major increase in heart disease and type 2 diabetes over the next 20 years.

The guidelines for prediabetes were set by experts so they could catch and treat as many people as possible to prevent more serious problems like heart attack, stroke, and type 2 diabetes. Testing is important, because those with prediabetes can do a great deal to delay and prevent type 2 diabetes from developing.

Should you be tested for prediabetes?

- If you are over 45 and your weight is normal, your doctor will decide if you should be tested based on your health history.
- Yes, if you are over age 45 and overweight.
- Yes, if you are younger than 45 and overweight and you have high blood pressure, low HDL cholesterol, high triglycerides, family history of diabetes, history of diabetes in pregnancy, or belong to an ethnic group at higher risk.

Your doctor can use any one of the following tests to screen for prediabetes.

- A1C is a blood test that gives a snapshot of the average amount of glucose in your blood over the last 3 months. Prediabetes A1C levels range from 5.7 to 6.4.
- Fasting blood glucose (FPG) requires fasting overnight. Blood glucose is measured before eating. A person has prediabetes when FPG measures 100 to 125.
- Oral glucose tolerance test (OGTT) also requires fasting overnight. Blood is tested before eating and again 2 hours after drinking a glucose-rich drink. OGTT values of 140 to 199 indicate prediabetes.

If your results are normal, testing should be done every 3 years. If your results indicate prediabetes, you should be retested yearly.

If untreated, people with prediabetes are likely to develop diabetes within 10 years. Without treatment, women tend to progress from prediabetes to diabetes faster than men. But this is not inevitable. With treatment and lifestyle changes, prediabetes can be reversed and may never develop into type 2 diabetes.

If you have prediabetes, losing 5% to 7% of your current weight and walking 2.5 hours a week can reduce your risk of developing diabetes by 58%. For people over age 60, the risk goes down over 70%.

You Should Know—

It is estimated that only 7% of those with prediabetes have been tested and are aware of the condition.

Increased testing and treatment for prediabetes could prevent millions of cases of type 2 diabetes and save billions in health care dollars.

SETTING YOUR WEIGHT LOSS GOALS

How much weight do I have to lose to control my diabetes?

Your health care team will help you set your specific weight loss goals, but any weight loss is beneficial—even a few pounds can be significant. A loss of between 10 and 20 pounds, which can be accomplished in 3 to 4 months, will improve type 2 diabetes remarkably. Your blood sugar will drop, your cholesterol and triglycerides will go down, you'll have more energy, and you'll look and feel better. You may even find you're able to reduce or possibly eliminate medication.

How much should I weigh?

There are many ways to determine your best weight or target weight, including weight charts, equations, even guesstimates. Your doctor, diabetes educator, or dietitian can help you with this step. But, a very easy way to "guess" at a good target weight is:

Multiply your weight at age 20 by 1.2
For example, if you weighed 135 pounds in your early 20s
$135 \times 1.2 = 162$ pounds

Your target weight should be 162 pounds or less. This may not be as thin as you wish to be, but it is a reasonable goal to shoot for and will give you health benefits.

You Should Know—

10% Is Great!

Losing 10% of your body weight—15 pounds for someone who weighs 150 pounds, 20 pounds for a person weighing 200 pounds, or 30 pounds if the scale tips in at 300 pounds—is all that is needed to significantly improve your health.

Lose 10% of your current body weight and you'll have:

- *Lower blood sugar*
- *Lower blood pressure*
- *Improved cholesterol levels*
- *Better sex*

How many calories should I eat every day?

As with target weight, your doctor may give you a daily calorie intake to aim for. Here's a way to determine how many calories to eat each day.

First you need to know your target weight, which you can get by using the equation above. Second, select an activity factor that fits your current activity level.

1. Your target weight is: ____
2. Your activity factor is: ____
   - 20 = Very active men
   - 15 = Moderately active men or very active women
   - 13 = Inactive men, moderately active women, and people over 55
   - 10 = Inactive women, repeat dieters, seriously overweight people
3. Target Weight × Activity Factor = Calories needed each day

For example, if your target weight is 162 and you are an inactive woman (factor 10), you need about 1600 calories a day.

162 pounds × 10 = 1620 calories

Eating 1600 calories each day will guarantee weight loss because you are getting only enough calories to support your target weight, not your current, heavier weight. Couple this reduced calorie intake with some added exercise and the pounds will come off even faster.

You Should Know—

Your Weight Loss Goals

Your target weight is: ____

Your daily calorie intake is: ____

Why is exercise so important?

Daily exercise helps control your blood sugar, maintain your target weight, and reduce your risk for heart disease. Research suggests that those with type 2 diabetes should aim for a goal of 90 to 150 minutes of exercise each week.

Everything counts—gardening, doing housework, bowling, and even walking around window shopping.

> **You Should Know—**
>
> *Taking an escalator up 3 flights of stairs burns 3 calories, walking 3 flights burns more than 20 calories.*

If you rarely exercise, start slowly.

- Try to be active every day.
- Start walking—even short walks. Park at the edge of the parking lot or walk around the mall once before shopping.
- Stop using the drive-thru at the bank and coffee shop.
- Walk in place during TV commercials.
- Aim for 30 minutes of activity each day; you can accumulate this by doing short periods of activity (10 minutes or less) throughout the day.

You Should Know—

Every Step Counts

People who consistently increased the number of steps they walked daily, over a 5-year period, to an ultimate goal of 10,000 steps reduced their risk for diabetes and improved insulin resistance. Keep walking.

LET'S TALK ABOUT FOOD

We know that when you are first diagnosed with diabetes, it's overwhelming. There are so many things to manage—your weight, your blood sugar, your food, your medication, how much you exercise. So, when it comes to food, let's take it slowly. We'll go step by step, and before you know it you'll be a pro at planning meals and choosing the right foods.

The first question everyone asks is, "What can I eat, now that I have diabetes?" The simple answer is "everything." No foods are off limits. It's when you eat and how much you eat that you need to watch.

Meal Planning

At first the idea of planning all your meals and snacks can be stressful. Relax. It isn't that hard. Start slowly. First, become accustomed to regular serving sizes, which are probably smaller than what you now eat. Stick with the smaller, regular sizes as often as you can. Next, work on spacing meals and snacks throughout the day, and try to keep to this schedule daily. Then work on making the best selections each time you eat.

That will probably involve counting calories and carbohydrates.

In the beginning, counting carbs is smart because it will help you learn a great deal about the foods you eat, and you'll become very skilled at making choices. Your certified diabetes educator or registered dietitian will be a great resource for meal planning and carb counting. We'll help get you started with both, as well.

Meal Planning Hints

Do: Eat regular meals and aim for the same amount of food at about the same time each day

- Choose regular serving sizes
- Eat moderately sized meals
- Choose foods with carbohydrate and fiber at each meal and each snack
- Include a good source of protein at each meal
- Choose foods low in fat
- Bring food with you so you don't miss a meal or snack

Go easy: On foods containing sugar
On foods containing saturated fat
On alcohol

Don't: Skip meals or snacks
Overeat

You Should Know—

When researchers compared people who ate on an irregular schedule to those who ate meals at regular times each day, they found that those with the regular meal pattern had lower blood sugar, lower cholesterol, and lower LDL (bad) cholesterol.

As we said earlier, you are the most important member of your health care team. Only you can decide what you can and will do to manage your diabetes.

The American Diabetes Association (ADA) recommends the following approach to managing diabetes:

Lose weight if needed
Be active daily
Eat a healthy diet

Lifestyle changes are not one-size-fits-all. The ADA further recommends that you consider:

Your life circumstances
Your culture
Your heritage
Your food likes and dislikes
Your willingness to make changes

Let's look at some good advice for healthy living—which works whether you have diabetes or not. If you didn't pay too much attention to what you ate or how much you exercised in the past, these guidelines will help you begin to make better choices.

Carbohydrates

Paying attention to carbohydrates is important. With diabetes, your body has limited ability to use carbs. It is important to eat the right kind, in the right amount, spaced out between meals and snacks.

- Include whole grain breads and cereals, fruits, vegetables, and lowfat milk in your meals and snacks.
- Keep track of the amount of carbohydrates you eat each day; include carbs at every meal and snack.
- It's OK to use low calorie and no calorie sweeteners.
- It's OK to eat sugar and foods containing sugar, but eat small amounts and count the sugar you eat in the day's total carbohydrate amount.
- Eat sugar and sugary foods with meals or snacks, not alone.

Fat

It is important to pay attention to fats, too. Having diabetes increases your risk for heart disease. Eating the right fats can help you control this risk.

- Eating less fat overall will help you lose weight and reduce your cholesterol.
- Eat more of the foods that contain "good" (monounsaturated) fats—like olive oil, avocado oil, grapeseed oil, canola oil, seeds, and nuts.
- Eat moderate amounts of the foods that contain polyunsaturated fat—including margarine, corn oil, vegetable oil, and salad dressing.

- Eat less of the foods that contain saturated fat—like meat, whole milk, butter, and cheese.

Protein

Some experts feel that adding more protein to your diet can help to manage diabetes more effectively and helps with weight loss.

- Eat lean protein sources like poultry without skin, lean beef and pork, fish, and lowfat or nonfat dairy products.
- Include some protein at every meal, but try to avoid very large portions.
- Eating eggs is fine; they are an excellent protein source.

Regular Serving Sizes

Most of us have portion perceptions that are out of whack—what we think of as a "normal" portion of food, whether we make it at home or eat it in a restaurant, is often much larger than it should be. At first, use measuring cups, spoons, or a kitchen scale to get used to the size of a normal portion. The following information will help you get started.

WHAT IS A SERVING?

Food	Serving Size
Breads, cereals, high carb foods	
bread	*1 slice*
roll, bun, or pita pocket	*½*
crackers	*4 to 6*
tortilla	*1 (6 inches across)*
cereal, cooked	*½ cup*
cereal, ready-to-eat	*¾ cup*
rice, cooked	*⅓ cup*
pasta, cooked	*½ cup*
popcorn	*3 cups*
Vegetables and fruits	
raw or cooked vegetables	*½ cup*
raw or cooked leafy greens	*1 cup*
green peas	*½ cup*
beans	*¼ cup*
potato	*1 small*
mashed potatoes	*½ cup*
French fries	*10 pieces*
fresh fruit	*1 small*
banana	*½ regular or 1 very small*
dried fruit	*2 tablespoons*
canned fruit	*½ cup*
juice	*½ cup*
Milk, yogurt, cheese	
nonfat or lowfat milk	*1 cup*
nonfat or lowfat yogurt	*1 cup*

(continued)

Food	Serving Size
cheese	*1 ounce or 1 slice*
cottage cheese	*½ cup*
ice cream	*½ cup*
Meat, poultry, fish	
cooked	*3 to 4 ounces*
Eggs	
egg, cooked	*1*
Fats	
butter or margarine	*1 teaspoon*
cream cheese	*2 tablespoons*
salad dressing	*2 tablespoons*
oil	*1 tablespoon*
peanut butter	*2 tablespoons*
Sugar	
sugar	*1 teaspoon*
honey	*1 teaspoon*
syrup	*2 tablespoons*

Eventually, you'll know just by looking how much you should be eating as a serving of food. Visual cues can be very useful as portion guides.

You Should Know—

Seeing Is Believing

These visual cues will help you keep portion sizes reasonable.

computer mouse	=	*4-ounce portion of meat, chicken, seafood* *or* *1 medium baked potato*
yo-yo	=	*a mini bagel or 100 calories (How many yo-yos fit into your bagel, muffin, or pastry?)*
music CD	=	*1 medium pancake or small waffle*
tennis ball	=	*medium piece of fresh fruit*
ping-pong ball	=	*2 ounces cheese* *or* *2 tablespoons salad dressing, gravy, sour cream*
quarter	=	*1 pat butter*

COUNTING CARBS

Everyone who has diabetes should know how to count carbs. Some people do it every day, some do it a few days a week to check on how they are doing, and others do it occasionally. Your certified diabetes educator (CDE) or registered dietitian (RD) will help you identify the system that is best for you.

You've got a great resource right in front of you. *The Diabetes Counter* has the carb counts for over 12,000 foods. You can look up any food you eat and know exactly how many carbs are in a serving.

The goals of carbohydrate counting are to:

- Learn which foods have carb
- Know how much carb is in each food
- Count up the carb in each meal
- Count up the carb in each snack
- Aim to eat the same amount of carb each day

Finding Carbohydrate Foods

You know that bread, pasta, cereal, and potatoes have carb. But did you know that fruits, vegetables, cakes, ice cream, candy, jelly, cookies, sugar, milk, and beans have carb, too? Some have more, some have less.

You Should Know—

Which Has More Carb?

Whole milk or skim milk?
White bread or whole wheat bread?
White sugar or brown sugar?
The carb count in each pair is the same.
The color of a food or the amount of fat does not change the amount of carb.

People are creatures of habit, and most people only regularly eat about 35 foods. A simple way to get familiar with the carb counts in foods is to list your favorites on the following chart, Carbs in My Favorite Foods. Then look up how much carb is in each food and check on pages 32–33 to be sure you are eating a normal portion size.

This might seem time consuming, but it is a really valuable exercise. This sheet will serve as a quick reference when you are planning meals and snacks. You may eventually make a number of these lists—one for each group of foods you eat. We've also had people tell us they make a list of possible options before going out to eat so they can make the best choices from a restaurant menu. There are many uses for a tool like this. You'll probably come up with your own interesting ways of using it.

CARBS IN MY FAVORITE FOODS

Food I Usually Eat	Normal Serving Size	Grams of Carbohydrate

Your Daily Carb Budget

An easy way to help you divide carbs into meals and snacks is to think about the amount of carb you can eat each day like a budget. If you had $40 a day and were told to buy 3 meals and 2 snacks, you would budget your money to cover all your food. It's the same idea with carbs. Your certified diabetes educator or registered dietitian will help you set up your carb budget.

We recommend that 40% to 60% of your daily calories come from carb. But people don't think in terms of percentages—you just want to know what foods you can eat and when. First we have to determine how much carb you can eat each day based on the amount of calories you are eating daily. On page 24 you figured out how many calories you needed each day. Find that number on the following chart, **My Daily Calories and Carbs,** and you'll find a target amount of carbs to eat. This number may vary slightly if you have already set up a carb budget with your diabetes educator, but the concept will remain the same.

MY DAILY CALORIES AND CARBS			
Calories Each Day	Grams of Carb Each Day		
	40% of Calories	50% of Calories	60% of Calories
1200	120	150	180
1300	130	160	195
1400	140	175	210
1500	150	190	225
1600	160	200	240
1700	170	215	255
1800	180	225	270
1900	190	240	285
2000	200	250	300
2100	210	265	315
2200	220	275	330
2300	230	290	345
2400	240	300	360
2500	250	315	375
2600	260	325	390
2700	270	340	405
2800	280	350	420

You Should Know—

Your Daily Carb Budget

Each day I can eat

Calories ____

Carbs ____

Carbohydrate-containing foods have the greatest impact on your blood sugar. Eat too many carbs and your blood sugar goes up; eat too few and your blood sugar may drop too low. Eat the right amount and your diabetes will be well controlled.

You Should Know—

Counting carbs counts toward managing your diabetes and keeping you healthy.

LET'S EAT—
PUTTING IT ALL TOGETHER

Okay, you are ready to take charge. You know how many calories you need each day. You know how much carb to eat each day. You are starting to understand how to identify foods with carb and why it is important to keep track of how much you eat. Now let's put all that information to use by planning meals and snacks for the day.

It's important to try to eat your meals and snacks at the same time each day. This timing helps your body use the carbs you eat and helps keep your blood sugar normal. If there is a long time between meals, your blood sugar could drop very low. If you eat fewer, large meals your blood sugar may go up too high.

> **You Should Know—**
>
> *Consistency in daily carb intake has been shown to be the best way to control blood sugar.*

What Is a Carb Choice?

1 carb choice = 15 grams of carbohydrate
1 slice of bread = 15 grams of carbohydrate

The easiest way to understand carb choices is to compare everything to a slice of bread, which contains 15 grams of carb, making it 1 carb choice. If you look up a food, such as a slice of apple pie, and you see that it has 45 grams of carb, it equals 3 slices of bread, or 3 carb choices. If that doesn't fit into your carb budget, you can eat half a slice of pie or pick something similar, like a baked apple, which is lower in carb. Other typical carb choices, all of which have 15 grams of carb, are on the following chart, **Carb Choices**.

CARB CHOICES

1 CARB CHOICE = 15 GRAMS OF CARBOHYDRATE

Breads and Cereals	Fruits	Vegetables
⅓ cup cooked rice	½ banana	⅓ cup beans
½ roll	1 small apple, orange, peach	½ cup green peas
1 (4-inch) pancake	4 fresh apricots	½ cup corn
½ cup cooked cereal	1 cup cut-up melon	½ cup plantain
¾ cup ready-to-eat cereal (unsweetened)	12 cherries	½ cup boiled or mashed potato
½ cup ready-to-eat cereal (sweetened)	18 grapes	1 cup winter squash
8 animal crackers	½ papaya	
6 saltines	½ cup unsweetened canned fruit	
3 cups popcorn	¾ cup fresh berries	
½ cup pasta	1 cup fresh strawberries	
	1¼ cups cubed watermelon	
	½ cup fruit juice	
	⅓ cup prune juice	

Planning Your Day

Let's assume you can eat 1800 calories a day. A person eating 1800 calories a day, whose daily meal plan aims for 50% of calories from carb, can eat 225 grams of carb each day. (See the chart on page 39, My Daily Calories and Carbs.) If you divide 225 by 15, you will find out how many carb choices you can eat.

225 ÷ 15 = 15 carb choices a day
Daily Carbs ÷ 1 Carb Choice = Number of Carb Choices allowed each day

If your daily meal plan calls for less carb or more carb, you can find the number of your daily carb choices the same way.

For example, 1800 calories a day with 40% carb calories equals 180 grams of carb daily.

180 ÷ 15 = 12 carb choices a day

1800 calories a day with 60% carb calories equals 270 grams of carb daily.

270 ÷ 15 = 18 carb choices a day

Trust us—the rest is simple. Here are some basic meal planning tips to help you get started.

- Divide your carb budget for the day between your meals and snacks
- Eat some carb at every meal
  Women: eat at least 2 to 3 carb choices at each meal
  Men: eat at least 3 to 4 carb choices at each meal

- Eat at least 1 carb at every snack; eat at least 2 snacks a day
- Include a protein choice or a fat choice at each meal or snack
- Do not eat carb alone—it will make your blood sugar rise too high
- Don't skip meals

The following Sample Day for Women and for Men uses the example we started above for a person eating 1800 calories a day, including 15 carb choices.

SAMPLE DAY 1800 CALORIES FOR WOMEN

Dividing Your Daily Carb Budget Between Meals and Snacks

Daily Carb Budget: 15 Carb Choices, or 225 grams Carb

Breakfast	3	*Carb choices*	=	45	*grams Carb*
AM Snack	1	*Carb choice*	=	15	*grams Carb*
Lunch	4	*Carb choices*	=	60	*grams Carb*
PM Snack	1	*Carb choice*	=	15	*grams Carb*
Dinner	4	*Carb choices*	=	60	*grams Carb*
Night Snack	2	*Carb choices*	=	30	*grams Carb*
Total	**15**	**Carb choices**	=	**225**	**total grams Carb**

The main difference between the Sample Day for Women and the Sample Day for Men is the way carbs are divided between meals and snacks. Women should eat 2 to 3 carb choices at each meal; men should eat 3 to 4 carb choices at each meal.

SAMPLE DAY 1800 CALORIES FOR MEN

Dividing Your Daily Carb Budget Between Meals and Snacks

Daily Carb Budget: 15 Carb Choices, or 225 grams Carb

Breakfast	4	*Carb choices*	=	60	*grams Carb*
AM Snack	1	*Carb choice*	=	15	*grams Carb*
Lunch	4	*Carb choices*	=	60	*grams Carb*
PM Snack	1	*Carb choice*	=	15	*grams Carb*
Dinner	4	*Carb choices*	=	60	*grams Carb*
Night Snack	1	*Carb choice*	=	15	*grams Carb*
Total	**15**	**Carb choices**	=	**225**	**total grams Carb**

Use the following box to divide your daily carb budget into a pattern you can follow for meals and snacks. Your diabetes educator may have you change this pattern depending on your medication and your blood sugar values. Or you may adjust the pattern if you are eating out or your activity schedule changes. The goal is to attempt to evenly divide the carbs you eat throughout the day and never go without food for long periods of time.

Dividing Your Daily Carb Budget Between Meals and Snacks

Your Calories per Day ____

Daily Carb Budget: ____ Carb Choices, or ____ grams Carb

Breakfast	____	*Carb choices*	=	____	*grams Carb*
AM Snack	____	*Carb choices*	=	____	*grams Carb*
Lunch	____	*Carb choices*	=	____	*grams Carb*
PM Snack	____	*Carb choices*	=	____	*grams Carb*
Dinner	____	*Carb choices*	=	____	*grams Carb*
Night Snack	____	*Carb choices*	=	____	*grams Carb*
Total	____	**Carb choices**	=	____	**total grams Carb**

To take this planning one step further, here is a sample day for a woman eating 1800 calories with a carb budget of 225 grams.

Sample Menu for a Woman

1800 Calories

Carb Budget 225 grams, or 15 Carb Choices

Food	Portion	Calories	Carbs
Breakfast Carb Budget			**45**
Pink grapefruit sections	½ cup	37	9
Fresh blueberries	¼ cup	20	5
Corn flakes	¾ cup	100	24
Nonfat milk	1 cup	86	12
Coffee + sugar substitute	as desired	0	0
Breakfast Totals		**243**	**50**

(continued)

Food	Portion	Calories	Carbs
Morning Snack Carb Budget			**15**
Apple	1 small	63	16
Cheddar cheese, lowfat	1 ounce	49	1
Morning Snack Totals		**112**	**17**
Lunch Carb Budget			**60**
Tuna salad	½ cup	192	10
Rye bread	2 slices	130	24
Swiss cheese	1 ounce	107	1
Tossed salad	1½ cups	32	7
Low calorie Italian dressing	2 tablespoons	32	2
Diet cola	1 can	0	0
Light flavored yogurt	1 package	100	16
Lunch Totals		**593**	**60**
Afternoon Snack Carb Budget			**15**
Graham crackers	2 squares	60	10
Lowfat cream cheese	1 tablespoon	60	2
Tea + sugar substitute	as desired	0	0
Afternoon Snack Totals		**120**	**12**
Dinner Carb Budget			**60**
Roast chicken w/skin	½ breast	142	0
Rice	⅔ cup	137	30
Cracked pepper	sprinkle	0	0
Butter	1 tablespoon	108	tr
Broccoli, cooked	1 cup	46	8
Vanilla ice cream (no sugar added)	¾ cup	165	21
Sparkling water	as desired	0	0
Dinner Totals		**598**	**59**
Evening Snack Carb Budget			**30**
Popcorn	2 cups	62	12
Nonfat milk	1 cup	86	12
Sugar free chocolate syrup	2 tablespoons	15	5
Evening Snack Totals		**163**	**29**
Day's Totals		**1829**	**227**

If the sample day was being planned for a man, the food choices would be very similar. Simply adjust the carb choices to reflect the way your individual carb budget is set up for the day. When you are first getting used to counting carbs and learning to manage diabetes, it is helpful to keep daily food records. Your diabetes educator may have already suggested this. It's also smart to check your food choices regularly to see if you are eating the calories and carbs that meet your treatment goals. The following Sample Daily Menu planning sheet will be a useful tool. Share the days you record with your diabetes educator to get feedback and fine-tune the management of your condition.

SAMPLE DAILY MENU

Date ____________________

_______ Calories Per Day

Daily Carb Budget: grams of Carb ____ or Carb Choices ____

Food	Portion	Calories	Carbs
Breakfast Carb Budget			______
Breakfast Totals		______	______
Morning Snack Carb Budget			______
Morning Snack Totals		______	______
Lunch Carb Budget			______
Lunch Totals		______	______
Afternoon Snack Carb Budget			______
Afternoon Snack Totals		______	______
Dinner Carb Budget			______
Dinner Totals		______	______
Evening Snack Carb Budget			______
Evening Snack Totals		______	______
Day's Totals		______	______

Considering Religious Fast Days

Embracing one's faith often reduces stress. Stress affects blood sugar. For some people, their faith helps them cope with diabetes. Many faiths have fast days. Though fasting may be part of your spiritual practice, it can create complications when managing diabetes.

Though all religions make exceptions from fasting for medical reasons, many people choose to fast anyway. Fasting and then eating a large meal when the fast ends puts you at risk for low blood sugar while fasting and high blood sugar after a large meal. Neither is good.

It is wise to discuss your fasting practice with both your doctor and your spiritual leader. Often a modification can be made to the fast requirements, or medical adjustments can be made to help you fast. For example, a Muslim who is managing diabetes might avoid eating from dawn to dusk during Ramadan but drink some fluids during the day to avoid very low blood sugar and dehydration. For many this compromise is acceptable.

If you fast, you should monitor your blood sugar more frequently. You may need to adjust your medication dosage. Be cautious of too much exercise and eating very large meals before and at the end of the fast. You will stay healthy if you develop a plan for fasting that takes into account activity, food, hydration, and medication.

EATING OUT

Whether it's a business lunch with clients, take-out on the way home from work, or a quick burger with your kids, eating out is part of the way we live. It's easy, quick and fun, and it can be healthy. Eating out, even regularly, can definitely fit into your diabetic meal plan.

You walk into a restaurant, you're shown to a table and handed a menu. Believe it or not, your key to successful eating out is right there in your hands. Read the menu carefully. Don't be afraid to ask for special options or substitutions. Many restaurants cater to diners' health needs. Some regularly offer "healthy" choices.

Menu selections that tend to have less calories and fat are:

au jus (in its own juice)
baked
boiled
broiled
cooked with lemon juice
cooked with wine
deviled
fresh
garden fresh
grilled
julienne
lean
marinara
poached
roasted
steamed
stir fry
without skin

Menu choices that have more calories are:

au gratin
battered
breaded
buttered
casserole
cheese sauce (mornay)
cream sauce (à la king)
creamed
creamy (béchamel)
crispy
deep fried
escalloped
fried
gravy
hollandaise
kiev
parmesan
parmigiana
pastry
pot pie
prime
remoulade
rich
scalloped
thermidor

When you eat out, simply apply the meal planning skills and carb counting strategies you use every day. All restaurants have low calorie and no calorie sweeteners. Most carry sugar free syrups and jelly, lowfat or nonfat salad dressings, nonfat milk, and diet drinks. Menu choices such as salads, grilled fish, broiled lean meats, vegetables, fresh fruit, and whole grain breads are readily available. Do not be afraid to take control, ask questions, suggest substitutions, and be creative in putting together a meal you'll enjoy that fits into your daily carb and calorie budget.

Let's Order

- *Don't be afraid to ask*
  Can you split a dinner between two?

Can your choice be broiled instead of fried?
Can you skip the potato and order double vegetables?
Can you swap French fries for a salad or sliced tomato?
Can the chef leave out the salt?

- *Avoid temptation*
  Stay away from all-you-can-eat buffets; it's too tempting to overeat
  Don't supersize your choice; large portions mean more carbs and calories
  Take a roll and ask that the bread basket be removed from the table
  Request no butter for the bread
  Keep the vegetable tray and give back the chips and dip
- *"Something to drink?"—"Water, thank you."*
  Choose calorie-free drinks—water, mineral water, club soda, unsweetened iced tea, diet soda
  Choose lower calorie drinks—wine, wine spritzers, fruit juice with club soda
  Limit alcohol; many drinks are packed with calories and carbs
- *Make an "appetizer" a meal*
  Order an appetizer or starter portion as an entree
  Ask if a lunch portion can be ordered at dinner
  Share a main dish and order extra vegetables
- *Play with your food*
  Trim away excess fat
  Remove skin from poultry

- *Put toppings on the side*
  This includes butter, gravy, salad dressing, sauce, sour cream, syrup, guacamole, grated cheese
  Use very small portions to enhance flavor and avoid piling on calories
  To get the flavor with fewer calories, try dipping your fork into the "extra" and then spearing a piece of food, rather than dunking each bite
- *Eat slowly*
  Enjoy the company—talk more, eat less
  Enjoy the ambiance of the restaurant
- *Eat until you feel fine, not full—be mindful of how your body feels*
  You don't have to clean your plate
  Ask for a doggie bag to take home
- *Be smart about dessert*
  Share with another person—or, better yet, with the whole table
  Order fresh fruit
  End the meal with a richly flavored coffee or interesting tea instead of dessert

You Should Know—

The Diabetes Counter *is a great eating out resource. In addition to 58 restaurant chains in Part Two, there are over 900 take-out choices listed.*

Think Before You Drink

As with many issues we have discussed, when it comes to alcohol, there is good news and bad news. The good news is that light to moderate use of alcohol lowers the risk for diabetes and raises your HDL (good) cholesterol. The bad news is that heavy drinking increases the risk for prediabetes and diabetes.

You Should Know—

1 Alcoholic Drink Equals

12 ounces light beer—1 bottle or can
1.5 ounces 80 proof distilled spirits—1 shot glass
1 ounce 100 proof distilled spirits—2 tablespoons
5 ounces wine—1 moderate-sized wineglass

Here are some things to consider when adding alcohol to your diabetic meal plans.

- Limit alcoholic drinks to 1 a day for women and 2 for men.
- Always drink alcohol with food, because drinking on an empty stomach can make your blood sugar drop too low.
- Alcohol by itself (gin, vodka, whiskey, rum) does not require insulin to be used for energy, so it does not cause blood sugar to go up.
- Mixed drinks, beer, and wine contain carb and may raise your blood sugar.

- Light beer is very low in carb and does not need to be counted into your daily carb budget, but don't overdo.
- Regular beer has more carb. One 12-ounce bottle should be counted as 1 carb choice in your daily carb budget.
- If you drink daily, the calories need to be added to your daily calorie intake. Alcohol calories do not need to be counted if you drink very infrequently.

You Should Know—

Binge drinking causes insulin resistance, which puts you at greater risk for type 2 diabetes and makes blood sugar harder to control.
Binge drinking = 5 or more drinks for men
or
4 or more drinks for women within 2 hours.

A Word About Tobacco

Many people use chewing tobacco. Surprisingly, the sugar content can affect blood sugar control. Pouch tobacco brands contain between 24% and 65% sugar; plug tobaccos have 13% to 50% sugar. A 1.2-ounce can contains 10 or more grams of sugar. If you use smokeless tobacco regularly, it could affect your blood sugar.

ALL ABOUT SUGAR

You are probably wondering why we haven't talked much about sugar up to now. In the past, people with diabetes were told they could not eat sugar because it would make their blood sugar go up too high. There is even a long-standing myth that eating too much sugar causes diabetes. It's not true.

> **You Should Know—**
>
> *Experts currently agree that people with diabetes can eat and enjoy moderate amounts of sugar.*

Research has shown that sugar has the same effect on blood sugar as any other carb you eat. Calorie for calorie, sugar raises blood sugar about the same amount as bread, pasta, or potatoes. You can eat sugar—and foods with sugar—as long as you count them in your total carb budget for the day.

You Should Know—

It's Amount, Not Type, That Counts

Research shows that it is the total amount of carb eaten at a meal that determines blood sugar levels after eating.

It doesn't matter if the carbs come from starches or sugars; it is the amount eaten that counts.

Natural Sugar Versus Added Sugar

Grains, fruits, vegetables, milk, and plain yogurt all contain sugars. These are *natural sugars* found in the food, along with vitamins, minerals, and fiber. In contrast, soda, candy, fruit drinks, cakes, cookies, ice cream, jelly, and syrup are full of added sugar. They offer little besides sweetness and calories.

Added sugars make up as much as 25% of our calories daily. Most of it comes from soda and sweetened fruit drinks. Cutting back on these sweetened drinks will cut your added sugar intake a good deal. To make the healthiest food choices, choose foods with natural sugars more often and foods with added sugars less often.

Go Easy with Sugar in a Glass

One out of every 5 calories we eat comes in liquid form—soda, fruit drinks, energy drinks, sports drinks, sweetened water, tea, iced tea, and coffee. You don't get the same feeling of fullness from liquid calories, and the more you are offered, the more you drink. Portion sizes have also increased dramatically over the last 25 years. We went from an 8-ounce soda bottle to a quart-sized glass with unlimited refills. Sweetened drinks come in 16-ounce bottles, double a standard serving size. A small coffee is now 10 ounces, and few of us ever order small.

Sweetened drinks load you up with sugar calories but let you down when it comes to all other nutrients and feeling satisfied.

Counting Sweets

As you choose different sweets, you need to know how each affects your carb budget for the day.

Sugars include table sugar, honey, brown sugar, molasses, fructose, cane syrup, corn syrup, maple syrup, raw sugar, powdered sugar, high fructose corn syrup (HFCS), fruit juice concentrate, brown rice syrup, date syrup, and agave syrup. Each of these sugars contains 4 calories per gram. You need to count these grams of sugar as part of your carb allowance in your daily carb budget.

When you look on a food label, the amount of sugar in the food is listed on the nutrition facts panel as part of the total carbohydrate. The best choices are those with more carb and less sugar.

You Should Know—

Sugar Counts

1 teaspoon sugar = 4 grams carb

Reduced calorie sweeteners are often found in low calorie and low sugar foods like chewing gum, candy, cookies, and desserts. They appear on labels as sorbitol, mannitol, xylitol, isomalt, lactitol, maltitol, erythritol, and trehalose. These sugar substitutes are called *sugar alcohols*. They are neither sugars nor alcohols but substances that are absorbed slowly by the body and add a sweet taste to foods. Sugar alcohols have little impact on blood sugar levels because they don't need insulin to be used in the body. Eating a lot of foods sweetened by sugar alcohols or chewing a lot of sugar free gum may cause gas and diarrhea in some people.

Sugar alcohols do contain carbs and calories—about half the calories in sugar. If you regularly eat foods with sugar alcohols, you need to count them in your carb budget for the day.

When you look at a food label, sugar alcohols may be listed on the nutrition facts panel under total carbohydrate (this is voluntary), but they must be listed in the ingredient list (this is required by law).

No calorie sweeteners are also called artificial sweeteners or nonnutritive sweeteners. They don't contain calories or carbs, and they don't affect your blood sugar. They are sometimes referred to as "free foods," and you can eat them as often as you wish. They must be listed on the food label in the ingredient list.

No Calorie Sweeteners

Generic name	Brand name
Acesulfame-K	*Sunett*
	Sweet & Safe
	Sweet One
Aspartame	*NutraSweet*
	Equal
	Sugar Twin
	AminoSweet
Luo han guo	*Monk Fruit*
	Fruit-Sweetness
Saccharin	*Sweet'N Low*
	Sweet Twin
	Necta Sweet
Stevia	*Truvia*
	Pure Via
	Pyure
	SweetLeaf
	Only Sweet
	Stevia In The Raw
Sucralose	*Splenda*

No calorie sweeteners all trigger slightly different taste receptors. You may need to try a few different ones to find the sweet taste you prefer.

Desserts

Just because you have diabetes does not mean you have to give up desserts. Instead of "give it up," think "downsize and negotiate." Eat a smaller portion, or trade dessert for a meal carb. Many desserts, like custard, rice pudding, or fruit-based sweets, are good for you and can be part of a healthy meal. Purely indulgent choices are not off-limits either—in those cases, just think small. Instead of a large candy bar, have a snack size. Try mini-cupcakes. With a little creative planning, there is a way to fit in your favorites.

- Small amounts of dried fruit can satisfy a sweet tooth.
- Eat smaller amounts of your favorites—a half cup of ice cream instead of a soup bowl full.
- When you eat out, split dessert with someone or, better yet, share with the whole table.
- Try lower calorie, lower sugar recipes.
- Buy lower sugar versions of favorites—but remember that low sugar doesn't always equal low calorie.
- Drink diet soda, sugar free drinks, and use no calorie sweeteners in coffee and tea.

Instead of Apple Pie, Try . . .

In a microwave safe serving dish, place
1 small apple, peeled and sliced
1 tablespoon raisins
1 teaspoon chopped walnuts
Pinch of cinnamon
1 package artificial sweetener
Cover with plastic wrap or wax paper and microwave on high for 1 minute 45 seconds.

Calories: 106 Carb: 23

A la mode, with ¼ cup light vanilla ice cream:

Calories: 150 Carb: 31

ALL ABOUT FIBER

Less than 4% of Americans eat enough fiber each day. Although nutrition guidelines recommend that we all eat at least 3 servings of whole grains a day, few of us do. Most eat less than 1 serving, and we all eat too few fruits, vegetables, and beans, the other fiber-rich foods. We average about 14 grams of fiber a day, only half of what we should be eating.

Fiber is the part of carbohydrates that you can't digest, which is why it has no calories. Although fiber is a carbohydrate, humans don't make the enzyme that digests fiber into simple sugar pieces so it can be absorbed into the bloodstream and used for energy in the body. Fiber does not affect your blood sugar.

The main sources of fiber are fruits, vegetables, beans, and whole grains—all good-for-you foods. Eating enough fiber each day offers important health benefits. Fiber:

- Lowers the risk for prediabetes by preventing insulin resistance
- Lowers the risk for type 2 diabetes by helping keep blood sugar levels normal

- Protects your heart by lowering blood pressure and reducing cholesterol
- Keeps your GI tract healthy
- Improves your immune system
- Protects you from some cancers, such as colon cancer
- Prevents and relieves constipation
- Helps you feel more satisfied after eating, which can help you maintain a healthy weight

Not bad for something that has no calories.

Fiber Tip

One easy way to add more fiber to your diet is to switch from white bread to whole wheat bread—the same amount of carbs per portion, with more fiber.

Figuring out how much fiber to eat each day is easy. Simply select your sex and age range on the following table and use that recommendation as your daily target fiber intake.

DAILY FIBER RECOMMENDATIONS

Men	Fiber
19–50 years	38 grams
50 and older	30 grams
Women	Fiber
19–50 years	25 grams
50 and older	21 grams
Pregnant	28 grams

You don't need to track your fiber intake daily, but you should be aware of which foods contain fiber. *The Diabetes Counter* lists fiber to help you find the best sources. Every so often, as you are adding up your daily carb intake, add up fiber as well to see if you are getting the recommended amount.

Fiber Tip

High fiber foods have 5 or more grams of fiber in a serving.
A good source of fiber has 2 or more grams of fiber in a serving.
Every gram of fiber you eat counts toward your daily goal.

If you normally eat little fiber—and that's the case for most of us—add foods rich in fiber slowly. Fiber-rich foods include: beans, berries, bran, fruits, oatmeal, popcorn, vegetables, and whole grains. Don't go overboard, because it takes your body a little time to adjust to the extra bulk passing through your digestive tract. At first, you may find you are a little gassy. This will pass as you adjust to the higher fiber intake. Be sure to drink plenty of fluids. Fiber soaks up fluids like a sponge. This not only helps you feel fuller longer but it also helps form soft, easily passed stools.

Add a Little Fiber to Your Life

- Eat whole fruits and vegetables instead of drinking juices.
- Don't peel! Eat the fiber-rich skins of cucumbers, apples, pears, potatoes, and zucchini.
- Eat more berries—blueberries, blackberries, raspberries, strawberries.
- Choose whole grains—brown rice, cornmeal, barley, cracked wheat, rye, whole wheat.
- Eat whole grain or high fiber cereals—oatmeal, oat flakes, bran, shredded wheat.
- Choose whole wheat bread, bagels, pasta, pretzels, crackers, and rolls.
- Eat beans, lentils, and peas a few times a week.
- Try soybeans in every form—soynuts, tofu, tempeh, edamame.
- Snack on fiber-rich fig newtons, graham crackers, popcorn, nuts, and seeds.
- Eat dried fruits and raisins.
- Sprinkle ground flaxseed, bran, or whole grain granola on cereal or yogurt for a healthy crunch.

- Experiment with higher fiber versions of old favorites, like brown rice instead of white rice, buckwheat noodles instead of regular noodles, or baked sweet potatoes instead of white potatoes.
- Have vegetarian meals a few times a week.

Mash It, Smash It, Break It Apart

Fiber is fiber no matter how you process or cook it. Canned, pureed pumpkin is a rich source of fiber, as is split pea soup, mashed sweet potatoes, cream of broccoli soup, or a fruit smoothie.

A Word About Fiber-Fortified Foods

Natural fiber sources are the best choices. Fiber naturally found in foods rarely causes problems. Vegetarians can eat as much as 80 grams of fiber a day, more than triple the daily recommendation for women and double that suggested for men.

Fiber added to foods, like a high fiber chocolate bar, does not help you feel fuller or less hungry between meals and is more likely to cause GI distress. Added fiber can cause gas, cramps, bloating, and diarrhea in some people, especially when eaten in large amounts. The easiest way to tell if the fiber in a food has been added is to look at the ingredient list. If you see inulin, fructan (also called fructooligosaccharides, or FOS), or methycellulose, there is added fiber in the food.

Chew on This

Eating naturally fiber-rich foods is a better choice than using fiber supplements. Fiber-rich foods are also rich in health-promoting antioxidants, vitamins, and minerals; supplements are not.

MONITORING DIABETES

Many diabetes experts believe that self-monitoring is the key to successfully managing diabetes, reducing risks, and minimizing complications. Your diabetes educator, doctor, and dietitian will help you learn how to best monitor your condition.

Counting carbs and keeping a record of what you eat is one self-monitoring tool. Monitoring your blood sugar is another important tool you will use.

You Should Know—

Lifestyle Counts

- *For some people, lifestyle changes may be more effective in managing type 2 diabetes than an intense focus on blood sugar levels.*
- *Reducing blood pressure, modest weight loss (5% of body weight), more exercise, a healthier diet, and smoking cessation may do more to slow the progression of the condition.*

Checking Blood Sugar

Blood sugar is checked 2 ways: self-monitoring and the A1C test. Your diabetes educator will tell you how often to check your blood sugar at home using a glucose monitor. At first, you may do it more often to be sure your medication and your diet are working together. Some people test 4 times a day, before each meal and at bedtime. If you have type 2 diabetes and your blood sugar is stable, you may test less frequently, 3 to 7 days a week before breakfast and randomly at other times during the day. At least 1 to 3 times a month you should test before each meal and at bedtime to be sure your levels are within range.

You Should Know—

When you regularly monitor your blood sugar, you will have better outcomes and your diabetes will be more effectively managed. Self-monitoring is important.

You may be asked to keep a blood sugar log and bring these records when you get a checkup. The numbers you record will help your doctor decide which type and how much of a drug or insulin you should be taking. They also give your diabetes educator information that will help in adjusting your daily carb budget.

Target Blood Sugar Values for People with Diabetes

Time to Check	Target Blood Sugar Values
Upon waking, before eating	90 to 130
Before meals (at least 3 hours since your last meal)	90 to 130
2 hours after eating	less than 160
Bedtime (if lower, have a bedtime snack)	110 to 150

You Should Know—

Blood Sugar Up, Mood Down

When blood sugar levels are poorly controlled you are more likely to experience depression, anxiety, anger, and an overall poorer quality of life.

A1C is a blood test that shows your average blood sugar level over the last 6 to 12 weeks. The higher the A1C number, the higher your blood sugar has been.

How does A1C measure your blood sugar? It measures a compound in your blood called *glycosylated hemoglobin*. Hemoglobin is found inside all red blood cells. When blood sugar is poorly controlled, too much glucose builds up in the blood. This extra glucose links up (or glycates) with hemoglobin to form glycosylated hemoglobin. Once cells are glycated, they stay that way. The more sugar in your blood, the higher the percentage of A1C cells you'll have. Since each A1C cell has a life span of about 3 months, measuring the percentage of glycosylated hemoglobin in your blood provides a snapshot of the levels of glucose in the blood over the last few months.

For most people with type 2, the A1C value should be below 7%; a value of 7% means your average blood sugar has been 150, which is very good. For younger adults with a long life expectancy and no current heart disease, an A1C goal of 6 to 6.5% might be considered. For people who have had type 2 for a long time, have other health issues, and may have a history of many incidents of low blood sugar (hypoglycemia), less strict A1C goals of 7.5 to 8% may be appropriate. You will set the goals that are right for you with the help of your doctor.

A1C tests should be done periodically throughout the year and are an excellent tool for monitoring long-term management of diabetes.

You Should Know—

Blood sugar below 70 is too low, and above 240 is too high.

Blood sugar equal to or over 200 increases your risk for infection and slows down wound healing.

Low Blood Sugar—Hypoglycemia

Though your goal is to keep your blood sugar level down, if it goes too low this can be a problem as well. The most common causes of low blood sugar are too much insulin or oral medication, eating too little food, exercising without eating extra food, or drinking alcohol on an empty stomach.

You Should Know—

Physical Signs of Low Blood Sugar

Sweating
Weakness
Hunger
Anxiety
Fast heartbeat
Irritability
Unable to think clearly
Headache
Drowsiness
Numbness or tingling around the lips

As you get older, the risk for hypoglycemia (low blood sugar) goes up. It can cause irregular heart rhythms, dizziness, falls, confusion, and put you at greater risk for infection. If you experience low blood sugar levels often, speak to your doctor, because your target blood sugars may be set too low, which is a major cause of low blood sugar in older adults.

If you ever think that your blood sugar is too low,

test yourself with your glucose monitor. If the level is 70 or lower, have one of these "quick fix" foods immediately to raise your blood sugar. Each equals 15 grams of carbohydrate, or 1 carb choice.

- glucose gel packet or glucose tablets equaling 15 grams of carb
- ½ cup fruit juice
- 1 cup milk
- 1 to 2 teaspoons sugar or honey
- ½ cup of regular soda
- ½ cup of regular Jell-O
- 2 tablespoons raisins
- 6 jelly beans
- 5 to 6 pieces of hard candy

Test your blood again in 15 minutes. If it is still below 70, eat another 15-gram carb choice. Wait 15 minutes and test your blood again. If it is an hour or more before your next meal, have a snack that contains both a carb and a protein. Good examples are:

- Peanut butter and crackers
- Cheese and crackers
- Half a ham or turkey sandwich
- Milk and cereal
- Hard or soft cooked egg and toast

It's a good idea to keep some of these "quick fix" choices in your house, desk drawer, or in the car when you drive long distances, just in case.

You Should Get a Round of Applause

Good diabetes control takes discipline,
effort, and commitment.
You need to monitor your diet, exercise,
blood glucose, and drugs.
Keep up the good work!

A WORD ABOUT THE GLYCEMIC INDEX

Decades ago, researcher David Jenkins at the University of Toronto coined the term *glycemic index* (GI). This index ranks carbohydrate foods. It shows how much a portion of a food raises blood sugar after being eaten, when compared to the rise in blood sugar after eating a reference food—either white bread or glucose. Foods with a high glycemic index raise blood sugar levels quickly. Foods with a low GI produce a much smaller rise in blood sugar levels, which helps keep blood sugar within a normal range.

The theory behind the glycemic index is correct. Some foods do raise blood sugar quickly; others do not. But in practice, it's not that simple.

The glycemic index measures the ability of foods to raise blood sugar when eaten alone. White bread has a very high glycemic index. But the glycemic index of food combinations can be very different. If you add peanut butter to white bread, the glycemic response goes down because peanut butter, a high fat food, has a low glycemic index. The same goes for a baked potato, another high glycemic food; top it with cheese sauce and broccoli, and the glycemic index plunges.

It gets even more complicated. Cooking pasta al dente is fine; overcook it, and its glycemic value goes up. Rice varieties vary as well. Swarna rice, the most widely grown variety in India, has a low glycemic index, but Doongara and basmati rice from Australia have medium glycemic values. Regular ice cream has a low glycemic index because the fat in it slows down the absorption of sugar. Even sugars vary. Glucose is high on the index, but fructose (fruit sugar) is low.

GLYCEMIC INDEX OF COMMON FOODS

High (greater than 70)	
Cornflakes	*119*
Rice cakes	*117*
Jelly beans	*114*
Carrots	*101*
White bread	*101*
Glucose	**100**
Wheat bread	*99*
Soda	*97*
Potato, white boiled	*96*
Sucrose	*92*
Rice, white cooked	*89*
Rice, brown cooked	*87*
Cheese pizza	*86*
Spaghetti	*83*
Pretzels	*83*
Pancakes	*80*
Popcorn	*79*
Corn	*78*
Banana over-ripe	*76*

(continued)

Honey	*74*
Orange juice	*74*
Watermelon	*72*
Moderate (between 56 and 69)	
Potato, white, with skin, baked	*69*
Peas	*68*
Pineapple, fresh	*66*
Orange	*62*
Bran cereal	*60*
Apple juice	*58*
Pumpernickel bread	*58*
Oatmeal	*58*
Potato chips	*56*
Low (55 and below)	
Banana ripe (all yellow)	*51*
Rye bread	*50*
Kidney beans	*42*
Kiwi fruit	*41*
Fish sticks	*38*
Nonfat milk	*37*
Peanut butter	*37*
Apple, golden delicious	*34*
Whole milk	*34*
Fructose (fruit sugar)	*32*
Lentils	*32*
Banana under-ripe	*30*
Peanuts	*23*

Source: Institute of Medicine of the National Academies. 2002. *Dietary Reference Intakes for Energy, Carbohydrate, Fiber, Fat, Fatty Acids, Cholesterol, Protein, and Amino Acids*. Part 1. The National Academies Press, and University of Sydney, Australia, June 2012.

You Should Know—

Drawbacks to the GI Approach

Values on GI tables vary depending on how the tests were measured.

People respond to foods differently, making GI results inconsistent from one person to another.

Studies comparing high GI diets versus low GI diets show inconsistent effects on A1C levels.

Bottom Line

Research into the health effects of the glycemic index is still evolving. Most experts agree that eating more high fiber foods and fewer processed foods is good. Low GI foods include nonstarchy vegetables, most fruits, and dairy products—all good choices for someone with diabetes. Using the index might help you "fine-tune" some of your carb choices, but exclusively eating-by-the-numbers could steer you away from otherwise healthy foods.

If you want to incorporate glycemic index choices into your carb budget for the day, that's fine. Some research has shown that this approach can give you a better blood sugar response.

You Should Know—

If you are considering using the glycemic index to help manage your diabetes, discuss the benefits with your diabetes educator, who can help you tailor this approach to your treatment goals.

WHERE TO GO FOR MORE INFORMATION

There are many resources available to help you learn more about diabetes, its treatment, and the newest research findings. Even food companies, drugstore chains, and pharmaceutical firms offer publications, newsletters, and recipes. Take advantage of all these resources, because they provide interesting and worthwhile information. You can start with the following well-known and reliable resources.

Academy of Nutrition and Dietetics
120 South Riverside Plaza
Suite 2000
Chicago, IL 60606-6995
www.eatright.org/programs/rdfinder/

American Association of Diabetes Educators
200 W. Madison Street
Suite 800
Chicago, IL 60606
www.diabeteseducator.org/DiabetesEducation/Find.html

American Diabetes Association
National Service Center
1701 North Beauregard Street
Alexandria, VA 22311
800-DIABETES (1-800-342-2383)
www.diabetes.org

Canadian Diabetes Association (CDA)
1400-522 University Avenue
Toronto, ON M5G 2R5
Canada
1-800-226-8464
www.diabetes.ca

Centers for Disease Control and Prevention
CDC-INFO
National Center for Chronic Disease Prevention
and Health Promotion
1600 Clifton Road
Atlanta, GA 30333
800-CDC-INFO (800-232-4636)
www.cdc.gov/diabetes

Diabetes Action Resource and Education Foundation
426 C Street, NE
Washington, DC 20002
202-333-4520
www.diabetesaction.org

Diabetes Care and Education Practice Group
Academy of Nutrition and Dietetics
www.dce.org/#2

dLife
101 Franklin Street
Westport, CT 06880
203-454-6985 or 886-354-3366
www.dlife.com

Indian Health Service
Division of Diabetes Treatment and Prevention
The Reyes Building
801 Thompson Avenue
Suite 400
Rockville, MD 20852
505-248-4182
www.ihs.gov/MedicalPrograms/Diabetes/

International Diabetes Federation
166 Chaussee de La Hulpe
B-1170 Brussels, Belgium
32-2-538 55 11
www.idf.org

Joslin Diabetes Center and Joslin Clinic
One Joslin Place
Boston, MA 02215
617-309-2400
www.joslin.org

National Diabetes Education Program (NDEP)
One Diabetes Way
Bethesda, MD 20814-9692
800-438-5383
www.ndep.nih.gov

National Diabetes Information Clearing House (NDIC)
1 Information Way
Bethesda, MD 20892-3560
800-860-8747
www.diabetes.niddk.nih.gov

USING YOUR DIABETES COUNTER

The Diabetes Counter lists the portion size, calories, fat, carbohydrate, sugar, and fiber values for more than 12,000 foods. Now you can compare the values in your favorite foods and, when necessary, choose substitutes before you go out to shop or eat. This will save you time and help you decide what to buy.

The carbohydrate and calorie values will help you stay within your carb and calorie budget for the day. Fat values have been included to help you plan lower fat meals to reduce your risk for heart disease. Sugar values were included to make you aware of which foods are high in sugar. Sugar is not counted separately but is part of your total carb budget for the day. Fiber values were included to make you aware of which foods are high in fiber. Fiber, like sugar, is found in foods that contain carbohydrates. It is a good idea to occasionally track your fiber intake for a day or two to see if you are meeting the requirements for your age and sex. (See page 66.)

The counter section of the book is divided into two parts—Part One: Brand Name, Nonbranded (Generic), and Take-Out Foods (page 93); and Part Two: Restaurant Chains (page 535). Each part lists foods or restaurant chains alphabetically.

In Part One, for each category you will find nonbranded (generic) foods listed first, in alphabetical order, followed by an alphabetical listing of brand name foods. The nonbranded listings will help you estimate calorie, fat, carbohydrate, fiber, and sugar values when you don't see your favorite brands. Large categories are divided into subcategories, such as canned, fresh, frozen, and ready-to-eat, to make it easier to find what you're looking for. Some categories have "see" and "see also" references to help you find related items.

Because we eat out so often, more than 900 take-out foods are listed in Part One. These are found in the take-out subcategory in many categories throughout Part One. Foods you take out or order in are rarely nutrition labeled.

Most foods are listed alphabetically. In some cases, though, foods are grouped by category. For example, a tuna sandwich is found in the SANDWICH category. Other group categories include:

ALCOHOL DRINKS: **Page 94**
Includes all alcoholic beverages and mixed drinks except beer, champagne, and wine, which have their own separate categories.

ASIAN FOOD: **Page 106**
Includes all types of Asian foods except egg rolls and sushi, which are found in the egg rolls and sushi categories.

DELI MEATS/COLD CUTS: **Page 253**
Includes all sandwich meats except chicken, ham, and turkey, which have their own separate categories.

DINNER: **Page 255**
Includes all prepared dinners listed by brand name, except pasta dinners, which are found in the pasta dinners category.

NUTRITION SUPPLEMENTS: **Page 358**
Includes all dieting aids, meal replacements, and drinks, except energy bars and energy drinks, which have their own separate categories.

SANDWICHES: **Page 440**
Includes popular sandwich, calzone, and panini choices.

SNACKS: **Page 460**

Includes a variety of snack items, such as pork rinds and cheese puffs.

SPANISH FOOD: **Page 481**

Includes all types of Spanish and Mexican foods except salsa and tortillas, which have their own separate categories

In Part Two, Restaurant Chains, 58 national and regional restaurant, coffee, doughnut, frozen yogurt, ice cream, pizza, sandwich, soup, and sushi chains are listed. Brand name foods are required by federal law to have nutrition information on labels, but restaurants are different. Currently, in most areas of the country restaurants provide this information voluntarily.

With *The Diabetes Counter* as your guide, you will never again wonder how much carbohydrate is in the foods you eat.

DEFINITIONS

as prep (as prepared): refers to food that has been prepared according to package directions

lean and fat: describes meat with some fat on its edges that is not cut away before cooking, or poultry prepared with skin and fat as purchased

lean only: refers to lean meat that is trimmed of all visible fat, or poultry without skin

not prep (not prepared): refers to food that has not been cooked and may require the addition of other ingredients to prepare

shelf-stable: refers to prepared products found on the supermarket shelf that are not canned or frozen but are packaged and ready-to-eat or are ready to be heated and do not require refrigeration

take-out: describes prepared dishes that you purchase ready-to-eat; those included serve as a guide to the calories, fat, carbohydrate, fiber, and sugar in products you may buy

ABBREVIATIONS

avg	=	average
diam	=	diameter
fl	=	fluid
frzn	=	frozen
g	=	gram
in	=	inch
lb	=	pound
lg	=	large
med	=	medium
mg	=	milligram
oz	=	ounce
pkg	=	package
prep	=	prepared
pt	=	pint
qt	=	quart
reg	=	regular
sec	=	second
serv	=	serving
sm	=	small
sq	=	square
tbsp	=	tablespoon
tr	=	trace
tsp	=	teaspoon
w/	=	with
w/o	=	without
<	=	less than

NOTES

cal = calories
fat = fat
carb = carbohydrates
sugar = sugar
fiber = fiber
All fat, carbohydrate, fiber, and sugar values are given in grams
— (dash) indicates that values are not available
tr (trace) = less than 1 gram of fat, carbohydrate, fiber, or sugar
0 (zero) indicates there are no calories, fat, carbohydrate, fiber, or sugar in that food

Discrepancies in figures are due to rounding of values, product reformulation, and reevaluation. The current labeling law allows rounding. Some of the data listed is analysis data, obtained directly from manufacturers, not from labels; therefore, some values may differ slightly from labels because the values have not been rounded.

PART ONE

Brand Name, Nonbranded (Generic), and Take-Out Foods

Natural Compounds in Foods Can Help Manage Diabetes

Here are some simple food options to help keep blood sugar under control.

Cinnamon Lowers Blood Sugar

Daily intake of 1 to 2 grams (½ to 1 teaspoon) of cinnamon lowers blood sugar after meals and helps with insulin resistance.

Green and black tea *help boost insulin activity and protect the eyes from damage.*

Buckwheat *lowers blood sugar.*

Cherries *lower blood sugar and help increase insulin production.*

Foods high in vitamin C, like citrus fruits, strawberries, watermelon, and orange juice *help prevent some complications from diabetes.*

FOOD	PORTION	CAL	FAT	CARB	SUGAR	FIBER
ABALONE						
breaded & fried	1 serv (3 oz)	162	6	9	tr	tr
steamed	1 serv (3 oz)	127	3	6	tr	0
ACAI						
Amafruits						
Acai Berry Puree frzn	1 pkg (3.5 oz)	80	6	4	0	3
ACAI JUICE						
Naked						
Acai Machine	8 oz	160	3	31	24	3
Ultra Lo-Gly						
Acai-Blue	1 bottle (10 oz)	45	0	11	10	0
ACEROLA						
fresh	1 (5 g)	2	tr	tr	–	tr
ACEROLA JUICE						
juice	1 cup	56	1	12	11	1
ADZUKI BEANS						
canned sweetened	½ cup	351	tr	81	–	–
dried cooked w/o salt	½ cup	147	tr	28	–	8
AGAVE (*see* SYRUP)						
AKEE						
fresh	3.5 oz	223	20	5	–	–
ALCOHOL DRINKS (*see also* BEER AND ALE, CHAMPAGNE, MALT, WINE)						
7&7	1 serv	178	0	19	–	0
alabama slammer	1 serv	103	tr	7	–	tr
amaretto sour	1 serv	295	tr	57	–	4
angel's kiss	1 serv	85	1	5	–	0
anisette	1 oz	111	0	11	–	0
antifreeze cocktail	1 serv	177	tr	31	–	tr
apricot brandy	1 oz	96	0	9	–	0

FOOD	PORTION	CAL	FAT	CARB	SUGAR	FIBER
apricot sour	1 serv	164	tr	8	–	tr
aquavit	1 oz	65	0	0	0	0
b 52	1 serv	247	4	25	–	0
b&b	1 serv	75	0	0	0	0
bahama breeze	1 serv	70	tr	9	–	tr
bahama mama	1 serv	153	tr	23	–	tr
bailey's & amaretto	1 serv	184	5	16	–	0
banana colada	1 serv	376	1	64	–	3
bay breeze	1 serv	173	tr	18	–	tr
bend me over	1 serv	242	tr	32	–	tr
benedictine	1 oz	104	0	11	–	0
betsy ross	1 serv	206	0	5	–	0
black devil	1 serv	220	tr	1	–	tr
black russian	1 serv	184	tr	12	–	0
bloody mary	1 serv	150	tr	5	–	1
blue whale	1 serv	222	tr	23	–	0
bourbon & soda	1 serv (4 oz)	105	0	0	0	0
bourbon sour	1 serv	166	tr	8	–	tr
brandy alexander	1 serv	266	6	12	–	0
brandy sour	1 serv	164	tr	8	–	tr
bushwacker	1 serv	286	5	27	–	tr
coffee liqueur	1 serv (1.5 oz)	175	tr	24	24	0
cognac	1 oz	67	0	tr	0	0
cosmopolitan martini	1 serv	126	tr	7	–	tr
creme de menthe	1 serv (1.5 oz)	186	tr	21	21	0
curacao liqueur	1 oz	81	0	9	–	0
daiquiri	1 serv (2 oz)	112	tr	4	3	tr
daiquiri banana	1 serv	277	tr	32	–	1
daiquiri frozen pineapple	1 serv	186	tr	28	–	2
dark & stormy	1 serv	64	0	0	0	0
doctor pepper	1 serv	95	0	12	–	0
fuzzy navel	1 serv	247	tr	10	–	tr

FOOD	PORTION	CAL	FAT	CARB	SUGAR	FIBER
gin	1 serv (1.5 oz)	110	0	0	0	0
gin & tonic	1 serv (7.5 oz)	171	0	16	–	–
gin ricky	1 serv	114	tr	1	–	tr
grasshopper	1 serv	275	5	26	–	0
happy hawaiian	1 serv	434	8	60	–	tr
harvey wallbanger	1 serv	198	tr	16	–	tr
head banger	1 serv	165	0	4	–	0
hot buttered rum	1 serv (8.8 oz)	316	12	4	4	tr
hot toddy	1 serv	188	1	13	–	5
hurricane	1 serv	205	tr	19	–	tr
kamikaze	1 serv	136	0	2	–	0
long island iced tea	1 serv	292	tr	7	–	0
lynchburg lemonade	1 serv	465	tr	85	–	1
mai tai	1 serv	165	tr	17	–	tr
manhattan	1 serv	171	tr	3	–	tr
margarita	1 serv	173	0	11	–	0
margarita strawberry	1 serv	106	tr	11	–	1
martini	1 serv (3 oz)	206	0	2	tr	0
martini apple	1 serv	147	tr	4	–	tr
martini rum	1 serv	131	0	tr	–	tr
mellow yellow	1 serv	95	0	4	–	0
mexican grasshopper	1 serv	638	19	52	–	0
mint julep	1 serv	136	tr	17	–	tr
mississippi mud	1 serv	496	12	46	–	0
mudslide	1 serv	566	10	46	–	0
narragansett	1 serv	168	0	2	–	0
nutcracker	1 serv	730	10	64	–	0
old fashioned	1 serv	223	tr	4	–	tr
orange crush	1 serv	461	tr	65	–	tr
pain killer	1 serv	277	tr	20	–	tr
peppermint pattie	1 serv	344	tr	37	–	0
pina colada	1 serv (4.5 oz)	245	3	32	31	tr

FOOD	PORTION	CAL	FAT	CARB	SUGAR	FIBER
planter's cocktail	1 serv	105	0	3	–	tr
planter's punch	1 serv	233	tr	34	–	4
presbyterian	1 serv	170	0	8	–	tr
purple passion	1 serv	215	tr	22	–	0
rob roy	1 serv	171	0	3	–	tr
rum	1 serv (1.5 oz)	97	0	0	0	0
rum boogie	1 serv	134	tr	12	–	tr
rum cola	1 serv	209	tr	21	–	tr
rum highball	1 serv	170	0	11	–	0
rum punch	1 serv	448	1	88	–	1
rum screwdriver	1 serv	166	tr	16	–	tr
rum sour	1 serv	156	tr	8	–	tr
rum swizzle	1 serv	187	0	15	–	0
rusty nail	1 serv	159	0	6	–	0
sake	1 serv (1 oz)	39	0	1	0	0
salty dog	1 serv	210	tr	19	–	tr
scotch & soda	1 serv	104	0	tr	–	tr
sea breeze	1 serv	207	tr	19	–	tr
sex on the beach	1 serv	190	tr	18	–	tr
slippery nipple	1 serv	142	2	11	–	0
sloe gin fizz	1 serv (2.5 oz)	132	0	4	–	0
snake bite	1 serv	362	0	22	–	0
tequila frozen screwdriver	1 serv	159	tr	17	–	1
tequila gimlet	1 serv	150	tr	6	–	1
tequila sour	1 serv	156	tr	8	–	tr
tequila stinger	1 serv	221	tr	14	–	0
tequila sunrise	1 serv (6.8 oz)	232	tr	24	–	0
tom collins	1 serv (7.5 oz)	121	0	3	–	–
vermouth cassis	1 serv	97	tr	5	–	tr
vodka	1 serv (1.5 oz)	97	0	0	0	0
vodka gimlet	1 serv	150	tr	6	–	1

FOOD	PORTION	CAL	FAT	CARB	SUGAR	FIBER
vodka sour	1 serv	138	tr	3	–	tr
vodka stinger	1 serv	378	tr	28	–	0
whiskey	1 serv (1.5 oz)	105	0	tr	–	0
whiskey 86 proof	1 jigger (1.5 oz)	105	0	tr	tr	0
whiskey sour	1 serv (3.5 oz)	162	tr	14	14	0
white russian	1 serv	290	8	17	–	0
zombie	1 serv	235	tr	10	–	tr
ALE (*see* BEER AND ALE)						
ALFALFA						
sprouts	½ cup	40	tr	1	tr	tr
ALLIGATOR						
cooked	3 oz	126	2	0	0	0
ALLSPICE						
ground	1 tsp	5	tr	1	–	tr
ALMONDS						
almond butter w/ salt	2 tbsp	203	19	7	2	1
almond butter w/o salt	2 tbsp	203	19	7	–	1
almond paste	¼ cup	260	16	27	21	3
chocolate covered	6 pieces (0.6 oz)	102	8	6	3	2
dry roasted w/ salt	¼ cup	206	18	7	2	4
dry roasted w/o salt	¼ cup	206	18	7	2	4
honey roasted	¼ cup	214	18	10	–	5
jordan almonds	6 (0.7 oz)	99	4	14	13	1
oil roasted w/ salt	¼ cup	238	22	7	2	4
oil roasted w/o salt	¼ cup	238	22	7	2	4
praline	17 pieces (1.4 oz)	210	12	21	17	3

FOOD	PORTION	CAL	FAT	CARB	SUGAR	FIBER
yogurt covered	6 pieces (0.8 oz)	122	8	10	8	1
Blue Diamond						
Thin-Shell Hint Of Salt Shelled	24 (1 oz)	170	15	5	1	3
Thin-Shell Unsalted Shelled	24 (1 oz)	170	15	5	1	3
Frito Lay						
Roasted Salted	3 tbsp (1 oz)	190	16	5	1	3
Kettle Brand						
Butter Salted	2 tbsp (1 oz)	180	17	6	0	2
Nut Harvest						
Lightly Roasted	2 tbsp	180	15	6	1	3
Planters						
Chocolate Lovers Dark Chocolate	11 pieces (1.4 oz)	220	17	18	13	3
Flavor Grove Chili Lime	1 oz	170	15	6	2	3
Flavor Grove Sea Salt & Olive Oil	1 oz	170	15	5	1	3
NUT-rition Bone Health Mix	¼ cup (1.2 oz)	170	10	19	11	2
Slivered	1 pkg (2 oz)	330	28	11	3	7
Smoked	1 pkg (1.5 oz)	250	22	8	2	5
Sante						
Chipotle	¼ cup (1 oz)	190	16	8	3	1
Wild Squirrel						
Almond Butter Chocolate Sunflower Seed	2 tbsp (1.1 oz)	200	17	7	2	4
Almond Butter Vanilla Espresso	2 tbsp (1.1 oz)	190	16	6	2	4
Wonderful						
Almond Accents Honey Roasted w/ Cranberries	1 tbsp (7 g)	35	2	3	2	1

FOOD	PORTION	CAL	FAT	CARB	SUGAR	FIBER
Almond Accents Original Oven Roasted	1 tbsp (7 g)	45	4	1	0	1
Almond Accents Oven Roasted No Salt	1 tbsp (7 g)	45	4	1	0	1
Almond Accents Sweet Roasted Pomegranate	1 tbsp (7 g)	40	3	3	1	1
AMARANTH						
grain cooked w/o salt	½ cup (4.6 oz)	125	2	23	–	3
grain uncooked	½ cup (3.4 oz)	358	7	63	2	7
leaves cooked w/o salt	1 cup (4.6 oz)	28	tr	5	–	–
leaves raw	1 cup (1 oz)	6	tr	1	–	–
ANCHOVY						
boneless	1 oz	60	3	0	0	0
canned in oil drained	1 can (2 oz)	94	4	0	0	0
fresh	1 (4 g)	8	tr	0	0	0
fresh fillets	3 (0.4 oz)	21	1	tr	–	–
Arroyabe						
In Olive Oil	1 oz	60	3	0	0	0
King Oscar						
Fillet In Olive Oil	⅓ can (0.6 oz)	25	2	0	0	0
ANGLERFISH						
raw	3.5 oz	72	1	0	0	0
ANISE						
seed	1 tsp	7	tr	1	–	tr
ANTELOPE						
roasted	4 oz	215	4	0	0	0
APPLE						
CANNED						
sliced sweetened	½ cup	68	1	17	15	2

FOOD	PORTION	CAL	FAT	CARB	SUGAR	FIBER
Dole						
Squish'ems	1 pkg	80	0	18	17	1
Jake & Amos						
Red Spiced Rings	1 (1 oz)	35	0	9	8	0
DRIED						
chopped	½ cup	104	tr	28	24	4
cooked w/o sugar	½ cup	73	tr	20	17	3
rings	5	78	tr	21	18	3
Del Monte						
Dried Apples	¼ cup (1.4 oz)	100	0	24	24	5
FRESH						
apple	1 sm	55	tr	15	11	3
apple	1 med	72	tr	19	14	3
apple	1 lg	110	tr	29	22	5
candied	1 sm (4.9 oz)	179	3	40	32	3
candied	1 med (6.5 oz)	234	4	52	42	4
candied	1 lg (9.8 oz)	357	6	79	64	6
w/ skin sliced	1 cup	57	tr	15	11	3
w/o skin sliced	1 cup	53	tr	14	11	1
Chiquita						
Apple Slices	1 pkg (2.2 oz)	30	0	8	5	2
Crunch Pak						
DipperZ Sweet Apples w/ Chocolate Dip	1 pkg (2.75 oz)	70	1	17	12	2
DipperZ Sweet Apples w/ Low Fat Caramel Dip	1 pkg (2.75 oz)	80	1	18	14	1
DipperZ Sweet Apples w/ Peanut Butter	1 pkg (2.75 oz)	150	11	13	8	2
DipperZ Sweet Apples w/ Yogurt Dip	1 pkg (2.75 oz)	150	11	13	8	2
DipperZ Tart Apples w/ Low Fat Caramel Dip	1 pkg (2.75 oz)	80	1	18	14	1

FOOD	PORTION	CAL	FAT	CARB	SUGAR	FIBER
FlavorZ Grape	1 pkg (2 oz)	30	0	7	5	tr
FlavorZ Peach Mango	1 pkg (2 oz)	35	0	8	5	tr
FlavorZ Strawberry Vanilla Cream	1 pkg (2 oz)	35	0	8	5	tr
Foodles Apples Granola & Yogurt	1 pkg (5 oz)	230	6	38	18	3
Snackers Apples w/ Caramel Dip & Chocolate	1 pkg (4.7 oz)	260	10	42	31	2
Snackers Apples w/ Grapes & Caramel	1 pkg (4.7 oz)	140	2	29	19	1
Snackers Apples w/ Pretzels & Cheese	1 pkg (4.7 oz)	240	10	29	9	2
Snackers Apples w/ Raisins & Pretzels	1 pkg (4.7 oz)	210	2	51	23	3
Dole						
Apple	1 med (5.4 oz)	80	0	22	16	4
Grapple						
Grape Flavored	1 med (6.4 oz)	95	0	25	19	4
Ready Pac						
Apples w/ Caramel Dip	1 pkg (6 oz)	200	0	52	34	2
Apples w/ Peanut Butter Dip	1 pkg (5.7 oz)	340	24	28	17	6
FROZEN						
sliced w/o sugar	½ cup	42	tr	11	–	2
REFRIGERATED						
Dole						
Fruit Crisp Apple Cinnamon	1 pkg (4 oz)	160	4	29	20	3
Parfait Apples & Creme	1 pkg (4.3 oz)	130	3	26	20	1
TAKE-OUT						
baked no sugar added	1 (5.6 oz)	90	tr	24	18	4
baked w/ sugar	1 (6 oz)	162	tr	42	37	4

FOOD	PORTION	CAL	FAT	CARB	SUGAR	FIBER
fried apple rings	1 serv (2.7 oz)	91	4	15	12	2
scalloped	½ cup (3.3 oz)	90	tr	24	20	2
APPLE JUICE						
cider	1 cup	117	tr	29	27	tr
juice + vitamin C & calcium	1 cup	117	tr	29	27	tr
mulled cider	1 serv	265	1	42	–	6
unsweetened w/o vitamin C	1 cup	117	tr	29	27	tr
Apple & Eve						
100% Juice	8 oz	110	0	26	22	–
Kedem						
100% Juice	8 oz	100	0	24	21	–
Minute Maid						
100% Juice	8 oz	100	0	28	26	–
Ocean Spray						
Juice	8 oz	100	0	28	28	–
Old Orchard						
100% Juice Apple Cider	8 oz	130	0	31	29	–
R.W. Knudsen						
Organic 100% Juice	8 oz	120	0	30	30	0
Smart Juice						
Organic 100% Juice	8 oz	117	0	29	27	tr
Snapple						
100% Juice Green Apple	8 oz	160	0	41	39	–
Juice Drink Apple	8 oz	110	0	27	27	–
TreeTop						
100% Juice	8 oz	120	0	29	26	–
Fiber Rich	8 oz	150	0	35	29	6
Grower's Best Apple Cider	8 oz	120	0	30	27	–

FOOD	PORTION	CAL	FAT	CARB	SUGAR	FIBER
Tropicana						
Trop50 Farmstand Apple	8 oz	50	0	12	12	0
APPLESAUCE						
sweetened	½ cup	97	tr	25	21	2
unsweetened	½ cup	52	tr	14	12	2
Beth's Farm Kitchen						
Chunky	2 tbsp (1 oz)	50	0	14	11	1
GoGo Squeeze						
Apple	1 pkg (3.2 oz)	60	1	14	13	1
Apple Banana	1 pkg (3.2 oz)	60	tr	14	11	1
Apple Cinnamon	1 pkg (3.2 oz)	50	tr	10	9	1
Apple Peach	1 pkg (3.2 oz)	60	tr	13	12	1
Seneca						
Apple Sauce	1 pkg (4 oz)	70	0	18	15	2
TreeTop						
Apple Sauce	1 pkg (4 oz)	70	0	18	15	2
APRICOT JUICE						
nectar	6 oz	106	tr	27	26	1
Ceres						
100% Juice	8 oz	130	0	32	28	0
APRICOTS						
canned in heavy syrup	½ cup	91	tr	23	20	3
canned in juice	½ cup	59	tr	15	13	2
canned in light syrup	½ cup	80	tr	21	19	2
canned in water	½ cup	33	tr	8	6	2
dried halves	6	51	tr	13	11	2
dried halves cooked w/o sugar	½ cup	106	tr	28	24	3
fresh	1	17	tr	4	3	1
fresh sliced	½ cup	40	tr	9	8	2
frozen sweetened	½ cup	119	tr	30	–	3

FOOD	PORTION	CAL	FAT	CARB	SUGAR	FIBER
Del Monte						
Halves Lite	½ cup (4.3 oz)	60	0	16	15	1
Mediterranean Dried	5 (1.4 oz)	100	0	24	18	4
Dole						
Fresh	3 (4 oz)	60	1	11	11	1
Fruit Bliss						
Soft Dried	1 pkg (1.76 oz)	135	0	31	18	3
ARROWHEAD						
corm boiled	1 med	9	tr	2	–	–
ARROWROOT						
raw	1 root (1.2 oz)	21	tr	4	–	tr
raw root sliced	1 cup	78	tr	16	–	2
ARTICHOKE						
CANNED						
hearts in oil	1 serv (3 oz)	100	7	9	1	4
Progresso						
Hearts	2	30	0	7	2	2
Hearts Marinated	2 (1.1 oz)	60	5	2	7	0
Reese						
Cocktail Artichokes Original	½ jar (5 oz)	50	0	9	2	2
Victoria						
Hearts	1 oz	25	1	12	0	0
FRESH						
cooked	1 med	60	tr	13	1	7
hearts cooked	½ cup	42	tr	9	1	5
FROZEN						
cooked	1 cup	42	tr	9	1	5
cooked w/o salt	1 pkg (9 oz)	108	1	22	2	11
TAKE-OUT						
stuffed	1 (8.8 oz)	397	14	54	6	10

FOOD	PORTION	CAL	FAT	CARB	SUGAR	FIBER
ASIAN FOOD (*see also* CURRY, DINNER, EGG ROLLS, SAUCE, SOY SAUCE, SUSHI)						
CANNED						
chow mein chicken w/o noodles	1 cup	194	8	10	6	2
FRESH						
wonton wrapper	1 (0.3 oz)	23	tr	5	–	tr
Nasoya						
Won Ton Wraps	8 (2.1 oz)	160	1	31	1	1
FROZEN						
Crazy Cuizine						
Korean Inspired BBQ Chicken	¼ pkg (5 oz)	240	10	16	16	0
Mandarin Orange Chicken	1 cup (5 oz)	260	7	35	14	0
Tangerine Beef	1 cup (5 oz)	360	18	38	18	1
Healthy Choice						
Sweet & Sour Chicken	1 pkg (11.9 oz)	420	9	71	25	6
Lean Cuisine						
Cafe Cuisine Chow Fun Beef	1 pkg (9 oz)	320	5	54	18	3
Cafe Cuisine Sweet & Sour Chicken	1 pkg (10 oz)	300	3	51	16	2
Cafe Cuisine Thai-Style Chicken	1 pkg (9 oz)	260	4	35	9	0
Simple Favorites Chicken Chow Mein	1 pkg (9 oz)	240	4	39	3	3
Newman's Own						
Skillet Meal General Paul's Chicken	½ pkg (10.9 oz)	400	16	47	20	5
Purely Asian Brand						
Broccoli Beef	½ pkg (11 oz)	400	22	32	8	8

FOOD	PORTION	CAL	FAT	CARB	SUGAR	FIBER
Mandarin Orange Chicken	½ pkg (12 oz)	450	10	73	47	7
Sweet & Sour Chicken	½ pkg (12 oz)	380	11	58	39	5
Quorn						
Kung Pao Chik'n	1 pkg (8.9 oz)	240	2	48	19	5
Tandoor Chef						
Chicken Tikka Masala	1 pkg (9.9 oz)	330	22	10	4	1
Vegetarian Plus						
Vegan Kung Pao Chicken	¼ pkg (2.5 oz)	205	7	32	4	6
Weight Watchers						
Chicken Teriyaki Stir Fry	1 pkg (11.8 oz)	340	6	49	13	5
SHELF-STABLE						
Dr. McDougall's						
Asian Entree Pad Thai Noodle Gluten Free as prep	1 pkg (2 oz)	200	2	42	2	2
Asian Entree Spicy Kung Pao Noodle as prep	1 pkg (2 oz)	220	2	42	5	2
Asian Entree Teriyaki Noodle as prep	1 pkg (2 oz)	200	1	43	8	3
Asian Entree Thai Peanut Noodles as prep	1 pkg (2 oz)	220	3	40	4	4
TAKE-OUT						
beef & broccoli	1 cup	221	12	10	3	3
beef w/ black bean sauce	1 serv (7 oz)	288	14	6	5	1
bo bia roll shrimp	1 (2.5 oz)	82	2	10	1	2
buddha's delight w/ cellophane noodles fat choi jai	1 serv (7.6 oz)	211	4	44	3	2

FOOD	PORTION	CAL	FAT	CARB	SUGAR	FIBER
bun baked red bean	1 (1.1 oz)	102	3	16	–	1
cha siu bao steamed buns w/ chicken filling	1 (2.3 oz)	160	3	26	4	tr
chicken masala	1 serv (8 oz)	430	25	8	–	0
chicken tandoori	1 serv (4 oz)	156	8	2	–	0
chicken tikka	1 serv (2.5 oz)	173	8	1	–	1
chinese garlic chicken	1 cup (5.7 oz)	290	19	8	3	1
chinese style fried egg noodles w/ seafood & lettuce	1 serv (14 oz)	694	37	63	1	8
chow mein beef w/o noodles	1 cup	271	15	12	4	3
chow mein chicken w/ noodles	1 cup (7.7 oz)	273	14	20	5	2
chow mein noodles	1 cup	237	14	26	tr	2
chow mein pork w/o noodles	1 cup	284	16	12	4	3
chow mein shrimp w/ noodles	1 cup (7.7 oz)	262	12	24	6	3
chow mein shrimp w/o noodles	1 cup	154	5	11	6	2
chow mein vegetable w/o noodles	1 cup	224	15	16	8	4
dim sum deep fried beancurd w/ shrimp	1 (1.1 oz)	77	6	2	–	1
dim sum deep fried yam	1 (2.4 oz)	201	12	23	–	2
dim sum meat filled	3 pieces (4 oz)	124	3	11	1	1
dim sum pork hash	1 (1.1 oz)	59	3	5	–	0
dim sum shrimp	3 (4 oz)	307	16	31	6	2
dim sum steamed chives & prawns	1 (1.2 oz)	48	2	5	–	1
egg foo yung beef	1 patty (6 oz)	243	16	7	3	1
egg foo yung chicken	1 patty (3 oz)	121	8	4	2	1

FOOD	PORTION	CAL	FAT	CARB	SUGAR	FIBER
egg foo yung pork	1 patty (3 oz)	125	8	4	2	1
egg foo yung shrimp	1 patty (3 oz)	153	12	3	2	1
filipino chicken adobo	1 serv (15 oz)	555	26	45	tr	1
foochow fish ball	1 (1 oz)	36	2	3	0	1
fried rice	1 cup	333	12	42	2	1
fried rice beef	1 cup	346	14	42	1	1
fried rice chicken	1 cup	329	12	42	1	1
fried rice pork	1 cup	335	13	42	1	1
fried rice shrimp	1 cup	323	12	42	2	1
general tsao's chicken	1 cup (5 oz)	296	17	16	5	1
green beans szechuan style	1 cup	176	12	16	3	6
indian style fried egg noodles w/ eggs tomato sauce & lime	1 serv (15 oz)	721	31	80	2	8
korean spicy shredded chicken	1 serv (5 oz)	258	16	5	5	2
kung pao beef	1 cup	410	30	9	2	2
kung pao chicken	1 cup (5.7 oz)	434	31	12	4	2
kung pao pork	1 cup	460	34	12	4	2
kung pao shrimp	1 cup (5.7 oz)	345	20	11	3	2
lemon chicken w/o vegetables	1 serv (6.6 oz)	503	28	26	3	1
lo mein beef	1 cup	286	11	31	3	3
lo mein chicken	1 cup (7 oz)	280	9	33	3	3
lo mein meatless	1 cup	234	6	38	3	3
lo mein pork	1 cup	314	14	34	3	3
lo mein shrimp	1 cup	236	7	33	2	4
moo goo gai pan chicken	1 cup (7.6 oz)	272	19	12	5	3
moo shu pork w/o pancake	1 cup	512	46	5	2	1
pad thai w/ chicken	1 cup (7 oz)	358	15	39	5	2

FOOD	PORTION	CAL	FAT	CARB	SUGAR	FIBER
pad thai w/ shrimp	1 cup (7 oz)	314	11	40	6	1
pakhoras	1 (2.5 oz)	163	8	16	–	4
paneer pakhora	1 (2.2 oz)	183	13	8	–	2
peking duck w/ pancakes & seafood sauce	1 serv (14 oz)	1871	121	157	39	5
pork w/ chinese cabbage	1 serv (4 oz)	120	8	1	0	1
sesame seed paste bun	1 (2.5 oz)	220	6	39	12	2
shrimp chips banh phong tom	6 med	214	14	20	1	tr
shrimp w/ lobster sauce	1 cup	298	12	8	2	1
shu mai chicken & vegetable dumplings	6 (3.6 oz)	160	5	18	6	1
sukiyaki beef	1 cup	165	7	6	4	1
sukiyaki chicken	1 serv (18 oz)	436	8	19	7	4
sweet & sour chicken w/o rice	1 cup	670	37	36	4	2
sweet & sour pork w/ rice	1 cup	268	6	40	10	2
sweet & sour pork w/o rice	1 cup	231	8	25	15	2
sweet & sour shrimp	1 cup	480	30	46	40	1
szechuan chicken	1 cup (5.7 oz)	180	9	9	2	2
szechuan shrimp & vegetables	1 cup	159	7	10	3	2
tempura hawaiian fish tofu vegetable	2 cups	285	22	13	9	2
tempura vegetable	8 pieces	90	6	8	1	1
teriyaki beef	1 cup	454	19	13	9	tr
teriyaki chicken	¾ cup	399	27	7	–	–
teriyaki chicken w/ rice	1 serv (11 oz)	430	6	77	10	1
teriyaki shrimp	1 cup	271	3	14	6	1
thai style pineapple rice w/ ham & pork floss	1 serv (7.7 oz)	408	14	60	22	6

FOOD	PORTION	CAL	FAT	CARB	SUGAR	FIBER
wonton fried meat filled	1 (0.7 oz)	54	3	5	tr	tr
wonton meat & shrimp boiled	1 (0.5 oz)	19	1	2	–	tr
ASPARAGUS						
CANNED						
spears	1	3	tr	tr	tr	tr
spears	1 cup	46	2	6	3	4
Del Monte						
Spears Tender Young	½ cup (4.3 oz)	20	0	3	0	1
Tips	½ cup (4.2 oz)	20	0	3	0	1
McSweet						
Pickled Spears	6 (1 oz)	25	0	6	6	0
FRESH						
cooked	½ cup	20	tr	4	1	2
spears cooked	4	13	tr	2	1	1
spears raw	4	10	tr	2	1	1
Dole						
Spears	5 med (2.8 oz)	15	0	3	2	2
FROZEN						
cooked	1 pkg (10 oz)	53	1	6	1	5
spears cooked	4	11	tr	1	tr	1
Seabrook Farms						
Spears	7 (2.9 oz)	20	0	3	2	2
ATEMOYA						
fresh	½ cup	94	1	24	–	–
AVOCADO						
california mashed	¼ cup	96	9	5	tr	4
california peeled & pitted	1	289	27	15	1	12
florida mashed	¼ cup	69	6	5	0	1
florida peeled & pitted	1	365	31	24	7	17

FOOD	PORTION	CAL	FAT	CARB	SUGAR	FIBER
Calavo						
Fresh	⅕ med (1 oz)	55	5	3	0	3
Dole						
Fresh	⅕ med (1 oz)	50	5	3	0	2
Margaritaville						
Guacamole Zesty Island Garlic	1 oz	40	4	3	0	2
Wholly Guacamole						
Classic	2 tbsp (1 oz)	60	5	3	0	2
Guacamole Snack Packs	1 pkg (2 oz)	100	10	5	0	3
TAKE-OUT						
guacamole	1 serv (2.2 oz)	105	10	5	1	2

BACON

FOOD	PORTION	CAL	FAT	CARB	SUGAR	FIBER
bacon grease	1 tbsp	116	13	0	0	0
beef breakfast strips cooked	3 strips	153	12	tr	0	0
gammon lean & fat grilled	4.2 oz	274	15	0	–	0
pan fried	3 strips	109	9	tr	–	0
turkey	2 (0.8 oz)	84	6	1	0	0
Dietz & Watson						
Gourmet	2 strips (0.5 oz)	70	6	1	1	0
Pancetta	⅙ pkg (0.5 oz)	50	5	0	0	0
Hormel						
Black Label Lower Sodium	2 slices (0.5 oz)	80	7	0	0	0
Microwave Ready	2 slices (0.5 oz)	80	7	0	0	0
Organic Prairie						
Uncured Hardwood Smoked	2 strips (2 oz)	270	27	1	1	0
Uncured Turkey	2 strips (1 oz)	40	1	0	0	0

FOOD	PORTION	CAL	FAT	CARB	SUGAR	FIBER
Oscar Mayer						
Bacon Bits	1 tbsp (7 g)	25	2	0	0	0
Fully Cooked	3 slices (0.5 oz)	70	5	0	0	0
Hardwood Smoked	2 slices (0.5 oz)	70	6	0	0	0
Lower Sodium	3 slices (0.5 oz)	70	6	0	0	0
Super Thick Applewood Smoked	0.6 oz	90	7	1	0	–
Turkey	0.5 oz	35	3	0	0	0
Turkey Lower Sodium	0.5 oz	35	3	0	0	0
BACON SUBSTITUTES						
bacon bits meatless	1 tbsp	33	2	2	0	1
meatless	1 strip	16	1	tr	0	tr
McCormick						
Bac'n Pieces	1 tbsp (7 g)	30	1	2	–	0
BAGEL						
cinnamon raisin	1 lg (4 in)	244	2	49	5	2
cinnamon raisin mini	1	71	tr	14	2	1
egg	1 lg (4.5 in)	364	3	69	–	3
low carb	1 (4 oz)	216	0	42	0	14
oat bran	1 lg (4 in)	227	1	47	1	3
onion mini	1 (1.4 oz)	100	0	20	1	1
plain	1 sm (3 in)	190	1	37	–	2
plain	1 med (3.5 in)	289	2	56	–	2
plain	1 lg (4.5 in)	360	2	70	–	3
Pepperidge Farm						
Bagel Flats Plain	1	100	1	22	3	5
Thomas'						
Bagel Holes Plain	3 (1.6 oz)	120	1	24	3	1
Bagel Thins Everything	1 (1.6 oz)	110	1	24	3	5
Udi's						
Gluten Free Plain	1 (3.5 oz)	280	9	43	5	3
Gluten Free Whole Grain	1 (3.5 oz)	280	9	43	4	3

FOOD	PORTION	CAL	FAT	CARB	SUGAR	FIBER
BAKING POWDER						
baking powder	1 tsp	2	0	1	0	0
low sodium	1 tsp	5	tr	2	0	tr
Davis						
Baking Powder	⅛ tsp (0.6 g)	0	0	tr	–	–
BAKING SODA						
baking soda	1 tsp	0	0	0	0	0
Arm & Hammer						
Baking Soda	¼ tsp	0	0	0	0	0
BALSAM PEAR (BITTER GOURD)						
leafy tips cooked w/o salt	1 cup	20	tr	4	1	1
leafy tips raw	1 cup	14	tr	2	–	–
pods raw sliced	1 cup	16	tr	3	–	3
pods sliced cooked w/ salt	1 cup	24	tr	5	2	3
BAMBOO SHOOTS						
canned sliced	½ cup	12	tr	2	1	1
fresh sliced cooked w/ salt	½ cup	7	tr	1	–	1
raw sliced	½ cup	20	tr	4	2	2
BANANA						
banana chips	1 oz	147	10	17	–	2
fresh	1 sm (6 in)	90	tr	23	12	3
fresh	1 med (7 in)	105	tr	27	14	3
fresh	1 lg (8 in)	121	tr	31	17	4
fresh baby	1 extra sm (<6 in)	72	tr	19	10	2
fresh mashed	½ cup	100	tr	26	14	3
fresh sliced	1 cup	134	1	34	18	4
green fried	1 (3.1 oz)	152	8	21	11	2

FOOD	PORTION	CAL	FAT	CARB	SUGAR	FIBER
green pickled	½ cup	240	22	11	6	1
green sliced fried	1 cup	323	18	45	24	5
powder	1 tbsp	21	tr	5	3	1
red ripe	1 (7 in)	93	tr	24	13	3
red ripe sliced	1 cup	134	1	34	18	4
whole dried	1 piece (1.2 oz)	130	1	33	22	2
Crispy Green						
Crispy Bananas	1 pkg (0.5 oz)	55	0	13	8	2
Crunchies						
Freeze Dried Organic	¼ cup (0.3 oz)	32	0	9	7	1
Crunchy N'Yummy						
Organic Freeze Dried	1 pkg (1 oz)	110	0	23	0	tr
Dole						
Fresh	1 med (4.4 oz)	110	0	29	15	3
TAKE-OUT						
batter dipped fried	1 sm (4 oz)	266	15	32	9	3
batter dipped fried sliced	1 cup	335	19	40	12	3
fried dwarf w/ cheese	1 (1.4 oz)	84	5	10	5	1
fritter	1 (2.3 oz)	197	5	36	14	2
BANANA JUICE						
R.W. Knudsen						
Sensible Sippers Organic	1 box (4.23 oz)	35	0	9	8	–
Snapple						
Juice Drink Go Bananas	8 oz	110	0	28	28	–
BARBECUE SAUCE						
barbecue	2 tbsp	52	tr	13	9	tr
low sodium	2 tbsp	52	tr	13	9	tr
Ali's All Natural						
Homestyle	2 tbsp	10	0	2	1	–
Raspberry Chipotle	2 tbsp	10	0	2	1	–

FOOD	PORTION	CAL	FAT	CARB	SUGAR	FIBER
Annie's Homegrown						
Organic	2 tbsp (1.2 oz)	45	1	9	5	–
Chef Hymie Grande						
Cascabel Express Barbecue Glaze	2 tbsp (1.2 oz)	30	0	7	5	1
Polapote Barbecue Glaze	2 tbsp (1.2 oz)	30	0	7	4	2
David's Unforgettables						
Balsamic Spicy	2 tbsp (1 oz)	70	5	6	5	0
Jake & Amos						
Apple Butter Barbecue Sauce	2 tbsp (0.5 oz)	30	0	7	7	0
OrganicVille						
Original No Added Sugar	2 tbsp (1 oz)	50	0	13	11	tr
Ribber City						
Kansas City	2 tbsp (1.1 oz)	40	0	11	9	0
Steel's						
No Sugar Added Gluten Free	2 tbsp (1.3 oz)	24	0	3	3	0
Walden Farms						
Original Calorie Free	2 tbsp (1 oz)	0	0	0	0	0
BARLEY						
flour	1 cup	511	2	110	1	15
pearled cooked	1 cup (5.5 oz)	193	1	44	tr	6
pearled uncooked	¼ cup	176	1	39	tr	8
BARRACUDA						
broiled	4 oz	239	14	tr	tr	0
cooked flaked	1 cup	287	16	1	tr	0
poached	4 oz	227	11	0	0	0
TAKE-OUT						
breaded & fried	4 oz	282	17	5	tr	tr

FOOD	PORTION	CAL	FAT	CARB	SUGAR	FIBER
BARRAMUNDI						
Australis						
Barramundi fresh or frzn	6 oz	140	2	0	0	0
Crispy Asian Sesame Panko	1 piece (4 oz)	240	11	24	2	1
Fast & Delicious Mediterranean Seafood	½ pkg (6 oz)	230	9	22	1	2
Fast & Delicious Rosemary Parmesan	½ pkg (6 oz)	230	11	17	2	2
Fast & Delicious Seafood Penne	½ pkg (6 oz)	250	11	22	3	1
Fast & Delicious Seafood Pomodoro	½ pkg (6 oz)	230	12	17	1	1
Fast & Delicious Seafood Risotto	½ pkg (6 oz)	250	15	14	1	1
Fast & Delicious Seafood Teriyaki	½ pkg (6 oz)	180	4	24	7	1
Fast & Delicious Seafood Veracruz	½ pkg (6 oz)	150	3	19	2	2
Lemon Herb Butter	1 piece (4.5 oz)	131	6	2	1	0
BASIL						
fresh chopped	2 tbsp	1	tr	tr	tr	tr
ground	1 tsp	4	tr	1	tr	1
leaves fresh	5	1	tr	tr	tr	tr
BASS						
breaded baked	4 oz	205	7	10	1	1
pickled mero en escabeche	2 oz	156	14	tr	tr	tr
striped baked	3 oz	105	3	0	0	0
striped bass farm raised	4 oz	110	3	0	0	0

FOOD	PORTION	CAL	FAT	CARB	SUGAR	FIBER
BAY LEAF						
crumbled	1 tsp	2	tr	tr	tr	tr
BEAN SPROUTS (*see* ALFALFA, SPROUTS)						
BEANS (*see also* INDIVIDUAL NAMES)						
CANNED						
baked beans plain	½ cup	119	tr	27	–	5
baked beans vegetarian	½ cup	119	tr	27	–	5
baked beans w/ franks	½ cup	184	9	20	–	9
baked beans w/ pork	½ cup	134	2	25	–	7
baked beans w/ pork & tomato sauce	½ cup	119	1	24	7	5
refried beans	½ cup	134	1	23	–	–
Bush's						
Boston Recipe	½ cup (4.6 oz)	150	1	31	11	5
Cocina Latina Frijoles A La Mexicana	½ cup (4.6 oz)	100	2	16	1	4
Cocina Latina Frijoles Charros Machacados	½ cup (4.6 oz)	130	3	19	1	5
Country Style	½ cup (4.6 oz)	160	1	33	16	5
Grillin' Beans Bourbon & Brown Sugar	½ cup (4.6 oz)	170	1	35	15	6
Grillin' Beans Steakhouse Recipe	½ cup (4.6 oz)	180	1	39	21	5
Grillin' Beans Sweet Mesquite	½ cup (4.6 oz)	160	1	32	13	5
Honey Baked	½ cup (4.6 oz)	160	1	32	14	6
Maple Cured Bacon	½ cup (4.6 oz)	140	1	28	11	5
Onion Baked	½ cup (4.6 oz)	140	1	29	12	5

FOOD	PORTION	CAL	FAT	CARB	SUGAR	FIBER
Original	½ cup (4.6 oz)	140	1	29	12	5
Refried Fat Free	½ cup (4.4 oz)	130	0	24	0	7
Refried Traditional	½ cup (4.4 oz)	150	3	24	0	7
Vegetarian Fat Free	½ cup (4.6 oz)	130	0	29	12	5
Goya						
Fiesta Baked Beans Original	½ cup (4.6 oz)	200	1	43	18	9
Hormel						
Kid's Kitchen Microwave Meals Beans & Wieners	1 pkg (7.7 oz)	310	13	37	14	7
Jake & Amos						
Four Bean Salad	2 tbsp	32	0	8	6	0
Van Camp's						
Beanee Weenee Original	1 can (7.75 oz)	240	8	29	8	8
FROZEN						
Lean Cuisine						
Simple Favorites Sante Fe Rice & Beans	1 pkg (10.4 oz)	290	5	50	8	4
TAKE-OUT						
baked beans	½ cup	191	7	27	–	7
barbecue beans	3.5 oz	120	tr	26	–	–
frijoles a la charra w/ pork tomatoes & chili peppers	1 cup	341	22	23	2	5
refried beans	½ cup	43	2	5	–	–
three bean salad	1 cup	114	5	15	2	5

BEAR

simmered	3 oz	220	11	0	0	0

FOOD	PORTION	CAL	FAT	CARB	SUGAR	FIBER
BEAVER						
roasted	4 oz	240	8	0	0	0
BEE POLLEN						
bee pollen	1 tsp (5 g)	16	tr	2	2	tr
BEECHNUTS						
dried	1 oz	163	14	10	–	–
BEEF (*see also* BEEF DISHES, JERKY, MEATBALLS, VEAL)						
CANNED						
corned beef	1 oz	71	4	0	0	0
Hormel						
Corned Beef	1 serv (2 oz)	120	6	0	0	0
Dried Beef	1 oz	50	2	1	1	0
FRESH						
arm pot roast trim 0 fat braised	3.5 oz	297	19	0	0	0
arm pot roast trim ⅛ in fat braised	3.5 oz	302	19	0	0	0
beef crumbles 70% lean pan browned	3 oz	230	15	0	0	0
bottom round roast trim 0 fat braised	4 oz	253	10	0	0	0
bottom round roast trim 0 fat roasted	3.5 oz	187	8	0	0	0
bottom round roast trim ½ in fat braised	4 oz	337	22	0	0	0
bottom round roast trim ⅛ in fat braised	4 oz	280	13	0	0	0
bottom round roast trim ⅛ in fat roasted	4 oz	247	13	0	0	0
bottom sirloin butt roast trim 0 fat roasted	3.5 oz	182	8	0	0	0

FOOD	PORTION	CAL	FAT	CARB	SUGAR	FIBER
brisket flat half trim ⅛ in fat braised	3.5 oz	298	19	0	0	0
brisket flat trim 0 fat braised	3.5 oz	221	9	0	0	0
brisket point half trim 0 fat braised	3.5 oz	358	29	0	0	0
brisket point half trim ¼ in fat braised	3.5 oz	404	22	0	0	0
brisket point half trim ⅛ in fat braised	3.5 oz	349	27	0	0	0
chuck boston cut roast trim 0 fat roasted	3.5 oz	207	11	0	0	0
chuck boston cut roast trim ¼ in fat roasted	3.5 oz	242	15	0	0	0
chuck bottom roast trim 0 fat braised	3.5 oz	334	24	0	0	0
chuck bottom roast trim ¼ in fat braised	3.5 oz	345	26	0	0	0
chuck fillet steak trim 0 fat broiled	4 oz	181	6	0	0	0
chuck top roast trim 0 fat broiled	4 oz	245	13	0	0	0
club steak trim ½ in fat broiled	4 oz	384	29	0	0	0
corned beef brisket cooked	3 oz	213	16	tr	0	0
crosscut shank trim ¼ in fat stewed	1 serv (6.8 oz)	510	28	0	0	0
delmonico steak trim ¼ in fat broiled	4 oz	409	33	0	0	0
entrecote steak trim ½ in fat broiled	4 oz	413	33	0	0	0
eye round roast trim 0 fat roasted	4 oz	190	5	0	0	0

FOOD	PORTION	CAL	FAT	CARB	SUGAR	FIBER
eye round roast trim ¼ in fat roasted	4 oz	283	17	0	0	0
filet mignon roast trim ¼ in fat roasted	4 oz	376	29	0	0	0
filet mignon roast trim ⅛ in fat roasted	4 oz	367	28	0	0	0
filet mignon trim 0 fat broiled	4 oz	247	13	0	0	0
filet mignon trim ⅛ in fat broiled	4 oz	303	19	0	0	0
ground 70% lean broiled	3.5 oz	273	18	0	0	0
ground 75% lean broiled	2.5 oz	195	13	0	0	0
ground 80% lean broiled	3 oz	234	15	0	0	0
ground 85% lean pan fried	3 oz	197	12	0	0	0
ground 90% lean pan fried	3 oz	173	9	0	0	0
ground 95% lean pan fried	3 oz	139	5	0	0	0
ground 97% lean irradiated	4 oz	160	8	0	0	0
ground lowfat w/ carrageenan raw	4 oz	160	7	tr	–	–
london broil trim 0 fat broiled	3.5 oz	188	8	0	0	0
london broil trim ¼ in fat broiled	4 oz	260	12	0	0	0
new york strip steak trim 0 fat broiled	4 oz	219	9	0	0	0
oxtails cooked	6 pieces (6.3 oz)	472	26	0	0	0

FOOD	PORTION	CAL	FAT	CARB	SUGAR	FIBER
porterhouse steak trim 0 fat broiled	1 lb	1252	87	0	0	0
porterhouse steak trim ¼ in fat broiled	1 lb	1492	117	0	0	0
porterhouse steak trim ⅛ in fat broiled	1 lb	1324	99	0	0	0
porterhouse steak trim ⅛ in fat broiled	4 oz	337	25	0	0	0
rib eye roast trim ¼ in fat roasted	3.5 oz	365	30	0	0	0
rib eye steak trim ⅛ in fat broiled	4 oz	221	9	0	0	0
rib roast trim ¼ in fat roasted	4 oz	406	33	0	0	0
rib steak trim ¼ in fat broiled	4 oz	388	31	0	0	0
round tip roast trim 0 fat roasted	4 oz	213	9	0	0	0
sandwich steaks thinly sliced	1 serv (2 oz)	173	15	0	0	0
shell steak trim ¼ in fat broiled	4 oz	366	27	0	0	0
shortribs lean & fat braised	1 serv (7.8 oz)	1060	94	0	0	0
skirt steak trim 0 fat broiled	4 oz	289	19	0	0	0
t-bone steak trim 0 fat broiled	4 oz	280	18	0	0	0
t-bone steak trim ¼ in fat broiled	1 lb	1388	103	0	0	0
t-bone steak trim ⅛ in fat broiled	1 lb	804	56	0	0	0
tip round roast trim ⅛ in fat roasted	4 oz	248	13	0	0	0

FOOD	PORTION	CAL	FAT	CARB	SUGAR	FIBER
top loin steak boneless trim ⅛ in fat broiled	4 oz	299	19	0	0	0
top round roast trim 0 fat braised	4 oz	237	7	0	0	0
top round roast trim ¼ in fat braised	4 oz	281	13	0	0	0
top round roast trim ¼ in fat roasted	4 oz	265	15	0	0	0
top round steak trim ¼ in fat pan fried	4 oz	314	17	0	0	0
top sirloin steak trim ⅛ in fat broiled	4 oz	275	16	0	0	0
top sirloin steak trim ⅛ in fat pan fried	4 oz	355	24	0	0	0
tri-tip roast trim 0 fat roasted	3.5 oz	218	12	0	0	0
tri-tip steak trim 0 fat broiled	4 oz	300	17	0	0	0
Dietz & Watson						
Prime Rib Seasoned	3 oz	150	8	0	1	0
Maverick Ranch						
Ground Beef 85% Lean not prep	4 oz	150	17	0	0	0
Ground Beef 96% Lean not prep	4 oz	130	5	0	0	0
NY Strip Steak not prep	4 oz	180	10	0	0	0
Ribeye Steak not prep	4 oz	215	15	0	0	0
Organic Prairie						
Grass Fed Ground	4 oz	240	17	0	0	0
READY-TO-EAT						
dried beef smoked chopped	1 oz	37	1	1	–	0
roast beef spread	¼ cup	127	9	2	tr	tr

FOOD	PORTION	CAL	FAT	CARB	SUGAR	FIBER
TAKE-OUT						
roast beef rare	2 oz	70	2	0	0	0
BEEF DISHES						
CANNED						
corned beef hash	3 oz	155	10	9	–	–
Dinty Moore						
Beef Stew	½ can	200	10	17	3	1
Hormel						
Beef Stew	1 pkg (7.5 oz)	150	6	15	2	2
Corned Beef Hash	1 cup (8.3 oz)	390	24	22	1	2
Corned Beef Hash 50% Reduced Fat	1 cup (8.3 oz)	290	12	24	2	2
Roast Beef Hash	1 cup (8.3 oz)	390	24	22	1	2
REFRIGERATED						
Hormel						
Beef Tips & Gravy	1 serv (4 oz)	170	8	4	3	1
TAKE-OUT						
beef bourguignonne	1 cup	339	12	10	3	1
beef satay + peanut sauce	2 skewers	253	16	6	4	1
bool kogi korean grilled beef	1 serv (5.2 oz)	256	15	5	3	tr
bool kogi korean marinated beef ribs	4 oz	190	10	6	4	0
bracciola	1 roll (4.7 oz)	276	14	8	1	1
bubble & squeak	5 oz	186	13	16	–	3
chipped beef on toast	1 slice (5 oz)	226	10	22	7	1
cornish pasty	1 (8 oz)	847	52	79	–	3
goulash w/ potatoes	1 cup	298	12	19	3	2
greek moussaka	1 serv (8.5 oz)	450	33	12	4	1
irish stew	1 cup (7 oz)	280	16	10	–	–
kebab indian	1 (5.4 oz)	553	40	2	–	–

FOOD	PORTION	CAL	FAT	CARB	SUGAR	FIBER
kheema	1 serv (6.7 oz)	781	71	1	–	tr
koftas	5	280	22	3	–	tr
meatloaf	1 lg slice (5 oz)	294	17	9	2	1
pepper steak	1 cup	317	20	5	2	1
pot roast w/ gravy	1 serv (6 oz)	320	10	4	0	0
samosa	2 (4 oz)	652	62	20	–	2
shepherds pie	1 serv (7 oz)	282	16	20	–	2
sloppy joes	1 serv (9 oz)	398	6	48	5	12
steak & kidney pie w/ top crust	1 slice (5 oz)	400	26	23	–	1
stew w/ potatoes & vegetables	1 cup	199	5	22	3	3
stroganoff	1 cup	394	25	15	2	1
swiss steak w/ sauce	1 serv (8 oz)	234	10	8	3	1
toad in the hole	1 (4.7 oz)	383	29	23	–	1
BEEFALO						
ground	3.5 oz	171	18	0	0	0
roasted	3.5 oz	188	6	0	0	0
t-bone steak	3.5 oz	111	3	0	0	0
BEER AND ALE						
alcohol free beer	7 oz	50	tr	11	5	–
ale brown	10 oz	77	0	8	–	0
ale pale	10 oz	88	0	12	–	0
beer cooler	1 (16 oz)	194	0	34	–	1
beer light	12 oz can	103	0	6	tr	0
beer regular	12 oz can	153	0	13	0	0
black & tan	1 serv (12 oz)	146	0	13	–	1
black velvet	1 serv (10 oz)	160	0	8	–	1
boilermaker	1 serv	216	0	13	–	1
lager	10 oz	80	0	4	–	0
lager & black	1 serv (14 oz)	241	0	39	–	–

FOOD	PORTION	CAL	FAT	CARB	SUGAR	FIBER
mead	1 serv	250	0	13	–	1
pilsener lager	7 oz	85	tr	13	2	–
shandy	1 serv	125	0	12	–	1
stout	10 oz	102	0	6	–	0
trojan horse	1 serv (16 oz)	189	0	35	–	–
Budweiser						
Beer	1 bottle (12 oz)	146	0	11	0	0
Bud Light	1 bottle (12 oz)	110	0	7	0	0
Select	1 bottle (12 oz)	99	0	3	0	0
Icehouse						
5.0	1 bottle (12 oz)	149	0	10	–	–
Keystone						
Light	1 bottle (12 oz)	103	0	5	–	–
Kilarney's						
Red Lager	1 bottle (12 oz)	197	0	23	–	–
Killian's						
Beer	1 bottle (12 oz)	163	0	14	–	–
Michelob						
Ultra	1 bottle (12 oz)	96	0	3	0	0
Weinhard's						
Amber Light	1 bottle (12 oz)	135	0	12	–	–
Blond Lager	1 bottle (12 oz)	161	0	14	–	–

FOOD	PORTION	CAL	FAT	CARB	SUGAR	FIBER
Hefeweizen	1 bottle (12 oz)	151	0	12	–	–
Pale Ale	1 bottle (12 oz)	147	0	13	–	–
BEET JUICE						
juice	7 oz	72	0	16	–	–
BEETS						
CANNED						
harvard	½ cup	90	tr	22	–	3
pickled	½ cup	74	tr	18	–	3
sliced	½ cup	37	tr	9	8	2
Butter Kernel						
Sliced	½ cup (4.2 oz)	40	0	8	6	1
Del Monte						
Pickled Sliced	½ cup (4.5 oz)	80	0	19	16	2
Sliced	½ cup (4.3 oz)	45	0	10	8	2
Jake & Amos						
Harvard	1 serv (4 oz)	90	0	23	20	1
FRESH						
greens cooked w/o salt	½ cup	19	tr	4	tr	2
sliced cooked	½ cup	37	tr	8	7	2
whole cooked	2 med (3.5 oz)	44	tr	10	8	2

BEVERAGES (*see* ALCOHOL DRINKS, BEER AND ALE, CHAMPAGNE, COFFEE, DRINK MIXERS, ENERGY DRINKS, FRUIT DRINKS, ICED TEA, MALT, MILKSHAKE, SMOOTHIES, SODA, TEA/HERBAL TEA, WATER, WINE, YOGURT DRINKS)

FOOD	PORTION	CAL	FAT	CARB	SUGAR	FIBER
BISCUIT						
MIX						
plain as prep	1 (2 oz)	190	7	27	–	1
Bisquick						
Heart Smart	⅓ cup (1.4 oz)	140	3	27	3	tr
REFRIGERATED						
plain baked	1 (1 oz)	93	4	13	tr	tr

FOOD	PORTION	CAL	FAT	CARB	SUGAR	FIBER
Immaculate Baking Co.						
Buttermilk	1 (2 oz)	170	7	23	4	0
TAKE-OUT						
buttermilk	1 lg (2.7 oz)	280	13	37	1	1
oatcakes	2 (4 oz)	115	5	16	–	1
plain	1 sm (1.2 oz)	127	6	17	tr	1
tea biscuit	1 (3 oz)	210	3	30	12	1
w/ egg	1 (4.8 oz)	373	22	32	–	1
w/ egg & bacon	1 (5.3 oz)	458	31	29	1	1
w/ egg & ham	1 (6.7 oz)	442	27	30	2	1
w/ egg & sausage	1 (6.3 oz)	581	39	11	1	1
w/ egg & steak	1 (5.2 oz)	410	28	21	–	–
w/ egg cheese & bacon	1 (5.1 oz)	477	31	33	–	–
w/ ham	1 (4 oz)	386	18	44	1	1
w/ sausage	1 (4.4 oz)	485	32	40	1	1

BISON (*see* BUFFALO)

BLACK BEANS

FOOD	PORTION	CAL	FAT	CARB	SUGAR	FIBER
dried cooked w/o salt	1 cup (6 oz)	227	1	41	–	15
Bush's						
Black Beans	½ cup (4.6 oz)	105	1	23	1	6
Reduced Sodium	½ cup (4.6 oz)	105	1	23	1	6
Progresso						
Black Beans	½ cup	100	1	17	–	5

BLACKBERRIES

FOOD	PORTION	CAL	FAT	CARB	SUGAR	FIBER
canned in heavy syrup	½ cup	118	tr	30	25	4
fresh	½ cup	31	tr	7	4	4
unsweetened frzn	½ cup	48	tr	12	8	4
Dole						
Fresh	1 cup (5.1 oz)	60	1	14	7	8
Marion frzn	1 cup (4.9 oz)	90	0	22	15	7

FOOD	PORTION	CAL	FAT	CARB	SUGAR	FIBER
BLACKBERRY JUICE						
canned	6 oz	65	1	13	13	tr
BLACKEYE PEAS						
CANNED						
cowpeas	1 cup (8.4 oz)	185	1	33	–	8
w/ pork	1 cup (8.4 oz)	199	4	40	–	8
Bush's						
Blackeye Peas	½ cup (4.6 oz)	75	0	15	0	3
Blackeye Peas w/ Bacon	½ cup (4.6 oz)	95	2	17	0	3
DRIED						
catjang cooked w/o salt	1 cup (6 oz)	200	1	35	–	6
cooked w/o salt	1 cup (5.8 oz)	160	1	34	5	8
FRESH						
cowpeas leafy tips chopped cooked w/o salt	1 cup (1.9 oz)	12	tr	1	–	–
TAKE-OUT						
blackeye peas & pork	1 cup (6.3 oz)	236	5	25	4	8
frijol de ojo negro guisados	1 cup (9.1 oz)	289	3	49	6	9
hopping john	1 cup (7.9 oz)	419	20	48	3	6
BLINTZE						
Golden						
Cheese	1 (2.1 oz)	80	2	13	5	2
Tofutti						
Mintz's Blintzes Dairy Free	1 (2 oz)	140	5	19	16	2
TAKE-OUT						
cheese	1 (2.7 oz)	160	9	15	4	tr
BLUEBERRIES						
canned in heavy syrup	½ cup	113	tr	28	26	2
fresh	½ cup	41	tr	11	7	2

FOOD	PORTION	CAL	FAT	CARB	SUGAR	FIBER
fresh	1 pt	229	1	58	40	10
frzn unsweetened	½ cup	40	1	9	7	2
Dole						
Blueberries frzn	1 pkg (3 oz)	50	1	10	7	2
Blueberries frzn	1 cup (4.9 oz)	70	1	17	12	4
Ocean Spray						
Fresh	1 cup	85	0	21	15	–
Top Crop						
Fresh	1 cup (4.9 oz)	80	0	19	9	5
BLUEFIN						
fillet baked	4.1 oz	186	6	0	0	0
BLUEFISH						
fresh baked	3 oz	135	5	0	0	0
BOAR						
wild roasted	3 oz	136	4	0	0	0
BOK CHOY (*see* CABBAGE)						
BONITO						
dried	1 oz	50	2	0	0	0
fresh	3 oz	117	4	0	0	0
BORAGE						
fresh chopped	1 cup	19	tr	3	–	–
BOTTLED WATER (*see* WATER)						
BOYSENBERRIES						
frzn unsweetened	½ cup	33	tr	8	5	4
in heavy syrup	½ cup	113	tr	29	–	3
BRAINS						
beef pan fried	3 oz	167	13	0	0	0
beef simmered	3 oz	123	9	0	0	0
lamb braised	3 oz	123	9	0	0	0

FOOD	PORTION	CAL	FAT	CARB	SUGAR	FIBER
lamb fried	3 oz	232	19	0	0	0
pork braised	3 oz	117	8	0	0	0
veal braised	3 oz	116	8	0	0	0
veal fried	3 oz	181	14	0	0	0
BRAN						
corn	1 cup (2.7 oz)	170	1	65	–	65
oat	½ cup (1.6 oz)	116	3	31	–	7
oat cooked	½ cup (3.8 oz)	44	1	13	–	3
rice	½ cup (2.1 oz)	187	12	29	–	12
wheat	½ cup (2 oz)	63	1	19	–	12
Mother's						
Oat Bran not prep	½ cup (1.4 oz)	150	3	25	1	6
BRAZIL NUTS						
dried unblanched	1 oz	186	19	4	–	–
BREAD						
CANNED						
boston brown	1 slice (1.6 oz)	88	1	19	5	2
FROZEN						
Kineret						
Challah Pull Apart	1 piece	140	3	25	2	3
Pepperidge Farm						
Garlic Toast	1 slice	150	7	18	2	1
Texas Toast Five Cheese	1 slice	150	7	17	1	2
Texas Toast Garlic	1 slice	140	7	17	2	tr
Tuscan Sourdough	2 in slice	170	7	22	1	1
Soul						
Naan Garlic	1 (3 oz)	340	6	62	0	2
Naan Tandoori	1 (3 oz)	320	6	57	0	2
Tandoor Chef						
Tandoori Naan	1 piece (3 oz)	182	2	37	0	3
MIX						
cornbread	1 piece (2 oz)	188	6	29	–	1

FOOD	PORTION	CAL	FAT	CARB	SUGAR	FIBER
READY-TO-EAT						
anadama	1 piece (1.1 oz)	87	1	16	3	1
baguette whole wheat	2 oz	140	0	29	tr	1
cassava	1 piece (3.5 oz)	299	1	71	3	3
challah	1 slice (1.4 oz)	115	2	19	1	1
cinnamon	1 slice (0.9 oz)	69	1	13	1	1
cracked wheat	1 slice (1.1 oz)	78	1	15	–	2
cuban bread	1 slice (1.1 oz)	83	1	16	1	1
french	1 slice (1.1 oz)	88	1	17	tr	1
italian	1 loaf (1 lb)	1255	4	256	–	–
navajo fry	1 piece	281	10	41	2	–
oat bran	1 slice (1.1 oz)	71	1	12	2	1
oatmeal	1 slice (0.9 oz)	73	1	13	2	1
pan criollo	1 piece (0.9 oz)	69	1	13	tr	tr
panettone	1 slice (0.9 oz)	86	2	15	5	1
pita	1 sm (1 oz)	77	tr	16	tr	1
pita	1 lg (2 oz)	165	1	33	1	1
pita whole wheat	1 sm (1 oz)	74	1	15	tr	2
pita whole wheat	1 lg (2.2 oz)	170	2	35	1	5
pumpernickel	1 slice (0.9 oz)	65	1	12	tr	2
raisin	1 slice (1.1 oz)	88	1	17	2	1
rye	1 slice (1.1 oz)	83	1	15	tr	2
seven grain	1 slice (1.1 oz)	80	1	15	3	2
wheat berry	1 slice (0.9 oz)	65	1	12	1	1
wheat bran	1 slice (1.3 oz)	89	1	17	3	1
wheat germ	1 slice (1 oz)	73	1	14	1	1
white cubed	1 cup	93	1	18	2	1
whole wheat	1 slice (1 oz)	69	1	13	6	2
Arnold						
Pocket Thins Flatbread 100% Whole Wheat	½ (1.5 oz)	100	2	20	2	5
Whole Grains 12 Grain	1 slice (1.5 oz)	110	2	21	3	3

FOOD	PORTION	CAL	FAT	CARB	SUGAR	FIBER
Farm To Market Bread						
100% Whole Wheat	1 slice	110	0	23	3	3
Grains Galore	1 slice (2 oz)	140	4	23	4	3
San Francisco Sour Dough	1 slice (1.4 oz)	90	0	19	0	1
Flatout						
Fold It Flatbread 5 Grain Flax	1 (1.7 oz)	100	3	17	1	8
Fold It Flatbread Traditional Country	1 (1.8 oz)	140	2	24	2	3
Light Original	1 (2 oz)	90	3	16	0	9
Light Sundried Tomato	1 (1.9 oz)	90	3	17	tr	9
Soft & No Crust Garden Spinach	1 (2 oz)	130	2	25	2	3
The Original	1 (2 oz)	130	2	24	2	3
Wrap Healthy Grain Harvest Wheat	1 (2 oz)	120	3	23	2	6
Wrap Healthy Grain Whole Grain White	1 (1.9 oz)	110	2	21	4	7
Wrap Mini Healthy Grain Harvest Wheat	1 (1 oz)	70	1	13	2	3
Food For Life						
Ezekiel 4:9 Flax Sprouted Grain Organic	1 slice (1.2 oz)	80	1	14	0	4
Garden Of Eatin'						
Pita Organic Bible Bread Original	1 (2 oz)	145	1	30	1	1
Gillian's Foods						
Gluten Free Cinnamon Raisin	1 slice (2 oz)	130	1	25	3	2
Kontos						
Pocket-Less Pita Whole Wheat	1 (2.8 oz)	210	2	38	4	4

FOOD	PORTION	CAL	FAT	CARB	SUGAR	FIBER
La Tortilla Factory						
Smart & Delicious Soft Wrap Multi Grain	1 (2.2 oz)	100	4	18	1	12
Smart & Delicious Soft Wrap Tomato Basil	1 (2.2 oz)	100	3	20	1	12
Smart & Delicious Soft Wrap Traditional	1 (2.2 oz)	90	3	20	tr	13
Smart & Delicious Soft Wrap Whole Grain	1 (2.2 oz)	170	4	28	1	5
Smart & Delicious Soft Wrap Whole Grain White	1 (2.2 oz)	100	3	23	0	13
Levy's						
Real Jewish Rye Everything	1 slice (1.1 oz)	90	2	16	1	tr
Manna Organics						
Banana Walnut Hemp	1 slice (2 oz)	140	3	27	12	2
Carrot Raisin	1 slice (2 oz)	130	0	27	10	5
Fig Fennel Flax	1 slice (2 oz)	120	2	26	8	5
Millet Rice	1 slice (2 oz)	130	0	28	9	5
Whole Rye	1 slice (2 oz)	150	0	32	7	5
Martin's						
Potato 100% Whole Wheat	1 slice (1.3 oz)	70	1	14	4	4
Matthew's						
Golden White	1 slice (1.1 oz)	90	1	18	2	tr
Honey 12 Grain	1 slice (1.1 oz)	80	2	15	3	1
Pepperidge Farm						
100% Whole Wheat	1 slice	100	2	20	3	4
15 Grain Whole Grain	1 slice	100	2	20	3	4
Ancient Grains	1 slice	100	2	20	3	4
Cinnamon Swirl	1 slice	80	2	15	4	tr
Cinnamon Swirl Raisin	1 slice	80	2	15	5	tr

FOOD	PORTION	CAL	FAT	CARB	SUGAR	FIBER
Deli Swirl	1 slice	80	1	14	tr	1
Farmhouse Hearty White	1 slice	120	2	22	4	1
Farmhouse Honey Wheat	1 slice (1.5 oz)	120	2	21	5	2
Farmhouse Oatmeal	1 slice (1.5 oz)	120	2	21	3	1
Farmhouse Sourdough	1 slice	120	2	22	2	1
Farmhouse Whole Grain White	1 slice	110	2	21	4	3
German Dark Wheat	1 slice	100	2	17	2	3
Goldfish 100% Whole Wheat	2 slices	100	2	21	3	4
Goldfish Soft White	2 slices	100	1	23	4	4
Hearty Oatmeal	1 slice	100	2	20	3	4
Italian w/ Sesame Seeds	1 slice	90	1	15	1	tr
Jewish Rye Party	5 slices	130	2	25	1	2
Jewish Rye Seeded	1 slice	80	1	15	1	2
Light Style Extra Fiber Wheat	1 slice	120	1	26	3	6
Pumpernickel	1 slice	80	1	15	1	1
Swirl Cinnamon Raisin 100% Whole Wheat	1 slice (1 oz)	80	1	13	4	2
Swirled White & Wheat	1 slice (1.5 oz)	110	2	22	4	2
Stonefire						
Naan Original	½ (2.2 oz)	190	5	30	2	1
Naan Whole Grain	½ (2.2 oz)	180	5	28	3	4
Pita Original	½ (1.6 oz)	120	1	24	2	1
Pita Whole Grain	½ (1.6 oz)	120	1	23	3	3
Tandoori Roti	½ (1.6 oz)	150	6	22	2	1
Tandoori Roti Whole Grain	½ (1.6 oz)	150	6	22	2	3
Tumaro's						
Deli Style Wraps Cracked Pepper	1 (2.1 oz)	100	3	21	1	12

FOOD	PORTION	CAL	FAT	CARB	SUGAR	FIBER
Deli Style Wraps Everything	1 (2.1 oz)	80	3	17	1	10
Deli Style Wraps Pumpernickel	1 (2.1 oz)	80	2	19	1	9
Deli Style Wraps Rye	1 (2.1 oz)	80	2	19	1	9
Deli Style Wraps Sour Dough	1 (2.1 oz)	80	2	17	1	9
Udi's						
Gluten Free Cinnamon Raisin	2 slices (2.1 oz)	160	4	29	10	1
Gluten Free Whole Grain	2 slices (2 oz)	140	4	22	3	1
Wonder						
100% Whole Wheat Soft	2 slices (1.6 oz)	110	2	20	3	3
Classic White	1 slice (1 oz)	70	1	14	2	0
Light White	1 slice (0.8 oz)	40	0	9	2	2
Smart White	1 slice (0.9 oz)	50	1	11	2	2
Texas Toast	1 slice (1.4 oz)	100	1	19	2	tr
Whole Grain White	2 slices (2 oz)	140	2	25	5	3
TAKE-OUT						
banana	1 slice (2 oz)	196	6	33	–	1
chapati as prep w/ fat	1 (1.6 oz)	95	2	18	1	3
chapati as prep w/o fat	1 (2.5 oz)	141	1	31	–	5
cornbread	1 piece (2.3 oz)	183	6	27	4	2
cornstick	1 (1.4 oz)	118	4	18	3	1
focaccia onion	1 piece (4.6 oz)	282	10	43	2	2
focaccia rosemary	1 piece (3.5 oz)	251	7	40	1	2
focaccia tomato olive	1 piece (4.7 oz)	270	8	42	1	2
garlic bread	1 slice (1 oz)	96	4	13	tr	1

FOOD	PORTION	CAL	FAT	CARB	SUGAR	FIBER
irish soda bread	1 slice (3 oz)	247	4	48	–	2
italian garlic	1 loaf (11 oz)	990	38	137	1	8
naan	1 bread (3.5 oz)	286	9	43	3	2
papadum fried	1 (6 g)	30	2	2	–	tr
paratha plain	1 (1.6 oz)	136	5	19	–	2
poori indian puffed bread	1 piece (1.3 oz)	112	4	16	tr	2
zucchini	1 slice (1.4 oz)	150	7	19	10	1
BREADCRUMBS						
dry seasoned	¼ cup	115	2	21	2	2
fresh	¼ cup	30	tr	6	tr	tr
plain	¼ cup	107	1	19	2	1
Gillian's Foods						
Plain Gluten Free	¼ cup (1.2 oz)	60	1	14	1	1
Kikkoman						
Panko	½ cup (1.1 oz)	110	1	24	2	tr
Progresso						
Italian Style	¼ cup (1 oz)	110	2	20	2	1
Panko Lemon Pepper	¼ cup (1 oz)	120	5	17	0	tr
Panko Plain	¼ cup (1 oz)	110	3	19	1	0
Plain	¼ cup (1 oz)	110	2	20	2	1
BREADFRUIT						
fresh	1 sm (13.5 oz)	396	1	104	42	19
fried	1 cup	379	21	52	21	9
raw	1 cup	227	1	60	24	11
BREADNUTTREE SEEDS						
dried	1 oz	104	tr	23	–	–
BREADSTICKS						
plain	1 sm	21	tr	3	tr	tr
plain	1 lg	41	1	7	tr	tr

FOOD	PORTION	CAL	FAT	CARB	SUGAR	FIBER
Stella D'Oro						
Sesame	1 (0.4 oz)	50	3	6	0	0
BREAKFAST BARS (*see* CEREAL BARS, ENERGY BARS)						
BREAKFAST DRINKS						
Carnation						
Breakfast Essential Classic French Vanilla	1 bottle (11.4 oz)	250	5	34	31	0
Breakfast Essentials Classic French Vanilla as prep w/ fat free milk	1 serv	220	0	39	1	0
Breakfast Essentials Rich Chocolate Milk as prep w/ fat free milk	1 serv	220	1	39	19	tr
Breakfast Essentials Rich Milk Chocolate	1 bottle (11.4 oz)	260	5	41	39	1
Breakfast Essentials Vanilla No Sugar Added as prep w/ fat free milk	1 serv	150	0	24	8	3
BROCCOFLOWER						
fresh flowerets cooked	1 cup (2.9 oz)	26	tr	5	3	3
fresh raw	1 cup (2.2 oz)	20	tr	4	2	2
head fresh raw	1 lg (18 oz)	158	2	31	15	16
BROCCOLI						
FRESH						
chinese broccoli (gai lan) cooked	1 cup (3 oz)	19	1	3	1	2
cooked w/o salt chopped	½ cup (2.7 oz)	27	tr	6	1	3
cooked w/o salt spear 5 in	1 (1.3 oz)	13	tr	3	1	1
raab cooked	½ cup (3 oz)	28	tr	3	1	2

FOOD	PORTION	CAL	FAT	CARB	SUGAR	FIBER
raw	1 bunch (1.3 lbs)	207	2	40	10	16
raw floweret	1 (0.4 oz)	3	tr	1	–	–
raw flowers	1 cup (2.5 oz)	20	tr	4	–	–
raw spear 5 in	1 (1.1 oz)	11	tr	2	1	1
Dole						
Broccoli	1 stalk (5.2 oz)	50	1	10	3	4
Broccoli Slaw	1 cup (3 oz)	25	0	5	2	2
Eat Smart						
Beneforte	1 serv (3 oz)	25	0	5	2	2
Florets	1 serv (3 oz)	25	0	4	2	2
Mann's						
Broccoli Wokly	1 serv (3 oz)	25	0	4	2	2
Broccolini	8 stalks (3 oz)	35	0	6	2	1
Ready Pac						
Microwave Broccoli Rabe as prep	½ cup (3 oz)	30	0	3	0	2
River Ranch						
Florets	¼ pkg (3 oz)	25	0	5	1	2
FROZEN						
chopped cooked w/o salt	1 cup (6.5 oz)	52	tr	10	3	6
spears cooked w/o salt	1 cup (6.5 oz)	52	tr	10	3	6
Dr. Praeger's						
Broccoli Bites	2 (2 oz)	110	4	17	2	2
Lisa's Organics						
Florets In Gorgonzola Bleu Cheese Sauce	½ pkg (4 oz)	60	3	4	1	2
Seabrook Farms						
Broccoli Raab	1 cup (2.9 oz)	25	0	4	tr	2
TAKE-OUT						
batter dipped & fried	3 pieces (1.4 oz)	58	4	5	1	1
w/ cheese sauce	1 cup (8 oz)	242	15	16	5	5

FOOD	PORTION	CAL	FAT	CARB	SUGAR	FIBER
BROWNIE						
brownie	1 (2 oz)	227	9	36	21	1
butterscotch	1 (1.2 oz)	151	8	19	12	tr
Betty Crocker						
Dark Chocolate as prep	1	170	7	25	17	tr
Fudge Low Fat as prep	1	140	3	28	19	1
Original Supreme as prep	1	160	6	26	18	tr
Triple Chunk as prep	1	180	8	25	18	1
Walnut as prep	1	170	9	22	15	tr
Warm Delights Hot Fudge	1 pkg (3 oz)	370	12	61	41	3
Fiber One						
Chocolate Fudge	1 (0.89 oz)	90	3	18	8	5
Chocolate Peanut Butter	1 (0.89 oz)	90	35	17	7	5
Foods By George						
Gluten Free	1/9 pkg (1.5 oz)	180	9	24	16	1
French Meadow Bakery						
Gluten Free Fudge	1 (2.82 oz)	350	16	48	34	2
Jiffy						
Fudge Mix as prep	1/8 pkg	160	7	24	15	tr
No Pudge!						
All Flavors as prep	1/12 pkg	120	0	51	22	1
Sans Sucre						
Blondie Mix as prep	1/8 pkg	130	0	25	0	0
Chocolate Fudge Mix as prep	1/8 pkg	130	3	25	0	tr
Milk Chocolate Mix as prep	1/8 pkg	130	3	25	1	0
Sheila G's						
Brownie Brittle Chocolate Chip	6 pieces (1 oz)	120	4	21	14	tr
Brownie Brittle Toffee Crunch	6 pieces (1 oz)	120	4	21	14	tr

FOOD	PORTION	CAL	FAT	CARB	SUGAR	FIBER
Brownie Brittle Traditional Walnut	6 pieces (1 oz)	120	4	20	13	tr
VitaBrownie						
Brownie	1 (2 oz)	100	2	25	10	10
Dark Chocolate Pomegranate	1 (2 oz)	100	2	21	11	6
BRUSSELS SPROUTS						
CANNED						
Jake & Amos						
Pickled Dill Brussels Sprouts	2 tbsp	10	0	1	0	0
FRESH						
cooked	6 pieces	45	1	9	2	3
Dole						
Brussels Sprouts	4 (2.9 oz)	30	0	6	1	3
Eat Smart						
Brussels Sprouts	1 serv (3 oz)	35	0	8	2	3
FROZEN						
cooked	1 cup	65	1	13	3	6
Green Giant						
Seasoned Steamers w/ Sea Salt & Black Pepper as prep	½ cup	70	3	8	2	3
BUCKWHEAT						
groats roasted cooked	1 cup (6 oz)	155	1	33	2	5
groats roasted uncooked	½ cup	292	3	61	–	9
Wolff's						
Kasha not prep	¼ cup (1.6 oz)	170	1	35	0	2
BUFFALO (*see also* HOT DOG, JERKY, SAUSAGE)						
burger	3 oz	202	13	0	0	0
chuck braised	4 oz	205	6	0	0	0

FOOD	PORTION	CAL	FAT	CARB	SUGAR	FIBER
top round steak broiled	3 oz	313	9	0	0	0
water buffalo roasted	3 oz	111	2	0	0	0
High Plains Bison						
Ribeye Steak	4 oz	215	14	1	0	0
BULGUR						
cooked	½ cup	76	tr	17	tr	4
uncooked	½ cup	239	1	53	tr	13
TAKE-OUT						
tabbouleh	1 cup	198	15	16	2	4
BURBOT (FISH)						
fresh baked	3 oz	98	1	0	0	0
BURDOCK ROOT						
cooked w/o salt	1 cup	110	tr	26	4	2
cooked w/o salt	1 root (5.8 oz)	146	tr	35	6	3
BUTTER						
clarified butter	1 tbsp (0.4 oz)	112	13	0	0	0
clarified butter	¼ cup (1.8 oz)	449	51	0	0	0
honey butter	1 tbsp (0.6 oz)	85	6	9	9	0
honey butter	¼ cup (2.5 oz)	338	23	36	35	tr
light butter whipped salted	1 tbsp (0.3 oz)	48	5	0	0	0
stick salted	1 tbsp (0.5 oz)	102	12	tr	tr	0
stick salted	¼ cup (2 oz)	407	46	tr	tr	0
stick salted	1 (4 oz)	810	92	tr	tr	0
stick unsalted	1 tbsp (0.5 oz)	102	12	tr	tr	0
stick unsalted	¼ cup (2 oz)	407	46	tr	tr	0
stick unsalted	1 (4 oz)	810	92	tr	tr	0

FOOD	PORTION	CAL	FAT	CARB	SUGAR	FIBER
whipped salted	1 tbsp (0.3 oz)	67	8	tr	tr	0
whipped salted	¼ cup (1.3 oz)	271	31	tr	tr	0
Breakstone's						
Salted	1 tbsp (0.5 oz)	100	11	0	0	0
Epicurean						
Scampi Butter	1 tbsp (0.5 oz)	90	10	1	–	–
Gopi						
Pure Ghee	1 tsp (5 g)	35	5	0	0	0
Karoun						
Unsalted	1 tbsp (0.5 oz)	100	11	0	0	–
Land O Lakes						
Butter Spread Cinnamon Sugar	1 tbsp (0.5 oz)	70	6	4	4	0
Honey	1 tbsp (0.5 oz)	90	8	4	3	0
Roasted Garlic w/ Oil	1 tbsp (0.5 oz)	90	10	0	0	0
Salted	1 tbsp (0.5 oz)	100	11	0	0	0
Plugra						
European Style Unsalted	1 tbsp (0.5 oz)	100	11	0	0	0
Straus						
Organic European Style Lightly Salted	1 tbsp (0.5 oz)	110	12	0	0	0
Organic European Style Sweet Butter	1 tbsp (0.5 oz)	110	12	0	0	0

BUTTER SUBSTITUTES

FOOD	PORTION	CAL	FAT	CARB	SUGAR	FIBER
stick	1 stick	811	91	1	–	–
Melt						
Rich & Creamy Organic	1 tbsp (0.5 oz)	80	9	0	0	0
Molly McButter						
Natural Butter	1 tsp (2 g)	5	0	1	–	0

FOOD	PORTION	CAL	FAT	CARB	SUGAR	FIBER
BUTTERBUR						
canned fuki chopped	1 cup	3	tr	tr	–	–
fresh fuki	1 cup	13	tr	3	–	–
BUTTERNUTS						
dried	1 oz	174	16	3	–	–
BUTTERSCOTCH (*see* CANDY)						
CABBAGE (*see also* COLESLAW)						
chinese bok choy shredded cooked w/o salt	1 cup	20	tr	3	1	2
chinese pe-tsai shredded cooked w/o salt	1 cup	17	tr	3	–	2
green raw shredded	1 cup	19	tr	4	2	2
green shredded cooked w/o salt	1 cup	34	tr	8	4	3
japanese pickled	½ cup	22	tr	4	1	2
red raw shredded	1 cup	22	tr	5	3	2
red shredded cooked w/o salt	1 cup	44	tr	10	5	4
savoy shredded cooked w/o salt	1 cup	35	tr	8	–	4
Aunt Nellie's						
Sweet & Sour Red	2 tbsp (1 oz)	20	0	5	4	0
Dole						
Shredded Red Fresh	1½ cups (3 oz)	25	0	6	3	2
Ready Pac						
Ready Fixin's Shredded Red	2 cups (3 oz)	25	0	6	3	2
River Ranch						
Angel Hair	1½ cups (3 oz)	25	0	5	3	2

FOOD	PORTION	CAL	FAT	CARB	SUGAR	FIBER
TAKE-OUT						
coleslaw w/ pineapple & dressing	1 cup (4.6 oz)	194	16	14	10	2
creamed	1 cup	158	10	13	7	2
kimchee	1 cup	32	tr	6	2	2
stuffed cabbage w/ rice & beef	1 (3.6 oz)	117	5	9	4	1
sweet & sour red cabbage	4 oz	61	3	8	–	3
CACTUS						
fresh cooked w/ fat	1 pad (1 oz)	11	1	1	tr	1
fresh cooked w/o fat	1 cup (5.2 oz)	22	tr	5	2	3
pricklypear fresh	1 cup (5.2 oz)	61	1	14	–	5
pricklypear fresh	1 (3.6 oz)	42	1	10	–	4
CAKE (*see also* CAKE MIX)						
battenburg cake	1 slice (2 oz)	204	10	28	–	1
cream puff shell	1 (2.3 oz)	239	17	15	–	–
crumpet	1 (2.3 oz)	131	1	31	–	2
dutch honey cake	1 slice (0.8 oz)	70	0	17	8	0
eccles cake	1 slice (2 oz)	285	16	36	–	1
madeira cake	1 slice (1 oz)	98	4	15	–	1
sponge	1 piece (1.3 oz)	110	1	23	14	tr
sponge cake dessert shell	1 (0.8 oz)	70	2	12	7	0
treacle tart	1 slice (2.5 oz)	258	10	42	–	1
turnover guava	1 (2.7 oz)	239	13	29	12	3
Athens						
Baklava	2 pieces (2 oz)	230	11	30	17	1
Balocco						
Il Panettone	1 (3.5 oz)	380	15	54	30	2

FOOD	PORTION	CAL	FAT	CARB	SUGAR	FIBER
Betty Crocker						
Warm Delights Cinnamon Swirl	1 (3.3 oz)	390	10	72	49	1
Coppenrath						
Mousse Cake Chocolate	⅛ cake (1.8 oz)	140	7	17	12	2
Mousse Cake Coconut	⅛ cake (1.8 oz)	140	8	15	11	2
Mousse Duets Chocolate	1 (3.2 oz)	290	15	32	25	2
Mousse Duets Lemon Chiffon	1 (3.2 oz)	280	16	31	23	tr
Do Goodie						
Gluten Free Banana Bread	1 slice (2 oz)	150	4	27	15	2
Gluten Free Cupcake Chocolate	1	290	14	41	31	1
Gluten Free Cupcake Vanilla	1	290	14	41	32	0
Earth Cafe						
Cheesecake Vegan Blueberry Thrill	1 slice (2 oz)	193	15	12	7	1
Cheesecake Vegan Coconut Carob	1 slice (2 oz)	206	16	13	8	1
Cheesecake Vegan Rockin' Raspberry	1 slice (2 oz)	194	15	12	7	2
Entenmann's						
Apple Puffs	1 (3 oz)	290	13	41	21	1
Blackout Iced	⅛ cake (2.2 oz)	210	8	34	23	1
Cheese Buns	1 (3 oz)	320	15	42	22	1
Chocolate Chip Iced	⅛ cake (2.5 oz)	330	18	40	31	tr

FOOD	PORTION	CAL	FAT	CARB	SUGAR	FIBER
Chocolate Fudge	⅛ cake (2.2 oz)	240	10	37	28	2
Cinnamon Swirl Buns	1 (3 oz)	320	14	45	21	2
Coffee Cake Cheese Filled Crumb	⅛ cake (2 oz)	210	10	28	13	tr
Danish Twist Cheese	⅛ cake (1.9 oz)	220	11	27	14	tr
Danish Twist Raspberry	⅛ cake (1.8 oz)	210	10	27	14	tr
Devil's Food Marshmallow Iced	⅛ cake (2.2 oz)	260	12	38	30	tr
Fudge Iced Golden Cake	⅛ cake (2.2 oz)	260	11	37	28	1
Lemon Crunch	⅛ cake (3 oz)	320	13	50	35	tr
Lemon Loaf	⅙ cake (2 oz)	210	10	28	17	0
Louisiana Crunch	⅛ cake (2.7 oz)	310	13	47	33	tr
Utlimate Super Cinnamons	½ bun (2.5 oz)	280	10	41	19	1
Vanilla Bean Iced	⅛ cake (2.2 oz)	290	17	36	28	0
Fiber One						
Toaster Pastry Blueberry	1 (1.8 oz)	180	4	36	15	5
Toaster Pastry Chocolate Fudge	1 (1.8 oz)	160	4	35	16	5
Foods By George						
Gluten Free Crumb Cake	⅑ cake (2.2 oz)	280	14	36	12	tr
Gluten Free Pound Cake	⅙ cake (2.7 oz)	290	12	35	16	tr
Kineret						
Babka Chocolate	1 piece (1 oz)	100	3	17	9	1

FOOD	PORTION	CAL	FAT	CARB	SUGAR	FIBER
Nature's Path						
Toaster Pastries Blueberry Organic	1 (1.8 oz)	210	5	40	18	1
Toaster Pastries Frosted Brown Sugar Maple Cinnamon Organic	1 (1.8 oz)	210	5	39	20	1
Toaster Pastries Frosted Chocolate Organic	1 (1.8 oz)	210	5	38	18	1
Toaster Pastries Frosted Strawberry	1 (1.8 oz)	210	4	40	19	1
Pepperidge Farm						
Coconut 3 Layer	⅛ cake	240	10	35	25	tr
German Chocolate 3 Layer	⅛ cake	240	10	34	23	1
Red Velvet 3 Layer	⅛ cake	230	11	32	25	0
Turnover Apple	1	260	13	31	11	1
Turnover Cherry	1	260	13	31	10	1
Prosperity						
Limoncello	1 serv (3.5 oz)	300	12	43	27	1
Weight Watchers						
Lemon Creme	1 (0.9 oz)	80	3	16	8	4
TAKE-OUT						
angelfood	1 slice (2 oz)	143	tr	33	17	tr
apple crisp	1 serv (8.6 oz)	384	8	76	49	4
apple turnover	1 (6.6 oz)	661	34	83	30	3
baklava	1 piece (2.7 oz)	334	23	29	10	2
basbousa namoura	1 piece (1 oz)	60	3	10	10	2
bean cake	1 cake (1.1 oz)	130	7	16	7	1
black forest chocolate cherry	1 piece (2.5 oz)	187	9	27	23	1

FOOD	PORTION	CAL	FAT	CARB	SUGAR	FIBER
boston cream pie	1 slice (3.2 oz)	232	8	39	33	1
cannoli w/ cannoli cream	1	369	21	42	28	–
carrot w/ icing	1 slice (4.7 oz)	543	28	70	52	2
cheesecake	1 slice (4.5 oz)	410	25	37	28	tr
cheesecake chocolate	1 slice (4.5 oz)	489	32	49	29	2
chinese moon cake	1 (4.8 oz)	458	6	92	49	4
cobbler pineapple	1 cup (7.6 oz)	414	10	80	45	2
coconut mochiko filipino cake	1 piece (2.7 oz)	252	12	35	11	2
coffeecake iced	1 piece (1.6 oz)	175	8	24	15	1
cream puff custard filled chocolate frosted	1 (3.9 oz)	293	18	27	7	1
éclair	1 (3.5 oz)	262	16	24	7	1
french apple tart	1 (3.5 oz)	302	15	37	15	2
fruitcake	1 slice (1.5 oz)	139	4	26	13	2
funnel cake	1 (3.2 oz)	276	14	29	4	1
gingerbread	1 piece (2.4 oz)	213	7	35	22	1
jelly roll	1 slice (1.8 oz)	146	2	28	20	tr
jelly roll lemon filled	1 slice (3 oz)	210	2	48	29	tr
napoleon	1 mini	123	9	9	1	tr
napoleon	1 (3 oz)	348	25	25	4	1
panettone	1/12 cake (2.9 oz)	300	12	43	21	2
petit fours	2 (0.9 oz)	120	7	15	12	0
pineapple upside down	1 piece (4.2 oz)	387	15	61	41	1
pound	1 slice (1 oz)	120	5	15	–	–

FOOD	PORTION	CAL	FAT	CARB	SUGAR	FIBER
pound fat free	1 slice (2 oz)	160	1	35	19	1
pumpkin bread w/ raisins	1 slice (2.1 oz)	178	4	34	22	1
red velvet cupcake w/ cream cheese frosting	1 sm	272	12	38	–	1
red velvet w/ cream cheese frosting	1/16 cake	520	24	70	–	1
sacher torte	1 slice (2.2 oz)	240	11	30	11	4
sacher torte chocolate + apricot jam	1 serv	430	12	23	–	–
strawberry shortcake	1 serv (4.1 oz)	211	5	40	35	1
strudel apple	1 piece (2.2 oz)	175	7	26	16	1
strudel cheese	1 piece (2.2 oz)	195	8	24	14	tr
strudel cherry	1 piece (2.2 oz)	179	6	29	18	1
strudel pineapple	1 piece (2.2 oz)	159	4	31	22	1
sweet potato w/ glaze	1 piece (2.7 oz)	275	12	39	26	1
tiramisu	1 piece (5.1 oz)	409	30	31	17	tr
tiramisu	1 cake (4.4 lbs)	5732	421	439	234	3
torte chocolate ganache	1 slice (3.5 oz)	400	26	40	24	6
trifle w/ cream	6 oz	291	16	34	–	1
white w/ coconut icing	1 slice (3.9 oz)	399	12	71	64	1
zucchini bread	1 slice (1.4 oz)	150	7	19	10	1

FOOD	PORTION	CAL	FAT	CARB	SUGAR	FIBER
CAKE ICING						
chocolate	¼ cup	269	7	53	51	1
vanilla	¼ cup	322	8	64	62	0
Betty Crocker						
HomeStyle Mix Fluffy White as prep	6 tbsp	100	0	24	23	–
Rich & Creamy Butter Cream	2 tbsp (1.3 oz)	140	5	15	19	–
Rich & Creamy Chocolate	2 tbsp (1.2 oz)	130	5	21	17	tr
Rich & Creamy Creamy White	2 tbsp (1.2 oz)	140	5	23	20	–
Rich & Creamy Lemon	2 tbsp (1.2 oz)	140	5	23	19	–
Rich & Creamy Vanilla	2 tbsp (1.2 oz)	140	5	23	19	–
Whipped Fluffy White	2 tbsp (0.8 oz)	100	5	15	14	–
Pillsbury						
Chocolate Fudge Sugar Free	2 tbsp (1 oz)	100	6	16	0	3
Creamy Supreme Buttercream	2 tbsp (1.2 oz)	150	6	24	22	0
Creamy Supreme Classic White	2 tbsp (1.2 oz)	150	6	24	0	0
Creamy Supreme Coconut Pecan	2 tbsp (1.2 oz)	160	10	17	16	tr
Creamy Supreme Milk Chocolate	2 tbsp (1.2 oz)	140	6	21	19	tr
Creamy Supreme Vanilla	2 tbsp (1.2 oz)	150	6	24	22	0
Easy Frost Chocolate Fudge	2 tbsp (1.2 oz)	140	6	21	19	tr
Easy Frost Cream Cheese	2 tbsp (1.2 oz)	150	6	24	22	0
Easy Frost Vanilla	2 tbsp (1.2 oz)	150	6	24	22	0

FOOD	PORTION	CAL	FAT	CARB	SUGAR	FIBER
Funfetti Pink Vanilla	2 tbsp (1.2 oz)	140	5	23	22	0
Vanilla Sugar Free	2 tbsp (1 oz)	100	6	17	0	3
Whipped Supreme Cream Cheese	1 tbsp (0.8 oz)	100	5	15	14	0
Whipped Supreme Strawberry	2 tbsp (0.8 oz)	110	5	15	14	0

CAKE MIX

Betty Crocker

FOOD	PORTION	CAL	FAT	CARB	SUGAR	FIBER
Gingerbread as prep	1 piece	220	6	39	19	–
Pineapple Upside Down as prep	⅙ cake	390	13	66	43	–
Pound Cake as prep	⅛ cake	260	8	45	26	–
SuperMoist Carrot as prep	1/12 cake	260	12	35	19	–
SuperMoist Chocolate as prep	1/12 cake	250	11	35	18	1
SuperMoist Devil's Food as prep	1/12 cake	260	12	35	18	1
SuperMoist Lemon as prep	1/12 cake	240	9	35	19	–
SuperMoist Milk Chocolate as prep	1/12 cake	240	9	35	19	tr
SuperMoist Spice as prep	1/12 cake	270	13	34	19	1
SuperMoist Vanilla as prep	1/12 cake	230	9	35	18	–
SuperMoist White as prep	1/12 cake	220	8	35	18	–
SuperMoist Yellow as prep	1/12 cake	230	9	35	19	–

Bisquick

FOOD	PORTION	CAL	FAT	CARB	SUGAR	FIBER
Heart Smart	⅓ cup (1.4 oz)	140	3	27	3	tr

FOOD	PORTION	CAL	FAT	CARB	SUGAR	FIBER
Jell-O						
No Bake Peanut Butter as prep	⅛ cake	360	21	42	27	0
No Bake Real Cheesecake as prep	⅛ cake	360	21	42	27	0
Jiffy						
Devil's Food as prep	⅕ cake	220	5	39	23	1
Krusteaz						
Honey Cornbread as prep	1 piece (2x2 in)	140	6	21	8	tr
Sans Sucre						
Apple Cinnamon Coffee Cake as prep	⅐ pkg	150	4	30	3	tr

CALZONE (*see* SANDWICHES)

CANADIAN BACON

FOOD	PORTION	CAL	FAT	CARB	SUGAR	FIBER
grilled	2 slices (1.6 oz)	87	4	1	0	0
Dietz & Watson						
Canadian Style	2 oz	70	2	1	1	0
Oscar Mayer						
Fully Cooked	3 slices (1.9 oz)	60	2	1	1	0

CANDY

FOOD	PORTION	CAL	FAT	CARB	SUGAR	FIBER
butterscotch	1 piece (6 g)	24	tr	6	–	–
candied cherries	1 (4 g)	12	tr	3	–	–
candied citron	1 oz	89	tr	23	–	–
candied lemon peel	1 oz	90	tr	23	–	–
candied orange peel	1 oz	90	tr	23	–	–
candied pineapple slice	1 slice (2 oz)	179	tr	45	–	–
candy corn	1 oz	105	0	27	–	–
caramels	1 piece (8 g)	31	1	6	–	–
caramels chocolate	1 piece (6 g)	22	tr	6	–	–

FOOD	PORTION	CAL	FAT	CARB	SUGAR	FIBER
carob bar	1 (3.1 oz)	453	28	42	–	–
dark chocolate	1 oz	150	10	16	–	–
fondant	1 piece (0.6 oz)	57	0	15	–	–
fondant chocolate coated	1 piece (0.4 oz)	40	1	9	–	–
fondant mint	1 oz	105	0	27	–	–
fruit pastilles	1 tube (1.4 oz)	101	0	25	–	–
fudge brown sugar w/ nuts	1 piece (0.5 oz)	56	1	11	–	–
fudge chocolate marshmallow	1 piece (0.7 oz)	84	3	14	–	–
fudge chocolate marshmallow w/ nuts	1 piece (0.8 oz)	96	4	15	–	–
fudge chocolate w/ nuts	1 piece (0.7 oz)	81	3	14	–	–
fudge peanut butter	1 piece (0.6 oz)	59	1	13	–	–
fudge vanilla w/ nuts	1 piece (0.5 oz)	62	2	11	–	–
gumdrops	10 sm (0.4 oz)	135	0	35	–	–
gumdrops	10 lg (3.8 oz)	420	0	108	–	–
hard candy	1 oz	106	0	28	–	–
jelly beans	10 lg (1 oz)	104	tr	26	–	–
jelly beans	10 sm (0.4 oz)	40	tr	10	–	–
lollipop	1 (6 g)	22	0	6	–	–
marzipan	1 oz	128	7	15	–	2
milk chocolate	1 bar (1.5 oz)	226	14	26	–	–
milk chocolate crisp	1 bar (1.45 oz)	203	11	28	–	–
milk chocolate w/ almonds	1 bar (1.45 oz)	215	14	22	20	–

FOOD	PORTION	CAL	FAT	CARB	SUGAR	FIBER
nougat nut cream	0.5 oz	49	4	8	–	–
peanut bar	1 (1.4 oz)	209	14	19	–	–
peanut brittle	1 oz	128	5	20	–	–
peanuts chocolate covered	1 cup (5.2 oz)	773	50	74	–	–
peanuts chocolate covered	10 (1.4 oz)	208	13	20	–	–
praline	1 piece (1.4 oz)	177	10	24	–	–
pretzels chocolate covered	1 oz	130	5	20	–	–
pretzels chocolate covered	1 (0.4 oz)	50	2	8	–	–
sesame crunch	20 pieces (1.2 oz)	181	12	18	–	–
taffy	1 piece (0.5 oz)	56	1	14	–	–
toffee	1 piece (0.4 oz)	65	4	8	–	–
truffles	1 piece (0.4 oz)	59	4	5	–	–
3 Musketeers						
Bar	1 (2.1 oz)	260	8	46	40	1
Fun Size	3 (1.6 oz)	190	6	34	30	1
Minis	7 (1.4 oz)	170	5	32	27	1
Mint	1 pkg (1.5 oz)	190	6	31	26	1
Altoids						
Cinnamon	3 (2 g)	10	0	2	2	–
Azature Chocolates						
Black Diamond Wild Treasure Cocoa	1 pkg (1 oz)	143	10	13	8	2
Green Diamond Poire William	1 pkg (1 oz)	130	7	15	11	1
Purple Diamond Chai	1 pkg (1 oz)	155	12	13	9	3

FOOD	PORTION	CAL	FAT	CARB	SUGAR	FIBER
Brach's						
Bridge Mix	15 pieces (1.4 oz)	190	10	26	21	1
Candy Corn	19 (1.4 oz)	140	0	36	32	–
Hard Candy Cinnamon	3 (0.6 oz)	70	0	16	14	–
Hard Candy Cinnamon Sugar Free	3 (0.6 oz)	35	0	17	0	–
Hard Candy Lemon Drops	4 (0.6 oz)	70	0	17	11	–
Hard Candy Lemon Drops Sugar Free	4 (0.6 oz)	35	0	17	0	–
Mandarin Orange Slices	3 (1.6 oz)	150	0	37	28	–
Milk Chocolate Stars	10 (1.3 oz)	190	10	24	22	1
Milk Maid Caramels	4 (1.3 oz)	150	4	25	15	0
Peanut Clusters	3 (1.4 oz)	210	15	20	16	2
Sour Gummi Bears	5 (1.3 oz)	120	0	28	24	–
Star Brites Peppermints	3 (0.5 oz)	60	0	15	11	–
Butterfinger						
Crisp Bar	1 (2.1 oz)	270	11	43	29	1
Original Bar	1 (2.1 oz)	270	11	43	29	1
Snackerz	1 pkg (1.3 oz)	170	8	23	15	2
Coco						
Brain Truffles Orange	1 (0.5 oz)	56	3	7	5	1
Preggers Truffles Dark Chocolate	1 (0.5 oz)	56	3	7	5	1
Coffee Spoons						
Flavored	1 (0.6 oz)	90	5	11	9	1
Dots						
Gumdrops Fruit	11 (1.4 oz)	130	0	33	21	–
Dove						
Cookies & Creme Silky Smooth	1 bar (1.3 oz)	210	12	22	20	0

FOOD	PORTION	CAL	FAT	CARB	SUGAR	FIBER
Dark Chocolate & Raspberry Swirl Promises Silky Smooth	1 bar (1.4 oz)	220	14	24	21	2
Dark Chocolate Silky Smooth	1 bar (1.4 oz)	220	13	24	19	3
Milk Chocolate Almond Promises Silky Smooth	1 bar (1.4 oz)	210	13	21	19	2
Milk Chocolate Covered Raisins & Peanuts Silky Smooth	22 pieces (1.4 oz)	210	12	23	20	2
Milk Chocolate Peanut Butter Promises Silky Smooth	1 bar	220	14	20	18	1
Milk Chocolate Silky Smooth	1 bar	220	13	24	22	1
Droste						
Pastilles Bittersweet Chocolate	8 (1.4 oz)	220	13	23	19	2
Elmer Chocolates						
Assorted	5 (2 oz)	240	10	41	35	1
Frankford						
Gold Coins Milk Chocolate	1 pkg (1.5 oz)	220	13	26	25	tr
Gimme						
Dark Chocolate Omega 3	1 pkg (1 oz)	130	7	19	14	2
Dark Chocolate Probiotics	1 pkg (1 oz)	130	7	20	14	2
Milk Chocolate Calcium	1 pkg (1 oz)	120	7	18	14	1
Ginger People						
Ginger Chews Peanut	2 (0.4 oz)	40	1	9	8	0
Ginger Chews Spicy Apple	2 (0.4 oz)	40	0	10	10	0
Gin-Gins	3 (0.3 oz)	35	0	8	7	0

FOOD	PORTION	CAL	FAT	CARB	SUGAR	FIBER
Godiva						
Gems Truffles Milk Chocolate	4 (1.5 oz)	200	13	20	18	tr
Guylian						
Twists Original Praline	2 (0.8 oz)	130	8	13	12	1
Hello Kitty						
Marshmallow Pop	1 (1.5 oz)	140	0	34	26	–
Hershey's						
Kisses Milk Chocolate	9 (1.4 oz)	200	12	25	23	1
Miniatures Special Dark	5 (1.4 oz)	190	13	24	18	3
Pieces All Flavors	51 (1.4 oz)	190	9	25	21	1
Pot Of Gold Assorted Milk & Dark Chocolate	4 (1.4 oz)	200	12	25	22	1
Jelly Belly						
Jelly Beans Cocktail Classics	1 pkg (0.75 oz)	80	0	20	15	–
Peas & Carrots	49 (1.4 oz)	140	0	37	29	–
Jer's						
Balls Peanut Butter Chocolate	1 piece (0.5 oz)	80	5	8	6	–
KitKat						
Bar Snack Size	3 (1.5 oz)	210	11	27	21	tr
Life Savers						
Gummies 5 Flavors	1 pkg (1.5 oz)	130	0	30	25	–
Variety	4 (0.5 oz)	45	0	11	9	–
Lindt						
Lindor Truffles Extra Dark Chocolate	3 pieces (1.3 oz)	230	19	15	11	2
M&M's						
Pretzel Fun Size	3 pkg (1.4 oz)	180	6	29	21	1
Manischewitz						
Fruit Slices	2 (1.3 oz)	90	0	24	23	0

FOOD	PORTION	CAL	FAT	CARB	SUGAR	FIBER
Maple Grove Farms						
Maple	5 pieces (1.5 oz)	160	0	42	37	–
Milky Way						
Bar	1 (2 oz)	260	10	41	35	1
Fun Size	2 (1.2 oz)	150	6	24	20	0
Midnight Bar	1 (1.76)	220	8	36	29	1
Midnight Minis	5 (1.4 oz)	180	7	29	24	1
Minis	5 (1.5 oz)	190	7	30	25	0
Simply Caramel Bar	1 (1.9 oz)	250	11	37	31	0
Mounds						
Bar Snack Size	1 (0.6 oz)	80	5	10	7	1
Raisinets						
Candy	¼ cup (1.6 oz)	190	8	32	28	1
Reese's						
Peanut Butter Cups Miniatures Dark Chocolate	5 (1.5 oz)	220	14	24	20	2
Ritter Sport						
Bar Cappuccino	1 (3.5 oz)	574	39	50	48	2
Bar Chocolate Marzipan	1 (3.5 oz)	484	27	53	52	5
Bar Chocolate & Cornflakes	1 (3.5 oz)	525	29	59	50	2
Bar Chocolate Butter Biscuit	1 (3.5 oz)	556	35	53	51	2
Bar Dark Chocolate	1 (3.5 oz)	525	33	51	49	7
Bar Milk Chocolate	1 (3.5 oz)	533	31	57	56	3
Bar Mousse Au Chocolat	1 (3.5 oz)	544	36	48	46	7
Bar White Chocolate Whole Hazelnuts	1 (3.5 oz)	562	38	48	44	2
Russell Stover						
All Dark Assorted	2 pieces (1.2 oz)	150	7	23	18	1

FOOD	PORTION	CAL	FAT	CARB	SUGAR	FIBER
Assorted Chocolates	2 pieces (1.1 oz)	160	7	22	18	1
Sadaf						
Halva Pistachio	1 oz	150	8	16	15	1
Skinny Cow						
Heavenly Crisp Bar	1 (0.8 oz)	110	4	14	9	1
Skittles						
Original	1 pkg (2.21 oz)	250	3	56	47	0
Snap Infusion						
Supercandy Bean Multi-Berry	1 pkg (1 oz)	90	0	23	18	0
Snickers						
Bar	1 bar (2 oz)	280	14	35	30	1
Fun Size	2 (1.2 oz)	160	8	21	17	1
Miniatures	4 (1.3 oz)	170	8	22	18	1
Sour Jacks						
Original	15 (1.3 oz)	140	0	33	26	0
Watermelon	15 (1.4 oz)	140	0	32	18	0
Starburst						
Jellybeans	¼ cup (1.5 oz)	150	0	37	29	0
Original	8 (1.4 oz)	160	4	33	23	0
SunRidge Farms						
Rainbow Drops Milk Chocolate	¼ cup (1.4 oz)	170	10	21	19	1
Surf Sweets						
Gummy Worms	4 (1.4 oz)	130	0	30	19	0
Terra Nostra						
Organic Bar Creamy Milk Raisins & Pecans	4 sections (1.2 oz)	180	11	18	17	1
Organic Bar Vegan Intense Dark	4 sections (1.2 oz)	180	12	15	9	4

FOOD	PORTION	CAL	FAT	CARB	SUGAR	FIBER
Organic Bar Vegan Ricemilk Choco	4 sections (1.2 oz)	190	14	18	16	0
Organic Bar Vegan Robust Dark Raisins & Pecans	4 sections (1.2 oz)	170	11	16	14	3
Twix						
Caramel Cookie	1 (1.8 oz)	250	12	34	24	1
Fun Size	1 (0.6 oz)	80	4	11	8	0
Welch's						
Licorice All Flavors	1 pkg (1.8 oz)	170	0	42	26	0
Licorice Filled All Flavors	½ pkg (1.8 oz)	170	9	42	26	0
Whitman's						
Assorted Chocolates	4 pieces (1.5 oz)	210	10	29	23	1
Wolfgang						
Cranberries Dipped In Dark Chocolate	2 (1 oz)	130	6	18	16	1
Wonka Exceptionals						
Bar Chocolate Waterfall	4 sq (1.4 oz)	210	13	23	22	tr
Bar Domed Dark Chocolate	4 sq (1.4 oz)	200	13	24	19	3
Fruit Jellies All Flavors	14 (1.5 oz)	130	0	34	26	–
Fruit Marvels All Flavors	10 (1.4 oz)	140	0	34	30	–
CANTALOUPE						
balls frzn	10 (4.7 oz)	46	tr	11	11	1
dried	3.5 pieces (1.4 oz)	140	0	34	32	1
fresh cubed	1 cup (5.6 oz)	54	tr	13	13	1
melon sm	⅛ (1.9 oz)	19	tr	4	4	1
melon med	⅛ (2.4 oz)	23	tr	6	5	1
melon large	⅛ (3.6 oz)	35	1	8	8	1
Crispy Green						
Freeze-dried	1 pkg (0.35 oz)	40	0	8	7	1

FOOD	PORTION	CAL	FAT	CARB	SUGAR	FIBER
Dole						
Fresh	¼ med (4.7 oz)	45	0	11	11	1
CANTALOUPE JUICE						
nectar	1 cup (8.8 oz)	155	tr	39	39	1
CAPERS						
capers canned	1 tbsp (0.3 oz)	2	tr	tr	tr	tr
Victoria						
Capers	2 tbsp (1 oz)	100	0	0	0	0
CARAWAY						
seed	1 tbsp	22	1	3	tr	3
CARDAMOM						
ground	1 tsp	6	tr	1	–	1
CARDOON						
fresh cooked w/o salt	1 serv (3.5 oz)	22	tr	5	–	2
fresh shredded	1 cup (6.2 oz)	30	tr	7	–	3
CARIBOU						
roasted	3 oz	142	4	0	0	0
CARISSA						
fresh	1	12	tr	3	–	–
CAROB						
carob mix	3 tsp	45	0	11	–	–
carob mix as prep w/ whole milk	9 oz	195	8	23	–	–
flour	1 cup	185	1	92	–	–
flour	1 tbsp	14	tr	7	–	–
CARP						
fresh cooked	3 oz	138	6	0	0	0
fresh cooked	1 fillet (6 oz)	276	12	0	0	0

FOOD	PORTION	CAL	FAT	CARB	SUGAR	FIBER
fresh raw	3 oz	108	5	0	0	0
roe raw	1 oz	37	tr	tr	–	–
roe salted in olive oil	2 tbsp (1 oz)	40	–	6	–	0
CARROT JUICE						
canned	1 cup (8.3 oz)	210	tr	22	9	2
CARROTS						
CANNED						
Allens						
Tiny Sliced	½ cup (4.5 oz)	45	0	11	3	3
Butter Kernel						
Sliced	½ cup (4.3 oz)	35	0	8	5	3
DRIED						
dehydrated	¼ cup (0.6 oz)	63	tr	15	7	4
FRESH						
baby raw	1 (0.5 oz)	6	tr	1	–	–
diced	½ cup (2.2 oz)	26	tr	6	3	2
medium raw	1 (2.1 oz)	25	tr	6	3	2
large raw	1 (2.5 oz)	30	tr	7	3	2
raw shredded	½ cup (1.9 oz)	23	tr	5	3	2
slices cooked w/o salt	½ cup (2.7 oz)	27	tr	6	3	2
small raw	1 (1.8 oz)	20	tr	5	2	1
Crunch Pak						
Baby Carrots w/ Ranch Dressing	⅕ pkg	50	3	7	5	2
DipperZ Carrot Sticks w/ Ranch Dip	1 pkg (2.75 oz)	50	2	8	4	2
Foodles Carrots Cheese & Pretzels	1 pkg (5 oz)	200	10	20	5	4
Dole						
Mini Cut	11 (3 oz)	30	0	8	4	2
Grimmway Farms						
Baby	3 oz	35	0	8	5	2
Carrot Chips	3 oz	35	0	8	5	2

FOOD	PORTION	CAL	FAT	CARB	SUGAR	FIBER
Carrot Creations Honey Brown Sugar & Cinnamon	¼ pkg (3 oz)	70	3	9	7	2
Carrot Creations Roasted Garlic & Savory Herbs	¼ pkg (3 oz)	70	5	8	5	2
Carrot Dippers	1 pkg (2.2 oz)	110	9	5	4	1
Shredded	3 oz	35	0	8	5	2
Ready Pac						
Baby Carrots	7 (3 oz)	40	0	9	5	2
FROZEN						
slices cooked w/o salt	1 cup (5.1 oz)	54	1	11	6	5
CASABA						
cubed	1 cup (6 oz)	46	tr	11	10	2
melon fresh	¼ (14 oz)	115	tr	27	23	4
CASHEWS						
butter w/ salt	1 tbsp (0.5 oz)	94	8	4	1	tr
butter w/o salt	1 tbsp (0.5 oz)	94	8	4	–	tr
dry roasted w/o salt	¼ cup (1.2 oz)	197	16	11	2	1
oil roasted w/o salt	¼ cup (1.1 oz)	187	15	10	2	1
raw	1 oz	157	12	9	2	1
Frito Lay						
Whole Salted	3 tbsp	180	15	8	2	1
Kettle Brand						
Butter Unsalted	2 tbsp (1 oz)	160	14	8	0	1
Nut Harvest						
Whole Sea Salted	2 tbsp (1 oz)	170	13	9	2	1
Planters						
Chocolate Lovers Milk Chocolate	10 pieces (1.5 oz)	230	16	20	15	1
Halves & Pieces	1 oz	160	13	9	2	1
Halves & Pieces Lightly Salted	1 oz	160	13	9	2	1

FOOD	PORTION	CAL	FAT	CARB	SUGAR	FIBER
Whole Honey Roasted	1 oz	150	11	11	5	1
Sante						
Cardamon Cashews	¼ cup (1 oz)	220	17	13	7	1
Yumnuts						
Chili Lime	¼ cup (1 oz)	170	13	7	2	3
Chocolate	¼ cup (1 oz)	160	11	12	6	2
Honey	¼ cup (1 oz)	170	12	10	6	1
CASSAVA						
diced cooked w/o fat	1 cup (4.6 oz)	213	tr	51	2	2
root raw	1 (14.3 oz)	653	1	155	7	7
TAKE-OUT						
fritter crab meat stuffed	1 (4.4 oz)	341	16	38	7	2
CATFISH						
channel breaded & fried	3 oz	194	11	7	–	–
wolfish atlantic baked	3 oz	105	3	0	0	0
CAULIFLOWER						
flowerets fresh	1 (0.5 oz)	3	tr	1	tr	tr
flowerets fresh cooked w/o salt	3 (2 oz)	12	tr	2	1	1
fresh	1 cup	25	tr	5	2	3
fresh cooked w/o salt	1 cup	29	1	5	3	3
fresh head small	1 (9.2 oz)	66	tr	14	6	7
frzn cooked w/o salt	1 cup	34	tr	7	2	5
green fresh	1 cup	20	tr	4	2	2
green fresh small head	1 (11.4 oz)	101	1	20	10	10
pickled	¼ cup	14	tr	3	2	1
pickled chow chow	¼ cup	74	1	16	15	1
Dole						
Fresh	1 cup (3.4 oz)	25	0	5	2	2
Jake & Amos						
Sweet Pickled Hot Cauliflower	1 tbsp	40	0	10	8	0

FOOD	PORTION	CAL	FAT	CARB	SUGAR	FIBER
Mann's						
Cauliettes Fresh	1 serv (3 oz)	20	0	4	2	2
River Ranch						
Florets Fresh	1 cup (3 oz)	20	0	5	2	2
Victoria						
Tangy	¼ cup (1 oz)	5	0	1	0	0
TAKE-OUT						
batter dipped fried	1 piece (0.9 oz)	55	4	4	tr	1
batter dipped fried	1 cup	178	13	12	1	2
w/ cheese sauce	1 cup	249	18	12	6	3
CAVIAR						
black or red	2 tbsp	81	6	1	0	0
CELERY						
fresh	1 lg stalk (2.2 oz)	9	tr	2	1	1
pickled	½ cup	10	tr	2	1	1
raw diced	½ cup	8	tr	2	1	1
seed	1 tsp	1	tr	tr	–	tr
strips	1 cup	17	tr	4	2	2
Dole						
Hearts	2 stalks (4 oz)	15	0	3	0	2
Ready Pac						
Sticks	5 (3 oz)	10	0	3	1	1
TAKE-OUT						
creamed	½ cup	87	6	7	4	1
stir fried	½ cup	30	2	3	2	1
stuffed w/ cheese	1 (5 inch)	38	3	1	tr	tr
CELERY JUICE						
juice	1 cup	42	tr	9	6	4

FOOD	PORTION	CAL	FAT	CARB	SUGAR	FIBER
CELERY ROOT						
fresh cooked w/o salt	1 cup (5.4 oz)	42	tr	9	–	2
fresh cut up	1 cup (5.4 oz)	66	tr	14	3	3
CELTUCE						
raw	3.5 oz	22	tr	4	–	–
CEREAL						
bran flakes	¾ cup	90	1	22	–	–
corn flakes	1¼ cups	110	tr	24	–	–
farina as prep w/ water	¾ cup	88	tr	19	–	2
granola	½ cup	285	15	32	–	6
oatmeal instant as prep w/ water	1 cup (8.2 oz)	138	2	24	–	4
oatmeal regular & quick as prep w/ water	¾ cup (6.1 oz)	149	2	19	–	3
oatmeal regular & quick not prep	⅓ cup (0.9 oz)	104	2	18	–	3
puffed rice	1 cup	56	tr	13	–	tr
puffed wheat	1 cup	44	tr	10	–	1
shredded mini wheats	1 cup	107	1	24	–	3
shredded wheat rectangular	1 biscuit (0.8 oz)	85	tr	19	–	2
Alpen						
High Fibre	1 serv (1.6 oz)	154	3	28	11	tr
No Sugar Added	1 serv (1.6 oz)	158	2	29	7	4
Annie's Homegrown						
Bunny O's Honey	¾ cup (1 oz)	110	1	25	7	1
Bunny O's Organic	¾ cup (1 oz)	120	2	24	2	1
Barbara's Bakery						
Organic Brown Rice Crisps Fruit Juice Sweetened	1 cup (1 oz)	120	1	25	1	1
Puffins Honey Rice Gluten Free	¾ cup (1 oz)	120	1	25	6	3

FOOD	PORTION	CAL	FAT	CARB	SUGAR	FIBER
Puffins Multigrain Gluten Free	¾ cup (1 oz)	110	0	25	6	3
Basic 4						
Whole Grain	1 cup (1.9 oz)	200	2	43	14	3
Bear Naked						
Cranberry Raisin	⅔ cup (2 oz)	210	5	41	15	4
Fit Vanilla Almond Crunch	¼ cup (1.1 oz)	120	3	22	4	2
Granola Fruit And Nut	¼ cup (1.1 oz)	140	7	17	6	2
Granola Heavenly Chocolate	¼ cup (1.1 oz)	130	4	21	7	2
Peak Flax Oats And Honey w/ Blueberries	¼ cup (1.1 oz)	130	4	22	7	2
Better Balance						
Protein Cereal All Flavors Gluten Free	1 oz	100	2	15	3	3
BetterOats						
Abundance Apple & Cinnamon	1 pkg (1.5 oz)	160	3	28	9	3
Good'N Hearty Maple & Brown Sugar	1 pkg (1.5 oz)	160	3	31	9	3
Lavish Dark Chocolate	1 pkg (1.5 oz)	160	3	33	12	3
MMM . . . Muffins Oatmeal Raisin Cookie	1 pkg (1.4 oz)	150	2	30	14	3
Oat Fit Cinnamon Roll	1 pkg (1 oz)	100	2	18	0	3
Oat Revolution! Cinnamon & Spice	1 pkg (1.6 oz)	170	3	35	15	3
Oat Revolution! Peaches & Cream	1 pkg (1.2 oz)	130	2	27	12	2
Oat Revolution! Thick & Hearty Classic	1 pkg (1.2 oz)	130	3	22	0	4
Boo Berry						
Cereal	3 cup (1.2 oz)	130	1	28	12	1

FOOD	PORTION	CAL	FAT	CARB	SUGAR	FIBER
Bready Brek						
Original	1 serv (1 oz)	108	3	18	tr	2
Cascadian Farm						
Organic Granola Berry Cobbler	⅔ cup (2.1 oz)	230	4	46	15	3
Organic Granola Oats & Honey	⅔ cup (1.9 oz)	230	6	42	14	3
Cheerios						
Banana Nut	¾ cup (1 oz)	120	1	26	12	0
Chocolate	¾ cup (1 oz)	100	2	22	9	2
Honey Nut	¾ cup (1 oz)	110	2	22	9	2
MultiGrain	1 cup (1 oz)	110	1	24	6	3
Whole Grain Oat	1 cup (1 oz)	100	2	20	1	3
Yogurt Burst Strawberry	¾ cup (1 oz)	120	2	24	9	2
Chex						
Chocolate	¾ cup (1.1 oz)	130	3	26	8	tr
Corn Gluten Free	1 cup (1.2 oz)	120	1	26	3	1
Multi-Bran	¾ cup (1.6 oz)	160	2	39	10	6
Wheat	¾ cup (1.6 oz)	160	2	38	5	5
Cinnamon Toast Crunch						
Cinnamon Sugar	¾ cup (1.1 oz)	130	3	25	9	2
CoCo Wheats						
Hot Cereal as prep w/ skim milk	1 serv	160	tr	24	0	1
Cocoa Puffs						
Cereal	¾ cup (1 oz)	100	2	23	11	2
Dr. McDougall's						
Organic Instant Oatmeal	1 pkg (1 oz)	120	2	21	0	3
Organic Maple 4 Grain	1 pkg (2.6 oz)	260	3	52	16	6
EnviroKidz						
Amazon Frosted Flakes Organic	⅔ cup (1.1 oz)	120	0	26	6	2
Gorilla Munch Organic	¾ cup (1 oz)	120	0	27	8	2

FOOD	PORTION	CAL	FAT	CARB	SUGAR	FIBER
Koala Crisp Organic	¾ cup (1.1 oz)	110	1	25	11	2
Panda Puffs Organic	¾ cup (1.1 oz)	130	3	24	7	2
Erewhon						
Aztec Crunchy Corn & Amaranth	1 cup (1 oz)	110	0	26	1	1
Barley Plus not prep	¼ cups (1.6 oz)	170	1	37	0	4
Brown Rice Cream not prep	¼ cup (1.6 oz)	170	1	36	0	1
Cocoa Crispy Brown Rice	1 cup (1.8 oz)	200	2	44	11	1
Crispy Brown Rice No Salt Added	1 cup (1 oz)	110	0	25	1	1
Crispy Brown Rice Original	1 cup (1 oz)	110	0	25	1	1
Organic Instant Oatmeal Apple Cinnamon not prep	1 pkg (1.2 oz)	130	2	24	4	3
Organic Instant Oatmeal w/ Oat Bran	1 pkg (1.8 oz)	130	3	25	tr	4
Rice Twice	¾ cup (1 oz)	120	0	26	8	0
Erin Baker's						
Granola Fruit & Nut	½ cup (1.6 oz)	190	8	25	10	4
Fiber One						
Honey Clusters	1 cup (1.8 oz)	160	2	44	6	13
Nutty Clusters & Almonds	1 cup (1.9 oz)	180	3	45	12	11
Original	½ cup (1 oz)	60	1	25	0	14
Raisin Bran Clusters	1 cup (2 oz)	170	1	45	13	11
Giddy Up & Go						
Granola Notoriously Nutty	¾ cup (2 oz)	250	11	32	11	5
Granola Seriously Seedy	¾ cup (2 oz)	230	10	32	11	5

FOOD	PORTION	CAL	FAT	CARB	SUGAR	FIBER
Glutenfreeda						
Granola Apple Almond Honey	¼ cup (1 oz)	150	11	10	7	2
Oatmeal Instant as prep	1 pkg (1.8 oz)	190	3	34	1	5
Kaia Foods						
Organic Granola Buckwheat Cinnamon Raisin	½ cup (2 oz)	230	10	34	12	6
Organic Granola Buckwheat Cocoa Bliss	½ cup (2 oz)	220	8	35	14	5
Kellogg's						
All-Bran Bran Buds	⅓ cup (1 oz)	80	1	24	8	13
All-Bran Complete Wheat Flakes	¾ cup (1 oz)	90	1	24	5	5
All-Bran Original	½ cup (1.1 oz)	80	1	23	6	10
Apple Jacks	1 cup (1 oz)	110	1	25	12	3
Corn Flakes	1 cup (1 oz)	100	0	24	3	1
Corn Pops	1 cup (1 oz)	120	0	27	9	3
Cracklin' Oat Bran	¾ cup (1.7 oz)	200	7	34	14	6
Crispix	1 cup (1 oz)	110	0	25	4	tr
Crunchmania Cinnamon Bun	1 pkg (1.8 oz)	220	7	37	12	2
Crunchy Nut Golden Honey Nut	⅓ cup (1.1 oz)	120	1	26	10	tr
Fiber Plus Antioxidants Cinnamon Oat Crunch	¾ cup (1.1 oz)	110	2	26	7	9
Froot Loops	1 cup (1 oz)	110	1	26	12	3
Frosted Flakes	¾ cup (1 oz)	110	0	27	11	tr
Frosted Mini-Wheat Crunch Brown Sugar	1 cup (2 oz)	200	2	44	12	5
Frosted Mini-Wheats Little Bites Original	1 cup (2 oz)	200	1	47	11	6

FOOD	PORTION	CAL	FAT	CARB	SUGAR	FIBER
Frosted Mini-Wheats Maple Brown Sugar	25 (2 oz)	190	1	47	12	6
Frosted Mini-Wheats Strawberry	25 (2 oz)	190	1	47	12	6
Granola Low Fat	½ cup (1.7 oz)	190	3	40	14	3
Honey Smacks	¾ cup (1.7 oz)	100	1	24	15	1
Krave Chocolate	¾ cup (1.1 oz)	120	4	24	11	3
Mueslix	⅔ cup (2 oz)	200	3	41	14	5
Product 19	1 cup (1 oz)	110	0	25	4	tr
Raisin Bran	1 cup (2 oz)	190	1	46	18	7
Raisin Bran Crunch	1 cup (1.9 oz)	190	1	45	19	4
Smart Start Original Antioxidants	1 cup (1.8 oz)	190	1	44	14	3
Smorz	1 cup (1.1 oz)	120	2	25	13	tr
Love Crunch						
Carrot Cake Organic	¼ cup (1.1 oz)	130	4	23	8	2
Dark Chocolate & Red Berries Organic	¼ cup (1.1 oz)	140	6	20	6	2
Lucky Charms						
Swirled	¾ cup (1 oz)	110	1	22	11	1
Malt-O-Meal						
Apple Zings	1 cup (1.2 oz)	130	1	30	16	1
Chocolate not prep	3 tbsp (1.2 oz)	130	0	27	7	1
Coco Roos	¾ cup (1 oz)	120	2	26	15	tr
Crispy Rice	1¼ cups (1.2 oz)	130	0	29	3	0
Golden Puffs	¾ cup (1 oz)	110	0	24	15	0
Honey Nut Scooters	1 cup (1 oz)	110	2	24	10	2
Mateys Marshmallow	1 cup (1 oz)	120	1	25	13	1
Original Cream Hot Wheat not prep	3 tbsp (1.2 oz)	130	0	27	0	1
Original not prep	3 tbsp (1.2 oz)	130	1	27	0	1
Tootie Fruities	1 cup (1.1 oz)	130	1	28	15	1

FOOD	PORTION	CAL	FAT	CARB	SUGAR	FIBER
McCann's						
Irish Oatmeal Instant Apples & Cinnamon not prep	1 pkg (1.2 oz)	130	2	27	12	3
Irish Oatmeal Instant Maple & Brown Sugar not prep	1 pkg (1.5 oz)	160	2	32	13	3
Irish Oatmeal Instant Regular not prep	1 pkg (1 oz)	100	2	18	1	3
Irish Oatmeal Quick Cooking not prep	½ cup (1.4 oz)	150	2	26	0	4
Irish Oatmeal Steel Cut not prep	¼ cup (1.4 oz)	150	2	26	0	4
Mom's Best Naturals						
Blue Pom Wheat-fuls	1 cup (1.9 oz)	210	1	45	11	6
Honey Grahams	¾ cup (1 oz)	130	3	25	10	1
Mallow Oats	1 cup (1 oz)	120	1	24	13	1
Raisin Bran	1 cup (2.1 oz)	230	2	49	20	6
Mother's						
Barley Hot Cereal not prep	⅓ cup (1.7 oz)	160	1	37	0	5
Peanut Butter Bumpers	1 cup (1.2 oz)	130	3	26	10	1
Rolled Oats not prep	½ cup (1.4 oz)	150	3	27	1	4
Toasted Oat Bran	¾ cup (1.1 oz)	120	2	24	5	3
Naked Granola						
Taste Of Seattle Nights	½ pkg (1.2 oz)	110	6	12	5	5
Nature's Path						
Corn Flakes Organic	¾ cup (1.1 oz)	110	0	24	3	2
Granola Hemp Plus Organic	¾ cup (1.9 oz)	260	10	36	10	5
Granola Peanut Butter Organic	¾ cup (1.9 oz)	260	11	35	9	4
Granola Pumpkin Flax Plus Organic	¾ cup (1.9 oz)	260	10	37	10	5

FOOD	PORTION	CAL	FAT	CARB	SUGAR	FIBER
Heritage Crunch Organic	¾ cup (1.9 oz)	230	3	44	6	6
Instant Oatmeal Flax Plus Organic	1 pkg (1.8 oz)	210	3	38	10	5
Instant Oatmeal Hemp Plus Organic	1 pkg (1.4 oz)	160	3	30	6	4
Instant Oatmeal Maple Nut Organic	1 pkg (1.8 oz)	210	4	38	11	4
Instant Oatmeal Optimum Cranberry Ginger Organic	1 pkg (1.4 oz)	150	2	30	10	3
Instant Oatmeal Original Organic	1 pkg (1.8 oz)	210	4	37	0	6
Kamut Puffs Organic	1 cup (0.5 oz)	50	0	11	0	2
Maple Pecan Crunch Flax Plus Organic	¾ cup (1.9 oz)	220	7	38	10	5
Millet Rice Flakes Organic	¾ cup (1.1 oz)	120	2	22	4	3
Optimum Blueberry Cinnamon Organic	1 cup (1.9 oz)	200	3	38	9	7
Optimum Cranberry Ginger Organic	¾ cup (1.9 oz)	190	3	41	13	8
Red Berry Crunch Flax Plus Organic	¾ cup (1.9 oz)	210	4	39	10	5
Rice Puffs Organic	1 cup (0.5 oz)	50	0	14	0	1
Shredded Oaty Bites Organic	¾ cup (1.1 oz)	110	2	23	5	2
New Morning						
Cocoa Crispy Rice	¾ cup (1 oz)	120	1	26	10	1
Oatios Original	1 cup (1 oz)	110	2	22	2	3
Oatmeal Crisp						
Crunchy Almond	1 cup (2.1 oz)	240	5	47	16	4
Post						
Grape-Nuts	½ cup (2 oz)	200	1	48	5	7

FOOD	PORTION	CAL	FAT	CARB	SUGAR	FIBER
Great Grains Raisins Dates & Pecans	¾ cup (2 oz)	200	4	40	14	5
Honey Bunches Of Oats	1 cup (1.8 oz)	200	2	42	14	2
Honey Bunches Of Oats Almonds	¾ cup (1.1 oz)	120	3	26	6	2
Selects Cranberry Almond Crunch	¾ cup (1.8 oz)	200	3	40	14	3
Shredded Wheat Spoon Size	1 cup (1.7 oz)	170	1	40	0	6
Quaker						
Instant Oatmeal Apples & Cinnamon	1 pkg (1.2 oz)	130	2	27	9	3
Instant Oatmeal Simple Harvest Multigrain Maple Brown Sugar w/ Pecans	1 pkg (1.48 oz)	160	4	30	9	4
Oatmeal	1 pkg (2.6 oz)	290	8	53	22	5
Oatmeal Cherry Pistachio as prep	1 pkg (2.6 oz)	290	8	49	19	5
Oatmeal Peach Almond	1 pkg (2.6 oz)	290	7	51	19	6
Oatmeal Summer Berry	1 pkg (2.5 oz)	250	3	51	14	7
Oatmeal Squares	1 cup (2 oz)	210	3	44	9	5
Ralston						
Enriched Wheat Bran Flakes	¾ cup (1 oz)	90	1	23	5	5
Shredded Wheat Frosted Bite Size	1¼ cups (1.9 oz)	190	1	46	11	5
Ready Brek						
Chocolate	1 serv (1 oz)	108	2	19	7	2
Reese's						
Puffs	¾ cup (1 oz)	120	3	22	10	1
Rice Krispies						
Cereal	1¼ cups (1.2 oz)	130	0	29	4	tr

FOOD	PORTION	CAL	FAT	CARB	SUGAR	FIBER
Simpli						
Instant Oatmeal Apricot Gluten Free	1 pkg (1.7 oz)	170	3	30	10	4
Instant Oatmeal Plain Gluten Free	1 pkg (1.4 oz)	150	3	27	0	4
Skinner's						
Raisin Bran	1 cup (1.9 oz)	190	1	42	8	6
Special K						
Original	1 cup (1.1 oz)	120	1	23	4	0
Protein Plus	¾ cup (1.1 oz)	120	1	19	7	3
Red Berries	1 cup (1.1 oz)	110	0	27	9	3
Total						
Cinnamon Crunch	1 cup (1.8 oz)	190	3	40	9	4
Raisin Bran	1 cup (1.9 oz)	160	1	40	17	5
Whole Grain	¾ cup (1 oz)	100	1	23	5	3
Trix						
Swirls	1 cup (1.1 oz)	120	2	28	11	1
Udi's						
Gluten Free Granola Au Naturel	¼ cup (1.1 oz)	120	4	19	5	3
Uncle Sam						
Honey Almond	¾ cup (1.9 oz)	230	6	37	5	6
Original	¾ cup (1.9 oz)	190	5	38	tr	10
Strawberry	¾ cup (2.1 oz)	240	5	40	7	8
Weetabix						
Crunchy Bran	1 serv (1.4 oz)	122	1	23	6	8
Multigrain	1 serv (1.3 oz)	127	1	26	2	4
Oatibix Bites	1 serv (1.4 oz)	148	3	27	6	4
Wheaties						
Cereal	¾ cup (1 oz)	100	1	22	4	3

FOOD	PORTION	CAL	FAT	CARB	SUGAR	FIBER
Yogi						
Granola Crisps Baked Cinnamon Raisin	½ cup	120	3	21	5	2
Granola Crisps Mountain Blueberry Flax	½ cup	110	3	21	5	2

CEREAL BARS (*see also* ENERGY BARS, FRUIT AND NUT BARS)

FOOD	PORTION	CAL	FAT	CARB	SUGAR	FIBER
Alpen						
Fruit & Nut	1	109	2	20	9	1
Light Chocolate & Fudge	1	63	1	11	5	5
Raspberry & Yogurt	1	120	3	22	11	1
Annie's Homegrown						
Organic Peanut Butter	1 (1 oz)	120	5	17	5	1
Bear Naked						
Grain-ola Tropical Fruit	1 (2 oz)	220	7	38	18	4
Cascadian Farm						
Organic Granola Oats & Cocoa	2 (1.4 oz)	190	8	26	9	3
Organic Granola Oats & Honey	2 (1.4 oz)	180	7	27	9	3
Organic Granola Peanut Butter	2 (1.4 oz)	190	8	26	9	3
Earnest Eats						
Almond Trail Mix	1 (1.94 oz)	210	9	31	14	1
Choco Peanut Butter	1 (1.94 oz)	230	10	32	14	4
Cran Lemon Zest	1 (1.94 oz)	210	9	32	14	4
EnviroKidz						
Crispy Rice Cheetah Berry Organic	1 (1 oz)	110	3	21	7	1
Crispy Rice Lemur Peanut Choco Drizzle Organic	1 (1 oz)	120	5	18	8	1

FOOD	PORTION	CAL	FAT	CARB	SUGAR	FIBER
Crispy Rice Panda Peanut Butter	1 (1 oz)	110	3	20	7	1
Fiber One						
Chewy Chocolate	1 (1 oz)	100	3	21	8	5
Chewy Strawberry PB&J	1 (1 oz)	110	4	20	7	5
Chocolate Caramel & Pretzel	1 (0.8 oz)	90	2	17	5	5
Oats & Caramel	1 (1.4 oz)	140	4	30	9	9
Oats & Chocolate	1 (1.4 oz)	140	4	29	10	9
Oats & Peanut Butter	1 (1.4 oz)	150	5	28	9	9
Fruition						
Blueberry	1 (1.7 oz)	160	2	34	21	4
Cran-Raspberry	1 (1.7 oz)	160	2	34	22	4
Lemon	1 (1.7 oz)	160	3	34	19	4
Fullbar						
Fit Chewy Brownie	1 (1.76 oz)	180	4	24	10	5
Gnu						
Flavor & Fiber Banana Walnut	1 (1.6 oz)	140	4	30	8	12
Flavor & Fiber Chocolate Brownie Bar	1 (1.6 oz)	140	4	30	9	12
Flavor & Fiber Cinnamon Raisin	1 (1.6 oz)	130	3	32	11	12
Flavor & Fiber Expresso Chip	1 (1.6 oz)	140	4	30	8	12
Flavor & Fiber Lemon Ginger	1 (1.6 oz)	130	4	32	10	12
Flavor & Fiber Orange Cranberry	1 (1.6 oz)	130	3	32	11	12
Flavor & Fiber Peanut Butter	1 (1.6 oz)	140	5	30	7	12
JK Gourmet						
Granola Bar Nuts & Cranberries	1 (1.6 oz)	230	18	16	10	3

FOOD	PORTION	CAL	FAT	CARB	SUGAR	FIBER
Granola Bar Roasted Nuts & Blueberries	1 (1.6 oz)	240	19	16	10	3
Granola Bar Roasted Nuts & Dates	1 (1.6 oz)	240	19	17	11	3
Jungle Grub						
Berry Bamboozle w/ Vanilla Icing Gluten Free	1 (0.9 oz)	100	4	14	8	1
Chocolate Chip Cookie Dough w/ Chocolate Coating Gluten Free	1 (0.9 oz)	100	4	13	8	4
Peanut Butter Groove w/ Vanilla Icing Gluten Free	1 (0.9 oz)	100	4	13	8	1
Kardea						
Lemon Ginger	1 (1.34 oz)	140	5	20	8	7
Kashi						
Granola Chewy Trail Mix	1 (1.2 oz)	140	5	20	6	4
TLC Chewy Granola Dark Mocha Almond	1 (1.2 oz)	130	4	21	6	4
Kellogg's						
FiberPlus Antioxidants Berry Yogurt Crunch	1 cup (1.9 oz)	180	1	46	12	10
Kind						
Peanut Butter Dark Chocolate + Protein	1 (1.4 oz)	180	12	17	11	2
Kraft						
MilkBite Chocolate	1 (1.2 oz)	140	6	18	10	3
MilkBite Mixed Berry	1 (1.2 oz)	140	5	18	10	3
MilkBite Oatmeal Raisin	1 (1.2 oz)	130	5	18	10	3
MilkBite Peanut Butter	1 (1.2 oz)	140	6	17	8	3
MilkBite Strawberry	1 (1.2 oz)	140	5	18	10	3

FOOD	PORTION	CAL	FAT	CARB	SUGAR	FIBER
Kudos						
Dove	1 (0.8 oz)	100	3	17	8	1
Snickers	1 (0.8 oz)	100	4	16	8	1
w/ M&Ms	1 (0.8 oz)	100	3	17	9	1
Nature Valley						
Chewy Trail Mix Fruit & Nut	1 (1.2 oz)	140	4	25	13	2
Crunchy Granola Peanut Butter	2 (1.5 oz)	190	7	28	11	2
Oats 'N Honey	2 (1.5 oz)	190	6	29	12	2
Protein Chewy Peanut Almond & Dark Chocolate	1 (1.4 oz)	190	12	14	6	5
Protein Chewy Peanut Butter Dark Chocolate	1 (1.4 oz)	190	12	14	6	5
Sweet & Salty Granola Almond	1 (1.2 oz)	160	7	22	12	2
Nature's Path						
Granola Bar Apple Pie Crunch Chia Plus Organic	2 (1.4 oz)	190	8	27	8	3
Granola Bar Honey Oat Crunch Flax Plus Organic	2 (1.4 oz)	190	7	28	9	3
Granola Bar Peanut Choco Organic	1 (1.2 oz)	150	6	22	11	2
Granola Bar Pumpkin-N-Spice Organic	1 (1.2 oz)	140	4	23	10	2
Granola Bar Sunny Hemp Organic	1 (1.2 oz)	140	4	24	11	3
Nutri-Grain						
Apple Cinnamon	1 (1.3 oz)	120	3	24	12	3
Mixed Berry	1 (1.3 oz)	120	3	24	11	3

FOOD	PORTION	CAL	FAT	CARB	SUGAR	FIBER
Planters						
Nut-rition Antioxidant Almonds Blueberries & Dark Chocolate	1 (1.2 oz)	160	8	18	9	2
Nut-rition Bone Health Honey Roasted Peanuts Cashews & Almonds	1 (1.2 oz)	160	9	18	8	2
Nut-rition Energy Honey Roasted Peanuts Almonds & Chocolate	1 (1.2 oz)	170	9	17	10	2
Nut-rition Heart Healthy Cranberry Almond Peanut	1 (1.2 oz)	160	8	19	9	3
ProBar						
Cran-Lemon Twister	1 (3 oz)	360	16	49	28	7
Kettle Corn	1 (3 oz)	390	20	47	17	8
Koka Moka	1 (3 oz)	360	18	47	21	7
Old School PB&J	1 (3 oz)	370	17	48	20	6
Superfood Slam	1 (3 oz)	380	19	46	17	7
Quaker						
Chewy Granola Chocolate Chip	1 (0.84 oz)	100	3	17	7	1
Chewy Granola w/ Protein Peanut Butter & Chocolate	1 (1 oz)	110	3	18	7	1
Soft Baked Banana Nut Bread	1 (1.5 oz)	140	4	26	11	5
Soft Baked Cinnamon Pecan Bread	1 (1.5 oz)	140	4	25	11	5
Rice Krispies						
Treats	1 (0.8 oz)	90	2	17	8	0
Rickland Orchards						
Greek Yogurt Granola Apple & Honey	1 (1.4 oz)	160	6	22	12	5

FOOD	PORTION	CAL	FAT	CARB	SUGAR	FIBER
Greek Yogurt Granola Blueberri Acai	1 (1.4 oz)	160	6	22	11	5
Greek Yogurt Granola Cranberri Almond	1 (1.4 oz)	160	6	22	12	5
Greek Yogurt Granola Orchard Peach	1 (1.4 oz)	160	6	22	8	5
Greek Yogurt Granola Peanut Butter	1 (1.4 oz)	170	8	17	8	5
Greek Yogurt Granola Strawberry	1 (1.4 oz)	150	4	23	8	5
Greek Yogurt Granola Toasted Coconut	1 (1.4 oz)	170	10	19	8	5
Rise Bar						
Breakfast Crunchy Cashew Almond	1 (1.4 oz)	190	12	19	11	3
Breakfast Crunchy Cranberry Apple	1 (1.4 oz)	160	7	25	19	3
South Beach						
Fiber Bar Granola Fudge Graham	1 (1.23 oz)	120	4	23	6	9
Protein Fit Cinnamon Raisin	1 (1.2 oz)	130	3	18	8	3
Snack Bar Fudgy Chocolate Mint	1 (0.98 oz)	100	4	14	5	6
Special K						
Granola Chocolatey Peanut Butter	1 (0.95 oz)	110	3	17	7	4
Lemon Twist	1 (1.6 oz)	160	4	25	11	5
Protein & Fiber Chocolatey Peanut Butter	1 (0.9 oz)	110	3	17	7	4
Raspberry Cheesecake	1 (0.8 oz)	90	2	17	7	3
Sweet & Savory						
Cocoa Pistachio	1 (3 oz)	390	22	42	17	7

FOOD	PORTION	CAL	FAT	CARB	SUGAR	FIBER
Tasty						
Carrot Cake	1 (1.2 oz)	110	2	24	14	3
Pumpkin Pie	1 (1.2 oz)	120	3	25	15	3
Weetabix						
Oaty Chocolate	1	67	2	12	3	6
Weetos	1	88	3	14	8	tr
Wings Of Nature						
Organic Cranberry Crunch	1 (1.4 oz)	170	10	18	9	2
Organic Espresso Coffee	1 (1.4 oz)	180	10	21	12	2
Zone Perfect						
Cookie Dough Chocolate Chip	1 (1.58 oz)	180	5	24	18	tr
Cookie Dough Oatmeal Raisin	1 (1.58 oz)	170	4	25	16	tr
Cookie Dough Peanut Butter	1 (1.58 oz)	190	7	22	16	1
Sweet & Salty Cashew Pretzel	1 (1.58 oz)	200	7	23	14	1
Sweet & Salty Trail Mix	1 (1.58 oz)	200	8	21	12	1

CHAMPAGNE

FOOD	PORTION	CAL	FAT	CARB	SUGAR	FIBER
champagne	1 serv (3.5 oz)	84	0	3	1	0
mimosa	1 serv	117	tr	12	–	tr
punch	1 serv (4 oz)	73	tr	8	6	0
sekt german champagne	1 serv (3.5 oz)	84	0	5	–	–

CHAYOTE

FOOD	PORTION	CAL	FAT	CARB	SUGAR	FIBER
fresh cooked	1 cup	38	1	8	–	–
raw	1 (7 oz)	49	1	11	–	–
raw cut up	1 cup	32	tr	7	–	–
Dole						
Fresh cooked	½ cup (2.8 oz)	17	0	4	0	2

FOOD	PORTION	CAL	FAT	CARB	SUGAR	FIBER
CHEESE (*see also* CHEESE DISHES, CHEESE SUBSTITUTES, COTTAGE CHEESE, CREAM CHEESE, CREAM CHEESE SUBSTITUTES, NEUFCHATEL)						
american	1 oz	93	7	2	–	–
american cheese spread	1 oz	82	6	2	–	–
beaufort	1 oz	115	9	tr	tr	0
bel paese	1 oz	112	9	0	0	0
blue	1 oz	100	8	1	–	–
blue crumbled	1 cup (4.7 oz)	477	39	3	–	–
bocconcini smoked	1 oz	90	6	1	0	0
brick	1 oz	105	8	1	–	–
brie	1 oz	95	8	tr	–	–
cacio di roma sheep's milk cheese	1 oz	130	10	0	0	0
caerphilly	1.4 oz	150	13	0	–	0
camembert	1 oz	85	7	tr	–	–
cantal	1 oz	105	9	tr	tr	0
caraway	1 oz	107	8	1	–	–
chabichou	1 oz	95	8	tr	tr	0
chaource	1 oz	83	7	tr	tr	0
cheddar	1 oz	114	9	tr	–	–
cheddar low sodium	1 oz	113	9	1	–	–
cheddar lowfat	1 oz	49	2	1	–	–
cheddar reduced fat	1.4 oz	104	6	0	–	0
cheddar shredded	1 cup	455	37	1	–	–
cheshire	1 oz	110	9	1	–	–
cheshire reduced fat	1.4 oz	108	6	tr	–	0
colby	1 oz	112	9	1	–	–
colby low sodium	1 oz	113	9	1	–	–
colby lowfat	1 oz	49	2	1	–	–
comte	1 oz	114	9	tr	tr	0
coulommiers	1 oz	88	7	tr	tr	0
crottin	1 oz	105	9	tr	tr	0
derby	1.4 oz	161	14	0	–	0
edam reduced fat	1.4 oz	92	4	tr	–	0

FOOD	PORTION	CAL	FAT	CARB	SUGAR	FIBER
emmentaler	1 oz	115	9	tr	–	–
feta	1 oz	75	6	1	–	–
fontina	1 oz	110	9	tr	–	–
frais	1.6 oz	51	3	3	–	0
gjetost	1 oz	132	8	12	–	–
gloucester double	1.4 oz	162	14	0	–	0
goat fresh	1 oz	23	2	tr	tr	0
goat hard	1 oz	128	10	1	–	–
gorgonzola	1 oz	107	9	tr	–	–
gouda	1 oz	101	8	1	–	–
grana padano parmesan shaved	1 tbsp	20	2	0	0	0
gruyere	1 oz	117	9	tr	–	–
lancashire	1.4 oz	149	12	0	–	0
leicester	1.4 oz	160	14	0	–	0
limburger	1 oz	93	8	tr	–	–
lymeswold	1.4 oz	170	16	tr	–	0
maroilles	1 oz	97	8	tr	tr	0
monterey	1 oz	106	9	tr	–	–
morbier	1 oz	99	8	tr	tr	0
mozzarella	1 oz	80	6	1	–	–
mozzarella fresh	1 oz	80	6	tr	0	0
mozzarella part skim	1 oz	72	5	1	–	–
muenster	1 oz	104	9	tr	–	–
parmesan grated	1 tbsp	23	2	tr	–	–
parmesan hard	1 oz	111	7	1	–	–
picodon	1 oz	99	8	tr	tr	0
pimento	1 oz	106	9	tr	–	–
pont l'eveque	1 oz	86	7	tr	tr	0
port du salut	1 oz	100	8	tr	–	–
provolone	1 oz	100	8	1	–	–
pyrenees	1 oz	101	8	tr	tr	0
quark 20% fat	1 oz	33	1	1	–	–
quark 40% fat	1 oz	48	3	1	–	–

FOOD	PORTION	CAL	FAT	CARB	SUGAR	FIBER
quark made w/ skim milk	1 oz	22	tr	1	–	–
queso anejo	1 oz	106	9	1	–	–
queso asadero	1 oz	101	8	1	–	–
queso chihuahua	1 oz	106	8	2	–	–
queso fresco	1 oz	41	2	1	–	0
queso manchego	1 oz	107	8	tr	–	0
queso panela	1 oz	74	5	1	–	0
raclette	1 oz	102	8	tr	tr	0
reblochon	1 oz	88	7	tr	tr	0
ricotta part skim	½ cup (4.4 oz)	171	10	6	–	–
ricotta whole milk	½ cup (4.4 oz)	216	16	4	–	–
romadur 40% fat	1 oz	83	6	tr	–	–
romano	1 oz	110	8	1	–	–
roquefort	1 oz	105	9	1	–	–
rouy	1 oz	95	8	tr	tr	0
saint marcellin	1 oz	94	8	tr	tr	0
saint nectaire	1 oz	97	8	tr	tr	0
saint paulin	1 oz	85	6	tr	tr	0
sainte maure	1 oz	99	8	tr	tr	0
selles sur cher	1 oz	93	8	tr	tr	0
stilton blue	1.4 oz	164	14	0	–	0
stilton white	1.4 oz	145	13	0	–	0
swiss	1 oz	107	8	1	–	–
swiss processed	1 oz	95	7	1	–	–
tilsit	1 oz	96	7	1	–	–
tome	1 oz	92	7	tr	tr	0
triple crème	1 oz	113	11	tr	tr	0
vacherin	1 oz	92	8	tr	tr	0
wensleydale	1.4 oz	151	13	0	–	0
whey cheese	1 oz	126	8	9	0	0
yogurt cheese	1 oz	80	7	0	0	0

FOOD	PORTION	CAL	FAT	CARB	SUGAR	FIBER
Athenos						
Blue Crumbled	¼ pkg (1.1 oz)	110	9	2	0	1
Feta Black Peppercorn	1 oz	80	6	1	0	0
Feta Crumbled Garlic & Herb	⅕ pkg (1.2 oz)	90	7	2	0	1
Gorgonzola Crumbled	2 tbsp (1.1 oz)	110	9	2	0	1
Boar's Head						
Imported Swiss	1 oz	110	8	tr	0	0
Cabot						
Cheddar Extra Sharp	1 oz	110	9	tr	0	0
Cheddar Horseradish	1 oz	110	9	tr	0	0
Cracker Barrel						
Baby Swiss	1 oz	110	9	0	0	0
Cheddar Extra Sharp 2% Milk	1 oz	90	6	1	0	0
Cheddar Extra Sharp Shredded 2% Milk	1 oz	80	6	1	0	0
Cheddar Sharp	1 oz	120	10	0	0	0
Cheddar Sharp Shredded	1 oz	110	9	1	0	0
White Cheddar Reduced Fat	1 oz	90	6	1	0	0
Dietz & Watson						
Aalsbruk Edam	1 oz	90	7	1	0	0
American Yellow	1 slice (1 oz)	110	8	0	0	0
Cheddar Sharp	1 oz	110	9	1	1	0
Danish Blue	1 oz	100	12	0	0	0
Danish Havarti	1 oz	110	9	1	1	0
Gorgonzola	1 oz	100	8	0	0	0
Muenster	1 slice (0.7 oz)	75	6	0	0	0
Easy Cheese						
American	2 tbsp (1.1 oz)	90	6	2	2	0
Cheddar	2 tbsp (1.1 oz)	90	6	2	2	0

FOOD	PORTION	CAL	FAT	CARB	SUGAR	FIBER
Finlandia						
Baby Muenster	1 oz	100	8	0	0	0
Double Gloucester Deli Slices	1 slice (0.8 oz)	83	7	1	0	0
Gouda Deli Slices	1 slice (0.8 oz)	79	6	0	0	0
Havarti Deli Slices	1 slice (0.8 oz)	86	7	0	0	0
Muenster Deli Slices	1 slice (0.8 oz)	86	7	0	0	0
Swiss Deli Slices	1 slice (0.8 oz)	86	7	0	0	0
Swiss Light Deli Slices	1 slice (0.8 oz)	57	3	0	0	0
Viola	2 tbsp (1 oz)	87	8	1	1	0
Galbani						
Precious Fresh Mozzarella Sliced	1 oz	90	6	0	0	0
Precious Sticksters Cheddar	1 (1 oz)	110	9	1	0	0
Precious Stringsters Mozzarella Part Skim	1 (1 oz)	80	6	1	0	0
Grana Padano						
PDO Cheese	1 oz	120	8	10	0	0
Hans All Natural						
Spread Cheddar & Jalapeno	2 tbsp (1 oz)	90	7	3	3	0
Spread Swiss Cheese & Almonds	2 tbsp (1 oz)	90	7	3	3	0
Karoun						
Ackawi	1 oz	110	8	0	0	0
Ani	1 in cube (1 oz)	110	8	0	0	0
Labne Kefir	2 tbsp (1 oz)	80	5	2	1	0
Paneer	1 oz	90	7	1	1	0
Kraft						
Big Slice Swiss	1 (0.8 oz)	90	7	0	0	0
Cheese Spread Pimento	2 tbsp	80	6	3	2	0

FOOD	PORTION	CAL	FAT	CARB	SUGAR	FIBER
Cheese Spread Roka Blue	2 tbsp	80	7	2	1	0
Cheese Spread Sharp Old English	2 tbsp (1.1 oz)	90	8	1	0	0
Fresh Take Cheese Breadcrumb Mix Italian Parmesan	1 oz	100	5	8	0	0
Fresh Take Cheese Breadcrumb Mix Southwest Three Cheese	1 oz	100	6	8	1	0
Grated 100% Parmesan	1 tsp (5 g)	20	2	0	0	0
Grated 100% Romano	1 tsp (5 g)	20	2	0	0	0
Grated Parmesan Reduced Fat	1 tsp (5 g)	20	1	2	0	0
Shredded Cheddar Fat Free	1 oz	45	0	2	0	0
Shredded Mexican Style Taco 2% Milk	1 serv (1 oz)	80	5	1	0	0
Shredded Mozzarella 2% Milk + Calcium	1 oz	70	5	1	0	0
Singles American	1 (0.7 oz)	60	4	2	1	0
Singles American 2% Milk	1 (0.7 oz)	45	3	2	2	0
Singles Pepper Jack	1 slice (0.7 oz)	80	6	0	0	0
Slices Havarti	1 (0.7 oz)	80	7	0	0	0
Slices Monterey Jack	1 (0.7 oz)	80	6	0	0	0
Laughing Cow						
Cinnamon Cream ⅓ Less Fat	1 wedge (0.7 oz)	45	4	2	1	0
Classic Cream ⅓ Less Fat	1 wedge (0.7 oz)	45	4	tr	tr	0
Creamy Swiss Light	1 wedge (0.7 oz)	35	2	1	1	0

FOOD	PORTION	CAL	FAT	CARB	SUGAR	FIBER
Creamy Swiss Original	1 wedge (0.7 oz)	50	4	1	1	0
Garden Vegetable ⅓ Less Fat	1 wedge (0.7 oz)	45	4	tr	1	0
Strawberries & Cream ⅓ Less Fat	1 wedge (0.7 oz)	45	4	2	1	0
Lifeway						
Farmer	2 tbsp (1.1 oz)	40	2	4	4	–
Farmer Lite	2 tbsp (1.1 oz)	25	1	2	1	–
Sweet Kiss Spread Peach	1 oz	50	2	6	6	–
Sweet Kiss Spread Plain	1 oz	50	2	5	5	–
Sweet Kiss Spread Raisins	1 oz	45	1	6	6	–
Molly McButter						
Natural Cheese	1 tsp (2 g)	5	0	1	–	0
Organic Valley						
American Singles Unprocessed Organic	1 slice	70	6	tr	tr	0
Pizza Zing						
Spicy Hot Cheese Shake	2 tsp	15	1	0	0	0
Polly-O						
Mozzarella Shredded Fat Free	1 oz	40	0	1	1	1
Mozzarella Shredded Part Skim	1 oz	80	5	1	0	0
Mozzarella Shredded Whole Milk	1 oz	90	7	1	0	0
String-Ums Mozzarella Part Skim	1 (1 oz)	80	6	0	0	0
Sara Lee						
Colby & Monterey Jack	3 slices (1.2 oz)	130	11	1	0	0

FOOD	PORTION	CAL	FAT	CARB	SUGAR	FIBER
Sargento						
Bistro Blends Shredded Italian Pasta Cheese	¼ cup (1 oz)	90	6	2	0	0
Cheddar Mild Shredded Reduced Sodium	¼ cup (1 oz)	110	9	1	0	0
Colby-Jack Sticks Reduced Sodium	1 (0.7 oz)	80	7	tr	0	0
Provolone Reduced Sodium	1 slice (0.7 oz)	70	5	0	0	0
String Light	1 piece (0.7 oz)	50	3	1	0	0
Smart Balance						
Creamy Cheddar Slices	1 (0.7 oz)	40	2	2	2	0
Fat Free Lactose Free Slices	1 (0.7 oz)	40	2	2	2	0
Sorrento						
Mozzarella Fresh	1 oz	90	6	0	0	0
Treasure Cave						
Feta Crumbled	¼ cup (1 oz)	80	6	1	0	tr
Yanni						
Grilling Cheese Original	1 oz	80	7	0	0	0
CHEESE DISHES						
Alexia						
Cheddar Bites	3 (1.2 oz)	110	6	8	0	0
Mozzarella Stix	2 pieces (1.3 oz)	120	6	10	1	1
Farm Rich						
Cheese Sticks	2 (2 oz)	170	9	14	1	0
Mozzarella Sticks Marinara Stuffed	2 (2.3 oz)	160	8	14	2	1
Mozzarella Bites	4 (1.8 oz)	150	6	13	4	1

FOOD	PORTION	CAL	FAT	CARB	SUGAR	FIBER
TAKE-OUT						
fondue	½ cup (3.8 oz)	247	15	4	–	–
fried mozzarella sticks	3 (4.6 oz)	503	32	20	2	1
souffle	1 serv (7 oz)	504	38	18	5	1
welsh rarebit	1 slice	228	16	14	–	1
CHEESE SUBSTITUTES						
mozzarella	1 oz	70	3	7	–	–
soya cheese	1.4 oz	128	11	tr	–	0
Daiya						
Cheddar Style Shreds	¼ cup (1 oz)	90	6	7	0	1
Mozzarella Style Shreds	¼ cup (1 oz)	90	6	7	0	1
Tofutti						
Better Ricotta Milk Free	¼ cup (2.2 oz)	100	7	8	0	1
Soy American	1 slice (0.7 oz)	80	6	2	–	0
Soy Mozzarella	1 slice (0.7 oz)	80	6	2	–	0
CHERIMOYA						
fresh	1	515	2	131	–	–
CHERRIES						
CANNED						
maraschino	1 (4 g)	7	tr	2	2	tr
maraschino	¼ cup (1.4 oz)	66	tr	17	16	1
sour in heavy syrup	½ cup	116	tr	30	28	1
sour in light syrup	½ cup	94	tr	24	–	1
sour water pack	½ cup	44	tr	11	9	1
sweet juice pack	½ cup	68	tr	17	15	2
sweet pitted in heavy syrup	½ cup	105	tr	27	25	2
sweet water pack	½ cup	57	tr	15	13	2

FOOD	PORTION	CAL	FAT	CARB	SUGAR	FIBER
Del Monte						
Sweet Dark Pitted In Heavy Syrup	½ cup (4.2 oz)	100	0	24	24	tr
Jake & Amos						
Brandied Sweet	½ cup (4.4 oz)	90	0	22	10	2
DRIED						
bing unsulfured	¼ cup	130	0	31	21	2
montmorency tart pitted	⅓ cup	160	1	36	24	2
rainier unsulfured	⅓ cup	140	1	32	30	2
tart	½ cup	200	1	49	41	2
yogurt covered	¼ cup	170	6	29	22	5
Raisinets						
Dark & Milk Chocolate	¼ cup (1.6 oz)	200	8	32	28	2
FRESH						
sour	1 cup	52	tr	13	9	2
sour pitted	1 cup	78	tr	19	13	3
sweet	20	86	1	22	17	3
Dole						
Cherries	1 cup (4.9 oz)	90	0	22	18	3
Domex Superfresh Growers						
Rainier	21 (5 oz)	90	0	19	16	3
FROZEN						
sour unsweetened	½ cup	36	tr	9	7	1
sweet sweetened	½ cup	115	tr	29	26	3
Dole						
Dark Sweet	1 cup (4.9 oz)	90	0	22	18	3

CHERRY JUICE

FOOD	PORTION	CAL	FAT	CARB	SUGAR	FIBER
tart cherry concentrate	1 cup	140	0	34	27	0
Cheribundi						
Skinny Cherry	8 oz	90	0	23	17	–
Tart Cherry	8 oz	130	0	32	28	–
Whey Cherry	8 oz	160	0	30	27	–

FOOD	PORTION	CAL	FAT	CARB	SUGAR	FIBER
Froose						
Cheerful Cherry	1 box (4.2 oz)	80	0	18	8	3
Old Orchard						
Very Cherre 100% Tart Cherry Juice	8 oz	130	0	31	21	–
Smart Juice						
Organic 100% Juice Tart Cherry	8 oz	140	0	32	24	1
CHERVIL						
seed	1 tsp	1	tr	tr	–	–
CHESTNUTS						
chinese steamed	3 (1 oz)	43	tr	10	–	–
creme de marrons	1 oz	73	tr	18	10	1
japanese roasted	1 oz	57	tr	13	–	–
ready-to-eat vacuum packed	5 (1 oz)	40	0	8	0	0
roasted	3 (1 oz)	70	1	15	3	1
Matiz						
Organic	7–8	86	1	17	12	5
CHEWING GUM						
bubble gum	1 block	20	tr	5	5	tr
stick	1 piece	7	tr	2	2	tr
sugarless	1 piece	5	tr	2	0	0
5 Gum						
Cobalt	1 piece	5	0	2	0	–
Big Red						
Gum	1 stick	10	0	2	2	–
Doublemint						
Gum	1 piece	10	0	2	2	–
Freedent						
Gum	1 piece	10	0	2	2	–

FOOD	PORTION	CAL	FAT	CARB	SUGAR	FIBER
Hubba Bubba						
Ouch! Bubble Gum	1 piece	5	0	1	0	–
Orbit						
Spearmint	1 piece	<5	0	1	0	0
Snap Infusion						
Citrus	1 piece (2.5 g)	5	0	2	0	0
Stride						
All Flavors	1 piece (1.9 g)	<5	0	1	0	–
Spark	1 piece (1.9 g)	5	0	1	0	–
Trident						
White Peppermint	2 pieces (3 g)	5	0	2	0	–
Vitamingum						
Fresh Sugar Free All Flavors	1 piece (3 g)	5	0	2	0	–
Sport Bubblegum	1 piece (6 g)	15	0	4	4	–
CHIA SEEDS						
dried	1 oz	134	7	14	–	–
Dole						
Chia & Fruit Clusters Cranberry Apple	12 (1 oz)	120	3	22	8	4
Chia & Fruit Clusters Mixed Berry	12 (1 oz)	120	3	22	8	4
Milled Seeds	5 tbsp (1 oz)	150	9	13	0	11
Whole Seeds	3 tbsp (1 oz)	150	9	13	0	11
Health Warrior						
Chia Bar Peanut Butter Chocolate	1 (0.9 oz)	100	5	15	4	3
Chia Seeds	1 tbsp (0.5 oz)	60	5	6	–	6
Spectrum						
Chia Seeds	1 tbsp (0.4 oz)	60	4	4	–	4
TruRoots						
Chia	1 tbsp (0.4 oz)	55	9	5	–	6

FOOD	PORTION	CAL	FAT	CARB	SUGAR	FIBER
CHICKEN (*see also* CHICKEN DISHES, CHICKEN SUBSTITUTES, DINNER, HOT DOG, MEATBALLS)						
CANNED						
chicken spread	1 serv (2 oz)	88	10	2	tr	tr
meat drained	1 can (5 oz)	230	10	1	0	0
w/ broth	½ can (2.5 oz)	117	6	0	0	0
Hormel						
Chunk White & Dark	2 oz	70	3	0	0	0
Premium Chunk Breast	2 oz	60	2	0	0	0
FRESH						
back w/ skin roasted bones removed	1 (3.7 oz)	318	22	0	0	0
back w/o skin roasted bones removed	1 (2.8 oz)	191	11	0	0	0
breast roasted diced	1 cup (5 oz)	231	5	0	0	0
breast w/ skin battered fried bones removed	½ breast (4.9 oz)	364	18	13	0	tr
breast w/ skin floured fried bones removed	1 (3.4 oz)	218	9	2	–	tr
breast w/ skin roasted bones removed	½ breast (3.4 oz)	193	8	0	0	0
breast w/ skin stewed bones removed	½ breast (3.9 oz)	202	8	0	0	0
breast w/o skin fried bones removed	½ breast (3 oz)	161	4	tr	0	0
breast w/o skin roasted bones removed	½ breast (3 oz)	142	3	0	0	0
breast w/o skin stewed bones removed	1 (3.3 oz)	143	3	0	0	0
broiler/fryer w/ skin roasted bones removed	½ (10.5 oz)	715	41	0	0	0
capon meat & skin roasted bones removed	½ (1.4 lbs)	1459	74	0	0	0

FOOD	PORTION	CAL	FAT	CARB	SUGAR	FIBER
cornish hen w/ skin roasted	½ (4.5 oz)	335	23	0	0	0
cornish hen w/ skin roasted	1 (9 oz)	668	47	0	0	0
cornish hen w/o skin roasted	½ (4 oz)	147	4	0	0	0
cornish hen w/o skin roasted	1 (7.7 oz)	295	9	0	0	0
dark meat w/o skin roasted diced	1 cup (5 oz)	287	14	0	0	0
drumstick w/ skin battered floured & fried bones removed	1 (1.7 oz)	120	7	1	–	0
drumstick w/ skin battered fried bones removed	1 (2.5 oz)	193	11	6	–	tr
drumstick w/ skin roasted bones removed	1 (1.8 oz)	112	6	0	0	0
drumstick w/ skin stewed bones removed	1 (2 oz)	116	6	0	0	0
drumstick w/o skin fried bones removed	1 (1.5 oz)	82	3	0	0	0
drumstick w/o skin roasted bones removed	1 (1.5 oz)	76	2	0	0	0
drumstick w/o skin stewed bones removed	1 (1.6 oz)	78	3	0	0	0
feet cooked	1 (1.2 oz)	73	5	tr	0	0
ground crumbled fried	3 oz	161	9	0	0	0
ground patty cooked	1 lg (2.8 oz)	190	11	0	0	0
ground patty cooked	1 med (2.1 oz)	142	8	0	0	0
ground patty cooked	1 sm (1.7 oz)	114	6	0	0	0
meat & skin stewed bones removed	¼ chicken (4.6 oz)	372	25	0	0	0

FOOD	PORTION	CAL	FAT	CARB	SUGAR	FIBER
neck w/ skin battered fried	1 (1.8 oz)	172	12	5	–	–
neck w/ skin fried	1 (1.3 oz)	120	9	2	–	–
neck w/ skin simmered	1 (1.3 oz)	94	7	0	0	0
roaster meat & skin roasted bones removed	¼ chicken (8.4 oz)	535	32	0	0	0
skin battered fried from ½ chicken	6.7 oz	749	55	44	–	–
skin floured fried from ½ chicken	2 oz	281	24	5	–	–
skin roasted from ½ chicken	2 oz	254	23	0	0	0
skin stewed from ½ chicken	2.5 oz	261	24	0	0	0
tail cooked	1 (1 oz)	84	5	3	0	tr
thigh w/ skin battered & fried bones removed	1 (3 oz)	238	14	8	–	tr
thigh w/ skin floured fried bones removed	1 (2.2 oz)	162	9	2	–	tr
thigh w/ skin roasted bones removed	1 (2.2 oz)	153	10	0	0	0
thigh w/ skin stewed bones removed	1 (2.4 oz)	158	10	0	0	0
thigh w/o skin fried bones removed	1 (1.8 oz)	113	5	1	–	0
thigh w/o skin roasted bones removed	1 (1.8 oz)	109	6	0	0	0
thigh w/o skin stewed bones removed	1 (1.9 oz)	107	5	0	0	0
wing w/ skin battered fried bones removed	1 (1.7 oz)	159	11	5	–	tr
wing w/ skin floured fried bones removed	1 (1.1 oz)	103	7	1	–	0

FOOD	PORTION	CAL	FAT	CARB	SUGAR	FIBER
wing w/ skin roasted bones removed	1 (1.4 oz)	100	7	0	0	0
wing w/o skin fried bones removed	1 (0.7 oz)	42	2	0	0	0
wing w/o skin roasted bones removed	1 (0.7 oz)	43	2	0	0	0
wing w/o skin stewed bones removed	1 (0.8 oz)	43	2	0	0	0
Coleman						
Organic Breast Boneless Skinless	4 oz	120	2	0	0	0
Organic Drumsticks	4 oz	180	10	0	0	0
Foster Farms						
Back & Necks	4 oz	340	31	0	0	0
Breast Skinless Boneless	4 oz	120	2	0	0	0
Drumsticks not prep	1 (2.8 oz)	130	7	0	0	0
Ground not prep	4 oz	210	14	0	0	0
Party Wings	5 (3.8 oz)	230	17	0	0	0
Thighs	1 (4.6 oz)	270	20	0	0	0
Perdue						
Oven Ready Roaster Bone-In Breast	4 oz	140	7	1	0	0
Rocky						
The Range Chicken Whole	4 oz	240	17	0	0	0
Rosie						
Organic Breast Boneless Skinless	4 oz	120	2	0	0	0
FROZEN						
breast roll roasted	2 oz	75	4	1	tr	0
fajita strips	1 (0.3 oz)	13	1	tr	0	0
patty cooked	1 (3.5 oz)	287	20	13	0	tr

FOOD	PORTION	CAL	FAT	CARB	SUGAR	FIBER
Bell & Evans						
Breaded Breast Nuggets	1 serv (4 oz)	220	9	13	2	1
Breasts Grilled	1 (2.75 oz)	90	1	1	0	0
Breasts Grilled Buffalo Style	1 (3 oz)	110	1	0	1	0
Burgers	1 (4 oz)	160	6	3	0	0
Chicken Tenders Gluten Free	1 serv (4 oz)	180	6	12	0	1
Wings Honey Barbeque	3 (4.6 oz)	160	8	6	6	0
Coleman						
Breast Nuggets Gluten Free	6 (2.7 oz)	130	6	10	1	0
Breast Strips	6 (2.7 oz)	130	3	14	1	1
Organic Prairie						
Breast Boneless Skinless	4 oz	150	2	1	1	tr
Ground	4 oz	200	12	1	–	–
Perdue						
Simply Smart Grilled Chicken Strips	3 oz	110	3	1	0	–
Simply Smart Lightly Breaded Chicken Strips	3 oz	140	5	6	0	–
Simply Smart Roasted Chicken Chunks	3 oz	120	2	2	1	–
Weaver						
Breast Nuggets	4 (2.8 oz)	190	11	13	0	1
Breast Strips	2 (2.7 oz)	190	12	10	0	0
Patties Breast	1 (2.9 oz)	200	11	13	0	1
Popcorn Chicken	12 pieces (2.9 oz)	200	10	19	0	1
Wings Buffalo Style	3 (2.9 oz)	160	10	3	0	0
READY-TO-EAT						
Dietz & Watson						
Breast Southern Fried	3 slices (1.9 oz)	70	2	1	1	0

FOOD	PORTION	CAL	FAT	CARB	SUGAR	FIBER
Foster Farms						
Breast Strips Grilled	3 oz	110	3	2	0	0
Cutlets Breaded	3 oz	180	8	14	tr	0
Perdue						
Short Cuts Chicken Breast Grilled Italian	½ cup (2.5 oz)	100	2	2	1	–
TAKE-OUT						
chicken tenders	4 (2.2 oz)	180	10	11	1	tr

CHICKEN DISHES

FOOD	PORTION	CAL	FAT	CARB	SUGAR	FIBER
CANNED						
Dinty Moore						
Chicken & Dumplings Big Bowl	½ pkg	220	7	29	1	1
Chicken & Noodles	1 can (7.5 oz)	190	9	19	2	1
Chicken Stew	½ can	220	11	17	3	2
Swanson						
Chicken A La King	1 can (10.5 oz)	320	19	20	3	2
FROZEN						
Crazy Cuizine						
Teriyaki Chicken	1 cup (5 oz)	240	8	23	21	3
TAKE-OUT						
arroz con pollo	1 serv (16 oz)	579	14	62	3	2
barbecued pulled chicken	1 serv (9 oz)	312	2	37	27	2
boneless breast w/ apple stuffing	1 serv (5 oz)	260	9	10	2	1
breast & wing breaded & fried	2 pieces (5.7 oz)	494	30	20	–	–
buffalo wing + sauce	2 (1.7 oz)	147	10	tr	tr	0
cacciatore breast + sauce	1 serv (5.9 oz)	323	18	9	3	1

FOOD	PORTION	CAL	FAT	CARB	SUGAR	FIBER
cacciatore drumstick + sauce	1 serv (3.2 oz)	172	9	5	2	1
cacciatore thigh + sauce	1 serv (3.8 oz)	204	11	6	2	1
cacciatore wing + sauce	1 serv (2.1 oz)	113	6	3	1	tr
chicharrones de pollo	3 (2.6 oz)	289	18	14	tr	1
chicken & dumplings	1 cup (8.6 oz)	368	19	22	1	1
chicken & noodles in cream sauce	1 cup (8 oz)	323	11	32	5	1
chicken a la king	1 cup (8.5 oz)	465	34	16	4	1
chicken cordon bleu + sauce	1 roll (8 oz)	504	29	11	1	1
chicken meatloaf	1 lg slice (5 oz)	243	9	11	3	1
chicken pie w/ top crust	1 slice (5.6 oz)	472	31	32	–	1
chicken satay + peanut sauce	2 skewers	239	12	6	4	1
chicken breast parmigiana	1 serv (5.8 oz)	278	14	13	3	1
chicken creole w/o rice	1 cup (8.6 oz)	187	4	8	5	2
chicken kiev breast meat	1 serv (9 oz)	653	34	11	1	1
chicken salad white meat	1 serv (4 oz)	300	21	1	0	0
creamed chicken	1 cup (8.5 oz)	388	23	14	8	tr
croquette	1 (2.2 oz)	159	9	8	2	tr
curry	1 cup (8.3 oz)	288	16	9	5	2
curry breast half + sauce	1 (7 oz)	244	14	8	4	2
curry drumstick + sauce	1 (3.7 oz)	129	7	4	2	1
curry thigh + sauce	1 (4.4 oz)	154	9	5	3	1
curry wing + sauce	1 (2.4 oz)	84	5	3	1	1
drumstick & thigh breaded & fried	2 pieces (5.2 oz)	431	27	16	–	–

FOOD	PORTION	CAL	FAT	CARB	SUGAR	FIBER
fricassee	1 cup (8.6 oz)	322	18	8	tr	tr
groundnut stew hkatenkwan	1 serv (15.7 oz)	576	40	18	3	4
jamaican jerk wings	4 wings (9.9 oz)	709	51	3	tr	tr
jambalaya w/ sausage & rice	1 cup (8.6 oz)	393	21	23	2	1
rotisserie seasoned breast w/ skin	1 serv (3.5 oz)	184	8	0	0	0
rotisserie seasoned breast w/o skin	1 serv (3.5 oz)	148	3	0	0	0
rotisserie seasoned thigh w/ skin	1 serv (3.5 oz)	233	16	0	0	0
rotisserie seasoned thigh w/o skin	1 serv (3.5 oz)	196	11	0	0	0
sancocho de pollo dominican chicken stew	1 serv	702	30	34	4	1
stew	1 cup (8.8 oz)	176	5	19	4	3
tandoori chicken breast	1 serv	260	13	5	–	–
tandoori chicken leg & thigh	1 serv	300	17	6	–	–
tetrazzini	1 cup (8.6 oz)	369	18	29	2	2
CHICKEN SUBSTITUTES						
Gardein						
Buffalo Wings	1 serv (3.5 oz)	120	3	8	1	2
Chick'n Filets	1 (3.5 oz)	120	2	7	1	2
Crispy Fingers	2 (3.2 oz)	160	5	12	1	2
Crispy Tenders	1 (1.8 oz)	90	2	9	0	1
Tuscan Breasts	1 (5.3 oz)	150	3	11	1	3
Quorn						
Chik'n Nuggets	3–4 (3 oz)	180	8	21	4	2
Chik'n Patties	1 (2.6 oz)	150	6	17	4	2

FOOD	PORTION	CAL	FAT	CARB	SUGAR	FIBER
Gruyere Chik'n Cutlet	1 (4 oz)	260	15	23	3	3
Naked Chik'n Cutlet	1 (2.4 oz)	80	3	5	1	2
Vegetarian Plus						
Vegan Half Chicken	¼ pkg (3 oz)	180	10	6	0	3
Veggie Patch						
Chick'n Nuggets	4 (2.7 oz)	170	7	20	1	2
CHICKPEAS						
CANNED						
chickpeas	1 cup	285	3	54	–	–
Progresso						
Chick Peas	½ cup (4.6 oz)	120	3	20	3	5
DRIED						
cooked	1 cup	269	4	45	–	–
Nutty Bean						
ChickPz Roasted Sea Salt	½ pkg (1 oz)	100	2	17	3	5
ChickPz Roasted Chai Vanilla	½ pkg (1 oz)	110	2	20	8	4
ChickPz Roasted Sweet & Sour Chipotle	½ pkg (1 oz)	100	2	19	7	4
ChickPz Roasted Tuscan Garlic & Herb	½ pkg (1 oz)	100	2	17	3	5
FROZEN						
Tandoor Chef						
Channa Masala	½ pkg (5 oz)	190	9	22	6	7
CHICORY						
endive fresh chopped	½ cup	4	tr	1	–	–
greens raw chopped	½ cup	21	tr	4	–	–
root raw	1 (2.1 oz)	44	tr	11	–	–
roots raw cut up	½ cup (1.6 oz)	33	tr	8	–	–
witloof head raw	1 (1.9 oz)	9	tr	2	–	–
witloof raw	½ cup (1.6 oz)	8	tr	2	–	–

FOOD	PORTION	CAL	FAT	CARB	SUGAR	FIBER
CHILI						
powder	1 tbsp	24	1	4	1	3
Bush's						
Chili Magic Chili Starter Texas Recipe	½ cup (4.6 oz)	110	1	19	2	5
Chili Magic Chili Starter Traditional Mild	½ cup (4.6 oz)	100	0	18	2	4
Frontera						
Chili Mix Chipotle Black Bean	½ cup	60	1	12	3	3
Chili Starter Green Chile White Bean	½ cup (4.4 oz)	80	2	14	2	4
Hormel						
Chili Mac	1 pkg (9.9 oz)	270	7	34	10	6
Chili No Beans	1 pkg (7.3 oz)	190	8	16	3	2
Chili No Beans Less Sodium	1 serv (8.3 oz)	220	9	18	3	3
Chili w/ Beans	1 serv (8.7 oz)	260	7	33	5	7
Chili w/ Beans Less Sodium	1 serv (8.7 oz)	260	7	33	5	7
Turkey Chili w/ Beans	1 serv (8.7 oz)	210	3	28	6	6
Vegetarian Chili w/ Beans	1 serv (8.7 oz)	190	1	35	6	10
Master Chili						
Chipotle Chicken No Bean	1 serv (8.3 oz)	230	10	18	7	3
Roasted Tomato w/ Bean	1 serv (8.3 oz)	210	6	25	7	7
Quorn						
Chili	1 pkg (8.9 oz)	160	3	26	7	7

FOOD	PORTION	CAL	FAT	CARB	SUGAR	FIBER
Stagg						
Chunkero	½ can	320	16	28	6	6
Classic	½ can	290	13	30	7	6
Ranch House Chicken	½ can	240	8	26	5	7
Silverado Beef	½ can	260	8	30	6	6
Turkey Ranchero	½ can	250	5	32	7	9
Vegetable Garden	½ can	200	1	37	9	8
Truitt Brothers						
Beef Natural Shredded	1 cup (9.4 oz)	240	5	32	4	7
Vegetarian	1 cup (9.4 oz)	220	2	42	5	10
TAKE-OUT						
chiles rellenos cheese filled	1 (5 oz)	365	30	8	5	1
chili con carne w/ beans	1 cup	264	11	22	6	7
chili con carne w/ beans & chicken	1 cup (8.9 oz)	218	7	19	6	6
chili con carne w/ beans & rice	1 cup	298	9	45	2	7
vegetarian chili	1 cup	272	7	35	7	11

CHILI PEPPER (*see* PEPPERS)

CHINESE FOOD (*see* ASIAN FOOD)

CHINESE PRESERVING MELON

FOOD	PORTION	CAL	FAT	CARB	SUGAR	FIBER
cooked	½ cup	11	tr	3	–	–

CHIPS (*see also* SNACKS)

FOOD	PORTION	CAL	FAT	CARB	SUGAR	FIBER
apple chips	10 (0.8 oz)	101	5	16	14	2
banana	1 oz	147	10	17	10	2
carrot	28 (1 oz)	95	tr	22	11	7
corn	1 oz	147	8	18	tr	2
plantain	1 oz	158	10	16	–	1
potato salted	1 oz	155	11	14	tr	1
potato sticks	½ cup (0.6 oz)	94	6	10	tr	1

FOOD	PORTION	CAL	FAT	CARB	SUGAR	FIBER
potato sticks	1 pkg (1 oz)	148	10	15	tr	1
potato unsalted	1 oz	152	10	15	tr	1
potato unsalted reduced fat	1 oz	138	6	19	tr	2
shrimp	4 sm (0.4 oz)	56	4	5	tr	tr
shrimp	4 med (0.9 oz)	141	9	13	tr	tr
shrimp	4 lg (1.4 oz)	219	14	20	1	tr
soy	1 oz	107	2	15	1	1
sweet potato	1 oz	141	7	18	2	1
taro	10 (0.8 oz)	115	6	16	1	2
tortilla lowfat baked	1 oz	118	2	23	tr	2
tortilla lowfat unsalted	1 oz	118	2	23	tr	2
tortilla white corn	1 oz	139	7	19	tr	2
tortilla yellow corn	1 oz	139	6	19	tr	1
Bachman						
Corn Jumbo Chipitos	16 (1 oz)	150	8	18	0	2
Potato Golden Ridges	22 (1 oz)	160	10	15	–	0
Tortilla Black Bean	1 oz	140	7	18	–	3
Tortilla Restaurant Style	11 (1 oz)	140	6	19	0	2
Tortilla Toasted Sweet Potato	11 (1 oz)	130	5	20	2	3
Beanfields						
Bean & Rice Naturally Unsalted	⅙ pkg (1 oz)	140	6	18	0	3
Bean & Rice Pico De Gallo	⅙ pkg (1 oz)	140	6	18	0	4
Bean & Rice Sea Salt	⅙ pkg (1 oz)	140	6	18	0	4
Bean & Rice Sea Salt & Pepper	⅙ pkg (1 oz)	140	6	18	0	4
Better Balance						
Protein Chips Gluten Free All Flavors	1 oz	110	4	14	0	3

FOOD	PORTION	CAL	FAT	CARB	SUGAR	FIBER
Betty Crocker						
Potato Kettle Cooked Lightly Salted	1 oz	120	5	15	0	1
Boulder Canyon						
Potato Honey Bar-B-Que	14 (1 oz)	140	7	17	2	1
Potato Sour Cream & Chive	14 (1 oz)	140	7	17	1	1
Potato Totally Natural	14 (1 oz)	140	8	17	0	1
Buffalo Nickel Wingers						
Potato Level 1: No Bull Barbecue	25 (1 oz)	120	4	19	2	1
Potato Level 3: Nacho Chiliehanga	25 (1 oz)	120	4	19	1	1
Potato Level 5: Fiery Buffalo Bleu	25 (1 oz)	120	4	19	1	1
Cape Cod						
Potato 40% Less Fat Aged Cheddar & Sour Cream	18 (1 oz)	140	6	18	0	1
Potato Chef's Recipe Feta & Rosemary	18 (1 oz)	140	7	18	0	1
Potato Original	19 (1 oz)	140	8	17	0	tr
Potato Original 40% Reduced Fat	19 (1 oz)	140	6	18	0	2
Potato Sea Salt & Cracked Pepper	18 (1 oz)	140	7	17	0	2
Potato Sour Cream & Green Onion	18 (1 oz)	140	8	16	tr	1
Potato Waffle Cut Sea Salt	17 (1 oz)	140	7	18	0	1
Whole Grain Toasted	10 (1 oz)	130	6	19	2	3
Corazonas						
Potato Lightly Salted	1 oz	130	6	18	0	2

FOOD	PORTION	CAL	FAT	CARB	SUGAR	FIBER
Potato Spicy Rio Habanero	1 oz	130	6	18	1	2
Tortilla Lightly Salted	14 (1 oz)	140	7	18	0	3
Tortilla Squeeze Of Lime	14 (1 oz)	140	7	17	0	3
Deep River Snacks						
Potato Kettle Cooked Asian Sweet & Spicy	1 oz	150	8	15	3	1
Potato Kettle Cooked Original Salted	1 oz	150	8	16	0	1
Potato Kettle Cooked Rosemary & Olive Oil	1 oz	150	8	16	1	1
Potato Kettle Cooked Salt & Vinegar	1 oz	150	8	15	0	1
Potato Zesty Jalapeno	1 oz	150	8	15	0	1
Doritos						
Tortilla Flamas	11 (1 oz)	140	8	16	0	1
Tortilla Nacho Cheese	11 (1 oz)	150	8	17	1	1
Tortilla Spicy Nacho	12 (1 oz)	140	7	19	1	1
Tortilla Toasted Corn	13 (1 oz)	140	7	18	0	1
Fritos						
Corn Lightly Salted	1 oz	160	10	16	0	1
Corn Original	32 (1 oz)	160	10	15	tr	1
Corn Scoops	10 (1 oz)	160	10	16	0	1
Frontera						
Tortilla Blue Corn	1/9 pkg (1 oz)	130	5	20	0	2
Tortilla Thick & Crunchy	1/9 pkg (1 oz)	130	5	20	0	2
Garden Of Eatin'						
Corn White Strips Mini	18 (1 oz)	140	6	19	0	2
Pita w/ Whole Grain Sea Salt	9 (1 oz)	120	3	21	1	2
Tortilla Blue Corn No Salt Added	16 (1 oz)	140	7	18	0	2
Tortilla Corn Sprouted Blues	11 (1 oz)	130	7	15	tr	3

FOOD	PORTION	CAL	FAT	CARB	SUGAR	FIBER
Tortilla Guac-A-Mole	9 (1 oz)	140	6	19	tr	2
Tortilla Key Lime Jalapeno	15 (1 oz)	140	7	18	0	3
Tortilla Little Soy Blues	13 (1 oz)	140	7	17	0	2
Tortilla Multi Grain Everything	16 (1 oz)	140	7	19	1	3
Tortilla Red	15 (1 oz)	140	7	18	0	1
Tortilla Salsa Red	15 (1 oz)	140	7	18	0	3
Tortilla Sweet Potato Corn	9 (1 oz)	140	7	17	1	1
Tortilla Tamari	8 (1 oz)	140	7	18	0	3
Tortilla Yellow	13 (1 oz)	140	7	18	0	2
Tortilla Popped Sea Salt	20 (1 oz)	110	3	19	1	3
Veggie Salt & Garlic	17 (1 oz)	140	6	19	1	2
Hawaiian Snacks						
Potato Kettle Style	13 (1 oz)	140	9	15	0	1
Potato Luau BBQ	13 (1 oz)	140	9	15	1	1
Potato Mango Habanero	13 (1 oz)	140	9	18	1	1
Hippie Chips						
Baked Potato Chive-Talkin' Sour Cream	1 pkg (0.7 oz)	90	3	14	1	tr
Baked Potato Haight AshBerry Jalapeno	1 pkg (0.7 oz)	90	3	15	2	tr
Baked Potato Memphis Blues Barbecue	1 pkg (0.7 oz)	90	3	15	2	tr
Baked Potato Sea Of Love Salt	1 pkg (1 oz)	125	4	21	0	1
Baked Potato Woodstock Ranch	1 pkg (0.7 oz)	90	3	14	1	tr
Kettle Brand						
Potato Baked Fully Loaded	13 (1 oz)	150	9	16	1	1

FOOD	PORTION	CAL	FAT	CARB	SUGAR	FIBER
Potato Baked Sea Salt & Vinegar	20 (1 oz)	120	3	20	0	2
Potato Baked Sour Cream And Onion	1 oz	120	4	20	1	2
Potato Krinkle Cut Buffalo Bleu	9 (1 oz)	150	9	16	1	1
Potato Krinkle Cut Salt & Fresh Ground Pepper	9 (1 oz)	140	9	16	0	1
Potato Krinkle Cut Sweet Chili Garlic	9 (1 oz)	150	9	16	1	1
Potato Krinkle Cut Zesty Ranch	9 (1 oz)	150	9	16	1	1
Potato New York Cheddar	13 (1 oz)	150	9	16	1	1
Potato Organic Country Style Barbeque	13 (1 oz)	150	9	16	1	2
Potato Reduced Fat Salt & Fresh Ground Pepper	13 (1 oz)	130	6	19	0	1
Potato Reduced Fat Sea Salt	13 (1 oz)	130	6	19	0	1
Potato Spicy Thai	13 (1 oz)	150	9	16	1	1
Potato Sweet Onion	13 (1 oz)	150	9	16	1	1
Potato Unsalted	13 (1 oz)	150	9	16	0	2
Tortilla Tias! Nacho Cheddar	12 (1 oz)	150	8	17	1	1
Tortilla Tias! Salsa Picante	12 (1 oz)	140	8	17	1	1
Tortilla Tias! Sweet Baja Barbeque	12 (1 oz)	140	8	17	1	1
Late July						
Organic Multigrain Dude Ranch	13 (1 oz)	120	5	17	0	2
Organic Multigrain Mild Green Mojo	13 (1 oz)	110	5	17	1	2

FOOD	PORTION	CAL	FAT	CARB	SUGAR	FIBER
Lay's						
Potato Balsamic Sweet Onion	15 (1 oz)	160	10	16	2	1
Potato Chipotle Ranch	15 (1 oz)	160	10	15	1	1
Potato Classic	15 (1 oz)	160	10	15	tr	1
Potato Garden Tomato & Basil	15 (1 oz)	160	10	16	2	1
Potato Kettle Cooked Crinkle Cut Spice Rubbed BBQ	15 (1 oz)	140	8	17	2	1
Potato Kettle Cooked Original	16 (1 oz)	160	9	16	tr	1
Potato Kettle Cooked Spicy Cayenne & Cheese	16 (1 oz)	150	9	16	1	1
Potato Lightly Salted	15 (1 oz)	160	10	16	tr	1
Potato Original Baked	15 (1 oz)	120	2	23	2	2
Potato Stax Sour Cream & Onion	12 (1 oz)	150	9	17	1	1
Potato Sweet Southern Heat Barbecue	15 (1 oz)	160	10	16	2	1
Potato Wavy Original	11 (1 oz)	160	10	15	tr	1
LesserEvil						
Potato Krinkle Sticks Cheddar	35 (1 oz)	120	5	18	0	1
Potato Krinkle Sticks Sea Salt	35 (1 oz)	120	5	19	0	1
Potato Krinkle Sticks Sour Cream & Onion	35 (1 oz)	120	5	19	0	1
Potato Krinkle Sticks Veggie	35 (1 oz)	120	5	18	0	1
Little Wings						
Multi Grain Hot Buffalo Wing w/ Bleu Cheese Drizzle	1 pkg (0.5 oz)	60	3	10	2	2

FOOD	PORTION	CAL	FAT	CARB	SUGAR	FIBER
Lundberg						
Organic Black Bean Rice Spicy	9 (1 oz)	140	6	18	1	1
Rice Chips Honey Dijon	9 (1 oz)	140	6	19	1	1
Rice Chips Original Sea Salt	9 (1 oz)	140	6	19	0	1
Rice Chips Sesame & Seaweed	9 (1 oz)	140	6	19	1	1
Margaritaville						
Tortilla Sea Salt	1 oz	140	7	16	0	0
Maui Style						
Potato	14 (1 oz)	150	9	16	tr	1
Shrimp Chips	1 oz	150	8	18	0	tr
Mediterranean Snacks						
Baked Lentil Cucumber Dill	22 (1 oz)	110	3	19	1	3
Baked Lentil Roasted Pepper	22 (1 oz)	110	3	19	2	3
Baked Lentil Rosemary	22 (1 oz)	110	3	19	1	3
Baked Lentil Sea Salt	22 (1 oz)	110	3	19	0	3
Multi Grain Original	16 (1 oz)	130	6	17	2	1
Veggie Medley	28 (1 oz)	130	7	15	1	1
Michael Season's						
Popped Black Bean Nacho	17 (1 oz)	120	4	20	1	3
Popped Black Bean Red Pepper	17 (1 oz)	120	4	20	1	3
Popped Black Bean Sea Salt	17 (1 oz)	120	4	20	1	3
Mrs. Cubbison's						
Tortilla Strips Southwest	1½ tbsp (0.2 oz)	30	2	4	0	0

FOOD	PORTION	CAL	FAT	CARB	SUGAR	FIBER
Popchips						
Potato Barbeque	19 (1 oz)	120	4	20	2	1
Potato Cheddar	20 (1 oz)	120	4	20	1	1
Potato Original	22 (1 oz)	120	4	20	0	1
Potato Parmesan Garlic	20 (1 oz)	120	4	20	1	1
Potato Salt & Pepper	11 (0.4 oz)	50	2	8	0	1
Potato Sea Salt & Vinegar	20 (1 oz)	120	4	20	1	1
Potato Sour Cream & Onion	20 (1 oz)	120	4	20	2	1
Tortilla Chili Limon	1 pkg (1 oz)	120	4	20	1	2
Tortilla Nacho Cheese	1 pkg (1 oz)	120	4	20	1	2
Tortilla Ranch	1 pkg (1 oz)	120	4	20	1	2
Rhythm						
Crispy Kale Bombay Curry	½ pkg (1 oz)	101	2	11	2	2
Crispy Kale Kool Ranch	½ pkg (1 oz)	100	5	10	1	2
Crispy Kale Zesty Nacho	½ pkg (1 oz)	106	5	12	2	2
Ruffles						
Baked Original Potato	9 (1 oz)	120	3	22	1	2
Original Potato	12 (1 oz)	160	10	15	tr	1
Reduced Fat Potato	13 (1 oz)	140	7	18	0	1
Reduced Fat Sea Salted Potato	1 oz	140	7	17	0	1
Santitas						
Tortilla Triangles White Corn	9 (1 oz)	140	6	19	0	2
Tortilla Triangles Yellow Corn	9 (1 oz)	140	6	19	0	2
Seneca						
Crispy Apple Apple Pie Ala Mode	12 (1 oz)	140	7	20	12	2
Crispy Apple Caramel	12 (1 oz)	140	7	20	12	2

FOOD	PORTION	CAL	FAT	CARB	SUGAR	FIBER
Crispy Apple Cinnamon	14 (1 oz)	150	7	18	8	4
Crispy Apple Original	12 (1 oz)	140	7	20	12	2
Crispy Apple Sour Apple	12 (1 oz)	150	9	18	9	3
Simply 7						
Hummus Chips Sea Salt	30 (1 oz)	130	5	19	2	tr
Lentil Chips Sea Salt	31 (1 oz)	140	6	18	0	tr
Snikiddy						
Fries Potato Bold Buffalo Gluten Free	1 oz	130	5	20	2	1
Fries Potato Classic Ketchup Gluten Free	1 oz	130	5	21	21	1
Fries Potato Original Gluten Free	1 oz	130	5	20	1	1
Fries Potato Southwest Cheddar Gluten Free	1 oz	130	5	20	2	1
Snyder's Of Hanover						
Tortilla Gluten Free MultiGrain	10 (1 oz)	150	7	19	2	3
Special K						
Popcorn Butter	28 (1 oz)	120	2	22	tr	tr
Popcorn Sweet & Salty	28 (1 oz)	120	3	23	2	tr
Stacy's						
Bagel Chips Everything	12 (1 oz)	130	4	19	1	1
Pita Chips Cinnamon Sugar	1 oz	140	5	20	6	1
SunChips						
Multigrain French Onion	15 (1 oz)	140	6	18	3	3
Multigrain Original	16 (1 oz)	140	6	19	2	3
The Whole Earth						
Tortilla Really Seedy Multigrain	9 (1 oz)	140	9	14	1	2
Tostitos						
Tortilla Baked Scoops	14 (1 oz)	120	3	22	0	2

FOOD	PORTION	CAL	FAT	CARB	SUGAR	FIBER
Tortilla Bite Size Rounds	24 (1 oz)	140	7	18	0	2
Tortilla Multigrain	8 (1 oz)	150	7	19	tr	2
Tortilla Scoops	12 (1 oz)	140	7	19	0	2
Umpqua Indian Foods						
Nana Crisps	⅕ pkg (1 oz)	120	6	15	3	tr
Veggie	¼ pkg (1 oz)	120	6	18	2	2
Want'ems						
Wonton Asian BBQ	16 (1 oz)	140	8	16	tr	1
Wonton Original	16 (1 oz)	140	8	16	0	1
Way Better Snacks						
Tortilla Black Bean Sprouted	11 (1 oz)	130	6	15	0	3
Tortilla Multi-Grain Sprouted	14 (1.25 oz)	170	9	19	0	4
Tortilla No Salt Naked Blues	11 (1 oz)	130	7	14	0	2
Tortilla Sweet Potato Sprouted	11 (1 oz)	130	7	16	0	2
Unbeatable Blues Sprouted	11 (1 oz)	130	7	14	0	2
Willamette Valley						
Granola Chips Honey Nut	⅙ pkg (1 oz)	110	2	23	5	3
Yogachips						
Organic Apple Chips Peach	1 pkg (0.35 oz)	35	0	9	7	tr
CHITTERLINGS						
pork cooked	3 oz	258	24	0	0	0
CHIVES						
freeze-dried	1 tbsp	1	tr	tr	–	–
fresh chopped	1 tsp	0	tr	tr	–	–
fresh chopped	1 tbsp	1	tr	tr	–	–

FOOD	PORTION	CAL	FAT	CARB	SUGAR	FIBER
CHOCOLATE (*see also* CANDY, CHOCOLATE SYRUP, COCOA, HOT CHOCOLATE, ICE CREAM TOPPINGS, MILK DRINKS)						
BAKING						
baking	1 oz	145	15	8	–	–
grated unsweetened	¼ cup	165	17	10	tr	6
liquid unsweetened	1 oz	134	14	10	0	5
mexican baking	1 sq (0.7 oz)	85	3	15	14	1
squares unsweetened	1 sq (1 oz)	145	15	9	tr	5
Baker's						
Semi-Sweet	0.5 oz	70	5	8	6	1
Unsweetened	0.5 oz	70	7	4	0	2
White	0.5 oz	80	5	9	9	0
CHIPS						
milk chocolate	1 cup (6 oz)	862	52	100	–	–
semisweet	1 cup (6 oz)	804	50	106	–	–
semisweet	60 pieces (1 oz)	136	9	18	–	–
Ghirardelli						
Semi-Sweet	32 (0.5 oz)	70	5	10	8	tr
MIX						
drink mix powder	2–3 heaping tsp	75	1	20	–	–
drink mix powder as prep w/ whole milk	9 oz	226	9	31	–	–
CHOCOLATE MILK (*see* MILK DRINKS)						
CHOCOLATE SYRUP						
chocolate fudge	1 cup (11.9 oz)	1176	46	200	–	–
chocolate fudge	1 tbsp (0.7 oz)	73	3	12	–	–
syrup	2 tbsp	82	tr	22	–	–
syrup	1 cup	653	3	177	–	–

FOOD	PORTION	CAL	FAT	CARB	SUGAR	FIBER
syrup as prep w/ whole milk	1 cup (9.9 oz)	254	8	36	32	1
Steel's						
No Sugar Added Fat Free	2 tbsp (1 oz)	50	0	17	0	0
CHUTNEY						
apple	1.2 oz	68	0	18	–	1
coconut	2 oz	87	9	1	1	3
fresh mint	2 oz	18	0	3	3	1
mango	¼ cup (2 oz)	227	5	43	16	10
tomato	1 oz	90	7	6	6	2
CILANTRO						
fresh	1 tsp (2 g)	<1	tr	tr	–	tr
fresh	¼ cup	1	tr	tr	tr	tr
fresh sprigs	5 (5 g)	1	tr	tr	tr	tr
CINNAMON						
cinnamon sugar	1 tsp	16	tr	4	4	tr
ground	1 tsp (2.6 g)	6	tr	2	tr	1
sticks	0.5 oz	39	tr	8	0	3
McCormick						
Grinder Cinnamon Sugar	1 tsp (3.5 g)	10	0	2	–	0
CISCO						
raw	3 oz	84	2	0	0	0
smoked	1 oz	50	3	0	0	0
CLAMS						
CANNED						
drained meat only	1 cup (5.6 oz)	227	3	9	0	0
liquid only	½ cup (4.2 oz)	2	tr	tr	0	0
smoked in oil	1 lg (2.1 oz)	113	7	2	0	0
Chicken Of The Sea						
Chopped	¼ cup	30	0	2	0	0
Whole Baby	¼ cup	30	0	1	0	0

FOOD	PORTION	CAL	FAT	CARB	SUGAR	FIBER
FRESH						
meat + liquid	1 cup (8 oz)	195	2	8	0	0
raw	1 sm (0.3 oz)	8	tr	tr	0	0
raw	1 med (0.5 oz)	12	tr	1	0	0
raw	1 lg (0.7 oz)	17	tr	1	0	0
raw	3 oz	73	1	3	0	0
steamed	20 sm (0.3 oz)	141	2	5	–	0
TAKE-OUT						
breaded & fried	10 sm (3.3 oz)	190	10	10	–	–
breaded & fried	12 med (5.3 oz)	286	12	18	1	1
casino	3 (3.2 oz)	108	4	9	2	1
stuffed	1 lg (1.8 oz)	104	6	7	1	1
CLEMENTINES						
Cuties						
Fresh	2 (6 oz)	80	1	17	13	4
Sunkist						
Fresh	2 (6 oz)	80	1	17	15	5
CLOVES						
ground	1 tsp	7	tr	1	tr	1
COCOA (*see also* HOT CHOCOLATE)						
cocoa butter	1 tbsp	120	14	0	0	0
powder unsweetened	1 tbsp	12	1	3	tr	2
CocoaVia						
Supplement Mix Dark Chocolate Unsweetened	1 pkg (0.27 oz)	30	1	5	–	1
Supplement Mix Summer Citrus	1 pkg (0.24 oz)	20	0	6	–	–
Honest CocoaNova						
Cherry Cacao	8 oz	50	0	13	13	–

FOOD	PORTION	CAL	FAT	CARB	SUGAR	FIBER
COCONUT						
dried sweetened shredded	¼ cup	116	8	11	10	1
dried toasted	1 oz	168	13	13	–	–
dried unsweetened	1 oz	187	18	7	2	5
fresh from 1 coconut	14 oz	1405	133	60	25	36
fresh shredded	¼ cup	71	7	3	1	2
Baker's						
Angel Flake Sweetened	0.5 oz	70	5	6	5	1
COCONUT JUICE						
coconut water fresh	½ cup	23	tr	4	3	1
creamed sweetened canned	½ cup	264	12	39	38	tr
milk canned	½ cup	276	29	7	4	3
Coco King						
Roasted w/ Pulp	1 can (11.75 oz)	130	0	29	26	1
w/ Pulp	1 can (11.85 oz)	130	2	30	28	–
CocoZona						
Coconut Water	1 bottle (14.5 oz)	70	0	18	16	0
KeVita						
Sparkling Probiotic Drink Organic	8 oz	5	0	1	1	–
Naked						
Coconut Water	1 box (11.2 oz)	60	0	14	11	0
Nature's Guru						
Instant Coconut Water Powder	1 pkg (0.5 oz)	50	0	11	11	0
Thai Kitchen						
Coconut Milk	⅓ cup (2.8 oz)	140	14	3	1	0

FOOD	PORTION	CAL	FAT	CARB	SUGAR	FIBER
Vita Coco						
Coconut Water	½ box (8.5 oz)	45	0	15	11	0
Coconut Water w/ Peach & Mango	½ box (8.5 oz)	60	0	15	11	0
Zico						
Coconut Water All Flavors	1 pkg (11 oz)	60	0	15	14	0

COD

FOOD	PORTION	CAL	FAT	CARB	SUGAR	FIBER
atlantic canned	3 oz	89	1	0	0	0
atlantic canned	1 can (11 oz)	327	3	0	0	0
atlantic dried	3 oz	246	2	0	0	0
atlantic fresh cooked	3 oz	89	1	0	0	0
atlantic fresh cooked	1 fillet (6.3 oz)	189	2	0	0	0
atlantic fresh raw	3 oz	70	1	0	0	0
pacific fresh baked	3 oz	95	1	0	0	0
roe canned	1 oz	34	1	tr	–	–
roe tarama	3.5 oz	547	55	6	tr	–
TAKE-OUT						
roe baked w/ butter & lemon juice	1 oz	36	1	tr	–	–

COFFEE (*see also* COFFEE BEVERAGES)

FOOD	PORTION	CAL	FAT	CARB	SUGAR	FIBER
INSTANT						
decaffeinated as prep	8 oz	2	0	0	0	0
decaffeinated powder	1 rounded tsp	4	0	1	0	0
regular powder	1 rounded tsp	4	tr	1	0	0
REGULAR						
brewed	8 oz	2	tr	0	0	0
roasted beans	1 oz	64	4	18	–	2

COFFEE BEVERAGES

FOOD	PORTION	CAL	FAT	CARB	SUGAR	FIBER
Bean & Body						
Coffee Anti-OX	1 can (8 oz)	100	2	20	19	0

FOOD	PORTION	CAL	FAT	CARB	SUGAR	FIBER
Coffee Energy	1 can (8 oz)	100	2	20	19	0
Coffee MarTeani	1 can (8 oz)	100	2	20	19	0
Coffee Rescue	1 can (8 oz)	100	2	20	18	0
Emmi						
Caffe Latte Cappuccino	1 pkg (7.7 oz)	140	4	20	19	0
Caffe Latte Vanilla	1 pkg (7.7 oz)	140	4	20	19	0
Health Is Wealth						
Nutriccino Vitamin Infused All Flavors	1 bottle (9.5 oz)	190	3	37	31	0
Vitamin Coffee Ener-G Infused Vanilla Latte	1 bottle (9.5 oz)	190	3	37	31	0
International Delight						
Iced Coffee All Flavors	8 oz	150	3	29	23	0
N.O. Brew						
Iced Coffee not prep	1 serv (2.6 oz)	10	0	1	0	0
Seattle's Best Coffee						
Iced Latte	1 can (9.5 oz)	130	2	25	23	0
Iced Latte Vanilla	1 can (9.5 oz)	130	2	25	24	0
Iced Mocha	1 can (9.5 oz)	130	2	24	24	0
TAKE-OUT						
cafe amaretto w/ alcohol	1 serv	192	9	15	–	0
cafe au lait	1 cup (8 oz)	77	4	6	7	–
cafe brulot	1 cup	48	0	3	3	–
cafe brulot w/ alcohol	1 serv	130	tr	16	–	3
cappuccino	1 cup (8 oz)	77	4	6	7	–
coffee con leche	1 cup (6 oz)	104	4	16	17	0
cuban coffee w/ rum & creme de cacao	1 (9 oz)	112	2	6	–	0
dutch coffee w/ gin	1 (7 oz)	181	10	6	5	0
espresso	1 cup (4 oz)	2	tr	0	0	0
french coffee w/ orange liqueur & kahlua	1 (8 oz)	232	10	24	–	0

FOOD	PORTION	CAL	FAT	CARB	SUGAR	FIBER
irish coffee	1 serv (8 oz)	209	11	5	4	0
italian coffee w/ strega	1 (7 oz)	163	10	12	10	0
latte w/ skim milk	1 serv (13 oz)	88	tr	12	11	0
latte w/ whole milk	1 serv (14 oz)	143	6	15	14	0
mocha	1 serv (17 oz)	403	9	69	54	2
puerto rican coffee w/ rum & kahlua	1 (8 oz)	166	10	9	–	0
turkish	1 cup (4 oz)	50	1	12	12	0

COFFEE WHITENERS

FOOD	PORTION	CAL	FAT	CARB	SUGAR	FIBER
Baileys						
Caramel	1 tbsp (0.5 oz)	40	2	6	5	0
French Vanilla	1 tbsp (0.5 oz)	40	2	6	5	0
Hazelnut	1 tbsp (0.5 oz)	35	2	5	5	0
Original Irish Cream	1 tbsp (0.5 oz)	40	2	5	5	0
Coffee-Mate						
Caramel Macchiato Liquid	1 tbsp (0.5 oz)	35	2	5	5	–
Natural Bliss Vanilla Liquid	1 tbsp (0.5 oz)	35	2	5	5	–
Original Liquid	1 tbsp (0.5 oz)	20	1	2	tr	–
Original Powder	1 tsp (2 g)	10	1	1	0	–
International Delight						
Caramel Macchiato	1 tbsp (0.5 oz)	40	2	7	6	0
Caribbean Cinnamon Crème	1 tbsp (0.5 oz)	45	2	6	6	0
English Almond Toffee	1 tbsp (0.5 oz)	45	2	6	6	0
French Vanilla	1 tbsp (0.5 oz)	45	2	6	6	0
Vanilla Caramel Cream	1 tbsp (0.5 oz)	35	2	6	6	0
Vanilla Latte	1 tbsp (0.5 oz)	40	2	7	6	0

COLESLAW

FOOD	PORTION	CAL	FAT	CARB	SUGAR	FIBER
Dole						
Classic Coleslaw	1½ cups (3 oz)	20	0	5	3	2

FOOD	PORTION	CAL	FAT	CARB	SUGAR	FIBER
Kit Creamy Coleslaw as prep	1½ cups (3.5 oz)	100	6	12	9	2
Eat Smart						
Broccoli Slaw	1 serv (3 oz)	25	0	5	2	3
Confetti Slaw	1 serv (3 oz)	25	0	5	2	2
Sunrise Slaw	1 serv (3 oz)	35	0	8	5	2
Mann's						
Broccoli Cole Slaw w/o Dressing	1 serv (3 oz)	25	0	5	2	3
Ready Pac						
Coleslaw	1½ cups (3 oz)	20	0	5	3	2
Coleslaw Mix as prep	1 cup (3.5 oz)	130	9	13	11	2
River Ranch						
Broccoli Slaw	1 cup (3 oz)	25	0	5	2	2
Three-Color Cole Slaw	1¼ cups (3 oz)	25	0	5	3	2
TAKE-OUT						
coleslaw w/ dressing	¾ cup	147	11	13	–	–
vinegar & oil coleslaw	3.5 oz	150	9	16	–	–
COLLARDS						
fresh cooked	½ cup	17	tr	4	–	–
frzn chopped cooked	½ cup	31	tr	6	–	–
raw chopped	½ cup	6	tr	1	–	–
Seabrook Farms						
Chopped Greens frzn	½ cup (3.1 oz)	30	0	2	1	2
COOKIES						
MIX						
chocolate chip	1 (0.56 oz)	79	4	10	–	–
oatmeal	1 (0.6 oz)	74	3	10	–	tr
oatmeal raisin	1 (0.6 oz)	74	3	10	–	tr
Betty Crocker						
Caramelita Bars as prep	1	190	8	28	17	1
Chocolate Chip as prep	2	170	8	21	13	tr

FOOD	PORTION	CAL	FAT	CARB	SUGAR	FIBER
Oatmeal as prep	2	160	7	22	11	tr
Peanut Butter as prep	2	50	7	20	12	–
Reese's Dessert Bar Mix No Bake as prep	1	180	10	20	13	1
Sugar as prep	2	160	8	21	12	0
Sunkist Lemon Bars as prep	1	140	4	24	17	–
Turtle Cookie Bars as prep	1	180	8	27	16	tr
READY-TO-EAT						
animal crackers	1 (2.5 g)	11	tr	2	–	–
animal crackers	1 box (2.4 oz)	299	9	51	–	–
animal crackers	11 (1 oz)	126	4	21	–	–
australian anzac biscuit	1	98	3	17	–	1
butter	1 (5 g)	23	1	3	–	tr
chocolate chip	1 (0.4 oz)	48	2	7	–	tr
chocolate chip	1 box (1.9 oz)	233	12	36	–	–
chocolate chip low sugar low sodium	1 (0.24 oz)	31	1	5	–	–
chocolate chip lowfat	1 (0.25 oz)	45	2	7	–	–
chocolate chip soft-type	1 (0.5 oz)	69	4	9	–	tr
chocolate w/ creme filling	1 (0.35 oz)	47	2	7	–	tr
chocolate w/ creme filling chocolate coated	1 (0.6 oz)	82	5	11	–	–
chocolate w/ creme filling sugar free low sodium	1 (0.35 oz)	46	2	7	–	–
chocolate w/ extra creme filling	1 (0.46 oz)	65	3	9	–	–
chocolate wafer	1 (0.2 oz)	26	1	4	–	–
cream cheese	1 (1.1 oz)	141	9	14	6	tr
digestive biscuits plain	2	141	7	21	–	1
fig bars	1 (0.56 oz)	56	1	11	–	1

FOOD	PORTION	CAL	FAT	CARB	SUGAR	FIBER
fortune	1 (0.28 oz)	30	tr	7	–	tr
fudge	1 (0.73 oz)	73	1	17	–	tr
gingersnaps	1 (0.24 oz)	29	1	5	–	–
graham	1 sq (0.24 oz)	30	1	5	–	–
graham chocolate covered	1 (0.49 oz)	68	3	9	–	–
graham honey	1 (0.24 oz)	30	1	5	–	tr
hermits	1 (1 oz)	117	5	18	10	1
jumbles coconut	1 (1 oz)	121	7	13	7	1
ladyfingers	1 (0.38 oz)	40	1	7	–	–
macaroons	1 (0.8 oz)	97	3	17	–	–
madeleines	1 (0.8 oz)	86	5	10	5	tr
marshmallow chocolate coated	1 (1.46 oz)	55	2	9	–	–
marshmallow pie chocolate coated	1 (1.4 oz)	165	7	26	–	–
molasses	1 (0.5 oz)	65	2	11	–	–
neapolitan tri-color cookie	1 (0.6 oz)	79	5	8	5	tr
oatmeal	1 (0.6 oz)	81	3	12	–	1
oatmeal soft-type	1 (0.5 oz)	61	2	10	–	tr
oatmeal raisin	1 (0.6 oz)	81	3	12	–	1
oatmeal raisin low sugar no sodium	1 (0.24 oz)	31	1	5	–	–
oatmeal raisin soft-type	1 (0.5 oz)	61	2	10	–	tr
peanut butter sandwich	1 (0.5 oz)	67	3	9	–	–
peanut butter sandwich sugar free low sodium	1 (0.35 oz)	54	3	5	–	–
peanut butter soft-type	1 (0.5 oz)	69	4	9	–	tr
pinenut cookies	1 (1.1 oz)	134	9	11	8	1
raisin soft-type	1 (0.5 oz)	60	2	10	–	–
reginette queen's biscuit	1 (0.8 oz)	86	3	13	4	tr
shortbread	1 (0.28 oz)	40	2	5	–	–
shortbread pecan	1 (0.49 oz)	79	5	8	–	tr

FOOD	PORTION	CAL	FAT	CARB	SUGAR	FIBER
spritz	1 (0.4 oz)	42	2	6	3	tr
sugar	1 (0.52 oz)	72	3	10	–	–
sugar low sugar sodium free	1 (0.24 oz)	30	1	5	–	–
sugar wafers w/ creme filling	1 (0.12 oz)	18	1	3	–	–
sugar wafers w/ creme filling sugar free sodium free	1 (0.14 oz)	20	1	3	–	–
toll house original	1 (0.8 oz)	105	6	13	9	tr
vanilla sandwich	1 (0.35 oz)	48	2	7	–	tr
vanilla wafers	1 (0.21 oz)	28	1	4	–	–
zeppole	1 (0.8 oz)	78	6	6	4	tr
6 Hour Energy						
Almond Cranberry Chocolate Chunk	½ (1.25 oz)	100	6	12	5	5
Almondina						
BranTreats w/ Cinnamon	4 (1 oz)	127	3	22	9	2
Gingerspice	4 (1 oz)	137	4	22	9	1
Sesame	4 (1 oz)	138	5	21	8	2
The Original	4 (1 oz)	133	4	22	10	1
The Original Chocolate Dipped	2	130	5	16	13	4
Anna's						
Chocolate Mint	6 (1 oz)	140	5	20	14	1
Vanilla Chocolate Chip	6 (1 oz)	140	6	20	8	0
Annie's Homegrown						
Bunny Ginger Gluten Free	29 (1 oz)	130	4	21	8	1
Bunny Gluten Free	27 (1 oz)	120	4	22	9	1
Bunny Grahams Chocolate	27 (1 oz)	130	5	21	9	2
Bunny Grahams Honey	28 (1 oz)	140	5	22	7	2

FOOD	PORTION	CAL	FAT	CARB	SUGAR	FIBER
Bahlsen						
Delice	6 (1.1 oz)	150	8	19	6	tr
Deloba	5 (1.2 oz)	170	8	23	12	tr
Hannover Waffeln	6 (1.1 oz)	180	10	19	7	0
Hit Cocoa Creme Filling	2 (1 oz)	150	8	18	8	1
Hit Creme Filling	2 (1 oz)	140	7	19	9	1
Nuss Dessert	3 (1 oz)	170	11	17	8	1
Barbara's Bakery						
Snackimals Chocolate Chip	10 (1 oz)	120	4	19	8	0
Bauducco						
Wafer Chocolate	4 (1.2 oz)	160	9	19	11	0
Wafer Vanilla	4 (1.2 oz)	140	8	19	11	0
Bear Naked						
Granola Soft Baked Fruit & Nut	1 (1 oz)	130	6	18	9	2
BelVita						
Breakfast Biscuits Blueberry	1 pkg (1.8 oz)	230	8	36	13	3
Breakfast Biscuits Chocolate	1 pkg (1.8 oz)	230	8	35	11	3
Breakfast Biscuits Cinnamon Brown Sugar	1 pkg (1.8 oz)	230	8	35	10	3
Breakfast Biscuits Golden Oat	1 pkg (1.8 oz)	230	8	35	11	3
Brent & Sam's						
Chocolate Chip	2 (0.8 oz)	110	6	15	10	1
Caveman Cookies						
Alpine	2 (1 oz)	150	9	16	14	2
Original	2 (1 oz)	130	7	15	13	1
Tropical	2 (1 oz)	140	10	13	10	2
Delacre						
Royal Moments Milk Chocolate Biscuits	2 (0.9 oz)	130	6	18	11	0

FOOD	PORTION	CAL	FAT	CARB	SUGAR	FIBER
Do Goodie						
Gluten Free Chocolate Chip	1	140	7	18	11	1
Gluten Free Oatmeal Raisin	1	120	4	21	13	1
Entenmann's						
Original Chocolate Chip	3 (1 oz)	140	7	20	11	tr
Erin Baker's						
Breakfast Banana Walnut	1 (3 oz)	300	8	52	17	5
Breakfast Caramel Apple	1 (3 oz)	280	4	55	21	5
Breakfast Double Chocolate Chunk	1 (3 oz)	300	6	53	19	6
Breakfast Oatmeal Raisin	1 (3 oz)	290	5	55	22	5
Breakfast Mini Fruit & Nut	1 (1 oz)	100	3	17	7	2
Fiber One						
Chocolate Chip	1 (0.89 oz)	90	3	18	8	5
Foods By George						
Gluten Free Biscotti	1 (0.8 oz)	90	5	11	6	1
Gamesa						
Animalitos	14 (1 oz)	110	1	25	7	tr
Emperador Vanilla Creme Sandwich	2 (0.9 oz)	120	4	19	9	0
Hawaianas Coconut	3 (1 oz)	130	4	22	9	tr
Sugar Wafers Chocolate	3 (1.2 oz)	160	7	23	15	0
Girl Scout						
Do-si-dos	2 (0.8 oz)	110	5	16	7	tr
Dulce De Leche	4 (1 oz)	160	8	20	9	0
Peanut Butter Sandwich	3 (1.2 oz)	160	6	26	8	tr
Samoas	2 (1 oz)	140	7	19	10	1
Savannah Smiles	5 (1 oz)	140	5	23	10	0

FOOD	PORTION	CAL	FAT	CARB	SUGAR	FIBER
Shout Outs!	4 (0.9 oz)	130	5	18	8	tr
Tagalongs	2 (0.9 oz)	140	9	13	8	tr
Thank U Berry Munch	2 (0.9 oz)	120	5	18	7	tr
Thin Mints	4 (1.1 oz)	160	8	22	10	tr
Trefoils	5 (1.2 oz)	160	8	22	7	tr
Glutenfreeda						
Kookies Sugar	1	142	7	19	11	0
Grandma's						
Chocolate Brownie	1 (1.4 oz)	190	8	27	14	2
Peanut Butter	1 (1.2 oz)	170	9	19	10	2
Vanilla Creme Sandwich	5 (1.4 oz)	190	9	27	12	tr
JK Gourmet						
Biscotti Almond Raisin	2 (1.1 oz)	150	11	11	6	2
Biscotti Dried Peach & Pistachio	3 (1.1 oz)	160	12	10	6	3
Jovial						
Checkerboard Organic	2 (0.9)	120	6	15	6	1
Chocolate Cream Filled Organic	2 (1.1 oz)	160	7	20	9	1
Crispy Cocoa Organic	3 (1 oz)	140	6	18	6	1
Fig Fruit Filled Organic	2 (1.1 oz)	130	4	23	12	1
Ginger Spice Organic	2 (1.1 oz)	150	6	21	7	1
Vanilla Cream Filled Organic	2 (1.1 oz)	160	7	21	10	1
Jules Destrooper						
Butter Crisp	2 (0.9 oz)	120	4	19	11	tr
Chocolate Thins	3 (1 oz)	150	7	19	14	tr
Kay's Naturals						
Protein + Cookie Bites All Flavors Gluten Free	1 oz	110	3	15	3	3
Keebler						
Vienna Fingers Reduced Fat	2 (1.1 oz)	140	5	24	12	tr

FOOD	PORTION	CAL	FAT	CARB	SUGAR	FIBER
Late July						
Organic Mini Sandwich Milk Chocolate	10 (1 oz)	130	6	19	8	1
Lotus						
Biscoff	4 (1.1 oz)	150	6	23	12	tr
LU						
Le Chocolatier	3 (1 oz)	150	9	17	12	1
Le Petit Beurre	4 (1.2 oz)	140	4	24	8	tr
Petit Ecolier Dark Chocolate	2 (0.9 oz)	130	6	17	9	1
Pim's Orange	2 (0.9 oz)	100	3	17	14	0
Lucy's						
Chocolate Chip Gluten Free Vegan	3	130	5	20	12	2
Cinnamon Thin Gluten Free Vegan	3	130	5	21	13	1
Oatmeal Gluten Free Vegan	3	120	5	18	9	1
Sugar Gluten Free Vegan	3	130	5	21	13	1
Mallomars						
Cookies	2 (0.9 oz)	120	5	18	12	1
Market Day						
Chocolate Chip Peanut Free	1 (1 oz)	150	9	17	9	0
Mary's Gone Crackers						
Chocolate Chip Gluten Free Organic	2 (0.9 oz)	130	6	19	9	2
Ginger Snaps Gluten Free Organic	3 (1.1 oz)	140	5	23	9	1
Miss Meringue						
Meringue Chocolate	1 pkg (1 oz)	100	0	24	23	1
Nabisco						
Grahams Original	8 (1.1 oz)	130	3	24	7	1

FOOD	PORTION	CAL	FAT	CARB	SUGAR	FIBER
Nairn's						
Oat Fruit & Cinnamon	2 (0.7 oz)	85	3	15	4	2
Oat Stem Ginger	2 (0.7 oz)	87	3	14	4	1
Napolitanke						
Lemon Orange	4 (0.7 oz)	108	6	13	7	–
Mocca	4 (0.7 oz)	101	5	13	7	–
New Morning						
Honey Grahams	2 (1.1 oz)	130	3	24	6	1
Newman's Own						
Fig Newmans Low Fat Organic	2 (1.1 oz)	110	2	23	12	tr
Newtons						
Fig Fat Free	2 (1 oz)	90	0	22	12	1
Fruit Thins Cranberry Citrus Oat	3 (1 oz)	140	5	22	7	1
Fruit Thins Fig And Honey	3 (1.1 oz)	140	5	21	7	2
Strawberry	2 (1 oz)	100	2	21	13	0
Nilla Wafers						
Cookies	8 (1 oz)	140	6	21	11	0
Nonni's						
Biscotti Bites Almond Dark Chocolate	3 (1 oz)	120	4	16	8	1
Biscotti Bites Classic Almond	4 (1 oz)	130	4	17	8	1
Biscotti Decadence	1 (0.8 oz)	100	4	16	9	1
Biscotti Originali	1 (0.7 oz)	90	3	14	7	0
Biscotti Salted Caramel	1 (0.8 oz)	100	4	16	11	0
Biscotti Triple Milk Chocolate	1 (0.8 oz)	110	5	17	10	1
Thinaddictives Cinnamon Raisin	1 pkg (0.7 oz)	100	3	14	7	1

FOOD	PORTION	CAL	FAT	CARB	SUGAR	FIBER
Thinaddictives Pistachio Almond	1 pkg (0.7 oz)	100	4	12	5	1
Oreo						
Golden Chocolate Creme	3 (1.2 oz)	170	7	25	12	tr
Reduced Fat	3 (1.2 oz)	150	5	27	14	1
Orion						
Choco Pie	1 (1 oz)	120	5	19	10	tr
Pepperidge Farm						
Bordeaux	4	130	5	19	12	tr
Brussels	3	150	7	20	11	1
Butter Chessmen	3	120	5	18	5	tr
Chesapeake Dark Chocolate Pecan	1 (0.9 oz)	130	6	17	10	0
Geneva	3	160	9	19	8	1
Homestyle Gingerman	4	130	4	22	13	tr
Homestyle Sugar	3	150	7	21	11	tr
Lemon	4 (1.1 oz)	160	8	21	8	0
Lexington Crispy Milk Chocolate Toffee Almond	1	130	7	17	10	1
Maui Crispy Milk Chocolate Coconut Almond	1	130	7	17	9	1
Milano	3	180	10	21	11	tr
Milano Melts Chocolate Creme	2	140	7	18	11	1
Milano Melts Dark Classic Creme	2	140	7	18	11	1
Pirouettes Chocolate Hazelnut	2	120	4	19	10	0
Sausalito Milk Chocolate Macadamia Nut	1	130	6	17	10	0

FOOD	PORTION	CAL	FAT	CARB	SUGAR	FIBER
Soft Baked Mystic Sugar	1 (1.1 oz)	140	5	22	9	1
Soft Baked Sanibel Snickerdoodle	1	140	5	22	9	tr
Soft Baked Santa Cruz Oatmeal Raisin	1	130	5	23	13	2
Tahiti	2	170	10	17	8	2
Tim Tam Chocolate Creme	2	190	10	24	18	tr
Verona Strawberry	3	140	5	22	9	tr
Simply Shari's						
Gluten Free Almond Shortbread	2 (1 oz)	120	6	15	7	0
Gluten Free Chocolate Chip	2 (1 oz)	120	6	17	9	1
Gluten Free Fudge Brownies	2 (1 oz)	130	7	16	10	1
Gluten Free Shortbread	2 (1 oz)	130	6	17	8	0
SnackWell's						
Creme Sandwich	2 (0.9 oz)	110	3	20	9	0
Special K						
Pastry Crisps Chocolatey Delight	1 (0.88 oz)	100	2	20	7	tr
Starbucks						
Madeleines Petite French Cakes	3 (1.8 oz)	230	11	32	19	tr
Stella D'Oro						
Margherite Combination	2 (1 oz)	130	5	19	7	tr
Swiss Fudge	3 (1.2 oz)	170	9	22	12	tr
Titan						
High Protein Chocolate Chip	1 (1.4 oz)	150	6	15	5	3
High Protein Oatmeal Raisin	1 (1.4 oz)	150	5	15	5	2

FOOD	PORTION	CAL	FAT	CARB	SUGAR	FIBER
High Protein Peanut Butter	1 (1.4 oz)	150	5	17	5	2
Voortman						
Shortbread	1 (0.6 oz)	90	5	12	4	0
Sugar Free Oatmeal	1 (0.7 oz)	70	4	10	0	tr
Walkers						
Shortbread Rounds	1 (0.6 oz)	90	5	10	3	0
WOW						
Chocolate Brownie	1 (1.4 oz)	161	9	20	15	1
Chocolate Chip Gluten Free	1 (1.4 oz)	170	8	25	14	1
Lemon Burst Gluten Free	1 (1.4 oz)	180	8	24	10	tr
Peanut Butter	1 (1.4 oz)	170	10	21	12	1
REFRIGERATED						
chocolate chip	1 (0.42 oz)	59	3	8	–	–
chocolate chip dough	1 oz	126	6	17	–	–
oatmeal	1 (0.4 oz)	56	3	8	–	–
oatmeal raisin	1 (0.4 oz)	56	3	8	–	–
peanut butter	1 (0.4 oz)	60	3	7	–	–
peanut butter dough	1 oz	130	7	15	–	–
sugar	1 (0.42 oz)	58	3	8	–	–
sugar dough	1 oz	124	6	17	–	–
TAKE-OUT						
biscotti w/ nuts chocolate dipped	1 (1.3 oz)	117	6	16	11	1
black & white	1 lg (3 oz)	302	9	52	31	1
finikia	1 (1.2 oz)	171	5	16	5	1
koulourakia butter cookie twist	1 (0.9 oz)	113	6	14	5	tr
linzer tart	1 (2.4 oz)	280	14	34	12	0

CORIANDER

leaf dried	1 tsp	2	tr	tr	tr	tr

FOOD	PORTION	CAL	FAT	CARB	SUGAR	FIBER
leaf fresh	¼ cup	1	tr	tr	–	–
seed	1 tsp	5	tr	1	–	1
CORN						
CANNED						
cream style	½ cup	93	1	23	–	–
w/ red & green peppers	½ cup	86	1	21	–	–
white	½ cup	66	1	15	–	–
yellow	½ cup	66	1	15	–	1
Butter Kernel						
Gold & White	½ cup (4.4 oz)	60	1	10	3	2
Whole Kernel No Salt Added	½ cup (4.4 oz)	70	1	10	3	2
Del Monte						
Cream Style No Salt Added	½ cup (4.4 oz)	60	1	14	7	2
Cream Style Sweet Corn	½ cup (4.4 oz)	70	1	14	6	4
Whole Kernel	½ cup (4.4 oz)	90	1	18	6	3
Whole Kernel No Salt Added	½ cup (4.4 oz)	90	1	18	6	3
Green Giant						
Cream Style Sweet	½ cup (4.5 oz)	90	1	19	7	1
Mexicorn	½ cup (3.3 oz)	90	1	19	6	1
Super Sweet Yellow & White	⅓ cup (2.6 oz)	60	1	12	3	1
Whole Kernel	½ cup (4.3 oz)	90	1	20	6	1
Jake & Amos						
Pickled Dill Baby Corn	2 tbsp	5	0	1	0	0
DRIED						
Crunchies						
Freeze Dried Corn Snack	⅓ cup (1 oz)	130	7	19	0	4
Freeze Dried Sweet Buttered	½ cup (1 oz)	100	2	21	5	3

FOOD	PORTION	CAL	FAT	CARB	SUGAR	FIBER
Sunrich Naturals						
Toasted Corn Cool Ranch	1 pkg (1 oz)	100	2	20	1	1
FRESH						
white cooked	½ cup	89	1	21	–	–
white raw	½ cup	66	1	15	–	–
yellow cooked	½ cup	89	1	21	–	–
yellow cooked	1 ear (2.7 oz)	83	1	19	–	–
yellow raw	1 ear (3 oz)	77	1	17	–	–
yellow raw	½ cup	66	1	15	–	–
FROZEN						
cooked	½ cup	67	tr	17	–	–
on the cob cooked	1 ear (2.2 oz)	59	tr	14	–	–
TAKE-OUT						
fritters	1 (1 oz)	62	2	9	–	1
on the cob w/ butter cooked	1 ear	155	3	32	–	–
scalloped	1 cup	257	11	34	11	3

CORN CHIPS (*see* CHIPS)

CORNISH HEN (*see* CHICKEN)

CORNMEAL

FOOD	PORTION	CAL	FAT	CARB	SUGAR	FIBER
cornmeal mush as prep w/ water	1 cup	223	1	47	tr	5
cornmeal yellow	½ cup (2.2 oz)	236	1	52	tr	1
whole grain blue	½ cup (1.9 oz)	201	3	41	0	5
yellow self-rising	½ cup (3 oz)	296	2	62	–	5
Quaker						
Instant Original not prep	1 pkg (1 oz)	100	0	22	0	1
Quick Grits not prep	¼ cup (1.3 oz)	130	1	29	0	2

FOOD	PORTION	CAL	FAT	CARB	SUGAR	FIBER
TAKE-OUT						
corn pone	1 piece (2.1 oz)	128	3	23	tr	2
fritter puerto rican style	1 (1.4 oz)	106	7	8	tr	tr
harina de maiz	1 cup (4 oz)	167	2	32	20	1
harina de maiz con coco	½ cup (4.6 oz)	383	27	36	21	3
hush puppies	1 (0.8 oz)	74	3	10	tr	1
johnnycake	1 piece (1.7 oz)	134	4	21	4	2
CORNSTARCH						
cornstarch	¼ cup (1.1 oz)	122	tr	29	0	tr
cornstarch	1 tbsp (0.3 oz)	34	0	8	0	tr
Clabber Girl						
Cornstarch Calcium Fortified	1 tbsp (0.4 oz)	35	0	8	–	–
Rumford						
Cornstarch Calcium Fortified	1 tbsp (0.4 oz)	35	0	8	–	–
COTTAGE CHEESE						
creamed small curd	½ cup (3.7 oz)	103	5	4	3	0
creamed large curd	½ cup (4 oz)	110	5	4	3	0
dry curd	½ cup (2.5 oz)	52	tr	5	1	0
lowfat 1%	½ cup (4 oz)	81	1	3	3	0
lowfat 1% lactose reduced	½ cup (4 oz)	84	1	4	3	1
Breakstone's						
2% Lowfat 30% Less Sodium	½ cup (4.4 oz)	90	3	6	4	0
2% Lowfat Small Curd	½ cup (4.4 oz)	100	3	6	4	0
4% Fat Small Curd	½ cup (4.4 oz)	120	5	6	5	0
Lactaid						
Lowfat	½ cup (4 oz)	80	1	7	3	0

FOOD	PORTION	CAL	FAT	CARB	SUGAR	FIBER
COTTONSEED						
kernels roasted	1 tbsp	51	4	2	–	–
COUSCOUS						
cooked	1 cup (5.5 oz)	176	tr	36	–	2
dry	1 cup (6.1 oz)	650	1	134	–	9
Bob's Red Mill						
Pearl not prep	⅓ cup (2 oz)	210	1	43	0	0
Pearl Tricolor not prep	⅓ cup (2 oz)	210	1	44	0	0
Pearl Whole Wheat not prep	⅓ cup (2 oz)	190	1	38	0	5
Lundberg						
Brown Rice Roasted Garlic & Olive Oil not prep	¼ pkg (1.6 oz)	150	2	34	1	2
Brown Rice Roasted Plain Original not prep	⅙ pkg (1.6 oz)	150	2	35	1	3
Near East						
Roasted Garlic & Olive Oil as prep	1 cup	220	5	40	1	2
CRAB						
CANNED						
blue	½ cup	67	1	0	0	0
blue drained	1 can (6.5 oz)	124	2	0	0	0
Chicken Of The Sea						
Fancy	⅓ can (2 oz)	40	0	2	0	0
Jumbo Lump	⅓ can (2 oz)	35	1	1	1	0
Wild Planet						
Dungeness	2 oz	62	1	tr	–	–
FRESH						
alaska king meat only steamed	3 oz	82	1	0	0	0
blue cooked flaked	1 cup (4 oz)	120	2	0	0	0

FOOD	PORTION	CAL	FAT	CARB	SUGAR	FIBER
dungeness steamed	3 oz	94	1	1	–	0
queen steamed	3 oz	98	1	0	0	0
Dockside Classics						
Crabcakes	1 (2.5 oz)	150	11	7	1	0
TAKE-OUT						
alaska king leg steamed	1 leg (4.7 oz)	130	2	0	0	0
baked	1 (3.8 oz)	160	2	4	–	–
cakes	2 (4.2 oz)	186	9	1	–	0
crab imperial	1 crab (6.8 oz)	289	15	6	3	0
crab salad	1 serv (5.5 oz)	285	21	3	1	1
crab thermidor	1 serv (6.4 oz)	456	37	8	tr	tr
deviled	1 serv (4.5 oz)	254	13	17	6	1
dungeness	1 crab (4.5 oz)	140	2	1	–	0
empanada de jueyes	1 (4.4 oz)	341	16	38	7	2
fried crab puffs	4 (3.2 oz)	323	18	30	tr	1
kenagi korean crab cooked	1 serv (3 oz)	71	tr	0	0	0
salmorejo de jueyes in tomato sauce	1 serv (4.5 oz)	215	14	3	1	tr
soft-shell breaded & fried	1 med (2.3 oz)	216	13	11	1	1
taco de jueyes	1 (4.2 oz)	266	14	18	1	2
CRACKER CRUMBS						
cracker meal	1 cup	440	2	93	tr	3
graham cracker crumbs	1 cup	355	8	65	26	2
Mary's Gone Crackers						
Just The Crumbs Gluten Free	½ cup (1.4 oz)	160	3	28	0	3

FOOD	PORTION	CAL	FAT	CARB	SUGAR	FIBER
CRACKERS						
melba toast round	1	12	tr	2	tr	tr
oyster cracker	¼ cup	48	1	8	tr	tr
saltines	1	13	tr	2	tr	tr
water biscuits	3	92	3	16	–	1
zwieback	1 oz	107	1	21	–	1
Annie's Homegrown						
Cheddar Bunnies Original	50 (1 oz)	140	6	19	1	0
Blue Diamond						
Nut-Thins Almond Country Ranch	16 (1 oz)	130	4	22	1	tr
Bran Crispbread						
GG Scandinavian	1 (0.4 oz)	12	0	7	0	5
Cheez-It						
Baby Swiss	25 (1 oz)	150	7	19	0	tr
Cheddar Jack	25 (1 oz)	140	7	17	0	tr
Colby	25 (1 oz)	150	8	18	0	tr
Crunchmaster						
Ancient Grains Cracked Pepper & Herb	14 (1 oz)	130	3	24	0	1
Crisps Cheezy Gluten Free	60 (1 oz)	120	3	23	2	2
Crisps Grammy Gluten Free	30 (1 oz)	130	2	25	5	1
Multi-Grain Sea Salt Gluten Free	16 (1 oz)	120	3	23	2	3
Multi-Seed Original Gluten Free	15 (1 oz)	140	5	20	0	2
Daelia's						
Biscuits For Cheese Almond w/ Raisins	4 (1 oz)	133	4	22	10	1

FOOD	PORTION	CAL	FAT	CARB	SUGAR	FIBER
Biscuits For Cheese Hazelnut w/ Figs	4 (1 oz)	133	5	20	9	1
Flatout						
Edge On Baked Flatbread Four Cheese	15 (1 oz)	130	5	15	1	5
Edge On Baked Flatbread Garlic Herb	15 (1 oz)	120	4	16	1	5
Kashi						
Heart To Heart Whole Grain	7 (1 oz)	120	4	22	0	4
TLC Toasted Asiago	15 (1.1 oz)	130	4	21	2	2
Keebler						
Club Original	4 (0.5 oz)	70	3	9	1	tr
Kim's Magic Pop						
Onion	1 (5 g)	15	0	3	0	0
Manischewitz						
Tam Tams Original	10 (1 oz)	110	4	16	1	0
Mary's Gone Crackers						
Herb Wheat & Gluten Free Organic	13 (1 oz)	140	5	21	0	3
Original Wheat & Gluten Free Organic	13 (1 oz)	140	5	21	0	3
Mediterranean Crackers						
Feta & Oregano	3 (0.6 oz)	91	5	11	1	0
Mediterranean Snacks						
Hummuz Crispz Olive Tapenade	14 (1 oz)	120	3	18	2	1
Hummuz Crispz Roasted Garlic	14 (1 oz)	120	3	18	2	1
Hummuz Crispz Roasted Red Pepper	14 (1 oz)	120	3	18	2	1
Lentil Cracked Pepper Gluten Free	22 (1 oz)	120	3	19	tr	3

FOOD	PORTION	CAL	FAT	CARB	SUGAR	FIBER
Lentil Sea Salt Gluten Free	18 (1 oz)	110	3	16	2	1
Nairn's						
Oatcake Fine	2 (0.5 oz)	70	3	10	0	1
Oatcake Rough	2 (0.8 oz)	91	4	14	tr	2
Pepperidge Farm						
Baked Naturals Cheese Crisps Four Cheese Medley	20	140	5	19	3	1
Baked Naturals Cracker Chips Simply Cheddar	27	130	4	24	4	2
Baked Naturals Cracker Chips Simply Multigrain	27	140	4	24	3	2
Baked Naturals Cracker Chips Simply Potato	26	140	5	22	3	2
Baked Naturals Wheat Crisps Toasted Wheat	17	140	5	21	5	2
Golden Butter	2	35	1	5	tr	0
Goldfish Cheddar	55	140	5	20	tr	tr
Goldfish Colors	55	140	5	20	tr	1
Goldfish Grahams Chocolate	37 (1.1 oz)	130	4	22	11	2
Goldfish Original	55	150	6	20	tr	tr
Goldfish Pretzel	43	130	3	24	tr	tr
Goldfish w/ Whole Grain Cheddar	55 (1.1 oz)	140	5	19	tr	2
Harvest Wheat	2	50	2	7	2	tr
Jingos Fiesta Cheddar	23	140	4	22	2	1
Jingos Lime & Sweet Chili	23	140	4	22	2	1
Pretzel Thins Simply Pretzel	11	110	0	21	2	1
Snack Sticks Toasted Sesame	12	140	5	20	1	2

FOOD	PORTION	CAL	FAT	CARB	SUGAR	FIBER
Premium						
Saltines Original	5 (0.5 oz)	60	2	11	0	0
Saltines Unsalted Tops	5 (0.5 oz)	70	2	13	0	0
Saltines w/ Whole Grain	6 (0.5 oz)	60	2	11	0	tr
Ritz						
Bites Cheese	13 (1 oz)	150	9	17	4	0
Reduced Fat	5 (0.5 oz)	70	2	11	1	0
Roasted Vegetable	5 (0.5 oz)	80	4	10	1	0
Special K						
Cracker Chips Cheddar	27 (1 oz)	110	3	22	1	3
Cracker Chips Sea Salt	30 (1 oz)	110	3	23	0	3
Cracker Chips Southwest Ranch	27 (1 oz)	110	3	22	1	3
Triscuit						
Fire Roasted Tomato	1 oz	120	4	20	0	3
Garden Herb	1 oz	120	4	20	0	3
Hint Of Salt	1 oz	130	5	19	0	3
Original	1 oz	120	5	19	0	3
Reduced Fat	1 oz	120	3	21	0	3
Rosemary & Olive Oil	1 oz	120	4	20	0	3
Thin Crisps Original	1 oz	130	5	21	0	3
Thin Crisps Quattro Formaggio	1.1 oz	140	5	22	1	3
Wellaby's						
Cheese Ups Classic Cheese Gluten Free	1 cup (1 oz)	122	5	18	0	tr
Cheese Ups Parmesan	1 cup (1 oz)	122	5	18	0	tr
Feta Oregano & Olive Oil Gluten Free	8 (1.1 oz)	130	59	19	1	1
Original Cheese Mini Gluten Free	8 (1.1 oz)	130	5	19	1	1
Wheat Thins						
Original	16 (1.1 oz)	140	5	22	4	2

FOOD	PORTION	CAL	FAT	CARB	SUGAR	FIBER
CRANBERRIES						
cranberry orange relish	¼ cup	118	tr	31	28	2
dried	½ cup	85	tr	23	18	2
fresh chopped	1 cup	13	tr	3	1	1
fresh whole	1 cup	11	tr	3	1	1
sauce	1 slice (2 oz)	86	tr	22	22	1
sauce	¼ cup	109	tr	27	26	1
Craisins						
Dried Cranberries	⅓ cup	130	0	33	26	–
Orange	⅓ cup	130	0	33	27	–
Dole						
Fresh Whole	1 cup (3.3 oz)	45	0	12	4	4
Ocean Spray						
Fresh	2 oz	30	0	6	2	–
Jellied Sauce	¼ cup (2.5 oz)	110	0	25	21	tr
Sarabeth's						
Relish	1 tbsp (0.7 oz)	45	0	36	31	3
Truitt Brothers						
Sauce Orchard Medley	⅓ cup (2.7 oz)	90	0	24	–	2
CRANBERRY BEANS						
canned	½ cup	108	tr	20	–	8
dried cooked w/o salt	½ cup	120	tr	22	–	9
CRANBERRY JUICE						
cranberry juice cocktail low calorie w/ vitamin C	8 oz	46	tr	11	11	0
cranberry juice cocktail w/ vitamin C	8 oz	137	tr	34	30	0
unsweetened	8 oz	116	tr	31	31	tr
Apple & Eve						
100% Juice	8 oz	130	0	32	30	–

FOOD	PORTION	CAL	FAT	CARB	SUGAR	FIBER
Ocean Spray						
100% Juice Cranberry Blend	8 oz	140	0	36	36	–
Cocktail Light	8 oz	40	0	10	10	–
Cran•Energy	8 oz	35	0	8	8	–
Diet	8 oz	5	0	2	2	–
White Cocktail Light	8 oz	40	0	10	10	–
Old Orchard						
Cranberry Naturals Classic Cranberry	8 oz	80	0	18	18	–
CRAYFISH						
cooked	3 oz	97	1	0	0	0
raw	8	24	tr	0	0	0
raw	3 oz	76	1	0	0	0
CREAM (*see also* WHIPPED TOPPINGS)						
clotted cream	2 tbsp (1 oz)	164	18	1	–	0
creme fraiche	2 tbsp (1 oz)	100	11	1	–	0
half & half	1 pkg (0.5 oz)	20	2	1	tr	0
half & half	1 tbsp (0.5 oz)	20	2	1	tr	0
half & half	¼ cup (2.1 oz)	79	7	3	tr	0
half & half fat free	4 oz	67	2	10	6	0
heavy whipping	½ cup (4.2 oz)	411	44	3	tr	0
heavy whipping	1 tbsp (0.5 oz)	52	6	tr	tr	0
heavy whipping whipped	½ cup (2.1 oz)	207	22	2	tr	0
light coffee	1 pkg (0.4 oz)	22	2	tr	tr	0
light coffee	1 tbsp (0.5 oz)	29	3	1	tr	0
light coffee	½ cup (4.2 oz)	234	23	4	tr	0
whipped pressurized can	4 tbsp (0.4 oz)	31	3	2	1	0

FOOD	PORTION	CAL	FAT	CARB	SUGAR	FIBER
whipped pressurized can	½ cup (1 oz)	77	7	4	2	0
Lactaid						
Half & Half	2 tbsp (1 oz)	40	3	1	1	0
Land O Lakes						
Half & Half Fat Free	2 tbsp (1.1 oz)	20	0	3	2	0
Straus						
Organic Half And Half	2 tbsp (1 oz)	35	3	1	1	0

CREAM CHEESE

FOOD	PORTION	CAL	FAT	CARB	SUGAR	FIBER
cream cheese	1 oz	99	10	1	–	–
cream cheese	1 pkg (3 oz)	297	30	2	–	–
Philadelphia						
⅓ Less Fat	2 tbsp (1.1 oz)	70	6	2	2	0
Fat Free	1 oz	30	0	2	1	0
Original	1 oz	100	9	1	1	0
Whipped Chive	2 tbsp (0.8 oz)	50	5	1	1	0

CREAM CHEESE SUBSTITUTES

FOOD	PORTION	CAL	FAT	CARB	SUGAR	FIBER
Tofutti						
Better Than Cream Cheese All Flavors	2 tbsp (1 oz)	60	5	2	0	0

CREAM OF TARTAR

FOOD	PORTION	CAL	FAT	CARB	SUGAR	FIBER
cream of tartar	1 tsp	8	0	2	0	0

CREPES

FOOD	PORTION	CAL	FAT	CARB	SUGAR	FIBER
basic crepe unfilled	1 (7 in)	112	6	11	2	tr
Ekizian						
Chickpea Crepe	7 in (1.5 oz)	212	13	16	3	3
Tandoor Chef						
Masala Dosa	1 (3 oz)	162	6	22	1	2

CROAKER

FOOD	PORTION	CAL	FAT	CARB	SUGAR	FIBER
atlantic breaded & fried	3 oz	188	11	6	–	–
atlantic raw	3 oz	89	3	0	0	0

FOOD	PORTION	CAL	FAT	CARB	SUGAR	FIBER
CROCODILE						
cooked	3 oz	78	1	0	0	0
CROISSANT						
apple	1 (2 oz)	145	5	21	–	1
butter	1 lg (2.4 oz)	272	14	31	8	2
butter mini	1 (1 oz)	114	6	13	3	1
cheese	1 (1.5 oz)	174	9	20	5	1
chocolate	1 (2 oz)	237	14	25	6	2
TAKE-OUT						
w/ egg & cheese	1 (4.5 oz)	368	25	24	–	–
w/ egg & sausage	1 (5 oz)	497	34	31	8	2
w/ egg cheese & bacon	1 (4.1 oz)	385	24	25	8	1
w/ egg cheese & ham	1 (5.1 oz)	402	24	25	8	1
w/ egg cheese & sausage	1 (5.6 oz)	539	39	26	8	1
w/ ham & cheese	1 (4 oz)	338	20	25	4	1
CROUTONS						
plain	1 cup (1 oz)	122	2	22	–	2
seasoned	1 cup (1.4 oz)	186	7	25	–	2
Chatham Village						
Cheese & Garlic	2 tbsp (7 g)	40	3	3	0	0
Mrs. Cubbison's						
Asiago Cheese Ciabatta	2 tbsp (0.2 oz)	30	2	4	0	0
Seasoned Texas Toast	2 tbsp (0.2 oz)	30	2	4	1	0
Pepperidge Farm						
Seasoned	6	30	1	5	tr	tr
Zesty Italian	6	30	1	5	tr	tr
CUCUMBER						
fresh peeled	1 sm (5.5 oz)	19	tr	3	2	1
fresh peeled	1 slice (7 g)	1	tr	tr	tr	0
fresh peeled	1 med (7.2 oz)	24	tr	4	3	1
fresh peeled sliced	1 cup (4.2 oz)	14	tr	3	2	1

FOOD	PORTION	CAL	FAT	CARB	SUGAR	FIBER
fresh w/ peel sliced	½ cup (1.8 oz)	34	tr	2	1	tr
fresh whole w/ peel	1 lg (10.6 oz)	45	tr	11	5	2
TAKE-OUT						
cucumber raita	1 serv (3.3 oz)	40	3	3	3	1
cucumber salad w/ onions + oil & vinegar	1 cup (5.6 oz)	183	15	11	8	1
cucumber salad w/ sour cream dressing	1 cup (4.7 oz)	63	5	3	2	1
kimchee	½ cup (1.8 oz)	36	2	4	3	tr
tzatziki	½ cup (3.4 oz)	72	6	4	3	1

CUMIN

FOOD	PORTION	CAL	FAT	CARB	SUGAR	FIBER
seed	1 tbsp (6 g)	22	1	3	tr	1
seed	1 tsp (2 g)	8	tr	1	tr	tr

CURRANT JUICE

FOOD	PORTION	CAL	FAT	CARB	SUGAR	FIBER
black currant nectar	7 oz	110	0	26	–	–
red currant nectar	7 oz	108	tr	26	–	–

CURRANTS

FOOD	PORTION	CAL	FAT	CARB	SUGAR	FIBER
black fresh	½ cup	36	tr	9	–	–
zante dried	½ cup	204	tr	53	–	–

CURRY

FOOD	PORTION	CAL	FAT	CARB	SUGAR	FIBER
curry powder	1 tsp	7	tr	1	tr	1
curry sauce mix	1 cup	120	6	14	–	–
curry sauce mix as prep w/ milk	1 cup	270	15	26	–	–
paste	1 tube (6 oz)	465	36	30	13	12
Kikkoman						
Sauce Thai Red Curry	¼ cup (2.2 oz)	90	6	7	4	0
Sauce Thai Yellow Curry	¼ cup (2.2 oz)	90	6	6	4	0
So-Yah!						
Creamy Coconut Curry	1 pkg (10 oz)	190	10	21	8	5
Red Vindaloo Curry	1 pkg (10 oz)	150	4	24	11	8

FOOD	PORTION	CAL	FAT	CARB	SUGAR	FIBER
Tandoor Chef						
Chicken Curry	1 pkg (9.9 oz)	330	19	8	3	1
Kofta Curry	½ pkg (5 oz)	100	7	6	2	1
Thai Kitchen						
Red Curry Paste	1 tbsp (0.5 oz)	15	0	3	1	0
TAKE-OUT						
beef curry	1 cup	432	31	14	6	3
beef kurma	1 serv (10.5 oz)	611	47	6	3	6
chicken curry ½ breast	1 serv	160	9	6	3	1
chicken curry boneless	1 serv (6.2 oz)	219	12	8	4	2
chicken curry leg & thigh	1 serv	180	10	7	3	1
chickpea curry	1 serv (8.3 oz)	305	15	23	1	15
eggplant curry	1 serv (8 oz)	241	19	12	–	5
lamb curry	1 cup	257	14	4	1	1
mixed vegetable curry	1 serv (7.7 oz)	398	33	22	–	–
pea & potato curry	1 serv (7 oz)	284	22	19	–	6
pork vindaloo curry	1 serv	620	47	3	–	–
potato curry	1 serv (5.5 oz)	791	60	35	5	14
sambhar dhal curry	1 serv (10 oz)	177	7	21	–	8
shrimp curry	1 cup (8.3 oz)	276	14	13	8	1
CUSK						
fillet baked	3 oz	106	1	0	0	0
CUSTARD						
MIX						
egg custard as prep w/ 2% milk	1 serv (3.5 oz)	112	3	18	5	0
egg custard as prep w/ whole milk	1 serv (3.5 oz)	122	4	18	5	0

FOOD	PORTION	CAL	FAT	CARB	SUGAR	FIBER
flan as prep w/ 2% milk	1 serv (3.5 oz)	103	2	19	–	0
flan as prep w/ whole milk	1 serv (3.5 oz)	113	3	19	–	0
Jell-O						
Flan as prep	¼ pkg	140	3	27	20	0
READY-TO-EAT						
Kozy Shack						
Flan Creme Caramel Gluten Free	1 pkg (4 oz)	140	3	27	27	0
TAKE-OUT						
baked	½ cup (5 oz)	147	6	16	16	0
flan	½ cup (5.4 oz)	222	6	35	35	0
flan de calabaza	1 serv (3.5 oz)	225	10	30	22	tr
flan de coco	½ cup (4.3 oz)	345	13	49	49	tr
flan de pina	1 serv (4.2 oz)	186	5	28	27	tr
flan de pini	½ cup (4.6 oz)	202	6	31	29	tr
puerto rican corn custard	½ cup (4.9 oz)	553	34	65	51	5
tocino del cielo heaven's delight	1 cup	856	21	156	154	0
zabaione	½ cup (2 oz)	135	5	13	–	0

CUTTLEFISH

FOOD	PORTION	CAL	FAT	CARB	SUGAR	FIBER
steamed	3 oz	134	1	1	–	–

DANDELION GREENS

FOOD	PORTION	CAL	FAT	CARB	SUGAR	FIBER
fresh cooked	½ cup	17	tr	3	–	–
raw chopped	½ cup	13	tr	3	–	–

FOOD	PORTION	CAL	FAT	CARB	SUGAR	FIBER
DANISH PASTRY						
READY-TO-EAT						
Entenmann's						
Pecan Danish Ring	⅛ ring (1.9 oz)	240	14	24	11	1
TAKE-OUT						
cheese	1 (2.5 oz)	266	16	26	5	1
cinnamon	1 (5 oz)	572	32	63	28	2
fruit	1 (5 oz)	527	27	68	39	3
lemon	1 (2.5 oz)	263	13	34	–	1
raisin nut	1 (2.3 oz)	280	16	30	17	1
DATES						
deglet noor chopped	¼ cup (1.3 oz)	104	tr	28	23	3
deglet noor dried	1 (7 g)	20	tr	5	5	1
jujube dried	1 oz	75	tr	19	–	2
jujube fresh	1 oz	30	tr	7	–	–
jujube preserved in sugar	1 oz	91	tr	22	–	–
medjool	1 (0.8 oz)	66	tr	18	16	2
Dole						
California Chopped	¼ cup (1.4 oz)	120	0	31	26	3
DEER (*see* JERKY, VENISON)						
DELI MEATS/COLD CUTS (*see also* BEEF, CHICKEN, HAM, MEAT SUBSTITUTES, TURKEY)						
barbecue loaf pork & beef	1 slice (0.8 oz)	40	2	1	–	0
beerwurst beef	2 oz	155	13	2	0	1
berliner pork & beef	1 slice (0.8 oz)	53	4	1	1	0
blood sausage	1 slice (0.9 oz)	95	9	tr	tr	0
bologna beef	1 slice (1 oz)	88	8	1	0	0
bologna beef & pork	1 slice (1 oz)	87	7	2	1	0

FOOD	PORTION	CAL	FAT	CARB	SUGAR	FIBER
bologna beef & pork lowfat	1 slice (1 oz)	64	5	1	0	0
bologna beef lowfat	1 slice (1 oz)	57	4	1	0	0
bologna beef reduced sodium	1 slice (1 oz)	88	8	1	0	0
braunschweiger pork	1 slice (1 oz)	92	8	1	0	0
corned beef brisket	2 oz	90	5	0	0	0
dutch brand loaf pork & beef	1 slice (1.3 oz)	104	9	1	0	tr
headcheese pork	1 slice (1.6 oz)	71	5	0	0	0
honey loaf pork & beef	1 slice (1 oz)	35	1	1	0	0
lebanon bologna beef	2 slices (1 oz)	105	6	tr	0	0
mortadella beef & pork	1 slice (0.5 oz)	47	4	tr	0	0
olive loaf pork	2 slices (2 oz)	134	9	5	0	0
pastrami beef	1 slice (1 oz)	41	2	tr	tr	tr
peppered loaf pork & beef	1 slice (1 oz)	41	2	1	0	0
pepperoni pork & beef	15 slices (1 oz)	135	12	1	tr	tr
picnic pork & beef loaf	1 slice (1 oz)	65	5	1	–	0
salami cooked beef & pork	1 slice (0.8 oz)	58	5	1	0	0
salami hard pork	3 slices (0.9 oz)	14	8	1	0	0
salami hard pork & beef less sodium	1 slice (1 oz)	113	9	2	2	tr
sandwich spread pork & beef	¼ cup	141	10	7	0	tr
summer sausage thuringer cervelat	2 oz	203	17	2	tr	0
Dietz & Watson						
Bologna Beef	3 slices (1.9 oz)	170	14	3	2	0
Mortadella	2 oz	150	14	2	0	0
Sopressata	1 oz	90	7	1	0	0

FOOD	PORTION	CAL	FAT	CARB	SUGAR	FIBER
Foster Farms						
Bologna Chicken	1 slice (1 oz)	60	5	tr	0	0
Hebrew National						
Bologna Beef	2 slices (2 oz)	170	15	1	0	0
Bologna Lean Beef	4 slices (2 oz)	90	5	2	–	–
Salami Beef	2 slices (2 oz)	150	13	1	0	0
Salami Lean Beef	4 slices (2 oz)	90	5	2	–	–
DILL						
seed	1 tsp	6	tr	1	–	tr
sprigs fresh	5 (0.3 oz)	0	tr	tr	–	–
weed dry	1 tbsp	8	tr	2	–	tr
DINNER (*see also* ASIAN FOOD, CURRY, PASTA DINNERS, POT PIE, SPANISH FOOD)						
Candle Cafe						
Ginger Miso Stir Fry	1 pkg (9 oz)	200	6	27	9	4
Seitan Piccata w/ Lemon Caper Sauce	1 pkg (9 oz)	210	4	32	6	4
Dinty Moore						
Big Bowl Scalloped Potatoes & Ham	½ can	280	16	23	1	2
Healthy Choice						
Bacon & Smokey Cheddar Chicken	1 pkg (8.6 oz)	240	6	28	2	3
Beef Tips Portabello	1 pkg (11.2 oz)	270	6	34	12	6
Country Breaded Chicken	1 pkg (10.6 oz)	340	9	52	15	6
Fire Roasted Tomato Chicken	1 pkg (11.6 oz)	310	5	46	18	6
Fresh Mixers Creamy Roasted Garlic Chicken	1 pkg (7.4 oz)	310	6	50	3	6
Fresh Mixers Steak Portobello	1 pkg (7.5 oz)	290	6	42	4	5

FOOD	PORTION	CAL	FAT	CARB	SUGAR	FIBER
Fresh Mixers Sweet Hickory BBQ Chicken	1 pkg (7.9 oz)	370	3	70	16	5
Grilled Chicken Monterey	1 pkg (10.9 oz)	320	8	43	12	6
Lemon Pepper Fish	1 pkg (10.6 oz)	300	5	49	15	5
Lunch Steamers Garlic Herb Shrimp	1 pkg (8.5 oz)	260	7	37	8	5
Lunch Steamers Lemon Herb Chicken	1 pkg (8.7 oz)	210	4	29	2	4
Lunch Steamers Rosemary Chicken & Sweet Potatoes	1 pkg (8.9 oz)	170	3	23	10	5
Pineapple Chicken	1 pkg (9 oz)	380	7	71	29	4
Portabella Spinach Parmesan	1 pkg (9.3 oz)	270	7	39	3	5
Salisbury Steak	1 pkg (8 oz)	170	5	18	2	4
Spicy Caribbean Chicken	1 pkg (8.5 oz)	310	2	56	16	5
Turkey Breast & Cranberries	1 pkg (10.7 oz)	250	4	36	12	6
Hormel						
Compleats Microwave Meals Beef Steak & Peppers w/ Noodles	1 pkg (9.9 oz)	210	5	22	4	2
Compleats Microwave Meals Chicken Breast & Dressing	1 pkg (9.9 oz)	270	7	29	3	2
Compleats Microwave Meals Chicken Breast & Gravy w/ Mashed Potatoes	1 pkg (9.9 oz)	200	3	24	3	2
Compleats Microwave Meals Homestyle Beef w/ Potatoes & Gravy	1 pkg (9.9 oz)	220	6	30	2	3

FOOD	PORTION	CAL	FAT	CARB	SUGAR	FIBER
Compleats Microwave Meals Meatloaf w/ Potatoes & Gravy	1 pkg (9.9 oz)	310	11	34	3	3
Compleats Microwave Meals Salisbury Steak w/ Slice Potato & Gravy	1 pkg (9.9 oz)	280	11	30	1	2
Compleats Microwave Meals Santa Fe Chicken w/ Rice & Beans	1 pkg (9.9 oz)	280	4	41	6	4
Compleats Microwave Meals Swedish Meatballs	1 pkg (9.9 oz)	350	18	32	4	1
Compleats Microwave Meals Tuna Casserole	1 pkg (9.9 oz)	240	7	26	3	2
Lean Cuisine						
Cafe Cuisine Chicken & Vegetables	1 pkg (10.5 oz)	220	4	29	5	3
Cafe Cuisine Chicken Marsala	1 pkg (8.1 oz)	250	9	29	4	2
Cafe Cuisine Lemon Pepper Fish	1 pkg (9 oz)	290	8	40	4	2
Cafe Cuisine Orange Chicken	1 pkg (9 oz)	300	7	46	11	2
Cafe Cuisine Roasted Garlic Chicken	1 pkg (8.8 oz)	170	6	11	3	0
Cafe Cuisine Steak Tips Portabello	1 pkg (7.5 oz)	150	4	14	4	3
Casual Cuisine Flatbread Melts Steakhouse Ranch	1 pkg (6.25 oz)	350	9	46	7	4
Comfort Classics Baked Chicken	1 pkg (8.6 oz)	240	7	30	4	2
Comfort Cuisine Beef Pot Roast	1 pkg (9 oz)	210	6	26	3	3

FOOD	PORTION	CAL	FAT	CARB	SUGAR	FIBER
Comfort Cuisine Meatloaf w/ Gravy & Whipped Potatoes	1 pkg (9.4 oz)	250	8	25	2	3
Comfort Cuisine Roasted Turkey Breast w/ Dressing	1 pkg (9.75 oz)	290	4	49	27	3
Comfort Cuisine Salisbury Steak w/ Mac & Cheese	1 pkg (9.5 oz)	260	8	23	3	3
Dinnertime Selects Balsamic Glazed Chicken	1 pkg (12 oz)	330	7	41	11	4
Dinnertime Selects Chicken Florentine	1 pkg (13.25 oz)	410	9	54	13	6
Dinnertime Selects Chicken Portabello	1 pkg (12 oz)	390	8	48	2	2
Dinnertime Selects Salisbury Steak	1 pkg (12.5 oz)	270	9	27	10	5
Market Creations Chicken Poblano	1 pkg (10.5 oz)	300	5	40	7	5
Market Creations Shrimp Scampi	1 pkg (10.5 oz)	250	7	32	4	4
Market Creations Sweet & Spicy Ginger Chicken	1 pkg (10.5 oz)	280	3	43	12	4
Simple Favorites Quesadilla BBQ Chicken	1 pkg (5 oz)	280	6	37	7	2
Simple Favorites Stuffed Cabbage	1 pkg (9.5 oz)	210	6	28	6	3
Simple Favorites Swedish Meatballs	1 pkg (9.1 oz)	290	8	35	4	3
Spa Cuisine Chicken In Peanut Sauce	1 pkg (9 oz)	280	6	35	5	5
Spa Cuisine Chicken Mediterranean	1 pkg (10.5 oz)	240	4	34	7	5

FOOD	PORTION	CAL	FAT	CARB	SUGAR	FIBER
Spa Cuisine Chicken Pecan	1 pkg (9 oz)	310	7	43	13	5
Spa Cuisine Lemon Chicken	1 pkg (9 oz)	290	9	40	8	5
Spa Cuisine Lemongrass Chicken	1 pkg (9.4 oz)	250	5	35	7	5
Spa Cuisine Rosemary Chicken	1 pkg (8.25 oz)	210	4	27	5	5
Spa Cuisine Salmon w/ Basil	1 pkg (9.5 oz)	210	5	25	2	5
Meal Mart						
Stuffed Cabbage Beef Hungarian Style	¼ pkg (2.5 oz)	210	5	30	12	2
Saffron Road						
Chicken Biryani	1 pkg (11 oz)	400	12	48	4	3
Chicken Tikka Masala w/ Basmati Rice	1 pkg (11 oz)	290	8	43	2	4
Lamb Saag w/ Basmati Rice	1 pkg (11 oz)	300	9	37	1	4
Lamb Vindaloo w/ Basmati Rice	1 pkg (11 oz)	340	7	54	2	5
Moroccan Lamb Stew	1 pkg (11 oz)	230	12	15	6	2
Simply Sensible						
Beef Pot Roast & Gravy w/ Mashed Potatoes	½ pkg (8.5 oz)	220	5	16	1	1
Beef Tips & Gravy w/ Brown Rice	1 cup (7 oz)	200	4	21	0	1
Zing Chicken & Brown Rice	1 cup (7 oz)	230	2	38	10	3
The Fillo Factory						
Fillo Pie Spinach & Cheese	⅕ pie (4.8 oz)	270	14	26	1	2

FOOD	PORTION	CAL	FAT	CARB	SUGAR	FIBER
Weight Watchers						
Smart Ones Chicken w/ Broccoli & Cheese	1 pkg (11.8 oz)	340	8	37	6	3
Zatarain's						
Blackened Chicken w/ Yellow Rice	1 pkg (10.5 oz)	470	13	71	3	3
Jambalaya w/ Sausage	1 pkg (12 oz)	500	14	79	3	3
Red Beans & Rice w/ Sausage	1 pkg (12 oz)	510	20	68	5	5
Rice Bowl Big Easy	1 pkg (10 oz)	430	12	56	3	5
Sausage & Chicken Gumbo w/ Rice	1 pkg (12 oz)	300	14	36	3	2

DIP

FOOD	PORTION	CAL	FAT	CARB	SUGAR	FIBER
shrimp cream cheese	¼ cup (2 oz)	152	14	2	1	tr
spinach sour cream	¼ cup	155	15	4	1	1
Cedar's						
Tzatziki Cucumber Garlic	2 tbsp (1 oz)	35	3	2	1	0
Cheez Whiz						
Original	1 serv (1.2 oz)	90	7	4	2	0
Fritos						
Bean	2 tbsp (1.2 oz)	35	1	5	0	2
Chili Cheese	2 tbsp (1.2 oz)	45	3	3	1	tr
Lay's						
Country Ranch Mix as prep w/ sour cream	2 tbsp (1.1 oz)	70	6	2	0	0
French Onion	2 tbsp (1.2 oz)	60	5	2	0	0
Salpica						
Chipotle Hummus Bean	2 tbsp (1 oz)	40	1	6	0	1
Cowgirl White Bean	2 tbsp (1 oz)	25	0	5	0	1
Salsa Con Queso	2 tbsp (1 oz)	20	1	4	4	0
Tostitos						
Creamy Spinach	2 tbsp (1.1 oz)	50	4	2	tr	tr

FOOD	PORTION	CAL	FAT	CARB	SUGAR	FIBER
Dip Creations Mix Freshly Made Guacamole as prep w/ avocados	2 tbsp (1.1 oz)	50	4	3	0	2
Zesty Bean & Cheese Medium	2 tbsp (1.2 oz)	45	2	5	tr	2
Victoria						
Artichoke	1 tbsp (1 oz)	30	2	2	2	1
Walden Farms						
Blue Cheese Calorie Free	2 tbsp (1 oz)	0	0	0	0	0
Ranch No Calorie	2 tbsp (1 oz)	0	0	0	0	0
Want'ems						
Sweet Chili Fusion	2 tbsp (1.1 oz)	50	0	12	11	0
Thai Mango Fusion	2 tbsp (1.1 oz)	40	0	9	8	0

DOCK

fresh cooked	3½ oz	20	1	3	–	–
raw chopped	½ cup	15	tr	2	–	–

DOUGHNUTS

chocolate glazed	1 med (1.5 oz)	175	8	24	13	1
chocolate w/ chocolate icing	1 med (2 oz)	218	12	26	13	1
creme filled	1 (3 oz)	307	21	26	12	1
custard filled	1 (2.3 oz)	235	16	20	9	1
french cruller glazed	1 med (1.4 oz)	169	8	24	14	1
jelly filled	1 (3 oz)	289	16	33	18	1
old fashioned plain	1 med (2 oz)	226	13	25	9	1
plain chocolate frosted	1 med (1.5 oz)	194	11	22	11	1
plain glazed	1 med (1.6 oz)	192	10	23	–	1
whole wheat sugared	1 med (1.6 oz)	162	9	19	10	1

FOOD	PORTION	CAL	FAT	CARB	SUGAR	FIBER
Entenmann's						
Crumb	1 (1.9 oz)	230	10	34	20	tr
Glazed	1 (2 oz)	250	13	32	20	tr
Mini Rich Frosted Chocolate	1 (1.1 oz)	170	12	14	8	0
Old Fashion Plain	1 (1.7 oz)	230	14	23	10	tr
Pop'Ems Cinnamon	4 (2 oz)	250	13	31	16	tr
Pop'Ems Glazed Crullers	2 (1.6 oz)	210	12	25	17	0
Pop'Ems Holes Rich Frosted	4 (2.1 oz)	320	23	28	17	tr
Rich Frosted	1 (1.9 oz)	240	19	27	16	tr
TAKE-OUT						
andagi okinawan doughnut	1 (0.7 oz)	84	5	10	–	0
malasada portuguese ball	1 (1.1 oz)	118	5	16	–	0

DRINK MIXERS

FOOD	PORTION	CAL	FAT	CARB	SUGAR	FIBER
whiskey sour mix not prep	1 pkg (0.6 oz)	64	0	16	–	–
whiskey sour mix	2 oz	55	0	14	–	0
Arizona						
Pina Colada Virgin Cocktail	8 oz	90	1	23	20	0
Go Cocktails!						
On-The-Go Sugar Free Appletini	1 pkg (1.9 g)	5	0	tr	0	0
On-The-Go Sugar Free Cosmo	1 pkg (2.2 g)	5	0	tr	0	0
On-The-Go Sugar Free Lemon Drop	1 pkg (2.5 g)	5	0	tr	0	0
On-The-Go Sugar Free Margarita	1 pkg (2.78 g)	5	0	tr	0	0

FOOD	PORTION	CAL	FAT	CARB	SUGAR	FIBER
Margaritaville						
Margarita Mix Mango	4 oz	120	0	29	26	–
Margarita Mix Original Lime	4 oz	110	0	27	26	–
Modmix						
Mojito	2 oz	50	0	13	13	0
Organic Citrus Margarita	2 oz	70	0	19	18	0
Organic French Martini	2 oz	50	0	13	12	0
Organic Lavender Lemon Drop	2 oz	55	0	14	13	0
Organic Pomegranate Cosmopolitan	2 oz	55	0	14	13	0
Organic Wasabi Bloody Mary	2 oz	20	0	4	3	0
Old Orchard						
Daiquiri Mixer Strawberry frzn as prep	8 oz	120	0	32	30	–
Margarita Mixer frzn as prep	8 oz	120	0	32	30	–
Pina Colada Mixer frzn as prep	8 oz	120	0	32	30	–
Prometheus Springs						
Capsaicin Spiced Elixir Citrus Cayenne	8 oz	70	0	17	17	–
Capsaicin Spiced Elixir Lychee Wasabi	8 oz	80	0	20	20	–
Capsaicin Spiced Elixir Mango Chili	8 oz	70	0	17	16	–
Capsaicin Spiced Elixir Spicy Pear	8 oz	70	0	17	16	–

DRUM

freshwater baked	3 oz	130	5	0	0	0
freshwater fillet baked	5.4 oz	236	10	0	0	0

FOOD	PORTION	CAL	FAT	CARB	SUGAR	FIBER
DUCK						
boneless roasted	½ duck (7.8 oz)	444	25	0	0	0
boneless w/o skin roasted	3.5 oz	201	11	0	0	0
boneless w/o skin roasted diced	1 cup (4.9 oz)	281	16	0	0	0
chinese pressed	3 oz	162	8	16	9	1
chinese pressed diced	1 cup (4.9 oz)	267	14	26	14	1
pekin breast boneless w/ skin roasted	1 (4.2 oz)	242	13	0	0	0
pekin breast w/o skin broiled	3 oz	133	2	0	0	0
pekin leg w/ skin w/o bone roasted	1 (3.2 oz)	200	10	0	0	0
pekin leg w/o skin & bone roasted	1 (2.6 oz)	134	5	0	0	0
w/ skin & bone roasted	½ duck (13 oz)	1287	108	0	0	0
w/ skin & bone roasted	1 serv (6 oz)	583	49	0	0	0
wing roasted bone removed	1 (1.1 oz)	101	8	0	0	0
TAKE-OUT						
breast battered & fried bone removed	½ (3.2 oz)	199	10	6	tr	tr
leg battered & fried bone removed	1 (2.5 oz)	155	8	5	tr	tr
DUMPLING						
Crazy Cuizine						
Potstickers Chicken w/ Sauce	8 (5 oz)	220	6	31	2	1
Potstickers Pork w/o Sauce	8 (5 oz)	240	8	32	1	1

FOOD	PORTION	CAL	FAT	CARB	SUGAR	FIBER
Fujisan						
Chicken Shumai Dumplings	3 (3 oz)	130	2	18	2	0
Healthy Choice						
Sweet Asian Potstickers Entree	1 pkg (9.9 oz)	340	5	66	14	5
Lean Cuisine						
Market Creations Pot Stickers Chicken	1 pkg (10 oz)	270	6	42	16	5
Simple Favorites Asian Pot Stickers	1 pkg (9 oz)	260	4	49	9	2
Panni						
Spaetzle Authentic German not prep	2 oz	200	2	39	0	2
Pepperidge Farm						
Apple	1	230	11	29	13	1
Peach	1	250	11	34	18	1
Saffron Road						
Manchurian Dumplings w/ Rice	1 pkg (11 oz)	340	11	50	5	2
TAKE-OUT						
apple	1 (6.7 oz)	661	34	83	30	3
bread dumpling	1 lg	330	10	28	–	–
cherry	1 (2.7 oz)	238	12	31	13	1
cornmeal	1 (2.8 oz)	134	4	20	1	2
fried pork	1 (3.5 oz)	338	21	25	1	1
fried puerto rican style	1 med (1.1 oz)	117	7	11	1	tr
gyoza potstickers vegetable	8 (4.9 oz)	210	4	34	7	5
peach	1 (2.7 oz)	253	12	33	12	1
piroshki meat filled	1 (3.4 oz)	348	22	25	tr	1
steamed meat	1 (1.3 oz)	41	1	4	tr	tr

FOOD	PORTION	CAL	FAT	CARB	SUGAR	FIBER
DURIAN						
fresh	3.5 oz	141	2	29	–	–
EDAMAME (*see* SOYBEANS)						
EEL						
fresh cooked	3 oz	200	13	0	0	0
fresh cooked	1 fillet (5.6 oz)	375	24	0	0	0
raw	3 oz	156	10	0	0	0
smoked	3.5 oz	330	28	0	0	0
EGG (*see also* EGG DISHES)						
CHICKEN						
fresh small	1 (1.3 oz)	54	4	tr	tr	0
fresh medium	1 (1.5 oz)	63	4	tr	tr	0
fresh large	1 (1.8 oz)	72	5	tr	tr	0
hard or soft cooked	1	77	5	1	1	0
pickled	1	72	5	1	1	0
poached	1	73	5	tr	tr	0
scrambled plain	1 (2 oz)	61	7	1	1	0
sunny side up	2	155	12	1	1	0
white raw	1 (1.1 oz)	17	tr	tr	tr	0
yolk raw	1 (0.5 oz)	55	4	1	tr	0
Egg-Land's Best						
Large	1 (1.8 oz)	70	4	0	0	0
Jake & Amos						
Pickled Red Beet Eggs	2 (5.3 oz)	200	8	21	21	0
Land O Lakes						
All Natural Brown Large ALA Omega-3	1 (1.8 oz)	70	5	0	0	0
Nature's Design						
Whole Peeled Egg	1 (1.5 oz)	70	4	1	–	–

FOOD	PORTION	CAL	FAT	CARB	SUGAR	FIBER
Pete & Gerry's						
Heirloom	1 (1.8 oz)	70	5	1	–	–
Safest Choice						
Pasteurized Fresh	1 lg (1.8 oz)	70	5	0	0	0
OTHER POULTRY						
duck 100 year old	1 (1 oz)	49	3	1	–	–
duck cooked	1 (2.5 oz)	129	10	1	1	0
duck preserved hard core	1 (1.8 oz)	80	6	1	0	0
duck preserved soft core	1 (1.8 oz)	80	6	1	0	0
duck salted	1 (1 oz)	54	4	2	–	–
goose cooked	1 (5 oz)	265	19	2	1	0
quail canned	1 (0.3 oz)	14	1	tr	tr	0
quail cooked	1 (0.5 oz)	24	2	0	0	0
turkey raw	1 (2.8 oz)	135	9	1	–	0

EGG DISHES

FOOD	PORTION	CAL	FAT	CARB	SUGAR	FIBER
Aunt Jemima						
Eggs & Sausage	1 pkg (6.2 oz)	320	21	17	3	2
Omelet Ham & Cheese	1 pkg (5.2 oz)	240	14	17	2	2
Scramble Ham & Egg	1 pkg (6.8 oz)	260	13	21	4	2
IHOP At Home						
Omelet Crisper Bacon & Cheese	1 (3.7 oz)	240	14	20	2	tr
Omelet Crisper Egg & Cheese	1 (3.7 oz)	210	12	20	2	tr
Omelet Crisper Sausage & Cheese	1 (3.7 oz)	230	13	20	2	tr
Weight Watchers						
Smart Ones Smart Morning Wrap Egg Sausage & Cheese	2 (4 oz)	240	8	32	2	7

FOOD	PORTION	CAL	FAT	CARB	SUGAR	FIBER
TAKE-OUT						
deviled	1 half	62	5	tr	tr	0
eggs benedict	2	825	64	26	3	2
omelet cheese	3 eggs	387	29	6	6	0
omelet mushroom	3 eggs	251	17	6	4	1
omelet mushroom & onion	3 eggs	294	20	7	5	1
omelet plain	3 eggs	338	25	4	4	0
omelet spanish	3 eggs	496	38	17	11	3
omelet spinach	3 eggs	279	19	6	4	1
omelet western	3 eggs	355	23	6	4	tr
salad	½ cup	353	34	2	1	0
scotch egg	1 (4.2 oz)	301	21	16	–	2
tortilla de amarillo omelet w/ plantain	3 eggs	536	35	43	21	3
EGG ROLLS						
egg roll wrapper fresh	1 (1.1 oz)	93	tr	19	–	1
Lean Cuisine						
Casual Cuisine Spring Rolls Fajita Chicken	½ pkg	200	7	20	3	2
Casual Cuisine Spring Rolls Garlic Chicken	½ pkg	200	8	24	4	2
Simple Favorites Eggroll Vegetable	1 pkg (9 oz)	320	4	62	12	2
TAKE-OUT						
chicken	1 (3 oz)	140	4	20	5	4
lobster	1 (4.8 oz)	270	7	43	4	6
lumpia vegetable & shrimp	2 (3 oz)	120	0	26	1	2
meat & shrimp	1 (4.8 oz)	320	12	41	3	4
pork & shrimp	1 (5 oz)	300	10	41	6	7
shrimp	1 (2.2 oz)	156	7	18	4	2
spicy pork	1 (3 oz)	200	9	23	3	3

FOOD	PORTION	CAL	FAT	CARB	SUGAR	FIBER
spring roll deep fried	1 (0.8 oz)	70	4	7	–	1
vegetable	1 (3 oz)	170	4	28	4	4
EGGNOG						
eggnog	1 cup	342	19	34	–	–
eggnog	1 qt	1368	76	138	–	–
eggnog flavor mix as prep w/ milk	9 oz	260	8	39	–	–
Lactaid						
Eggnog	½ cup (4 oz)	170	9	20	19	0
Straus						
Organic	4 oz	160	10	13	13	0
Turkey Hill						
EggNog	½ cup (4.2 oz)	190	9	23	23	0
Light Vanilla	½ cup (4.2 oz)	150	5	23	22	0
TAKE-OUT						
eggnog	1 cup	306	22	16	–	0
EGGPLANT						
cubed cooked w/ oil	1 cup	133	8	17	6	5
pickled	½ cup	33	tr	7	3	2
slices grilled	1 (2 oz)	36	2	5	2	1
Victoria						
In Vinegar	¼ cup (1 oz)	5	0	1	1	1
TAKE-OUT						
baba ghannouj	¼ cup	55	4	5	–	–
caponata	2 tbsp (1 oz)	30	2	3	2	–
iman bayildi eggplant w/ onion & tomato	1 serv (15.6 oz)	345	28	25	6	2
indian eggplant runi	1 serv	180	14	13	1	1
moussaka	1 serv (9 oz)	372	24	18	6	5

FOOD	PORTION	CAL	FAT	CARB	SUGAR	FIBER
papoutsaki little shoes	1 serv (15.5 oz)	245	16	15	1	1
tempura	1 serv (1.5 oz)	118	10	5	0	1
ELDERBERRIES						
fresh	1 cup	105	1	27	–	–
ELDERBERRY JUICE						
elderberry	7 oz	76	0	16	–	–
ELK						
eye of round roasted	3.5 oz	151	3	1	0	0
ground cooked	3.5 oz	143	3	0	0	0
ENERGY BARS (*see also* CEREAL BARS, FRUIT AND NUT BARS, NUTRITION SUPPLEMENTS)						
Bora Bora						
Organic Island Brazil Nut Almond	1 (1.4 oz)	200	12	18	10	2
Glenny's						
Fruit & Nut Mixed Nut	1	230	16	14	6	3
Granola Gourmet						
Chocolate Espresso	1 (1.23 oz)	150	6	20	10	3
Ultimate Berry	1 (1.2 oz)	150	6	19	9	3
Ultimate Cran-Orange	1 (1.2 oz)	140	5	19	11	3
Ultimate Fudge Brownie	1 (1.3 oz)	150	6	19	10	3
Halo						
Honey Graham	1 (1.3 oz)	150	5	24	8	2
Nutty Marshmallow	1 (1.3 oz)	150	6	22	9	2
Rocky Road	1 (1.3 oz)	160	8	20	9	2
S'Mores	1 (1.3 oz)	150	5	25	13	2
Journey						
Coconut Curry	1 (1.75 oz)	220	11	28	10	5
Hickory Barbecue	1 (1.75 oz)	170	6	27	6	4
Pizza Marinara	1 (1.75 oz)	170	6	27	5	4

FOOD	PORTION	CAL	FAT	CARB	SUGAR	FIBER
LaraBar						
Pineapple Upside Down Cake	1 (1.6 oz)	180	7	27	10	4
Luna						
Blueberry Bliss	1 (1.7 oz)	180	5	27	13	3
Chocolate Raspberry	1 (1.7 oz)	170	5	27	13	5
Fiber Chocolate Raspberry	1 (1.4 oz)	110	4	25	11	7
Fiber Vanilla Blueberry	1 (1.4 oz)	110	3	25	11	7
Mini LemonZest	1 (0.7 oz)	80	2	11	6	1
Mini White Chocolate Macadamia	1 (0.7 oz)	80	3	10	5	1
Nutz Over Chocolate	1 (1.7 oz)	180	6	25	10	3
Protein Chocolate Peanut Butter	1 (1.6 oz)	190	8	19	12	3
Protein Cookie Dough	1 (1.6 oz)	170	6	21	14	1
Protein Mint Chocolate Chip	1 (1.6 oz)	170	5	20	13	3
Vanilla Almond	1 (1.7 oz)	190	6	25	11	3
Marathon						
Snickers Chewy Chocolatey Peanut	1 (1.9 oz)	210	8	26	15	5
Snickers Crunchy Dark Chocolate	1 (1.6 oz)	150	5	22	9	7
Snickers Crunchy Multi-Grain	1 (1.9 oz)	220	7	31	17	3
Muscle Milk						
Light Chocolate Peanut Caramel	1 (1.59 oz)	170	6	18	9	4
Nogii						
No Gluten High Protein Peanut Butter & Chocolate	1 (2 oz)	230	8	20	10	2

FOOD	PORTION	CAL	FAT	CARB	SUGAR	FIBER
Premier						
Protein Bar Double Chocolate Crunch	1 (2.5 oz)	270	6	26	9	2
Protein Bar Yogurt Peanut Crunch	1 (2.5 oz)	290	8	24	10	1
Quest						
Cravings Protein Peanut Butter Cups	2 (1.8 oz)	240	17	10	1	3
Natural Protein Chocolate Peanut Butter	1 (2.1 oz)	160	5	25	1	17
Natural Protein Cinnamon Roll	1 (2.1 oz)	170	6	24	1	17
Natural Protein Peanut Butter & Jelly	1 (2.1 oz)	210	10	21	2	17
Natural Protein Vanilla Almond Crunch	1 (2.1 oz)	200	9	22	1	18
Rise Bar						
Energy + Cherry Almond	1 (1.6 oz)	200	11	23	11	3
Protein + Almond Honey	1 (2.1 oz)	280	16	20	13	4
Protein + Crunchy Carob Chip	1 (2.1 oz)	260	15	22	13	5
SoyJoy						
Soy & Fruit Blueberry	1 (1.1 oz)	140	6	17	12	4
Think5						
Red Berry	1 (2.5 oz)	240	4	48	7	3
Titan						
High Protein Chocolate Peanut Butter Crunch	1 (2.8 oz)	320	13	32	5	1
High Protein Cookies And Cream	1 (2.8 oz)	330	9	34	5	tr

FOOD	PORTION	CAL	FAT	CARB	SUGAR	FIBER
ENERGY DRINKS						
Arizona						
Energy Low Carb	1 can (8 oz)	10	0	3	3	–
Rx Energy Fast Shot Natural Green Tea	1 bottle (2 oz)	10	0	3	3	–
Sports Orange	8 oz	50	0	14	13	0
Bai						
Antioxidant Infusion Jamaica Blueberry	8 oz	70	0	18	18	–
Antioxidant Infusion Kenya Peach	8 oz	70	0	17	17	–
Antioxidant Infusion Mango Kauai	8 oz	70	0	18	18	–
Bing						
Energy Drink	1 can (12 oz)	40	0	10	10	–
Cytomax						
Performance Drink Cool Citrus	1 pkg (1.4 oz)	140	0	35	19	0
EX						
Aqua Vitamins Lemon Lime	1 bottle (16.9 oz)	110	0	27	26	–
Chillout	1 can (8.4 oz)	80	0	20	20	–
Pure Energy	1 can (8.4 oz)	70	0	17	15	–
Slim Energy	1 can (8.4 oz)	20	0	5	2	–
Facedrink						
The Social Drink	1 bottle (2.5 oz)	3	0	1	0	–
Fever						
Stimulation Beverage All Flavors	8 oz	130	0	31	31	–
Fitness Edge						
Tropical Orange	1 bottle (12 oz)	170	2	17	15	1

FOOD	PORTION	CAL	FAT	CARB	SUGAR	FIBER
Gatorade						
G Fit 03 Recover	1 pouch (11 oz)	120	2	14	10	1
G Series Fit 02 Perform	8 oz	10	0	2	2	–
G2 Natural Perform	8 oz	20	0	5	5	–
Healthy Shot						
High Protein All Flavors	1 bottle (2.5 oz)	110	0	17	16	0
Hero						
Energy Shot	1 bottle (2 oz)	0	0	0	0	0
Honeydrop						
Alive Blood Orange & Honey	8 oz	40	0	11	10	–
Strong Blueberries & Honey	8 oz	40	0	11	10	–
Mamma Chia						
All Flavors	8 oz	120	4	20	14	6
Nawgan						
Berry Caffeine Free	1 can (11.5 oz)	40	0	10	10	–
Torocco Orange	1 can (11.5 oz)	45	0	15	11	–
Ocean Spray						
Cranergy Cranberry	8 oz	35	0	8	8	–
Cranergy Pomegranate Cranberry Lift	8 oz	35	0	9	9	–
Cranergy Raspberry Cranberry Lift	8 oz	20	0	9	9	–
Palo						
Mamajuana	7 oz	50	0	15	13	–
Phase III Recovery						
Chocolate	1 bottle (14.5 oz)	330	5	36	32	3
Vanilla	1 bottle (14.5 oz)	320	5	34	33	1

FOOD	PORTION	CAL	FAT	CARB	SUGAR	FIBER
Premier						
Nitro Shot	1 (1.8 oz)	75	0	15	15	0
Rocket Shot Berry Blast	1 (1.8 oz)	30	0	7	7	–
Pyure						
O.E.O. Shot All Flavors	1 bottle (2 oz)	0	0	0	0	0
Recharge						
Lemon as prep	8 oz	10	0	1	tr	–
Tropical as prep	8 oz	10	0	1	tr	–
Red Bull						
Original	1 can (8.3 oz)	110	0	28	27	–
Sugar Free	1 can (8.3 oz)	10	0	3	0	–
Scheckter's						
Organic Energy	1 can (8.4 oz)	112	0	28	26	–
Organic Energy Lite	1 can (8.4 oz)	78	0	20	17	–
SoCal						
Just Chill	1 can (8.4 oz)	50	0	12	12	–
Solixir						
Blackberry	1 can	50	0	12	11	–
Orange	1 can	55	0	13	12	–
Pomegranate	1 can	60	0	14	13	–
Svelte						
Protein Drink All Flavors	1 bottle (15.9 oz)	260	10	35	9	5
Unwind						
All Flavors	1 can (12 oz)	40	0	10	10	–
ENGLISH MUFFIN						
READY-TO-EAT						
crumpets	1 (1.5 oz)	80	0	16	1	tr
plain	1 (2 oz)	129	1	25	2	2
whole wheat	1 (2.3 oz)	134	1	27	5	4
Foods By George						
Gluten Free Multigrain	1 (3.6 oz)	220	5	39	4	2
Gluten Free No-Rye Rye	1 (3.6 oz)	210	4	40	4	2

FOOD	PORTION	CAL	FAT	CARB	SUGAR	FIBER
Matthew's						
Golden White	1 (2.1 oz)	140	2	28	2	0
Pepperidge Farm						
100% Whole Wheat	1	140	2	26	4	3
Original	1	130	2	25	1	1
Thomas'						
10 Grain	1 (2.1 oz)	130	1	29	2	6
100% Whole Wheat	1 (2 oz)	120	1	23	2	3
Corn	1 (2.1 oz)	150	1	29	3	1
Honey Wheat	1 (2 oz)	130	1	26	2	1
Light Multi-Grain	1 (2 oz)	100	1	25	tr	8
Multi-Grain	1 (2 oz)	150	3	27	3	2
Original	1 (2 oz)	120	1	25	1	1
Raisin Cinnamon	1 (2.1 oz)	140	1	29	8	1
TAKE-OUT						
w/ butter	1 (2.2 oz)	189	6	30	–	–
w/ cheese & sausage	1 (4 oz)	365	22	27	2	1
w/ egg cheese & canadian bacon	1 (4.9 oz)	307	13	30	3	1
w/ egg cheese & sausage	1 (5.8 oz)	472	30	29	2	tr
EPAZOTE						
fresh	1 tbsp (1 g)	<1	0	tr	–	tr
fresh sprig	1 (2 g)	1	tr	tr	–	tr
EPPAW						
raw	½ cup	75	1	16	–	–
FALAFEL						
Falafel Republic						
Traditional	3 (3 oz)	210	7	26	1	6
Veggie Patch						
Falafel	4 (3 oz)	180	9	21	3	6

FOOD	PORTION	CAL	FAT	CARB	SUGAR	FIBER
TAKE-OUT						
falafel	1 (1.2 oz)	57	3	5	–	–
FAT (*see also* BUTTER, BUTTER SUBSTITUTES, MARGARINE, OIL)						
bacon grease	1 tbsp	116	13	0	0	0
beef shortening	1 tbsp	115	13	0	0	0
beef suet	1 oz	242	27	0	0	0
chicken	1 tbsp (0.4 oz)	115	13	0	0	0
duck	1 tbsp (0.4 oz)	113	13	0	0	0
goose	1 oz	257	29	0	0	0
goose	1 tbsp	115	13	0	0	0
lamb new zealand	1 oz	182	19	0	0	0
lard	1 cup (7.2 oz)	1849	205	0	0	0
lard	1 tbsp (0.5 oz)	115	13	0	0	0
meat pan drippings	½ tbsp	124	14	0	0	0
pork raw	1 oz	230	25	0	0	0
salt pork	1 cube (1 oz)	215	23	0	0	0
shortening	1 tbsp	113	13	0	0	0
shortening	1 cup	1812	205	0	0	0
turkey	1 tbsp	116	13	0	0	0
ucuhuba butter	1 tbsp	120	14	0	0	0
whale blubber	1 oz	248	28	0	0	0
More Than Gourmet						
Duck Rendered	1 tbsp (0.5 oz)	130	14	0	0	0
Spectrum						
Organic Shortening	1 tbsp (0.5 oz)	110	13	0	0	0
Shortening Butter Flavor Organic	1 tbsp (0.4 oz)	110	12	0	0	0
FAVA BEANS						
canned	½ cup	91	tr	16	–	–
fava fresh cooked	½ cup	94	tr	17	2	5

FOOD	PORTION	CAL	FAT	CARB	SUGAR	FIBER
Progresso						
Fava Beans	½ cup (4.6 oz)	110	1	17	–	5
FEIJOA						
fresh	1 (1.75 oz)	25	tr	5	–	–
puree	1 cup	119	2	26	–	–
FENNEL						
fresh bulb	1 (8.2 oz)	73	tr	17	–	7
fresh sliced	1 cup	27	tr	6	–	3
leaves	1 oz	7	tr	1	–	1
seed	1 tsp	7	tr	1	–	1
stir fried	1 cup	85	6	9	5	3
FENUGREEK						
seed	1 tsp	12	tr	2	–	1
FIBER						
apple fiber	0.5 oz	40	1	15	0	7
Spectrum						
Flax Fiber Prebiotic	1 tbsp (0.3 oz)	25	1	5	–	5
FIDDLEHEAD FERNS						
fresh	3.5 oz	34	tr	6	–	–
FIG JUICE						
Smart Juice						
Organic 100% Juice	8 oz	131	0	35	29	1
FIGS						
calimyrna	3 (5.4 oz)	120	0	28	11	4
canned in heavy syrup	½ cup	114	tr	30	27	3
canned in light syrup	½ cup	87	tr	23	20	2
canned water pack	½ cup	66	tr	17	15	3
dried california	½ cup (3.5 oz)	200	1	58	–	17
dried cooked	½ cup	139	1	36	30	5

FOOD	PORTION	CAL	FAT	CARB	SUGAR	FIBER
dried small	1 (1.4 oz)	30	tr	8	7	1
fresh large	1 (2.2 oz)	47	tr	12	10	2
Fruit Bliss						
Soft Dried	2–3 (1.5 oz)	110	0	26	20	5
Jenny						
Kalamata Crown Natural Sundried	4 (1.5 oz)	120	0	28	21	5
FIREWEED						
leaves chopped	¼ cup (0.2 oz)	6	tr	1	–	1
plant	1 (0.8 oz)	23	1	4	–	2
FISH (*see also* INDIVIDUAL NAMES, FISH SUBSTITUTES, SUSHI)						
FROZEN						
breaded fillet	1 (2 oz)	155	7	14	–	–
sticks	1 stick (1 oz)	76	3	7	–	–
Dr. Praeger's						
Fillets Lightly Breaded	1 (2.1 oz)	100	4	12	1	0
Fish Sticks Potato Crusted	3 (2.3 oz)	120	6	7	0	tr
Gorton's						
Grilled Fillets Lemon Pepper	1 (3.8 oz)	90	3	0	0	0
TAKE-OUT						
amuk bok kum korean stir fried fish cake	1 cup (7.6 oz)	267	7	31	–	3
fish cake	1 (4.7 oz)	166	7	6	–	–
jamaican brown fish stew	1 serv	426	22	9	–	2
kedgeree	5.6 oz	242	11	15	–	1
mousse	1 serv (3.5 oz)	185	14	3	tr	tr
stew	1 cup (7.9 oz)	157	4	10	–	–
taramasalata	2 tbsp	124	14	1	–	–

FOOD	PORTION	CAL	FAT	CARB	SUGAR	FIBER
FISH OIL						
cod liver	1 tbsp	123	14	0	0	0
herring	1 tbsp	123	14	0	0	0
menhaden	1 tbsp	123	14	0	0	0
salmon	1 tbsp	123	14	0	0	0
sardine	1 tbsp	123	14	0	0	0
shark	1 oz	270	29	0	0	0
whale beluga	1 oz	256	29	0	0	0
whale bowhead	1 oz	252	28	0	0	0
Genesis Today						
Omega-3 Vitamin Super Chews	1	20	0	4	3	–
Nordic Naturals						
Nordic Omega-3 Gummies Tangerine Treats	2 pieces	20	0	4	3	–
Omega 3-6-9 Junior	2 pieces	9	1	0	0	0
Omega-3 Effervescent as prep	1 pkg (9.7 g)	39	2	3	–	–
FISH PASTE						
fish paste	2 tsp	15	1	tr	–	0
FISH SUBSTITUTES						
Vegetarian Plus						
Vegetarian Fish Fillets	1 (2 oz)	220	19	4	0	2
FLAXSEED						
Carrington Farms						
Organic Flax Paks	1 pkg (0.4 oz)	50	5	3	0	3
Spectrum						
Ground Organic	2 tbsp (0.5 oz)	80	5	5	tr	4

FOOD	PORTION	CAL	FAT	CARB	SUGAR	FIBER
FLOUNDER						
FRESH						
cooked	1 fillet (4.5 oz)	148	2	0	0	0
cooked	3 oz	99	1	0	0	0
FROZEN						
Beacon Light						
Fillets Wild Caught baked	3 oz	100	1	0	0	0
TAKE-OUT						
breaded & fried	3.2 oz	211	11	15	–	–
stuffed w/ crab	1 piece (7.6 oz)	332	11	14	2	1
FLOUR						
all-purpose enriched bleached	½ cup (2.2 oz)	228	1	48	tr	2
all-purpose self-rising	½ cup (2.2 oz)	221	1	46	tr	2
all-purpose unbleached	½ cup (2.2 oz)	228	1	48	tr	2
arrowroot	½ cup (2.2 oz)	228	tr	56	–	2
bread flour	½ cup (2.4 oz)	247	1	50	tr	2
buckwheat whole groat	½ cup (2.1 oz)	201	2	42	2	6
cake	½ cup (2.4 oz)	248	1	53	tr	1
carob	½ cup (1.8 oz)	114	tr	46	25	21
carob	1 tbsp (0.2 oz)	13	tr	5	3	2

FOOD	PORTION	CAL	FAT	CARB	SUGAR	FIBER
chickpea besan	½ cup (1.6 oz)	178	3	27	5	5
peanut lowfat	½ cup (1.1 oz)	128	7	9	–	5
potato	½ cup (2.8 oz)	286	tr	66	3	5
rice brown	½ cup (2.8 oz)	287	2	60	1	4
rice white	½ cup (2.8 oz)	289	1	63	tr	2
rye dark	½ cup (2.2 oz)	207	2	44	1	15
rye light	½ cup (1.8 oz)	187	1	41	1	7
soy lowfat	½ cup (1.5 oz)	165	4	15	5	7
triticale whole grain	½ cup (2.3 oz)	220	1	48	–	10
whole wheat	½ cup (2.1 oz)	203	1	44	tr	7
Azukar Organics						
Coconut	3.5 oz	413	9	65	9	39
Ceresota						
100% Whole Wheat	¼ cup (1 oz)	100	1	21	0	3
All Purpose Unbleached	¼ cup (1 oz)	100	0	22	tr	tr
Heckers						
100% Whole Wheat	¼ cup (1 oz)	100	1	21	0	3
All Purpose Unbleached	¼ cup (1 oz)	100	0	22	tr	tr
JK Gourmet						
Almond	¼ cup (1 oz)	170	14	6	1	3
Jovial						
Organic Einkorn	⅓ cup (1 oz)	100	1	20	0	2

FOOD	PORTION	CAL	FAT	CARB	SUGAR	FIBER
King Arthur						
Whole Wheat Unbleached	¼ cup (1.1 oz)	110	1	23	0	4
Lundberg						
Brown Rice	¼ cup (1.1 oz)	110	2	22	1	2
Manischewitz						
Potato Starch	1 tbsp (0.4 oz)	30	0	8	0	0
Pillsbury						
All Purpose	¼ cup (1.1 oz)	110	0	23	tr	tr
Bread Flour	¼ cup (1.1 oz)	110	0	22	0	tr
Self Rising	¼ cup (1.1. oz)	100	0	22	0	tr
Whole Wheat	¼ cup (1.1 oz)	110	1	22	tr	3
Simpli						
Whole Oat Gluten Free	¼ cup (1.1 oz)	110	3	17	0	3
FOOD COLORS						
blue	1 tsp	0	0	0	0	0
orange	1 tsp	0	0	0	0	0
red	1 tsp	<1	0	tr	0	0
yellow	1 tsp	tr	0	0	0	0
FRENCH BEANS						
dried cooked	1 cup	228	1	43	–	17
FRENCH FRIES (*see* POTATO)						
FRENCH TOAST						
french toast frzn	1 slice (2 oz)	126	4	19	–	2
Aunt Jemima						
Cinnamon Sticks	4 (3.1 oz)	270	10	41	11	1
Homestyle	2 slices (4.1 oz)	220	5	37	7	1
Whole Grain	2 slices (4 oz)	210	5	34	8	3
Farm Rich						
Toast Sticks	4 (3.7 oz)	270	11	39	7	1

FOOD	PORTION	CAL	FAT	CARB	SUGAR	FIBER
Toast Sticks Cinnamon Sprinkle	4 (3.7 oz)	290	10	45	15	2
IHOP At Home						
Breakfast Sandwich Canadian Bacon	1 (4.3 oz)	200	8	22	5	tr
Breakfast Sandwich Maple Sausage	1 (4.8 oz)	290	16	23	5	tr
Stuffed Pastries Apple Cinnamon	1 (2.1 oz)	180	6	28	10	tr
Stuffed Pastries Blueberry	1 (2.1 oz)	200	9	27	6	1
Stuffed Pastries Cream Cheese	1 (2.1 oz)	210	9	28	10	tr
Jimmy Dean						
French Toast Duos	1 serv (3.2 oz)	210	10	19	8	1
French Toast Griddlers Sandwich	1 (3.6 oz)	210	8	27	6	0
Van's						
Cinnamon Wheat Free	2 slices (2.8 oz)	190	4	39	12	1
Sticks	2 (2.8 oz)	190	5	33	9	1
Weight Watchers						
Smart Ones French Toast w/ Turkey Sausage	1 pkg (4.4 oz)	280	8	38	18	2
TAKE-OUT						
plain	1 slice	151	7	16	–	–
sticks	5 (4.9 oz)	513	29	58	–	3
w/ butter	2 slices	356	19	36	–	–

FOOD	PORTION	CAL	FAT	CARB	SUGAR	FIBER
FROG LEGS						
TAKE-OUT						
as prep w/ seasoned flour & fried	1 (0.8)	70	5	15	–	–
FRUCTOSE						
liquid	1 oz	84	0	23	23	0
powder	1 tsp (4.2 g)	15	0	4	4	0
powder	¼ cup (1.7 oz)	180	0	49	45	0
FRUIT AND NUT BARS (*see also* CEREAL BARS, ENERGY BARS)						
Cavewoman Bars						
Baklava	1 (2 oz)	190	9	33	26	5
PB&J	1 (2 oz)	210	7	36	27	4
Pineapple Upside Down Cake Raw	1 (2 oz)	190	6	39	31	4
Goodnessknows						
Nutty Apple	1 (1.2 oz)	150	7	21	12	2
Very Cranberry	1 (1.2 oz)	150	7	21	11	2
Kind						
Apple Cinnamon Nut	1 (1.4 oz)	180	10	22	12	5
Blueberry Vanilla & Cashew	1 (1.4 oz)	180	9	24	11	2
Blueberry Pecan + Fiber	1 (1.4 oz)	180	10	23	12	5
Mango Macadamia	1 (1.4 oz)	190	12	20	15	3
Mini Bar Almond & Apricot	1 (0.8 oz)	110	7	13	7	3
Mini Bar Almond & Coconut + Omega-3	1 (0.8 oz)	107	6	12	8	2
Mini Bar Cranberry Almond + Antioxidants	1 (0.8 oz)	115	8	12	7	2
Mini Bar Fruit & Nut Delight	1 (0.8 oz)	108	6	12	7	2
Pomegranate Blueberry Pistachio + Antioxidants	1 (1.4 oz)	170	8	24	13	4

FOOD	PORTION	CAL	FAT	CARB	SUGAR	FIBER
Orchard Bar						
Blueberry Pomegranate & Almond	1 (1.6 oz)	180	6	26	19	2
Pineapple Coconut & Macadamia	1 (1.6 oz)	190	7	25	18	2
Strawberry Raspberry & Walnut	1 (1.6 oz)	190	7	26	18	2
Pure						
Organic Apple Cinnamon	1 (1.7 oz)	190	8	28	20	3
Organic Chocolate Almond	1 (1.7 oz)	190	8	25	17	5
Organic Cranberry Orange	1 (1.7 oz)	190	8	27	19	3
Organic Peanut Raisin Crunch	1 (1.5 oz)	200	12	18	9	5
Organic Superfruit Nutty Crunch	1 (1.5 oz)	190	11	22	12	5
Organic Wild Blueberry	1 (1.7 oz)	190	8	26	19	3

FRUIT AND VEGETABLE DRINKS

FOOD	PORTION	CAL	FAT	CARB	SUGAR	FIBER
EarthWise						
Orange Carrot Mango	8 oz	110	0	30	27	0
It Tastes RAAW						
Passion Fruit Wheatgrass	8 oz	100	0	23	21	1
Pineapple Cucumber	8 oz	105	0	25	24	1
Strawberry Purple Carrot	8 oz	100	0	24	23	6
Naked						
Berry Veggie	8 oz	130	1	37	18	5
Green Machine	8 oz	140	0	33	28	0
Orange Carrot	8 oz	120	0	29	26	1

FOOD	PORTION	CAL	FAT	CARB	SUGAR	FIBER
Ocean Spray						
100% Juice Fruit & Veggie Tropical Citrus	8 oz	130	0	32	27	–
100% Juice Fruit & Veggie Tropical Citrus Light	8 oz	60	0	15	11	–
Smart Juice						
Organic 100% Juice Pomegranate Purple Carrot	8 oz	137	0	35	33	0

FRUIT DRINKS (*see also* INDIVIDUAL NAMES, SMOOTHIES, VEGETABLE JUICE, YOGURT DRINKS)

FOOD	PORTION	CAL	FAT	CARB	SUGAR	FIBER
FROZEN						
Dole						
Orange Peach Mango not prep	¼ cup	120	0	29	23	0
MIX						
Aquafull						
Pomegranate Orange Dietary Supplement	1 pkg (9 g)	30	0	8	–	4
Crystal Light						
Fusion Fruit Punch as prep	8 oz	5	0	0	0	0
Immunity Cherry Pomegranate as prep	8 oz	5	0	1	0	–
Strawberry Orange Banana as prep	8 oz	5	0	0	0	0
READY-TO-DRINK						
fruit punch	6 oz	87	tr	22	–	–
Apple & Eve						
Mango Passion 100% Juice	8 oz	120	0	30	26	–

FOOD	PORTION	CAL	FAT	CARB	SUGAR	FIBER
Capri Sun						
Super V All Flavors	1 pkg (6 oz)	70	0	18	14	3
Dole						
Orange Peach Mango	8 oz	120	0	29	27	–
Paradise Blend	8 oz	120	0	29	24	0
Pina Colada	8 oz	120	0	29	24	0
Strawberry Kiwi	8 oz	120	0	31	26	0
Fave						
Orange Tangerine Pineapple	8 oz	60	1	12	12	0
Strawberry Banana Kiwi	8 oz	60	0	13	12	0
Fizzy Lizzy						
Raspberry Lemon	1 bottle (12 oz)	120	0	28	28	–
Genesis Today						
Boost Pomegranate Berry 100% Juice	8 oz	130	0	31	27	1
Honest Ade						
Superfruit Punch	8 oz	48	0	12	12	–
Honest Kids						
Organic Tropical Tango Punch	1 pkg (6.75 oz)	40	0	10	10	–
Minute Maid						
Citrus Punch	8 oz	90	0	26	25	–
Enhanced Mango Tropical	1 bottle	120	0	28	25	4
Fruit Punch	8 oz	90	0	25	25	–
Pomegranate Blueberry 100% Juice	8 oz	120	1	31	29	–
Tropical Punch	8 oz	90	0	25	25	–
Moto Bar						
Strawberry Kiwi	8 oz	110	0	28	28	0

FOOD	PORTION	CAL	FAT	CARB	SUGAR	FIBER
Naked						
Peach Guava Reduced Calorie 100% Juice	8 oz	100	0	25	20	0
Pomegranate Acai	8 oz	160	1	36	31	0
Power-C Machine	8 oz	120	0	29	23	0
Protein Zone	8 oz	220	2	34	28	0
Protein Zone Double Berry	8 oz	220	2	35	29	0
Red Machine 100% Juice	8 oz	170	5	31	25	3
Ocean Spray						
Blueberry Pomegranate	8 oz	120	0	30	30	–
Cran-Apple Light	8 oz	40	0	10	10	–
Cran-Cherry	8 oz	120	0	30	30	–
Ruby Tangerine	8 oz	110	0	28	28	–
White Cran-Peach	8 oz	110	0	27	27	–
Old Orchard						
100% Juice Acai Pomegranate	8 oz	130	0	31	29	–
100% Juice Berry Blend	8 oz	130	0	31	29	–
100% Juice Cherry Pomegranate	8 oz	130	0	31	29	–
Cranberry Grape Cocktail	8 oz	31	0	6	6	–
Healthy Balance Apple Kiwi Strawberry Cocktail	8 oz	31	0	6	6	–
Pomegranate Blueberry Acai Cocktail	8 oz	31	0	6	6	–
Very Cherre 100% Juice Tart Cherry Cranberry	8 oz	130	0	31	21	–
R.W. Knudsen						
Razzleberry 100% Juice	8 oz	120	0	28	27	0

FOOD	PORTION	CAL	FAT	CARB	SUGAR	FIBER
Sensible Sippers Organic Fruit Punch	1 box (4.23 oz)	30	0	7	7	–
Snapple						
100% Juice Fruit Punch	8 oz	170	0	42	40	–
Juice Drink Acai Blackberry	8 oz	110	0	27	27	–
Juice Drink Cranberry Raspberry	8 oz	100	0	26	26	–
TreeTop						
Apple Berry	8 oz	120	0	31	28	–
Apple Cranberry 100% Juice	8 oz	120	0	30	23	–
Apple Fruit Punch 100% Juice	8 oz	120	0	29	25	–
Apple Grape 100% Juice	8 oz	130	0	32	26	–
Apple Pear 100% Juice	1 box (3.5 oz)	100	0	25	21	–
Kiwi Strawberry 100% Juice	1 bottle (10 oz)	130	0	32	30	–
Ochango 100% Juice	1 bottle (10 oz)	170	0	42	33	–
Orange Passionfruit 100% Juice	8 oz	110	0	26	24	–
Pineapple Orange 100% Juice	8 oz	120	0	29	23	–
V8						
V-Fusion Black Cherry Pomegranate	1 can (8.4 oz)	60	0	14	12	0
V-Fusion Cranberry Blackberry	8 oz	110	0	27	26	–
V-Fusion Tangerine Raspberry	1 can (8.4 oz)	60	0	14	13	0
Welch's						
Sparkling Mango Passion Fruit	8 oz	130	0	32	31	–

FOOD	PORTION	CAL	FAT	CARB	SUGAR	FIBER
FRUIT MIXED (*see also* INDIVIDUAL NAMES, FRUIT AND NUT BARS)						
CANNED						
fruit cocktail in heavy syrup	½ cup	93	tr	24	–	–
fruit cocktail juice pack	½ cup	56	tr	15	–	–
fruit cocktail water pack	½ cup	40	tr	10	–	–
fruit salad in heavy syrup	½ cup	94	tr	24	–	–
fruit salad in light syrup	½ cup	73	tr	19	–	–
fruit salad juice pack	½ cup	62	tr	16	–	–
fruit salad water pack	½ cup	37	tr	10	–	–
mixed fruit in heavy syrup	½ cup	92	tr	24	–	–
tropical fruit salad in heavy syrup	½ cup	110	tr	29	–	–
Del Monte						
Citrus Salad	½ cup (4.4 oz)	50	0	12	8	1
Fruit Cocktail Lite	½ cup (4.4 oz)	60	0	15	14	1
Mixed Fruit Chunks In Mango Passion Fruit Juice	1 pkg (6 oz)	120	0	29	20	3
Snack Cups Cherry Mixed Fruit	1 pkg (4 oz)	70	0	18	15	–
Superfruit Peach Chunks Pomegranate & Orange Juice	1 pkg (6 oz)	100	0	26	12	3
Superfruit Pear Chunks In Acai & Blackberry Juice	1 pkg (6 oz)	120	0	31	24	3
Tropical Fruit	1 pkg (4 oz)	70	0	18	16	–
Tropical Fruit Salad In 100% Juice	½ cup (4.4 oz)	80	0	21	20	1

FOOD	PORTION	CAL	FAT	CARB	SUGAR	FIBER
Dole						
Cherry Mixed Fruit In Fruit Juice	1 pkg (4 oz)	70	0	17	16	1
Tropical Fruit In Fruit Juice	1 pkg (4 oz)	60	0	15	14	1
DRIED						
mixed	11 oz pkg	712	1	188	–	–
Crunchies						
Freeze Dried Mixed Fruit	¼ cup (7 g)	25	0	6	4	1
Fruit Bliss						
Soft Dried Medley	¼ pkg (1.5 oz)	90	0	22	14	3
FROZEN						
mixed fruit sweetened	1 cup	245	tr	61	–	–
REFRIGERATED						
Del Monte						
Fruit Naturals Mixed Berries	1 pkg (6 oz)	100	1	25	20	3

FRUIT SNACKS

FOOD	PORTION	CAL	FAT	CARB	SUGAR	FIBER
fruit leather	1 bar (0.8 oz)	81	1	18	–	–
fruit leather pieces	1 pkg (0.9 oz)	92	2	21	–	–
fruit leather pieces	1 oz	97	2	22	–	–
fruit leather rolls	1 sm (0.5 oz)	49	tr	12	–	–
fruit leather rolls	1 lg (0.7 oz)	73	1	18	–	–
Annie's Homegrown						
Orchard Fruit Bites Grape	1 pkg (0.6 oz)	60	0	15	12	1
Orchard Fruit Bites Strawberry	1 pkg (0.6 oz)	60	0	15	12	1
Organic Bunny Fruit Snacks Lemonade	1 pkg (0.6 oz)	70	0	18	10	–
Organic Bunny Fruit Tropical Treat	1 pkg (0.8 oz)	70	0	18	10	–

FOOD	PORTION	CAL	FAT	CARB	SUGAR	FIBER
Dole						
Real Fruit Bites Apple	1 pkg (0.7 oz)	80	2	16	11	0
Froose						
All Flavors	1 pkg (0.9 oz)	70	0	19	9	3
FruitziO						
Apples & Strawberries	1 pkg (0.9 oz)	100	0	23	19	2
Apricots	1 pkg (0.35 oz)	40	0	9	7	1
Peach	1 pkg (0.35 oz)	40	0	9	7	1
Strawberries	1 pkg (0.9 oz)	100	0	22	17	3
Funky Monkey						
Applemon	1 pkg (0.42 oz)	40	0	11	9	1
Bananamon	1 pkg (0.42 oz)	45	0	11	9	1
Carnaval Mix	1 pkg (0.42 oz)	45	0	11	9	1
Jivealime	1 pkg (0.42 oz)	45	0	11	8	1
MangoOJ	1 pkg (0.42 oz)	35	0	10	8	1
Pink Pineapple	1 pkg (0.42 oz)	45	0	11	9	1
Purple Funk	1 pkg (0.42 oz)	50	0	11	8	1
Juicefuls						
Berry Mania	1 pkg (0.9 oz)	80	0	19	11	–
Kaia Foods						
Fruit Leather Lime Ginger	1 (1 oz)	50	0	12	7	2
Fruit Leather Vanilla Pear	1 (1 oz)	60	0	15	9	3
Kettle Valley						
100% Fruit Bar All Flavors	1 (0.7 oz)	70	0	16	12	1
Fruit Twists All Flavors	1 (0.6 oz)	60	0	15	12	1
Mott's						
Medleys Assorted Fruit	1 pkg (0.8 oz)	80	0	19	12	–
Revolution Foods						
Organic Mashups Strawberry Banana	1 pkg (3.2 oz)	60	0	13	9	1

FOOD	PORTION	CAL	FAT	CARB	SUGAR	FIBER
Sun-Rype						
Fruit Bar Mango Strawberry	1 (1.3 oz)	120	0	31	27	3
Fruit Bar Strawberry	1 (1.3 oz)	130	0	32	29	2
Tasty						
All Flavors	1 pkg (0.8 oz)	130	0	32	17	0
That's It						
Bar 1 Apple + 3 Apricots	1 (1.2 oz)	100	0	27	23	3
Bar 1 Apple + 10 Cherries	1 (1.2 oz)	100	0	26	22	3
Bar 1 Apple + 1 Pear	1 (1.2 oz)	100	0	27	24	3
The Good Bean						
The Fruit & No-Nut Bar Apricot Coconut	1 (1.4 oz)	130	5	25	12	5
The Fruit & No-Nut Bar Chocolate Berry	1 (1.4 oz)	140	5	25	11	5
The Fruit & No-Nut Bar Fruit & Seeds Trail Mix	1 (1.4 oz)	130	5	25	11	5
TreeTop						
Fruit Snacks All Natural	1 pkg (0.9 oz)	80	0	18	15	–
Welch's						
Mixed Fruit	1 pkg (0.9 oz)	80	0	19	11	0
Mixed Fruit Reduced Sugar	1 pkg (0.9 oz)	70	0	18	8	–
GARLIC						
clove	1	4	tr	1	tr	tr
fresh chopped	1 tbsp	18	tr	4	tr	tr
powder	1 tsp	9	tr	2	1	tr
Garlic It!						
Caramelized	1 tbsp (0.5 oz)	80	8	2	0	0
Dijon	1 tbsp (0.5 oz)	80	8	2	0	0
Savory Basil	1 tbsp (0.5 oz)	80	8	2	0	0

FOOD	PORTION	CAL	FAT	CARB	SUGAR	FIBER
Thai Peanut	1 tbsp (0.5 oz)	90	9	2	0	0
Tomato Curry	1 tbsp (0.5 oz)	50	3	7	6	tr
Jake & Amos						
Sweet Pickled Garlic	1 oz	36	0	9	7	0
McSweet						
Pickled	8 pieces (1 oz)	40	0	5	tr	0
Rinaldo's Organic						
Gold Nuggets	1 tsp	10	1	1	0	0
Victoria						
Chopped In Water	1 tsp (5 g)	0	0	1	0	0
GEFILTE FISH						
sweet	1 piece (1.5 oz)	35	1	3	–	–
Manischewitz						
In Jelly	1 (2.2 oz)	70	2	4	0	0
Jellied Reduced Sodium	1 (2.2 oz)	70	2	4	0	0
Pieces In Liquid	7 (2 oz)	45	2	2	0	0
GELATIN						
MIX						
Jell-O						
Apricot as prep	1 serv	80	0	19	19	–
Cherry as prep	1 serv	80	0	19	19	–
Lime as prep	1 serv	80	0	19	19	0
Margarita as prep	1 serv	80	0	19	19	–
Orange as prep	1 serv	80	0	19	19	–
Orange Sugar Free as prep	1 serv	10	0	0	0	0
Peach Sugar Free as prep	1 serv	10	0	0	0	0
Watermelon as prep	1 serv	80	0	18	19	0
READY-TO-EAT						
Del Monte						
Mixed Fruit In Cherry Gel	1 pkg (4.5 oz)	90	0	23	20	0

FOOD	PORTION	CAL	FAT	CARB	SUGAR	FIBER
Dole						
Mixed Fruit In Cherry Gel Sugar Free	1 pkg (4.3 oz)	60	0	14	5	1
Mixed Fruit In Peach Gel	1 pkg (4.3 oz)	100	0	24	22	1
Pineapple In Lime Gel	1 pkg (4.3 oz)	90	0	23	22	1
Jell-O						
Cherry & Black Cherry	1 pkg (3.2 oz)	10	0	0	0	0
Raspberry & Orange Sugar Free	1 pkg (3.2 oz)	10	0	0	0	0
Strawberry	1 pkg (3.5 oz)	70	0	17	17	–
Strawberry Sugar Free	1 pkg (3.2 oz)	10	0	0	0	0
Kozy Shack						
Gel Treats Sugar Free Strawberry	1 pkg (3.5 oz)	10	0	2	0	0
Smart Gels Cherry	1 pkg (3.5 oz)	80	0	21	20	0
Smart Gels Orange	1 pkg (3.5 oz)	80	0	24	22	0
Smart Gels Strawberry	1 pkg (3.5 oz)	80	0	24	22	0
Smart Gels Sugar Free Orange	1 pkg (3.5 oz)	5	0	1	0	0
Tropical	1 pkg (3.5 oz)	80	0	21	20	0
Tropical Sugar Free	1 pkg (3.5 oz)	5	0	1	0	1
Snack Pack						
Gels Cherry No Sugar Added	1 pkg (3.5 oz)	10	0	2	0	tr
Gels Strawberry	1 pkg (3.5 oz)	100	0	25	22	0
GIBLETS						
capon simmered	1 cup (5 oz)	238	8	0	0	0
chicken fried	1 cup (5 oz)	402	20	6	–	0
chicken simmered	1 cup (5 oz)	289	17	1	0	0
turkey simmered	1 cup (5 oz)	243	7	3	–	–
GINGER						
ground	1 tsp	6	tr	1	tr	tr
pickled	1 tbsp (0.3 oz)	9	0	2	–	0

FOOD	PORTION	CAL	FAT	CARB	SUGAR	FIBER
preserved	1.5 oz	34	0	8	7	1
root fresh	5 slices	9	tr	2	tr	tr
root fresh sliced	¼ cup	19	tr	4	tr	1
GINKGO NUTS						
canned	1 oz	32	tr	6	–	–
dried	1 oz	99	tr	21	–	–
raw	1 oz	52	tr	11	–	–
GINSENG						
dried	1 oz	90	tr	20	–	2
fresh	1 oz	28	tr	6	–	tr
GIZZARDS						
chicken simmered	1 cup (5 oz)	212	4	0	0	0
turkey simmered	1 (3 oz)	103	3	tr	0	0
Foster Farms						
Chicken Gizzards & Hearts fresh	4 oz	150	8	0	0	0
GNOCCHI						
spinach	12 (4 oz)	220	1	50	2	5
Racconto						
Potato Whole Wheat as prep w/o salt	1 cup (5.8 oz)	248	0	60	tr	8
Solterra						
Original Potato	¼ pkg (3 oz)	100	0	22	1	2
Spinach	¼ pkg (3 oz)	100	0	24	1	2
GOAT						
diced boiled	1 cup (4.7 oz)	190	4	0	0	0
fried boneless	3 oz	130	4	0	0	0
ribs cooked	3 (4.8 oz)	196	4	0	0	0
roasted boneless	3 oz	122	3	0	0	0
TAKE-OUT						
stew puerto rican style	1 cup (6.2 oz)	460	31	4	2	1

FOOD	PORTION	CAL	FAT	CARB	SUGAR	FIBER
GOJI BERRIES						
dried	1 oz	106	3	19	–	2
GOOSE						
boneless roasted	2.7 oz	231	17	0	0	0
meat only raw	6.5 oz	298	13	0	0	0
w/ skin & bone roasted	1 serv (6.6 oz)	573	41	0	0	0
wild boneless roasted diced	1 cup (4.9 oz)	426	31	0	0	0
GOOSEBERRIES						
canned in light syrup	1 cup	184	1	47	–	6
fresh	1 cup	66	1	15	–	7
GRAINS						
Village Harvest						
Wheatberry & Barley	½ cup	260	3	57	0	10
Whole Grain Creations w/ Cranberries & Almonds	¾ cup (4.3 oz)	220	4	44	6	6
Whole Grain Medley Farro & Red Rice	1 cup (5 oz)	290	3	60	0	4
GRAPE JUICE						
bottled unsweetened	1 cup	154	tr	38	38	tr
Fizzy Lizzy						
Yakima Grape	1 bottle (12 oz)	120	0	30	30	–
Kedem						
Organic	8 oz	140	0	35	33	–
Manischewitz						
Concord Purple	8 oz	160	0	40	39	–
Minute Maid						
100% Juice Grape Blend	8 oz	150	0	39	34	–

FOOD	PORTION	CAL	FAT	CARB	SUGAR	FIBER
Old Orchard						
100% Juice	8 oz	130	0	31	29	–
100% Juice White	8 oz	130	0	31	29	–
R.W. Knudsen						
100% Juice	8 oz	130	0	32	31	tr
Snapple						
100% Juice Grape	8 oz	170	0	43	41	–
Grapeade	8 oz	100	0	26	26	–
TreeTop						
Vineyard Grape 100% Juice	1 bottle (10 oz)	160	0	40	33	–
Welch's						
100% White	8 oz	160	0	39	38	–
Concord Grape Light	8 oz	45	0	12	11	–
Fruit Fizz Concord Grape Blast	1 can (8.4 oz)	70	0	20	18	–
Healthy Start 100% Juice	8 oz	140	0	38	36	–
White Light Juice Beverage	8 oz	45	0	12	11	–
GRAPE LEAVES						
canned	1 (4 g)	3	tr	tr	–	–
fresh raw	1 (3 g)	3	tr	1	tr	tr
Galil						
Stuffed	5 (4.2 oz)	200	11	23	2	3
TAKE-OUT						
dolmas w/ beef & rice	1 (0.7 oz)	50	4	2	1	1
dolmas w/ lamb & rice	1 (0.7 oz)	56	4	3	1	1
dolmas w/ rice	1 (2 oz)	92	6	8	2	2
GRAPEFRUIT						
CANNED						
sections juice pack	½ cup (4.4 oz)	46	tr	11	11	1

FOOD	PORTION	CAL	FAT	CARB	SUGAR	FIBER
sections light syrup	½ cup (4.5 oz)	76	tr	20	19	1
sections water pack	½ cup (4.3 oz)	44	tr	11	11	1
Del Monte						
Fruit Bowls Grapefruit Duo	½ cup (4.4 oz)	60	0	16	14	1
Red In Light Syrup	½ cup (4.4 oz)	90	0	21	17	1
FRESH						
pink or red	½ (4.6 oz)	52	tr	13	8	2
sections pink or red	1 cup (8.1 oz)	97	tr	25	16	4
sections white	1 cup (8.1 oz)	76	tr	19	17	3
white	½ (4.1 oz)	39	tr	10	9	1
Ocean Spray						
Sweet Ruby	½ med (5.4 oz)	60	0	16	10	6
Sunkist						
Fresh	½ med (5.4 oz)	60	0	15	11	2

GRAPEFRUIT JUICE

FOOD	PORTION	CAL	FAT	CARB	SUGAR	FIBER
canned sweetened	1 cup (8.8 oz)	115	tr	28	28	tr
canned unsweetened	1 cup (8.7 oz)	94	tr	22	22	tr
pink fresh	1 cup (8.7 oz)	96	tr	23	–	–
white fresh	1 cup (8.7 oz)	96	tr	23	22	tr
Apple & Eve						
Ruby Red	8 oz	130	0	32	32	–
Fizzy Lizzy						
Grapefruit	1 bottle (12 oz)	100	0	25	25	–
Minute Maid						
100% Juice + Calcium frzn not prep	2 oz	100	0	25	20	–
Ruby Red	8 oz	130	0	34	32	–
Ocean Spray						
100% Juice Pink	8 oz	100	0	23	23	–

FOOD	PORTION	CAL	FAT	CARB	SUGAR	FIBER
100% Juice White	8 oz	90	0	21	17	–
Ruby Drink Light	8 oz	40	0	10	10	–
Old Orchard						
Ruby Red Cocktail	8 oz	31	0	6	6	–
GRAPES						
muscadine	10–12 (3.5 oz)	76	0	14	–	3
scuppernongs	10–12 (3.5 oz)	68	0	12	–	3
seedless red or green	1 cup	110	tr	29	24	1
seedless red or green	20	69	tr	18	15	1
thompson seedless in heavy syrup	½ cup	93	tr	25	24	1
thompson seedless water pack	½ cup	49	tr	13	12	1
with seeds red or green	1 cup	106	tr	28	24	1
with seeds red or green	20	80	tr	21	18	1
Crunch Pak						
Sweet Seedless	⅕ pkg	40	0	10	9	tr
Dole						
Fresh	26 (4.4 oz)	90	0	23	20	1
Sunkist						
Fresh	1 cup (5.3 oz)	110	0	27	23	1
GRAVY						
CANNED						
beef	1 can (10 oz)	155	7	14	–	–
beef	1 cup	124	6	11	–	–
chicken	1 cup	189	14	13	–	–
mushroom	1 cup	120	6	13	–	–
turkey	1 cup	122	5	12	–	–
Campbell's						
Beef	¼ cup (2 oz)	25	1	3	tr	0
Mushroom	¼ cup (2.1 oz)	20	1	3	1	0

FOOD	PORTION	CAL	FAT	CARB	SUGAR	FIBER
Heinz						
HomeStyle Classic Chicken	¼ cup (2 oz)	15	0	3	0	0
HomeStyle Rich Mushroom	¼ cup (2.1 oz)	20	1	3	0	0
Homestyle Savory Beef	¼ cup (2 oz)	25	1	4	0	0
Roasted Turkey Fat Free	¼ cup (2.1 oz)	20	0	3	0	0
Manischewitz						
Beef Savory	¼ cup (2.1 oz)	20	1	3	0	0
Chicken Reduced Sodium	¼ cup (2.1 oz)	20	1	3	0	0
Chicken Classic	¼ cup (2.1 oz)	20	1	3	0	0
Roasted Turkey	¼ cup (2.1 oz)	25	1	3	0	0
MIX						
au jus as prep w/ water	1 cup	32	1	4	–	–
brown as prep w/ water	1 cup	75	2	13	–	–
chicken as prep	1 cup	83	2	14	–	–
mushroom as prep	1 cup	70	1	14	–	–
onion as prep w/ water	1 cup	77	1	16	–	–
pork as prep	1 cup	76	2	13	–	–
turkey as prep	1 cup	87	2	15	–	–
Bournvita						
Extract	2 heaping tsp	34	1	7	–	–
Bovril						
Extract	1 heaping tsp	9	0	tr	–	0
Loney's						
Brown as prep	¼ cup (2.1 oz)	15	0	3	0	0
Turkey as prep	¼ cup (2.1 oz)	20	0	4	0	0
Marmite						
Extract	1 heaping tsp	9	0	tr	–	–
TAKE-OUT						
au jus	1 cup	62	6	1	tr	tr
giblet gravy	¼ cup	45	3	3	tr	tr

FOOD	PORTION	CAL	FAT	CARB	SUGAR	FIBER
GREAT NORTHERN BEANS						
canned	1 cup	299	1	55	–	13
dried cooked	1 cup	209	1	37	–	12
GREEN BEANS						
CANNED						
drained	1 cup	27	tr	6	1	3
Butter Kernel						
Cut	½ cup (4.2 oz)	20	0	4	2	2
Cut No Salt Added	½ cup (4.2 oz)	20	0	4	2	2
Del Monte						
Cut	½ cup (4.2 oz)	20	0	5	1	2
Cut No Salt Added	½ cup (4.2 oz)	20	0	4	2	2
French Style	½ cup (4.2 oz)	20	0	4	2	2
McSweet						
Dilly Beans Whole	5 (1 oz)	30	0	7	6	tr
FRESH						
cooked w/o salt	1 cup	44	tr	10	2	4
raw	1 cup	34	tr	8	2	4
raw whole beans	10	17	tr	4	1	2
Ready Pac						
Fast 'N Fresh as prep	1 cup (3 oz)	30	0	7	1	3
FROZEN						
cooked	1 cup	38	tr	9	2	4
Lisa's Organics						
Whole In Garlic Oil Sauce	½ pkg (4 oz)	60	2	8	4	3
TAKE-OUT						
casserole w/ mushroom sauce	1 cup	108	6	11	3	3
pickled	½ cup	19	tr	4	1	2
GROUNDCHERRIES						
fresh	½ cup	37	tr	8	–	–

FOOD	PORTION	CAL	FAT	CARB	SUGAR	FIBER
GROUPER						
cooked	3 oz	100	1	0	0	0
cooked	1 fillet (7.1 oz)	238	3	0	0	0
raw	3 oz	78	1	0	0	0
GUAVA						
fresh	1 (1.9 oz)	37	1	8	5	3
fresh cut up	1 cup (5.8 oz)	112	2	24	15	9
fresh strawberry	1 (6 g)	4	tr	1	–	tr
fresh strawberry cut up	1 cup (8.6 oz)	168	1	42	–	13
guava paste	1 piece (1.1 oz)	90	tr	23	23	tr
GUAVA JUICE						
nectar canned	8 oz	143	tr	37	31	3
GUINEA HEN						
boneless w/o skin raw	½ hen (9.3 oz)	290	7	0	0	0
w/ skin raw	½ hen (12 oz)	545	22	0	0	0
HADDOCK						
fresh broiled	4 oz	127	1	0	0	0
roe raw	1 oz	37	tr	tr	–	–
smoked	1 oz	33	tr	0	0	0
TAKE-OUT						
breaded & fried	4 oz	229	10	10	1	1
HAGGIS						
scottish haggis	1 serv (6.4 oz)	473	32	31	3	5
HALIBUT						
atlantic & pacific cooked	3 oz	119	2	0	0	0
atlantic & pacific cooked	½ fillet (5.6 oz)	223	5	0	0	0
atlantic & pacific raw	3 oz	93	2	0	0	0

FOOD	PORTION	CAL	FAT	CARB	SUGAR	FIBER
greenland baked	5.6 oz	380	28	0	0	0
greenland baked	3 oz	203	15	0	0	0
HAM						
boneless extra lean roasted	3 oz	123	5	1	0	0
boneless roasted	3 oz	151	8	0	0	0
canned extra lean roasted	3 oz	116	4	tr	–	0
canned lean roasted	3 oz	142	7	tr	–	0
center slice lean & fat roasted	3 oz	173	11	tr	–	0
deviled	¼ cup	188	17	1	0	0
ham salad spread	2 tbsp	65	5	3	0	0
patty grilled	1 patty (2 oz)	205	19	1	0	0
prosciutto	4 slices (1.3 oz)	72	3	tr	0	0
sliced	3 slices (2.9 oz)	137	7	3	0	1
sliced extra lean	3 slices (2.2 oz)	69	2	2	0	0
westphalian smoked	1 oz	105	10	0	0	0
whole roasted	3 oz	207	14	0	0	0
Dietz & Watson						
Boneless Old Fashioned	3 oz	110	5	1	1	0
Smoked	2 oz	80	3	1	1	0
Steak Our Traditional	5 oz	100	3	2	2	0
Hormel						
Chunk Ham canned	2 oz	90	6	0	0	0
Jones						
Steak Extra Lean	3 oz	100	4	2	–	–
Organic Prairie						
Hardwood Smoked Bone In Spiral Cut	3 oz	110	3	tr	tr	0

FOOD	PORTION	CAL	FAT	CARB	SUGAR	FIBER
TAKE-OUT						
croquette	1 (2.2 oz)	149	9	8	2	tr
salad	½ cup	287	23	5	–	tr
spam musubi	1 serv (6 oz)	253	6	42	–	1
thick slice fried	1 (2.2 oz)	140	9	tr	0	0

HAMBURGER

FOOD	PORTION	CAL	FAT	CARB	SUGAR	FIBER
Al Fresco						
Chicken Burger Buffalo Style	1 (3.4 oz)	130	7	2	1	0
Chicken Burger Sweet Italian	1 (3.4 oz)	140	8	1	0	0
Farm Rich						
Cheeseburgers Mini Bacon	2 (2.2 oz)	150	7	14	2	1
Foster Farms						
Cheeseburgers Mini Chicken w/ BBQ Sauce	1 (1.3 oz)	90	4	9	1	0
TAKE-OUT						
cheeseburger + condiments	1 reg (4.5 oz)	347	17	28	5	1
double hamburger + condiments	1 reg (5.8 oz)	384	19	30	7	2
single patty + condiments	1 reg (4 oz)	299	11	35	8	2

HAMBURGER SUBSTITUTES (*see also* MEAT SUBSTITUTES)

FOOD	PORTION	CAL	FAT	CARB	SUGAR	FIBER
Asherah's Gourmet						
Organic Vegan Burger Chipotle	1 (4 oz)	180	5	30	3	5
Organic Vegan Burgers Original	1 (4 oz)	180	5	30	3	5

FOOD	PORTION	CAL	FAT	CARB	SUGAR	FIBER
Boca						
All American Flame Grilled	1 (2.5 oz)	120	5	5	0	4
Dr. Praeger's						
Veggie Burger California Slider	1 (1.6 oz)	80	4	8	1	2
Harmony Valley						
Vegetarian Hamburger Mix as prep	1 (3 oz)	120	5	8	1	4
Quorn						
Classic Burger	1 (2.1 oz)	90	3	7	1	3
Vegan Burger	1 (2.1 oz)	100	4	9	1	2
Sunshine						
Organic Garden Burger	1 (2.6 oz)	250	13	14	2	3
Veggie Bites						
Garlic Portabella	1 (2.5 oz)	120	6	8	1	4
HAZELNUTS						
chocolate hazelnut spread	2 tbsp (1.3 oz)	200	11	23	20	2
chopped	¼ cup (1 oz)	181	17	5	1	3
ground	¼ cup (0.7 oz)	118	11	3	1	1
whole	¼ cup (1.2 oz)	212	21	6	1	3
whole nuts	21 (1 oz)	178	17	5	1	3
Fundelina						
Choco-Hazelnut Spread All Flavors	2 tbsp (1.3 oz)	200	11	23	21	2
Kettle Brand						
Butter Unsalted	2 tbsp (1 oz)	180	17	5	1	3
HEART						
beef simmered	3 oz	140	4	tr	0	0
chicken cooked	1 (3 g)	5	tr	0	0	0
chicken diced simmered	½ cup	134	6	tr	–	0

FOOD	PORTION	CAL	FAT	CARB	SUGAR	FIBER
lamb braised	3 oz	157	7	2	–	0
pork braised	1 (4.5 oz)	191	7	1	–	0
turkey simmered	½ cup	94	3	tr	0	0
veal braised	3 oz	158	6	tr	–	0
HEARTS OF PALM						
canned	1 (1.2 oz)	9	tr	2	–	1
canned	½ cup	20	tr	3	–	2
HEMP						
Manitoba Harvest						
Organic Pro Fiber	4 tbsp (1 oz)	127	3	14	0	14
Organic Protein Dark Chocolate	4 tbsp (1 oz)	120	3	17	6	9
HERBAL TEA (*see* TEA/HERBAL TEA)						
HERBS/SPICES (*see also* INDIVIDUAL NAMES)						
cajun seasoning	1 tbsp	19	1	3	–	1
chinese five spice	1 tsp	7	tr	2	–	tr
garam masala	1 tsp	8	tr	1	–	–
poultry seasoning	1 tsp	5	tr	1	tr	tr
pumpkin pie spice	1 tsp (1.7 g)	6	tr	1	tr	tr
Emeril's						
Original Essence	½ tsp (2 g)	0	0	tr	–	–
McCormick						
Grill Mates Rub Applewood	2 tsp	15	0	3	1	0
Meat Tenderizer Seasoned	¼ tsp (1 g)	0	0	0	0	0
Perfect Pinch Salt Free Original	¼ tsp	0	0	0	0	0
Modern Day Masala						
Organic Garam Masala	1 tsp (3 g)	10	0	2	–	1

FOOD	PORTION	CAL	FAT	CARB	SUGAR	FIBER
Mrs. Dash						
Grilling Blend Steak	¼ tsp (0.7 g)	0	0	0	0	0
Seasoning Blends Caribbean Citrus	¼ tsp (0.7 g)	0	0	0	0	0
Old Bay						
Seasoning	¼ tsp (0.6 g)	0	0	0	0	0
Seasoning 30% Less Sodium	¼ tsp (0.6 g)	0	0	0	0	0
Ribber City						
Rib-A-Dub-Rub Dry Rub Seasoning	¼ tsp (0.8 oz)	3	0	1	0	0
HERRING						
atlantic baked	4 oz	230	13	0	0	0
dried salted	1 fillet (1.4 oz)	161	9	0	0	0
pickled	1 oz	74	5	3	–	0
pickled in cream sauce	1 oz	72	5	2	tr	0
roe	1 tbsp	39	2	tr	0	0
smoked kippered	1 oz	62	4	0	0	0
TAKE-OUT						
breaded fried	1 serv (4 oz)	225	14	9	1	1
HIBISCUS						
flowers dried sweetened	⅓ cup	100	0	23	21	2
HICKORY NUTS						
dried	1 oz	187	18	5	–	–
HOMINY						
white canned	1 cup	119	1	24	3	4
yellow canned	½ cup	115	1	23	–	4
Bush's						
Golden	½ cup (4.6 oz)	60	0	13	0	3
HONEY						
honey	¼ cup (3 oz)	258	0	70	70	tr

FOOD	PORTION	CAL	FAT	CARB	SUGAR	FIBER
honey	1 tbsp (0.7 oz)	64	0	17	17	–
orange blossom	1 tbsp	60	0	17	16	0
wild honey	1 tbsp	60	0	17	16	–
Maple Grove Farms						
Honey Maple Spread	2 tbsp (1.5 oz)	160	0	42	37	–
Steel's						
Sugar Free	1 tbsp (0.5 oz)	24	0	11	0	0
SueBee						
Honey	1 tbsp (0.7 oz)	60	0	17	16	–
HONEYDEW						
balls frzn	1 cup (8 oz)	83	tr	21	19	2
fresh cut up	1 cup	61	tr	15	14	1
fresh wedge	⅛ melon (4.5 oz)	45	tr	11	10	1
whole fresh	1 (35 oz)	360	1	91	81	8
Dole						
Fresh	1/10 med (4.7 oz)	50	0	12	11	1
HORSE						
roasted	3 oz	149	5	0	0	0
HORSERADISH						
japanese wasabi	¼ tsp	1	–	tr	–	0
sauce	1 tbsp	7	tr	2	1	1
wasabi root raw	1 (5.9 oz)	184	1	40	–	13
wasabi root raw sliced	½ cup (2.3 oz)	71	tr	15	–	5
Dietz & Watson						
Cranberry Horseradish Sauce	1 tsp (5 g)	10	1	1	1	0
Manischewitz						
Sauce Original	1 tsp (5 g)	15	2	1	1	0
Zatarain's						
Prepared	1 tbsp (0.5 oz)	15	0	2	0	0

FOOD	PORTION	CAL	FAT	CARB	SUGAR	FIBER
HOT CHOCOLATE						
mix not prep	1 pkg (1 oz)	111	1	23	18	1
mix w/ no calorie sweetener as prep w/ water	8 oz	72	1	14	7	2
mix w/ sugar as prep w/ nonfat milk	8 oz	209	1	30	29	1
mix w/ sugar as prep w/ water	8 oz	138	1	29	23	1
Nestle						
Hot Cocoa Rich Milk Chocolate as prep w/ water	1 pkg (0.7 oz)	80	3	14	12	tr
Hot Cocoa Mix Fat Free as prep	1 pkg	20	0	4	4	tr
TAKE-OUT						
chocolate caliente w/ lowfat milk	1 serv (8.4 oz)	221	9	27	25	1
chocolate caliente w/ whole milk	1 serv (8.4 oz)	276	17	25	23	1
hot chocolate	1 cup (8.7 oz)	192	6	30	24	3
mexican hot chocolate	1 cup	173	6	20	–	1
HOT DOG (*see also* HOT DOG SUBSTITUTES)						
beef	1 (1.5 oz)	149	13	2	2	0
beef & pork	1 (1.5 oz)	137	12	1	0	1
beef lowfat	1 (2 oz)	133	11	1	0	0
chicken	1 (1.5 oz)	116	9	3	0	0
fat free	1 (2 oz)	62	1	6	0	0
low sodium	1 (2 oz)	180	16	1	0	0
lowfat	1 (2 oz)	88	6	3	0	0
pork and beef cheese smokie	1 (1.5 oz)	141	12	1	1	0
turkey	1 (1.5 oz)	102	8	1	0	0

FOOD	PORTION	CAL	FAT	CARB	SUGAR	FIBER
Abeles&Heymann						
Beef Uncured Reduced Fat & Sodium	1 (1.7 oz)	120	9	1	0	0
Al Fresco						
Chicken Uncured	1 (1.5 oz)	60	3	0	0	0
Applegate Farms						
The Great Uncured Beef	1 (2 oz)	110	8	0	0	0
The Great Uncured Chicken	1 (1.7 oz)	70	4	0	0	0
The Great Uncured Turkey	1 (1.7 oz)	60	4	1	0	0
Uncured Beef	1 (1.5 oz)	70	6	0	0	0
Uncured Big Apple	1 (2 oz)	110	9	1	0	0
Dietz & Watson						
Black Forest Wieners	1 (2 oz)	180	16	0	0	0
Gourmet Lite	1 (2 oz)	60	2	5	1	0
Super Franks	1 (3.2 oz)	270	24	3	3	0
Foster Farms						
Chicken	1 (2 oz)	140	12	1	tr	0
Corn Dog Chili Cheese	1 (2.6 oz)	190	9	21	4	1
Corn Dog Extreme Cheese	1 (2.6 oz)	200	10	22	4	0
Corn Dogs Honey Crunchy	1 (2.6 oz)	180	9	19	6	0
Corn Dogs Mini	4 (2.7 oz)	210	12	18	0	1
Turkey	1 (2 oz)	140	12	1	tr	0
Hebrew National						
Beef	1 (1.7 oz)	150	14	1	0	0
Beef 97% Fat Free	1 (1.6 oz)	40	1	3	0	0
Beef Franks In A Blanket	5 (2.8 oz)	300	24	12	tr	1
Beef Jumbo	1 (3 oz)	270	25	2	0	0
Organic Prairie						
Beef Uncured	1 (1.5 oz)	120	11	0	0	0

FOOD	PORTION	CAL	FAT	CARB	SUGAR	FIBER
Oscar Mayer						
Turkey Uncured	1 (2 oz)	120	9	3	1	–
State Fair						
Classic Corn Dog	1 (2.7 oz)	210	10	23	7	0
Corn Dog Beef	1 (2.7 oz)	220	10	25	8	0
Corn Dog Mini	6 (3 oz)	230	12	25	6	1
TAKE-OUT						
corndog	1	460	19	56	–	–
w/ bun chili	1	297	13	31	–	–
w/ bun plain	1	242	15	18	–	–

HOT DOG SUBSTITUTES

FOOD	PORTION	CAL	FAT	CARB	SUGAR	FIBER
Morningstar Farms						
Veggie Dogs	1 (1.4 oz)	50	1	4	2	tr

HUMMUS

FOOD	PORTION	CAL	FAT	CARB	SUGAR	FIBER
Athenos						
Artichoke & Garlic	2 tbsp (0.9 oz)	50	3	4	1	1
Cucumber Dill	2 tbsp (0.9 oz)	50	3	5	1	1
Greek Style	2 tbsp (0.9 oz)	50	3	5	1	1
Original	2 tbsp (0.9 oz)	50	3	5	1	1
Roasted Red Pepper	2 tbsp (0.9 oz)	50	3	5	1	1
Cedar's						
Artichoke Spinach	2 tbsp (1 oz)	70	4	5	1	1
Fountain Of Health						
Traditional	1 oz	70	5	6	1	1
Margaritaville						
Cilantro Jalapeno	1 oz	70	5	4	1	1
Island Lemon	1 oz	70	6	4	1	1
Nasoya						
Super Classic Original	2 tbsp (1 oz)	50	3	2	1	1
Sabra						
Classic Singles	1 (2 oz)	150	11	9	1	3
Greek Olive	2 tbsp (1 oz)	70	6	4	0	1

FOOD	PORTION	CAL	FAT	CARB	SUGAR	FIBER
Roasted Pine Nut	2 tbsp (1 oz)	80	7	4	0	1
Spinach & Artichoke	2 tbsp (1 oz)	70	6	4	0	1
TAKE-OUT						
hummus	¼ cup (2.2 oz)	109	5	12	tr	3

HYACINTH BEANS

FOOD	PORTION	CAL	FAT	CARB	SUGAR	FIBER
dried cooked	1 cup	228	1	40	–	–

ICE CREAM AND FROZEN DESSERTS (*see also* ICES AND ICE POPS, SHERBET, YOGURT FROZEN)

FOOD	PORTION	CAL	FAT	CARB	SUGAR	FIBER
chocolate	½ cup (4 fl oz)	143	7	19	13	–
dixie cup chocolate	1 (3.5 fl oz)	125	6	16	11	–
dixie cup strawberry	1 (3.5 fl oz)	112	5	16	9	–
dixie cup vanilla	1 (3.5 fl oz)	116	6	14	9	–
freeze dried ice cream chocolate strawberry & vanilla	1 pkg (0.75 oz)	158	5	24	10	1
strawberry	½ cup (4 fl oz)	127	6	18	10	–
vanilla	½ cup (4 fl oz)	132	7	16	10	–
vanilla soft serve	½ cup	111	2	19	–	–
Arctic Zero						
Chocolate	½ cup (2.6 oz)	37	0	7	6	2
Chocolate Coated Bars All Flavors	1 (2 oz)	85	5	7	5	1
Coffee	½ cup (2.6 oz)	37	0	6	5	2
Mint Chocolate Cookie	½ cup (2.6 oz)	37	0	6	5	2
Pumpkin Spice	½ cup (2.6 oz)	45	0	7	7	2
Vanilla Maple	½ cup (2.6 oz)	37	0	7	7	2
Carvel						
Cake Original Ice Cream	⅙ cake (3.2 oz)	250	13	27	21	1

FOOD	PORTION	CAL	FAT	CARB	SUGAR	FIBER
Clemmy's						
Bar Sugar Free Cherry Vanilla	1 (1.9 oz)	70	3	16	0	5
Bar Sugar Free Chocolate Fudge	1 (2.2 oz)	70	3	18	0	5
Bar Sugar Free Orange Creme	1 (2 oz)	70	3	16	0	5
Butter Pecan Sugar Free	½ cup (2.6 oz)	180	14	19	0	5
Chocolate Sugar Free	½ cup (2.6 oz)	160	11	20	0	5
Ice Cream Os Sugar Free	1 (1.75 oz)	100	7	12	0	2
Peanut Butter Chocolate Chip Sugar Free	½ cup (2.6 oz)	200	15	20	0	5
Toasted Almond Sugar Free	½ cup (2.7 oz)	180	13	22	0	5
Vanilla Bean Sugar Free	½ cup (2.5 oz)	150	11	19	0	5
Dove						
Miniatures Dark Chocolate Variety Pack	5 (3.1 oz)	320	21	31	24	3
Miniatures Milk Chocolate Variety Pack	5 (3.1 oz)	340	22	32	29	1
Mint Chocolate Chunk	½ cup (2.4 oz)	180	11	17	14	1
Unconditional Chocolate	½ cup	200	12	23	17	2
Vanilla Chocolate Chunk	½ cup (2.3 oz)	180	11	17	15	0
Good Karma						
Organic Rice Divine Bar Chocolate Chocolate	1 (2.4 oz)	200	13	22	12	1
Organic Rice Divine Chocolate Chip	½ cup (2.6 oz)	170	9	23	13	2

FOOD	PORTION	CAL	FAT	CARB	SUGAR	FIBER
Organic Rice Divine Coconut Mango	½ cup (2.6 oz)	150	6	23	14	1
Organic Rice Divine Key Lime Pie	½ cup (2.6 oz)	140	6	23	13	1
Haagen-Dazs						
Bailey's Irish Cream	½ cup (3.6 oz)	260	17	21	21	0
Bar Vanilla & Almonds	1 (3 oz)	310	22	22	20	tr
Caramel Cone	½ cup (4 oz)	320	19	32	27	0
Chocolate Chip Cookie Dough	½ cup (3.6 oz)	310	20	29	24	0
Chocolate Peanut Butter	½ cup (3.8 oz)	360	24	27	24	2
Five Mint	½ cup (3.6 oz)	220	12	24	23	0
Strawberry	½ cup (3.7 oz)	250	16	23	22	tr
Healthy Choice						
Bar Fudge	1 (2.2 oz)	80	2	13	4	4
Bar Low Fat Sorbet & Cream	1 (2.2 oz)	80	1	18	12	tr
Sandwich Vanilla	1 (2.4 oz)	150	2	30	14	0
Julie's						
Organic Gluten Free Sandwich Vanilla	1 (2.6 oz)	220	11	30	20	1
Lactaid						
Butter Pecan	½ cup (4 oz)	170	11	16	11	0
Chocolate	½ cup (2.5 oz)	160	8	19	13	0
Vanilla	½ cup (4 oz)	150	8	16	12	0
Lifeway						
Frozen Kefir Tart And Tangy Mango	½ cup (2.5 oz)	90	1	18	16	0

FOOD	PORTION	CAL	FAT	CARB	SUGAR	FIBER
Frozen Kefir Tart And Tangy Original	½ cup (2.5 oz)	90	1	18	16	0
Frozen Kefir Tart And Tangy Pomegranate	½ cup (2.5 oz)	90	1	18	16	0
Frozen Kefir Tart And Tangy Strawberry	½ cup (2.5 oz)	90	1	18	16	0
Magnum						
Classic	1 bar (2.7 oz)	240	16	22	21	tr
Dark	1 bar (2.7 oz)	240	17	20	18	2
Double Caramel	1 bar (3.2 oz)	320	20	32	29	1
White	1 bar (2.7 oz)	250	16	23	23	0
Skinny Cow						
Bar Dippers Vanilla & Caramel	1	80	3	11	7	2
Bar Truffle Caramel	1	100	2	19	12	3
Bar Truffle French Vanilla	1	100	2	18	12	3
Cone Chocolate w/ Fudge	1	150	3	29	17	3
Cone Vanilla w/ Caramel	1	150	3	29	18	3
Fudge Bar	1	100	1	22	13	4
Sandwich Chocolate Peanut Butter	1	150	2	30	15	3
Sandwich Cookies 'N Cream	1	150	2	31	15	3
Sandwich Vanilla	1	140	2	30	15	3
Sandwich Vanilla No Sugar Added	1	140	2	30	5	5
Stonyfield Farm						
Gotta Have Java	1 serv (4 oz)	250	16	22	20	0
Strawberry Licious	1 serv (4 oz)	220	13	23	21	0
Vanilla Chai	1 serv (4 oz)	240	16	21	20	0

FOOD	PORTION	CAL	FAT	CARB	SUGAR	FIBER
Straus						
I'm Organic Coffee	4 oz	240	15	19	19	0
I'm Organic Raspberry	½ cup (4 oz)	230	14	19	19	1
I'm Organic Vanilla Bean	4 oz	240	15	19	19	0
Organic Brown Sugar Banana	½ cup (3.2 oz)	250	11	32	31	0
Tofutti						
Cuties Chocolate	1 (1.3 oz)	130	1	16	9	0
Cuties Vanilla	1 (1.3 oz)	130	6	17	9	0
Flowers Chocolate Covered	1 (1.4 oz)	180	8	23	19	2
Marry Me Dessert Bars	1 bar (2.5 oz)	168	8	22	18	tr
Yours Truly Cones	1 (2.6 oz)	220	13	24	21	2
Weight Watchers						
Smart Ones Sundae Chocolate Fudge Brownie	1 (2.3 oz)	140	3	26	14	tr
Smart Ones Sundae Turtle	1 (2.2 oz)	130	3	23	10	0
TAKE-OUT						
cone vanilla light soft serve	1 (4.6 oz)	164	6	24	–	–
gelato chocolate hazelnut	½ cup (5.3 oz)	370	29	26	21	2
gelato vanilla	½ cup (3 oz)	211	15	18	18	0
ice cream pie no crust	1 slice (3.4 oz)	218	14	21	18	1
mud pie	⅛ pie (8 oz)	698	32	96	64	3
sundae caramel	1 (5.4 oz)	303	9	49	–	–
sundae hot fudge	1 (5.4 oz)	284	9	48	–	–
sundae strawberry	1 (5.4 oz)	269	8	45	–	–

ICE CREAM CONES AND CUPS

FOOD	PORTION	CAL	FAT	CARB	SUGAR	FIBER
brown sugar cone	1 (10 g)	40	tr	8	3	tr

FOOD	PORTION	CAL	FAT	CARB	SUGAR	FIBER
wafer cone	1	17	tr	3	tr	tr
waffle cone	1 lg	121	2	23	2	1
ICE CREAM TOPPINGS						
butterscotch	2 tbsp (1.4 oz)	103	tr	27	–	–
caramel	2 tbsp (1.4 oz)	103	tr	27	–	–
marshmallow cream	1 oz	88	tr	23	–	–
marshmallow cream	1 jar (7 oz)	615	tr	157	–	–
nuts in syrup	2 tbsp	184	9	24	15	1
pineapple	1 cup (11.5 oz)	861	–	226	–	–
pineapple	2 tbsp (1.5 oz)	106	tr	28	9	tr
strawberry	1 cup (11.5 oz)	863	1	225	–	–
strawberry	2 tbsp (1.5 oz)	107	tr	28	–	–
Smucker's						
Plate Scrapers Chocolate Fudge	2 tbsp (1.4 oz)	120	3	22	14	tr
Steel's						
Sugar Free Fudge Sauce	2 tbsp (0.9 oz)	110	6	13	10	1
ICED TEA						
MIX						
Crystal Light						
Antioxidant Sugar Free Green Tea Raspberry as prep	8 oz	5	0	1	0	–
On The Go White Peach Tea as prep	8 oz	5	0	0	0	0
Pure Sugar Free Mixed Berry as prep	8 oz	15	0	4	3	0
READY-TO-DRINK						
Arizona						
Black & White	8 oz	50	0	14	14	0

FOOD	PORTION	CAL	FAT	CARB	SUGAR	FIBER
Diet Black Tea Peach	8 oz	0	0	tr	tr	0
Green Tea Lemonade	8 oz	50	0	14	13	0
Organic Green Tea	8 oz	50	0	14	13	0
Honest Tea						
Assam Black	8 oz	17	0	5	5	–
Green Dragon	8 oz	30	0	8	8	–
Green Tea Zero Calorie Passion Fruit	8 oz	0	0	0	0	0
Half & Half	8 oz	48	0	12	12	–
Heavenly Lemon Tulsi	8 oz	30	0	8	8	–
Jasmine Green Energy	8 oz	17	0	5	5	–
Just Green	8 oz	0	0	0	0	0
Pearfect White	8 oz	35	0	9	9	–
White Mango Acai	8 oz	35	0	9	9	–
Ito En						
Dark Green Tea Oi Ocha	8 oz	0	0	0	0	0
Golden Oolong	8 oz	0	0	0	0	0
Green Tea Jasmine	8 oz	0	0	0	0	0
Green Tea Oi Ocha	8 oz	0	0	0	0	0
Sencho Shot Japanese Green Tea	1 can (6.4 oz)	0	0	0	0	0
Lipton						
Diet Green Tea w/ Citrus	8 oz	0	0	0	0	0
Diet Green Tea w/ Watermelon	8 oz	0	0	0	0	–
Green Tea 100% Natural Citrus	8 oz	70	0	19	18	–
Green Tea 100% Natural Passionfruit Mango	8 oz	50	0	13	13	–
Old Orchard						
Green Tea w/ Lemon & Honey	8 oz	45	0	12	12	0
Red Tea w/ Currant	8 oz	45	0	12	12	–

FOOD	PORTION	CAL	FAT	CARB	SUGAR	FIBER
POM						
Green Tea Pomegranate Lychee	8 oz	70	0	18	17	–
Pomegranate Blackberry	8 oz	80	0	20	18	–
Rooibee Red Tea						
Lemon Honey	1 bottle (12.5 oz)	80	0	21	20	–
Peach	1 bottle (12.5 oz)	80	0	21	21	–
Unsweet	1 bottle (12.5 oz)	0	0	0	0	0
Snapple						
Black Tea Lemon	8 oz	80	0	21	21	–
Diet Lemon Tea	8 oz	10	0	0	0	–
Diet Lemonade Iced Tea	8 oz	10	0	2	2	–
Diet Peach	8 oz	0	0	0	0	–
Diet Plum-A-Granate	8 oz	5	0	0	0	0
Green Tea Mango Metabolism	8 oz	60	0	15	15	–
Peach	8 oz	90	0	23	23	–
Red Tea Pomegranate Raspberry	8 oz	80	0	21	21	–
White Tea Apple Plum	8 oz	80	0	21	21	–
Spindrift						
Sparkling Half & Half	8 oz	80	0	21	20	0
Tea Of A Kind						
All Flavors	8 oz	10	0	3	3	–
Teas' Tea						
Green Hoji	8 oz	0	0	0	0	0
Lemongrass Green	8 oz	0	0	0	0	0
Pure Black	8 oz	0	0	0	0	0
Pure Green	8 oz	0	0	0	0	0

FOOD	PORTION	CAL	FAT	CARB	SUGAR	FIBER
ICES AND ICE POPS						
Del Monte						
Fruit Chillers Arctic Strawberry Cup	1 (4.5 oz)	170	0	45	26	2
Fruit Chillers Frosty Peach Cup	1 (4.5 oz)	170	0	45	26	2
Fruit Chillers Grape Berry Blast Tube	1	55	0	13	11	1
Fruit Chillers Strawberry Snow Storm Tube	1	55	0	13	11	1
Dole						
Fruit Bars Strawberry	1 (2.75 oz)	90	0	23	22	0
Super Fruit Bars Acai Blueberry	1 (2.75 oz)	90	0	22	21	0
Haagen-Dazs						
Fat Free Sorbet Mango	½ cup (4 oz)	120	0	37	36	0
Minute Maid						
Soft Frozen Lemonade Lemon	1 pkg	70	0	19	13	–
Soft Frozen Limeade Cherry	1 pkg	70	0	19	13	–
Power Of Fruit						
Fruit Bar Banana Berry	1 (1.75 oz)	27	tr	7	5	1
Fruit Bar Original	1 (1.75 oz)	28	tr	7	5	1
Fruit Bar Tropical	1 (1.75 oz)	30	tr	8	6	1
INDIAN FOOD (*see* ASIAN FOOD)						
JACKFRUIT						
canned in syrup	½ cup (3.1 oz)	82	tr	21	–	1
fresh sliced	1 cup (5.8 oz)	157	1	38	31	3
JALAPENO (*see* PEPPERS)						

FOOD	PORTION	CAL	FAT	CARB	SUGAR	FIBER
JAM/JELLY/PRESERVES						
apple butter	1 tbsp (0.6 oz)	31	tr	8	6	tr
jam all flavors	1 tbsp (0.7 oz)	56	tr	14	10	tr
jam all flavors	1 pkg (0.5 oz)	39	tr	10	7	tr
jam apricot	1 tbsp (0.7 oz)	48	tr	13	9	tr
jam diet all flavors	1 tbsp (0.5 oz)	18	tr	8	5	tr
jelly all flavors	1 tbsp (0.7 oz)	51	0	13	10	tr
jelly reduced sugar all flavors	1 tbsp (0.7 oz)	34	tr	9	9	tr
jelly diet all flavors	1 tbsp (0.7 oz)	25	tr	10	7	1
orange marmalade	1 tbsp (0.7 oz)	49	0	13	12	tr
preserves all flavors	1 tbsp (0.7 oz)	56	tr	14	10	tr
Beth's Farm Kitchen						
Apple Butter	2 tbsp (1 oz)	15	0	4	3	1
Jam Gooseberry	2 tbsp (1 oz)	45	0	11	10	1
Marmalade Bitter Orange	2 tbsp (1 oz)	40	0	10	10	0
Bonne Maman						
Jelly Muscat Grape	1 tbsp (0.7 oz)	50	0	13	13	–
Orange Marmalade	1 tbsp (0.7 oz)	50	0	13	13	–
Preserves Apricot	1 tbsp (0.7 oz)	50	0	13	13	–
Preserves Cherry	1 tbsp (0.7 oz)	50	0	12	13	–
Preserves Golden Plum Mirabelle	1 tbsp (0.7 oz)	50	0	12	12	–
Jake & Amos						
Jam Fig	1 tbsp (0.5 oz)	35	0	9	8	0
Jam Hot Pepper	1 tbsp	43	0	9	8	–
Jam Rhubarb	1 tbsp (0.7 oz)	40	0	12	11	0
Jenkins Jellies						
Fiery Figs Pepper Jelly	1 tbsp (0.7 oz)	50	0	12	11	–
Guava Brava	1 tbsp (0.7 oz)	50	0	12	11	–
Hell Fire Pepper Jelly	1 tbsp (0.7 oz)	40	0	11	10	1
Passion Fire Pepper Jelly	1 tbsp (0.7 oz)	45	0	11	12	–

FOOD	PORTION	CAL	FAT	CARB	SUGAR	FIBER
Sarabeth's						
Spreadable Fruit Chunky Apple	1 tbsp (0.7 oz)	30	0	7	7	–
Spreadable Fruit Orange Apricot Marmalade	1 tbsp (0.7 oz)	30	0	8	8	–
Spreadable Fruit Pineapple Mango	1 tbsp (0.7 oz)	35	0	9	9	0
Spreadable Fruit Strawberry Peach	1 tbsp (0.7 oz)	30	0	8	7	–
Spreadable Fruit Strawberry Rhubarb	1 tbsp (0.7 oz)	40	0	10	9	tr
Smucker's						
Jam Blackberry	1 tbsp (0.7 oz)	50	0	13	12	–
Jam Concord Grape	1 tbsp (0.7 oz)	50	0	13	12	–
Jam Red Plum	1 tbsp (0.7 oz)	50	0	13	12	–
Jam Seedless Red Raspberry	1 tbsp (0.7 oz)	50	0	13	12	–
Jelly Apple	2 tbsp (0.7 oz)	50	0	13	12	–
Jelly Concord Grape	1 tbsp (0.7 oz)	50	0	13	12	–
Jelly Strawberry	1 tbsp (0.7 oz)	50	0	13	12	–
Orange Marmalade Low Sugar	2 tbsp (0.7 oz)	25	0	6	5	–
Preserves Apricot Low Sugar	1 tbsp (0.6 oz)	25	0	6	5	–
Simply Fruit Black Cherry	1 tbsp (0.7 oz)	40	0	10	8	–
Simply Fruit Peach	1 tbsp (0.7 oz)	40	0	10	8	–
Simply Fruit Strawberry	1 tbsp (0.7 oz)	40	0	10	8	–
Trappist						
Jelly Hot Pepper	1 tbsp (0.7 oz)	50	0	13	13	–
Welch's						
Grape Jelly	1 tbsp (0.7 oz)	50	0	13	13	–

FOOD	PORTION	CAL	FAT	CARB	SUGAR	FIBER
Natural Spread Concord Grape	1 tbsp (0.6 oz)	30	0	8	8	–
Natural Spread Strawberry	1 tbsp (0.6 oz)	30	0	8	8	–

JAPANESE FOOD (*see* ASIAN FOOD, SUSHI)

JELLY (*see* JAM/JELLY/PRESERVES)

JELLYFISH

FOOD	PORTION	CAL	FAT	CARB	SUGAR	FIBER
pickled	½ cup (1 oz)	10	tr	0	0	0

JERKY

FOOD	PORTION	CAL	FAT	CARB	SUGAR	FIBER
beef	1 oz	122	8	3	3	1
pork	1 oz	122	8	3	3	1
venison	1 oz	119	7	4	4	0
Jerky For Life						
Beef Steak Black Pepper & Garlic	¼ pkg (1 oz)	50	2	0	0	0
Beef Steak Jalapeno	¼ pkg (1 oz)	50	2	tr	0	–
King Kalibur						
Black Angus Beef Sticks	1 (1.2 oz)	93	5	4	4	0
Krave						
Beef Chili Lime	1 oz	50	2	3	2	0
Beef Pineapple Orange	1 oz	80	2	8	6	0
Beef Sweet Chipotle	1 oz	80	2	9	7	0
Pork Smoky Grilled Teriyaki	1 oz	70	2	9	8	0
Turkey Basil Citrus	1 oz	100	0	16	16	0
Matador						
Beef Original	1 pkg (1.4 oz)	110	2	8	7	0
Snack Stick Original	1 (1 oz)	150	13	2	0	0
Oh Boy! Oberto						
Beef Hickory	1 oz	80	1	6	6	0
Beef Original	1 oz	80	1	6	5	0

FOOD	PORTION	CAL	FAT	CARB	SUGAR	FIBER
Beef Peppered	1 oz	80	1	6	5	0
Original Thin	1 pkg (1.2 oz)	90	2	3	1	0
Pepperoni Bite Size Sticks	6 (1.1 oz)	160	13	3	1	0
Smok-A-Roni	2 (1 oz)	140	12	2	1	0
Sticks Original	1 pkg (1 oz)	130	10	2	0	0
Tender Style	1 pkg (0.4 oz)	45	3	2	1	0
Ostrim						
Stick Beef & Ostrich	1 (1.5 oz)	80	2	3	2	–
Perky Jerky						
Beef	1 pkg (1 oz)	90	2	6	5	0
Turkey	1 pkg (1 oz)	50	0	2	2	0
Sunrich Naturals						
Fruit Bar Sour Apple	1 (0.7 oz)	70	0	16	12	1
Fruit Bar	1 (0.7 oz)	70	0	16	12	1
Umpqua Indian Foods						
Brew Pub Steak Jerky Beef Flavored	¼ pkg (1 oz)	90	3	6	5	–
Steak Jerky Original	¼ pkg (1 oz)	60	2	0	0	0
JICAMA						
fresh	1 sm (12.8 oz)	139	tr	32	7	18
raw sliced	1 cup	46	tr	11	2	6
JUJUBE						
dried	1 oz	82	tr	21	–	–
JUTE						
cooked	1 cup	32	tr	6	1	2
KALE						
chopped cooked w/o salt	1 cup	36	1	7	2	3
fresh cooked w/ fat	1 cup	69	4	7	2	2

FOOD	PORTION	CAL	FAT	CARB	SUGAR	FIBER
scotch chopped cooked w/o salt	1 cup	36	1	7	–	2

KEFIR

FOOD	PORTION	CAL	FAT	CARB	SUGAR	FIBER
kefir	8 oz	98	2	12	12	0
Green Valley						
Organic Lactose Free Blueberry Pom Acai	1 pkg (6 oz)	150	3	25	19	0
Organic Lactose Free Plain	8 oz	90	3	10	4	0
Helios						
Organic Blueberry	8 oz	160	2	25	21	3
Organic Nonfat Plain w/ Omega 3s	8 oz	80	0	10	10	0
Organic Plain	8 oz	120	5	12	10	2
Organic Raspberry	8 oz	160	4	26	23	2
Lifeway						
BioKefir Shot Digestion Vanilla	1 bottle (3.5 oz)	60	0	10	9	2
BioKefir Shot Heart Health Black Cherry	1 bottle (3.5 oz)	60	0	10	10	–
BioKefir Shot Heart Health Blackberry	1 bottle (3.5 oz)	60	0	10	10	–
Greek Style	8 oz	210	14	12	12	–
Lowfat Blueberry	8 oz	140	2	20	20	–
Lowfat Cappuccino	8 oz	140	2	20	20	–
Lowfat Pomegranate	8 oz	140	2	20	20	–
Nonfat Peach	8 oz	180	0	33	30	3
Nonfat Plain	8 oz	90	0	12	12	–
Nonfat Raspberry	8 oz	150	0	27	27	–
Organic Lowfat Plain	8 oz	110	2	12	12	–
Organic Lowfat Wildberry	8 oz	160	2	25	21	3
Original	8 oz	150	8	12	12	0

FOOD	PORTION	CAL	FAT	CARB	SUGAR	FIBER
Plain Lowfat	8 oz	110	2	12	12	–
Plain Whole Milk	8 oz	160	8	12	12	–
Probugs Goo-Berry Pie	1 bottle (5 oz)	130	5	15	13	2
Probugs Frozen Kefir Pop Goo-Berry Pie	1 (1.9 oz)	70	1	13	12	–
Probugs Frozen Kefir Pop Orange Creamy Crawler	1 (1.9 oz)	70	1	13	12	–
Probugs Frozen Kefir Pop Strawnana Split	1 (1.9 oz)	70	1	13	12	0
Slim6 Mixed Berry	8 oz	110	2	8	6	2
Slim6 Plain	8 oz	110	2	8	6	2
The Greek Gods						
Honey & Strawberry	8 oz	230	3	38	37	0
Plain	8 oz	140	3	17	17	0
Vanilla Honey	8 oz	220	3	38	38	0
Yakult						
Drink	1 bottle (2.7 oz)	50	0	12	11	0

KETCHUP

FOOD	PORTION	CAL	FAT	CARB	SUGAR	FIBER
banana	1 tsp	10	0	2	2	0
ketchup	1 pkg (0.2 oz)	6	tr	2	–	tr
ketchup	1 tbsp	15	tr	4	3	0
low sodium	1 tbsp	15	tr	4	3	0
Annie's Homegrown						
Organic	1 tbsp (0.6 oz)	15	0	5	4	–
Del Monte						
Tomato	1 tbsp (0.6 oz)	15	0	4	4	0
Fischer & Wieser						
Chipotle Chili	1 tbsp (0.7 oz)	15	0	3	2	–
Heinz						
No Salt Added	1 tbsp (0.6 oz)	20	0	5	4	0
Reduced Sugar	1 tbsp (0.6 oz)	5	0	1	1	0

FOOD	PORTION	CAL	FAT	CARB	SUGAR	FIBER
Hunt's						
Ketchup	1 tbsp (0.6 oz)	20	0	5	4	0
Ketchup No Salt Added	1 tbsp (0.6 oz)	25	0	6	4	0
OrganicVille						
No Added Sugar	1 tbsp (0.6 oz)	20	0	4	3	0
Walden Farms						
Calorie Free	1 tbsp (0.5 oz)	0	0	0	0	0
KIDNEY						
beef simmered	3 oz	134	4	0	0	0
lamb braised	3 oz	116	3	1	–	0
pork braised	3 oz	128	4	0	0	0
veal braised	3 oz	139	5	0	0	0
KIDNEY BEANS						
canned	½ cup	108	1	19	2	6
dried cooked w/o salt	½ cup	112	tr	20	tr	6
Vitarroz						
Light Red	½ cup (4.2 oz)	100	0	17	1	5
KIWI						
fresh	1 med (2.6 oz)	46	tr	11	7	2
fresh	1 lg (3.2 oz)	56	tr	13	8	3
KNISH						
Gabila's						
Potato	1 (4.5 oz)	180	3	36	tr	2
TAKE-OUT						
cheese	1 (2.1 oz)	205	12	19	tr	1
meat	1 sm (1.8 oz)	174	11	13	tr	1
meat	1 lg (5.6 oz)	524	32	38	1	2
potato	1 sm (2.1 oz)	213	12	21	tr	1
potato	1 lg (6.3 oz)	616	35	56	2	2

FOOD	PORTION	CAL	FAT	CARB	SUGAR	FIBER
KOHLRABI						
raw sliced	1 cup	36	tr	8	4	4
sliced cooked w/o salt	1 cup	48	tr	11	5	2
TAKE-OUT						
creamed	1 cup	150	9	14	6	1
KRILL						
fresh	1 oz	22	1	tr	–	0
KUMQUATS						
canned in syrup	1	13	tr	3	3	1
fresh	1	13	tr	3	2	1
LAMB						
cubed lean & fat braised	4 oz	253	10	0	0	0
cubed lean broiled	4 oz	211	8	0	0	0
ground broiled	4 oz	321	22	0	0	0
leg roasted	4 oz	213	15	0	0	0
loin chop lean & fat broiled	1 chop (4 oz)	222	16	0	0	0
rib chop lean & fat broiled	1 chop (1.6 oz)	165	14	0	0	0
rib roast baked	4 oz	386	31	0	0	0
shank lean & fat braised	4 oz	360	20	0	0	0
shoulder chop lean & fat cooked	1 chop (5.5 oz)	274	20	0	0	0
shoulder w/ bone braised	4 oz	231	17	0	0	0
LAMB DISHES						
TAKE-OUT						
keema w/ coconut milk	1 serv (8 oz)	380	28	18	9	6
moussaka	4 in sq (16 oz)	659	43	32	10	8
shepherd's pie	1 (21.3 oz)	742	31	76	9	9

FOOD	PORTION	CAL	FAT	CARB	SUGAR	FIBER
stew w/ potatoes & vegetables	1 cup	260	6	29	3	4
LAMBSQUARTERS						
chopped cooked w/ salt	1 cup	58	1	9	–	4
LECITHIN						
lecithin	1 tbsp	104	14	0	0	0
LEEKS						
chopped cooked w/o salt	¼ cup	8	tr	2	–	tr
cooked	1 (4.4 oz)	38	tr	9	–	1
freeze dried	1 tbsp	1	0	tr	–	0
LEMON						
fresh	1 med (4 oz)	22	tr	12	–	5
peel	1 tsp	1	0	tr	tr	tr
peel	1 tbsp	3	tr	1	tr	1
wedge	1 (7 g)	2	tr	1	tr	tr
Sunkist						
Fresh	1 med (2 oz)	15	0	5	2	2
LEMON CURD						
lemon curd made w/ egg	2 tsp	29	1	4	–	0
LEMON JUICE						
bottled	1 tbsp	3	tr	1	tr	tr
bottled	1 oz	6	tr	2	1	tr
fresh	1 oz	8	0	3	1	tr
from 1 lemon	1.6 oz	12	0	4	1	tr
from wedge	6 g	1	0	1	tr	0
Italian Volcano						
Organic	2 tbsp (1 oz)	9	0	2	1	0
Izze						
Esque Sparkling Limon	1 bottle (12 oz)	50	0	12	11	–

FOOD	PORTION	CAL	FAT	CARB	SUGAR	FIBER
KeVita						
Sparkling Probiotic Drink Lemon Ginger Organic	8 oz	45	0	11	9	–
Volcano						
Organic Lemon Burst	2 tbsp (1 oz)	0	0	1	0	0
LEMONADE						
MIX						
Crystal Light						
Sugar Free as prep	8 oz	5	0	0	0	0
READY-TO-DRINK						
EarthWise						
Harvest Lemonade	8 oz	100	0	26	25	0
Honest Ade						
Classic Zero Calorie	8 oz	0	0	0	0	0
Minute Maid						
Just 15 Calories	8 oz	15	0	4	2	–
Lemonade	8 oz	110	0	29	28	–
Pink Light	8 oz	15	0	4	3	–
Santa Cruz						
Organic Peach	8 oz	100	0	25	25	0
Organic Strawberry	8 oz	90	0	23	22	–
Simply						
Lemonade	8 oz	120	0	30	28	–
Spindrift						
Sparkling	8 oz	80	0	21	19	0
Sunkist						
Sparkling	8 oz	110	0	30	29	–
Tropicana						
Trop50 Raspberry	8 oz	50	0	12	12	–
V8						
V-Fusion Strawberry	1 can (8.4 oz)	60	0	14	11	0

FOOD	PORTION	CAL	FAT	CARB	SUGAR	FIBER
Welch's						
Sparkling	8 oz	140	0	36	35	–
LEMONGRASS						
fresh	1 tbsp	5	tr	1	–	–
LENTILS						
dried cooked	1 cup	230	1	40	4	16
TruRoots						
Organic Sprouted Green not prep	¼ cup (1.4 oz)	140	1	25	1	7
TAKE-OUT						
lentil loaf	1 slice (1.6 oz)	83	4	10	1	3
yemiser selatta ethiopian lentil salad	1 serv (3 oz)	115	7	11	1	2
LETTUCE (*see also* SALAD)						
arugula	6 leaves (0.4 oz)	3	tr	tr	tr	tr
arugula shredded	1 cup	5	tr	1	tr	tr
boston	1 head (5.7 oz)	21	tr	4	2	2
boston chopped	6 leaves	7	tr	1	1	1
cornsalad field salad	1 cup (1.9 oz)	7	tr	1	–	1
iceberg	1 lg head (26.5 oz)	106	1	22	15	9
iceberg	6 med leaves	7	tr	1	1	1
iceberg shredded	1 cup	10	tr	2	1	1
looseleaf outer leaves	6 (5 oz)	22	tr	4	1	2
looseleaf shredded	1 cup	5	tr	1	tr	1
red leaf	6 leaves (3.6 oz)	16	tr	2	tr	1
red leaf shredded	1 cup	4	tr	1	tr	tr
romaine	3 leaves (3 oz)	14	tr	3	1	2
romaine heart	6 leaves (1.3 oz)	6	tr	1	tr	1
romaine shredded	1 cup	8	tr	2	1	1

FOOD	PORTION	CAL	FAT	CARB	SUGAR	FIBER
Dole						
Just Lettuce	1½ cups (3 oz)	15	0	3	1	1
Romaine Chopped	1½ cups (3 oz)	15	0	3	2	1
Mann's						
Green Leaf Singles	6 leaves (3 oz)	15	0	3	2	2
Ready Pac						
Baby Arugula	4 cups (3 oz)	20	0	3	2	1
Shredded Iceberg	1 cup (3 oz)	10	0	3	1	1
Simply Lettuce	2½ cups (3 oz)	15	0	3	1	1
River Ranch						
Iceberg Shreds	2 cups (3 oz)	10	0	3	2	1
LILY ROOT						
dried	1 oz	89	1	21	–	tr
fresh	1 oz	32	tr	8	–	tr
LIMA BEANS						
CANNED						
lima beans	½ cup	95	tr	18	–	6
Del Monte						
Green	½ cup (4.4 oz)	80	0	15	0	4
DRIED						
cooked	½ cup	150	tr	20	1	5
LIME						
fresh	1 (2.4 oz)	20	tr	7	1	1
wedge	1 (8 g)	2	tr	1	tr	tr
Sunkist						
Fresh	1 med (2.4 oz)	20	0	7	0	2
LIME JUICE						
bottled	1 oz	6	tr	2	tr	tr
fresh	1 oz	8	tr	3	1	tr
from 1 lime	1.1 oz	11	tr	4	1	tr
Honest Ade						
Limeade	8 oz	48	0	12	12	–

FOOD	PORTION	CAL	FAT	CARB	SUGAR	FIBER
Minute Maid						
Limonada Limeade	8 oz	120	0	33	31	–
Sunkist						
Cherry Limeade	8 oz	120	0	30	29	–
Volcano						
Organic Lime Burst	2 tbsp (1 oz)	0	0	1	0	0
Welch's						
Sparkling Limeade Raspberry	8 oz	140	0	34	33	–

LING

blue raw	3.5 oz	83	1	0	0	0
fresh baked	3 oz	95	1	0	0	0
fresh fillet baked	5.3 oz	168	1	0	0	0

LINGCOD

baked	3 oz	93	1	0	0	0
fillet baked	5.3 oz	164	2	0	0	0

LIQUOR (*see* ALCOHOL DRINKS, BEER AND ALE, CHAMPAGNE, MALT, WINE)

LIVER (*see also* PATE)

beef braised	1 slice (2.4 oz)	130	4	3	0	0
beef pan-fried	1 slice (2.8 oz)	142	4	4	0	0
chicken fried	3 oz	146	5	1	0	0
chicken simmered	3 oz	142	6	1	0	0
duck raw	1 (1.5 oz)	60	2	2	–	0
goose raw	1 (3.3 oz)	125	4	6	–	0
lamb braised	3 oz	187	7	2	–	0
lamb fried	3 oz	202	11	3	–	0
moose braised	3 oz	132	4	3	–	–
pork braised	3 oz	140	4	3	–	0
turkey simmered	1 liver (2.9 oz)	227	17	1	0	0
veal braised	1 slice (2.8 oz)	154	5	3	0	0
veal pan fried	1 slice (2.4 oz)	129	4	3	0	0

FOOD	PORTION	CAL	FAT	CARB	SUGAR	FIBER
Organic Prairie						
Beef	2 oz	80	2	2	0	0
TAKE-OUT						
calves liver w/ onions	1 serv (5 oz)	177	4	10	2	1
LOBSTER						
northern cooked	1 cup	142	1	2	–	–
northern cooked	3 oz	83	1	1	–	–
northern raw	3 oz	77	1	tr	–	–
northern raw	1 lobster (5.3 oz)	136	1	1	–	–
spiny steamed	3 oz	122	2	3	–	–
spiny steamed	1 (5.7 oz)	233	3	5	–	–
TAKE-OUT						
newburg	1 cup	485	27	13	–	–
LOGANBERRIES						
fresh	½ cup (2.5 oz)	40	tr	9	6	4
frzn thawed	½ cup (2.6 oz)	40	tr	10	6	4
LONGANS						
fresh	1	2	0	tr	–	–
LOQUATS						
fresh	1 sm (0.5 oz)	6	tr	2	–	tr
fresh	1 lg (0.7 oz)	9	tr	2	–	tr
fresh cubed	½ cup (2.6 oz)	35	tr	9	–	1
LOTUS						
root raw sliced	10 slices	45	tr	14	–	–
root sliced cooked	10 slices	59	tr	14	–	–
seeds dried	1 oz	94	1	18	–	–
LOX (*see* SALMON)						
LUPINES						
dried cooked	1 cup	197	5	16	–	–

FOOD	PORTION	CAL	FAT	CARB	SUGAR	FIBER
LYCHEES						
canned in syrup	½ cup (4.4 oz)	114	tr	29	28	1
canned in syrup	1 (0.7 oz)	19	tr	5	5	tr
dried	1 (2.5 g)	7	tr	2	2	tr
fresh	1 (0.3 oz)	6	tr	2	1	tr
fresh cut up	½ cup (3.3 oz)	63	tr	16	14	1
MACADAMIA NUTS						
dry roasted w/ salt	11 nuts (1 oz)	200	22	4	2	1
oil roasted	1 oz	204	22	4	–	–
MACE						
ground	1 tsp	8	1	1	–	tr
MACKEREL						
CANNED						
jack	1 can (12.7 oz)	563	23	0	0	0
jack	1 cup	296	12	0	0	0
Chicken Of The Sea						
Jack In Water	⅓ cup	90	4	0	0	0
FRESH						
atlantic cooked	3 oz	223	15	0	0	0
atlantic raw	3 oz	174	12	0	0	0
jack baked	3 oz	171	9	0	0	0
jack fillet baked	6.2 oz	354	18	0	0	0
king baked	3 oz	114	2	0	0	0
king fillet baked	5.4 oz	207	4	0	0	0
pacific baked	3 oz	171	9	0	0	0
pacific fillet baked	6.2 oz	354	18	0	0	0
spanish cooked	3 oz	134	5	0	0	0
spanish fillet cooked	1 (5.1 oz)	230	9	0	0	0
spanish raw	3 oz	118	5	0	0	0

FOOD	PORTION	CAL	FAT	CARB	SUGAR	FIBER
SMOKED						
atlantic	3.5 oz	296	24	0	0	0
MAHI MAHI						
fresh baked	4 oz	192	13	1	tr	0
MALANGA						
dasheen mashed	1 cup	226	tr	53	1	8
dasheen pieces boiled	1 cup	212	tr	50	1	8
pieces fried	1 cup	304	11	52	1	8
root raw	1 (10.7 oz)	299	1	72	–	5
MALT						
malt liquor	1 bottle (12 oz)	148	0	13	tr	tr
nonalcoholic	1 bottle (12 oz)	133	tr	29	29	0
MALTED MILK						
chocolate as prep w/ milk	1 cup	179	5	27	15	1
chocolate flavor powder	3 heaping tsp (0.7 oz)	79	1	18	5	1
natural flavor as prep w/ milk	1 cup	186	6	24	22	tr
natural flavor powder	3 heaping tsp (0.7 oz)	87	2	16	12	tr
MAMMY APPLE						
fresh	1	431	4	106	–	–
MANGO						
dried	1 slice (5 g)	16	tr	4	4	tr
dried	½ cup (1.8 oz)	74	tr	41	38	3
fresh	1 (7.3 oz)	135	1	35	31	4
fresh sliced	½ cup (3 oz)	54	tr	14	12	2
pickled	1 slice (1 oz)	38	tr	10	9	tr

FOOD	PORTION	CAL	FAT	CARB	SUGAR	FIBER
Crispy Green						
Crispy Mangoes	1 pkg (0.35 oz)	40	0	8	7	1
Crunchies						
Freeze Dried	¼ cup (6 g)	20	0	5	3	1
Crunchy N'Yummy						
Organic Freeze Dried	1 pkg (1 oz)	100	0	20	0	tr
Dole						
Chunks frzn	¾ cup (4.9 oz)	90	0	24	21	2
Fresh	½ (3.6 oz)	70	0	18	15	2
MANGO JUICE						
nectar canned	1 cup (8.8 oz)	128	tr	33	31	1
It Tastes RAAW						
Mango Guarana	8 oz	90	0	25	25	0
Naked						
Mighty Mango	8 oz	150	0	36	30	0
Old Orchard						
Nectar Cocktail	8 oz	75	0	17	17	–
Snapple						
Juice Drinks Mango Madness	8 oz	100	0	26	25	–
TreeTop						
100% Juice	8 oz	190	0	47	34	3
Ultra Lo-Gly						
Mango Mojito	1 bottle (10 oz)	35	0	8	7	0
Welch's						
Mango Twist Cocktail	8 oz	150	0	38	37	–
MANGOSTEEN						
canned in syrup	½ cup (3.4 oz)	72	1	18	–	2
Nature's Guru						
Instant Mangosteen Fruit Powder	1 pkg (0.9 oz)	70	0	18	3	0

FOOD	PORTION	CAL	FAT	CARB	SUGAR	FIBER
Xango						
Single Supplement	1 pkg (1 oz)	13	0	3	3	–
MARGARINE						
margarine butter blend	1 tbsp (0.5 oz)	101	11	tr	0	0
squeeze	1 pkg (0.2 oz)	36	4	0	0	0
squeeze liquid	1 tbsp (0.5 oz)	102	11	0	0	0
stick	1 stick (4 oz)	810	91	1	0	0
stick	1 tbsp (0.5 oz)	100	11	tr	0	0
tub diet	1 tbsp (0.5 oz)	26	3	tr	0	0
tub fat free	1 tbsp (0.5 oz)	27	tr	1	0	0
tub light	1 tbsp (0.5 oz)	59	7	tr	–	0
tub salted	1 tbsp (0.5 oz)	101	11	tr	0	0
whipped salted	1 tbsp (0.3 oz)	67	8	tr	0	0
Blue Bonnet						
Light Stick	1 tbsp (0.5 oz)	50	5	0	0	0
Soft Spread	1 tbsp (0.5 oz)	60	6	0	0	0
Soft Spread Light	1 tbsp (0.5 oz)	40	5	0	0	0
Sticks	1 tbsp (0.5 oz)	70	8	0	0	0
Brummel & Brown						
Spread w/ Natural Yogurt	1 tbsp (0.5 oz)	45	5	0	0	0
I Can't Believe It's Not Butter						
Original	1 tbsp (0.5 oz)	70	8	0	0	0
Original Soft	1 tbsp (0.5 oz)	70	8	0	0	0
Original Squeeze	1 tbsp (0.4 oz)	60	7	0	0	0
Spray	2 sprays (1 g)	0	0	0	0	0
Olivio						
Original Olive Oil	1 tbsp (0.5 oz)	80	8	0	0	0

FOOD	PORTION	CAL	FAT	CARB	SUGAR	FIBER
Parkay						
Original Spread	1 tbsp (0.4 oz)	70	7	0	0	0
Spray	5 sprays (1 g)	0	0	0	0	0
Squeeze	1 tbsp (0.5 oz)	70	8	0	0	0
Stick	1 tbsp (0.5 oz)	80	9	0	0	0
Promise						
Buttery Spread	1 tbsp (0.5 oz)	80	8	0	0	0
Smart Balance						
Butter Blend Stick	1 tbsp (0.5 g)	100	11	0	0	0
Buttery Spread 37% Light	1 tbsp (0.5 oz)	45	5	0	0	0
Buttery Spread Low Sodium	1 tbsp (0.4 oz)	65	7	0	0	0
Buttery Spread Omega Plus	1 tbsp (0.5 oz)	80	9	0	0	0
Buttery Spread Omega-3 w/ Extra Virgin Olive Oil	1 tbsp (0.4 oz)	60	7	0	0	0
Buttery Spread w/ Flax Oil	1 tbsp (0.5 oz)	80	9	0	0	0
Spray Buttery Burst w/ Organic Soy	5 sprays (1 g)	0	0	0	0	0
MARINADE (*see* SAUCE)						
MARIONBERRY JUICE						
TreeTop						
Grower's Best 100% Juice	8 oz	130	0	33	30	–
MARJORAM						
dried	1 tsp	2	tr	tr	tr	tr
MARLIN						
raw	3 oz	110	3	0	0	0

FOOD	PORTION	CAL	FAT	CARB	SUGAR	FIBER
MARSHMALLOW						
chocolate coated	1 (0.4 oz)	41	1	8	6	tr
coconut coated	1 (0.4 oz)	33	1	7	5	tr
marshmallow regular	1 (0.3 oz)	23	tr	6	4	0
miniatures	1 cup (1.8 oz)	159	tr	41	29	tr
miniatures	10 (0.3 oz)	22	tr	6	4	0
MATZO						
brie	1 piece (0.5 oz)	54	3	5	3	tr
egg	1 (1 oz)	109	1	22	–	1
matzo ball	1 med (1.2 oz)	48	2	6	tr	tr
plain	1 (1 oz)	111	tr	23	–	1
whole wheat	1 (1 oz)	98	tr	22	–	3
Manischewitz						
Egg	1 (1.2 oz)	100	0	20	0	0
Everything	1 (1 oz)	80	0	16	1	0
Farfel	¼ cup (0.6 oz)	70	0	14	1	0
Matzo	1 (1 oz)	110	0	24	0	0
Matzo Meal	¼ cup (1 oz)	110	0	23	1	1
Matzo Meal Whole Grain	¼ cup (1 oz)	120	1	24	1	4
Whole Wheat	1 (1 oz)	110	1	21	0	3
MAYONNAISE						
diet	1 tbsp	36	3	3	1	0
imitation	1 tbsp	35	3	2	1	0
mayonnaise	1 tbsp	99	11	1	tr	0
Baconnaise						
Lite	1 tbsp (0.5 oz)	30	3	2	0	0
Cains						
All Natural	1 tbsp (0.5 oz)	100	11	0	0	0
Fat Free	1 tbsp (0.5 oz)	10	0	2	1	0

FOOD	PORTION	CAL	FAT	CARB	SUGAR	FIBER
Light	1 tbsp (0.5 oz)	50	5	2	1	0
Sandwich Spread	1 tbsp (0.5 oz)	70	7	2	2	0
w/ Olive Oil	1 tbsp (0.5 oz)	50	5	1	tr	0
Dietz & Watson						
Mixed Pepper Mayo	1 tbsp (0.5 oz)	100	11	1	0	0
Hellman's						
Light	1 tbsp (0.5 oz)	35	4	tr	–	–
Miracle Whip						
Original	1 pkg (0.4 oz)	35	3	2	1	–
Nasoya						
Nayonaise Original	1 tbsp (0.5 oz)	35	4	1	0	0
Smart Balance						
Omega Plus Light	1 tbsp (0.5 oz)	50	5	2	–	–
Spectrum						
Canola Squeeze	1 tbsp (0.5 oz)	100	11	0	0	0
Canola Squeeze Light Eggless Vegan	1 tbsp (0.5 oz)	35	4	0	0	0

MEAT SUBSTITUTES (*see also* BACON SUBSTITUTES, CHICKEN SUBSTITUTES, HAMBURGER SUBSTITUTES, MEATBALL SUBSTITUTES, SAUSAGE SUBSTITUTES, TURKEY SUBSTITUTES)

FOOD	PORTION	CAL	FAT	CARB	SUGAR	FIBER
Gardein						
BBQ Pulled Shreds	1 serv (4.5 oz)	160	2	16	10	1
Beefless Tips	1 serv (3.5 oz)	120	3	7	0	3
Seasoned Bites	1 serv (4.4 oz)	130	3	8	0	2
Quorn						
Beef-Style Grounds	⅔ cup (3 oz)	90	2	9	1	5
Viana						
Veggie Doner Kebab	½ cup (3 oz)	210	14	3	2	2

FOOD	PORTION	CAL	FAT	CARB	SUGAR	FIBER
MEATBALL SUBSTITUTES						
meatless	2 (1.3 oz)	71	3	3	tr	2
Franklin Farms						
Portabella Veggiballs Gluten Free	3 (3 oz)	140	1	18	3	4
Morningstar Farms						
Meal Starters Veggie Meatballs	5 (2.8 oz)	130	5	7	tr	3
Nate's						
Classic	3 (1.5 oz)	90	5	5	tr	2
Savory Mushroom	3 (1.5 oz)	100	5	6	tr	2
Zesty Italian	3 (1.5 oz)	90	5	4	tr	2
Quorn						
Meatless Meatballs	3–4 (2.4 oz)	90	2	7	1	1
Veggie Patch						
Meatless	4 (3 oz)	120	5	7	1	4
MEATBALLS						
beef cocktail	1 (0.2 oz)	18	1	0	0	0
beef	1 med (1 oz)	74	5	0	0	0
beef	1 lg (1.5 oz)	111	7	0	0	0
chicken cocktail	1 (0.2 oz)	12	tr	1	tr	0
chicken	1 med (1 oz)	47	2	2	1	tr
chicken	1 lg (1.5 oz)	71	3	3	1	tr
turkey med	1 (1 oz)	47	2	2	1	tr
venison	1 (1.5 oz)	69	3	3	1	tr
Al Fresco						
Chicken Teriyaki Ginger	4 (3 oz)	200	8	11	8	0
Chicken Tomato & Basil	4 (3 oz)	160	9	4	2	0
Coleman						
Chicken Buffalo Style	4	160	12	1	0	0
Chicken Chipotle Cheddar	4 (2.6 oz)	180	14	1	0	0

FOOD	PORTION	CAL	FAT	CARB	SUGAR	FIBER
Chicken Italian w/ Parmesan	7 (2.6 oz)	150	10	1	0	1
Chicken Pesto Parmesan	4 (2.6 oz)	170	12	1	0	0
Chicken Spinach Fontina Cheese & Roasted Garlic	4 (2.6 oz)	130	9	0	0	0
Chicken Sun-Dried Tomato Basil & Provolone	4 (2.6 oz)	150	9	2	0	0
Dinty Moore						
Meatball Stew	½ can	250	15	19	3	1
Farm Rich						
Original	6 (3 oz)	240	20	3	1	2
Turkey	5 (3.1 oz)	150	9	4	1	2
Foster Farms						
Turkey	3 (2.9 oz)	150	7	8	tr	0
Hans All Natural						
Chicken Buffalo Style	4	160	12	1	0	0
Chicken Sweet Basil Parmesan	4	170	12	1	0	0
Mom Made						
Bite-Size Turkey	9 (3 oz)	140	4	9	1	0
Saffron Road						
Lamb Koftis w/ Rice	1 pkg (11 oz)	340	11	45	8	4
Shady Brook						
Turkey Meatballs Appetizer Size + Sweet & Sour Sauce	6 + 2 tbsp sauce	235	10	17	11	tr
TAKE-OUT						
albondigas w/ sauce	3 + sauce (5.3 oz)	372	27	11	3	1

FOOD	PORTION	CAL	FAT	CARB	SUGAR	FIBER
porcupine w/ tomato sauce	3 + sauce	160	7	14	3	1
swedish w/ cream sauce	3 + sauce (4.7 oz)	215	12	9	2	tr
sweet & sour	3 + sauce (4.5 oz)	188	11	8	1	1

MEXICAN FOOD (*see* SALSA, SPANISH FOOD, TORTILLA)

MILK

FOOD	PORTION	CAL	FAT	CARB	SUGAR	FIBER
CANNED						
condensed sweetened	1 cup (10.7 oz)	982	27	166	166	0
condensed sweetened	1 tbsp (0.7 oz)	61	2	10	10	0
evaporated nonfat	1 cup (9 oz)	200	1	29	29	0
evaporated nonfat	1 tbsp (0.5 oz)	12	tr	2	2	1
Borden						
Sweetened Condensed	2 tbsp (1.4 oz)	130	3	22	22	0
Meyenberg						
Goat Evaporated	4 oz	145	8	10	10	–
DRIED						
buttermilk	1 tbsp (0.2 oz)	25	tr	3	3	0
buttermilk	¼ cup (1 oz)	111	2	14	14	0
nonfat instant	1 pkg (3.2 oz)	326	1	47	47	0
nonfat instant	1 tbsp (0.6 oz)	61	tr	9	9	0
whole milk	¼ cup (1.1 oz)	159	9	12	12	0
Meyenberg						
Goat Powdered	1 scoop (1 oz)	90	0	11	11	0
REFRIGERATED						
1%	1 cup (8.6 oz)	102	3	12	13	0
2%	1 cup (8.6 oz)	122	5	11	12	0
buffalo	7 oz	224	16	10	–	–
buttermilk lowfat	1 cup (8.6 oz)	98	2	12	12	0
camel	7 oz	160	8	10	–	–

FOOD	PORTION	CAL	FAT	CARB	SUGAR	FIBER
donkey	7 oz	86	2	12	–	–
fat free	1 cup (8.6 oz)	83	tr	12	12	0
goat	1 cup (8.6 oz)	168	10	11	11	0
human	1 cup (8.6 oz)	172	11	17	7	0
indian buffalo	1 cup (8.6 oz)	237	17	13	–	0
mare	7 oz	98	4	12	–	–
sheep	1 cup (8.6 oz)	265	17	13	–	0
whole	1 cup (8.6 oz)	146	8	11	14	0
Horizon						
Fat Free	8 oz	90	0	12	12	0
Lowfat 1%	8 oz	100	3	12	12	0
Reduced Fat 2%	8 oz	120	5	12	12	0
Whole	8 oz	150	8	12	12	0
Lactaid						
Fit & Creamy Lowfat	8 oz	120	3	12	12	0
Whole	8 oz	160	8	12	12	0
Meyenberg						
Goat Low Fat	8 oz	89	2	9	9	–
Goat Whole	8 oz	142	7	11	11	–
Over The Moon						
Fat Free	8 oz	120	0	17	16	0
Low Fat	8 oz	120	3	14	13	0
Smart Balance						
Fat Free w/ Omega-3s & Vitamin E	1 cup (8 oz)	120	0	15	15	–
Straus						
Organic Cream Top Whole	8 oz	150	8	11	11	0
Organic Fat Free	8 oz	90	0	12	12	0
Organic Whole Milk	8 oz	170	7	14	7	0
MILK DRINKS						
chocolate milk	1 cup (8.8 oz)	208	8	26	24	2
chocolate milk lowfat	1 cup (8.8 oz)	158	3	26	25	1

FOOD	PORTION	CAL	FAT	CARB	SUGAR	FIBER
DrSears						
Cool Fuel Chocolate	1 pkg (8 oz)	190	6	25	9	4
Cool Fuel Chocolate Banana	1 pkg (8 oz)	190	6	28	9	4
Cool Fuel Vanilla	1 pkg (8 oz)	190	6	28	9	4
Lactaid						
Chocolate Milk 1% Fat	8 oz	150	3	24	23	tr
MojoMilk						
Chocolate Mix not prep	1 pkg (4.5 g)	20	1	4	2	0
Probiotic Chocolate Milk not prep	1 pkg (4.5 g)	20	1	4	2	0
Over The Moon						
Chocolate Milk Fat Free	8 oz	150	0	27	25	tr
Rockin' Recovery						
Intense Recovery Protein Fortified Lowfat Milk Chocolate	1 bottle (12 oz)	300	5	48	44	1
Intense Recovery Protein Fortified Lowfat Milk Vanilla	1 bottle (12 oz)	280	4	45	42	0
Muscle Builder Protein Fortified Milk Chocolate	1 bottle (12 oz)	190	5	12	6	3
Muscle Recovery Protein Fortified Lowfat Milk Chocolate No Sugar Added	1 bottle (12 oz)	240	4	35	23	1
Refuel Protein Fortified Lowfat Milk Strawberry	1 bottle (12 oz)	280	4	45	42	0
TruMoo						
Chocolate Milk Fat Free	8 oz	130	0	24	22	0
Chocolate Milk Lowfat	8 oz	150	3	24	22	0
Strawberry Milk Fat Free	8 oz	130	0	23	22	0

FOOD	PORTION	CAL	FAT	CARB	SUGAR	FIBER
MILK SUBSTITUTES						
soy milk	1 cup	79	5	4	–	–
Good Karma						
Flax Milk Original	8 oz	60	3	11	11	0
Flax Milk Unsweetened	8 oz	25	3	1	0	0
Flax Milk Vanilla	8 oz	60	3	11	11	0
Whole Grain Rice Original Organic	8 oz	100	3	19	9	3
Whole Grain Rice Vanilla Organic	8 oz	120	3	26	13	3
Pacific Foods						
7 Grain Original Organic	1 cup (8 oz)	140	2	27	16	1
Almond Original Unsweetened Organic	8 oz	35	3	2	0	0
Hazelnut Original	8 oz	110	4	18	14	1
Hemp Original	8 oz	140	5	20	14	1
Oat Original Organic	1 cup (8 oz)	130	3	24	19	2
Rice All Natural Plain	1 cup (8 oz)	130	2	27	14	0
Soy Original Unsweetened Organic	1 cup (8 oz)	90	5	4	2	2
Soy Ultra Plain	1 cup (8 oz)	120	4	11	8	1
Pearl						
Organic Soymilk Coffee	8 oz	150	4	24	22	0
Organic Soymilk Green Tea	8 oz	110	4	13	10	1
Organic Soymilk Original	8 oz	110	4	12	9	1
Simpli						
Naked Oat Vanilla	8 oz	100	3	18	10	2
Sol						
Sunflower Original	8 oz	70	4	9	7	1
Sunflower Unsweetened	8 oz	45	4	2	0	1
Sunflower Vanilla	8 oz	90	4	14	12	1

FOOD	PORTION	CAL	FAT	CARB	SUGAR	FIBER
Sunrich Naturals						
Soymilk Original Plain	8 oz	110	5	11	9	1
Soymilk Vanilla	8 oz	130	5	14	11	1
Vitasoy						
Organic Lite Plus Original	8 oz	60	2	6	5	0
Organic Lite Plus Vanilla	8 oz	80	2	12	11	0
Organic Mint Chocolate	8 oz	160	4	27	24	1
Organic Original	8 oz	90	4	9	7	1
Organic Vanilla	8 oz	110	4	14	12	1
MILKFISH (AWA)						
baked	4 oz	215	10	0	0	0
MILKSHAKE						
chocolate	1 serv (10.6 oz)	357	8	63	63	1
malted milk shake	1 serv (10 oz)	402	14	62	58	1
vanilla	1 (11 oz)	351	9	56	56	0
Special K						
Protein Shake Dark Chocolate	1 bottle (10 oz)	190	5	29	18	5
MILLET						
cooked	1 cup (6.1 oz)	207	2	41	–	2
MINERAL WATER (*see* WATER)						
MISO						
dried	1 oz	86	3	10	–	1
miso	½ cup	284	8	39	–	7
MOLASSES						
blackstrap	1 tbsp (0.7 oz)	47	0	12	–	–
molasses	¼ cup (3 oz)	244	tr	63	47	0
molasses	1 tbsp (0.7 oz)	58	tr	15	11	0

FOOD	PORTION	CAL	FAT	CARB	SUGAR	FIBER
MONKFISH						
baked	3 oz	82	2	0	0	0
MOOSE						
roasted	4 oz	142	1	0	0	0
MOTH BEANS						
dried cooked	1 cup	207	1	37	–	–
MOUSSE						
TAKE-OUT						
chocolate	½ cup	454	32	32	30	1
fish timbale	1 cup	329	25	3	1	0
MUFFIN						
MIX						
Betty Crocker						
Banana Nut as prep	1	120	3	22	10	0
Blueberry as prep	1	120	3	23	11	–
Cornbread Muffin as prep	1	160	6	24	5	tr
Fiber One Banana Nut as prep	1	170	7	27	12	5
Fiber One Blueberry as prep	1	160	6	30	13	5
Lemon Poppyseed as prep	1	200	8	29	17	–
Jiffy						
Banana as prep	1	170	6	27	10	tr
Bran w/ Dates as prep	1	160	6	24	9	2
Corn as prep	1	170	6	27	7	tr
Oatmeal as prep	1	170	6	27	8	tr
VitaMuffin						
Deep Chocolate as prep	1 (2 oz)	100	2	26	11	9
Golden Corn as prep	1 (2 oz)	100	0	24	7	5

FOOD	PORTION	CAL	FAT	CARB	SUGAR	FIBER
READY-TO-EAT						
Do Goodie						
Gluten Free Banana Nut	1	180	9	24	20	1
Foods By George						
Gluten Free Blueberry	1 (2.8 oz)	220	8	33	11	1
Udi's						
Gluten Free Double Chocolate	1 (4 oz)	350	15	52	32	3
Uncle Wally's						
Apple Cinnamon Rich & Moist	1 (4 oz)	380	18	51	29	1
Blueberry Rich & Moist	1 (4 oz)	370	18	49	27	1
Cheesecake Rich & Moist	1 (4 oz)	390	19	50	27	0
Chocolate Passion Fat Free	½ (2 oz)	120	0	28	16	0
Corn Rich & Moist	1 (4 oz)	400	18	55	27	1
Cranberry Apple Smart Portion	1 (1.1 oz)	80	1	17	9	2
Cranberry Orange Supreme Fat Free	½ (2 oz)	140	0	32	19	1
Fiber One Banana Chocolate Chip	1 (2.3 oz)	180	5	36	19	7
Fiber One Wild Blueberry & Oats	1 (2.3 oz)	170	4	33	16	7
Honey Raisin Bran Fat Free	½ (2 oz)	140	0	32	19	1
My Sweet Multi Bran Sugar Free	1 (2 oz)	120	3	28	1	1
Pineapple Coconut Rich & Moist	1 (4 oz)	390	19	51	19	1
Sweet Chocolate Dreams Sugar Free	1 (2 oz)	130	3	29	1	1

FOOD	PORTION	CAL	FAT	CARB	SUGAR	FIBER
Wild Blueberry Bliss Fat Free	½ (2 oz)	110	0	25	14	1
VitaMuffin						
Banana Nut	1 (2 oz)	100	2	19	3	5
Banana Nut Sugar Free	1 (2 oz)	90	3	21	0	5
VitaTop						
Apple Crumb	1 (2 oz)	100	1	25	7	8
BlueBran	1 (2 oz)	100	1	20	9	5
CranBran	1 (2 oz)	100	1	22	11	5
Deep Chocolate	1 (2 oz)	100	2	26	11	9
Golden Corn	1 (2 oz)	100	1	27	9	10
Raisin Bran	1 (2 oz)	100	1	22	11	5
TAKE-OUT						
blueberry	1 (5 oz)	546	27	69	38	2
corn	1 lg (5 oz)	424	12	71	10	5
oat bran	1 lg (5 oz)	375	10	67	11	6
pumpkin w/ raisins & nuts	1 med (4 oz)	351	8	67	43	2
MULBERRIES						
fresh	½ cup (2.5 oz)	30	tr	7	6	1
fresh	20 (1 oz)	13	tr	3	2	1
MULLET						
striped cooked	3 oz	127	4	0	0	0
striped raw	3 oz	99	3	0	0	0
MUNG BEANS						
dried cooked	1 cup	213	1	39	–	–
TruRoots						
Organic Sprouted not prep	¼ cup (1.4 oz)	140	1	30	1	7
MUNGO BEANS						
dried cooked	1 cup	190	1	33	–	–

FOOD	PORTION	CAL	FAT	CARB	SUGAR	FIBER
MUSHROOMS						
CANNED						
caps	8 (1.6 oz)	12	tr	2	1	1
caps pickled	6 (0.8 oz)	5	tr	1	tr	tr
chanterelle	3.5 oz	12	1	tr	–	6
pickled	1 cup	33	tr	5	2	1
pieces	½ cup	20	tr	2	1	1
straw	1 cup	58	1	8	–	5
Jake & Amos						
Pickled Dill Mushrooms	1 serv (1 oz)	5	0	1	0	tr
Victoria						
Marinated	¼ cup (1 oz)	20	2	1	0	0
DRIED						
chanterelle	1 oz	25	tr	tr	–	17
shiitake	1 (3.6 g)	11	tr	3	tr	tr
tree ear	½ cup (0.4 oz)	36	tr	10	–	–
wood ear mok yee	½ cup (0.4 oz)	25	tr	8	–	4
FRESH						
brown italian or crimini sliced	1 cup	19	tr	3	1	tr
brown italian or crimini whole	1 (0.7 oz)	5	tr	1	tr	tr
chanterelle	3.5 oz	11	tr	tr	–	6
enoki raw	1 lg (5 g)	2	tr	tr	tr	tr
enoki sliced	1 cup	29	tr	5	tr	2
enoki whole	1 cup	28	tr	5	tr	2
maitake diced	1 cup	26	tr	5	1	2
maitake whole	1 (6.6 g)	2	tr	tr	tr	tr
morel	3.5 oz	9	tr	0	–	7
oyster	1 sm (0.5 oz)	5	tr	1	tr	tr
oyster sliced	1 cup	30	tr	6	1	2
portabella raw	1 cap (3 oz)	22	tr	4	2	1
portabella sliced grilled	1 cup (4.2 oz)	42	1	6	0	3

FOOD	PORTION	CAL	FAT	CARB	SUGAR	FIBER
shiitake cooked	4 (2.5 oz)	40	tr	10	3	2
shiitake pieces cooked	1 cup	81	tr	21	5	3
white	1 (0.6 oz)	4	tr	1	tr	tr
white sliced cooked	1 cup	28	tr	4	0	2
white sliced raw	½ cup	8	tr	1	1	tr
Dole						
Raw	½ cup (1.2 oz)	9	0	1	0	0
FROZEN						
Farm Rich						
Breaded	5 (3 oz)	120	2	23	0	1
TAKE-OUT						
battered fried	1 lg (0.6 oz)	39	3	3	1	tr
creamed	1 cup	171	11	15	7	3
stuffed	1 (0.8 oz)	67	4	6	1	1
MUSKRAT						
roasted	3 oz	199	10	0	0	0
MUSSELS						
blue raw	3 oz	73	2	3	–	–
blue raw	1 cup	129	3	6	–	–
fresh blue cooked	3 oz	147	4	6	–	–
MUSTARD						
dry mustard	1 tsp	15	1	1	–	–
hot chinese	1 tsp	3	tr	tr	tr	tr
organic yellow	1 tsp	5	0	0	0	0
seed	1 tsp	15	1	1	tr	1
yellow prepared	1 tbsp	3	tr	tr	tr	tr
Annie's Homegrown						
Organic Dijon	1 tsp (5 g)	5	0	1	–	–
Beaver						
Chinese Extra Hot	1 tsp (5 g)	10	1	1	–	–
Hickory Bacon	1 tsp (5 g)	10	0	1	0	0

FOOD	PORTION	CAL	FAT	CARB	SUGAR	FIBER
Dietz & Watson						
Champagne Dill	1 tsp (5 g)	5	0	0	0	0
Yellow	1 tsp (5 g)	0	0	0	0	0
Gold's						
New York Deli	1 tsp (5 g)	0	0	0	0	0
Gulden's						
Spicy Brown	1 tsp	5	0	0	0	0
Inglehoffer						
Organic Honey	1 tsp (5 g)	10	0	3	2	–
Organic Stone Ground	1 tsp (5)	10	0	1	–	–
Wasabi	1 tsp (5 g)	10	1	1	–	–
Jack & Amos						
Sweet Dipping	1 tbsp (0.5 oz)	30	1	5	4	0
OrganicVille						
Stone Ground No Sugar Added	1 tbsp (5 g)	5	0	0	0	0
Zatarain's						
Creole	1 tsp (7 g)	10	1	tr	0	0
MUSTARD GREENS						
canned	1 cup	23	tr	3	tr	3
fresh as prep w/ fat	1 cup	50	3	3	tr	3
fresh chopped boiled w/o salt	1 cup	21	tr	3	tr	3
fresh raw chopped	1 cup	15	tr	3	1	2
frozen chopped boiled w/o salt	1 cup	28	tr	5	tr	4
NAVY BEANS						
canned	1 cup	296	1	54	–	–
dried cooked	1 cup	259	1	48	–	–
NECTARINE						
fresh	1 sm (4.5 oz)	57	tr	14	10	2

FOOD	PORTION	CAL	FAT	CARB	SUGAR	FIBER
fresh	1 lg (5.5 oz)	69	1	16	12	3
fresh sliced	1 cup (5 oz)	63	tr	15	11	2
Dole						
Fresh	1 med (5 oz)	60	0	15	11	2
NEUFCHATEL						
neufchatel	1 pkg (3 oz)	215	19	3	3	0
neufchatel	1 oz	72	6	1	1	0
Philadelphia						
⅓ Less Fat	1 oz	70	6	1	1	0
NONI JUICE						
Snapple						
Juice Drink Low Calorie Metabolism Noni Berry	8 oz	15	0	2	1	–
NOODLES						
cellophane	1 cup	492	tr	121	–	–
chow mein	1 cup (1.6 oz)	237	14	25	–	2
egg	1 cup (38 g)	145	2	27	–	–
egg cooked	1 cup (5.6 oz)	213	2	40	–	2
japanese soba cooked	1 cup (4 oz)	113	tr	24	–	–
japanese somen cooked	1 cup (6.2 oz)	231	tr	48	–	–
korean acorn noodles not prep	2 oz	195	tr	41	–	tr
rice cooked	1 cup (6.2 oz)	192	tr	44	–	2
spinach/egg cooked	1 cup (5.6 oz)	211	3	39	–	4
Krasdale						
Egg Wide not prep	1 cup (2 oz)	210	2	41	2	2
Light 'N Fluffy						
Egg Extra Wide not prep	⅙ pkg (2 oz)	210	3	40	2	2
Manischewitz						
Egg Fine not prep	1½ cups (2 oz)	210	3	39	2	2

FOOD	PORTION	CAL	FAT	CARB	SUGAR	FIBER
Whole Grain Yolk Free Extra Wide not prep	1¼ cups (2 oz)	180	1	40	2	6
Yolk Free Medium	1¾ cups (2 oz)	210	1	40	2	2
NoOodle						
All Natural	1 serv (1.6 oz)	0	0	1	tr	0
Pennsylvania Dutch						
Fine Egg not prep	1 cup (2 oz)	220	3	40	2	2
Ronzoni						
Healthy Harvest Whole Grain Extra Wide not prep	2 oz	180	1	41	0	6
Streit's						
Egg Wide not prep	1¾ cups (2 oz)	210	3	39	2	2

NUT BUTTER (*see also* INDIVIDUAL NUT NAMES, PEANUT BUTTER)

FOOD	PORTION	CAL	FAT	CARB	SUGAR	FIBER
NuttZo						
Original Omega-3 Multi-Nut	2 tbsp (1.1 oz)	180	16	7	1	3

NUTMEG

FOOD	PORTION	CAL	FAT	CARB	SUGAR	FIBER
ground	1 tsp	12	1	1	1	1
nutmeg butter	1 tbsp	120	14	0	0	0

NUTRITION SUPPLEMENTS (*see also* CEREAL BARS, ENERGY BARS, ENERGY DRINKS)

FOOD	PORTION	CAL	FAT	CARB	SUGAR	FIBER
BANa						
Hydration Drink	1 bottle (16.9 oz)	0	0	1	–	–
Be Happy						
Health Guard	1 bottle (2 oz)	40	0	10	9	0
Cirku						
Beverage Mix Summer Citrus	1 pkg (0.23 oz)	15	0	3	–	–

FOOD	PORTION	CAL	FAT	CARB	SUGAR	FIBER
Joint Juice						
Cranberry Pomegranate	1 bottle (8 oz)	20	0	5	2	–
Easy Shot Glucosamine Chondroitin	2.5 tbsp (1.25 oz)	15	0	3	2	–
Easy Shot Hyal-Joint	2.5 tbsp (1.25 oz)	15	0	3	2	–
On The Go Blueberry Acai	1 pkg (6 g)	20	0	4	–	–
Mix1						
Lean Performance All Fruit Flavors	1 bottle (11 oz)	90	1	10	7	3
Lean Performance Chocolate or Vanilla	1 bottle (11 oz)	90	1	14	9	3
Nutrition Shake All Flavors	1 bottle (11 oz)	200	3	29	22	3
Orgain						
Organic Meal Replacement All Flavors	1 pkg (11 oz)	255	7	32	12	2
Premier						
Protein Shake Chocolate	1 (11 oz)	160	3	5	1	3
Protein Shake Strawberry	1 (11 oz)	160	3	3	1	2
Protein Shake Vanilla	1 (11 oz)	160	3	3	1	2
Special K						
Protein Meal Bar Chocolate Caramel	1 (1.59 oz)	170	5	25	15	5

NUTS MIXED (*see also* INDIVIDUAL NUT NAMES)

FOOD	PORTION	CAL	FAT	CARB	SUGAR	FIBER
dry roasted w/ peanuts salted	¼ cup	203	18	9	–	3
dry roasted w/ peanuts w/o salt	¼ cup	203	18	9	–	3
mixed nuts chocolate covered	¼ cup (1.5 oz)	240	17	20	17	2

FOOD	PORTION	CAL	FAT	CARB	SUGAR	FIBER
oil roasted w/o peanuts salted	¼ cup	221	20	8	2	2
oil roasted w/o peanuts w/o salt	¼ cup	221	20	8	–	2
Frito Lay						
Deluxe Mixed	¼ cup	170	16	6	1	2
Planters						
Bar Big Triple Nut	1 (1.6 oz)	220	12	22	12	3
Lightly Salted	1 oz	170	15	5	1	2
Mixed	1 oz	170	15	5	1	2
Nut-rition Men's Health	28 (1 oz)	170	15	5	1	3
Unsalted	1 oz	170	15	5	1	2
Simple Squares						
Nut & Honey Bar Rosemary	1 (1.6 oz)	230	17	16	10	3
Nut & Honey Bar Sage	1 (1.6 oz)	230	17	16	10	3
Whole Food Bar Cinnamon Clove	1 (1.6 oz)	230	17	16	9	3
OCTOPUS						
dried boiled	3 oz	144	2	4	0	0
fresh steamed	3 oz	139	2	4	0	0
smoked	1 oz	40	1	1	0	0
Matiz						
Pulpo In Olive Oil	½ pkg (2 oz)	107	5	3	0	0
TAKE-OUT						
ensalada de pulpo	1 cup	299	21	10	4	2
OHELOBERRIES						
fresh	1 cup	39	tr	10	–	–
OIL						
almond	1 tbsp	120	14	0	0	0
almond	1 cup	1927	218	0	0	0
apricot kernel	1 tbsp	120	14	0	0	0

FOOD	PORTION	CAL	FAT	CARB	SUGAR	FIBER
apricot kernel	1 cup	1927	218	0	0	0
avocado	1 cup	1927	218	0	0	0
avocado	1 tbsp	124	14	0	0	0
babassu palm	1 tbsp	120	14	0	0	0
butter oil	1 cup	1795	204	0	0	0
butter oil	1 tbsp	112	13	0	0	0
canola	1 cup	1927	218	0	0	0
canola	1 tbsp	124	14	0	0	0
coconut	1 tbsp	117	14	0	0	0
corn	1 cup	1927	218	0	0	0
corn	1 tbsp	120	14	0	0	0
cottonseed	1 tbsp	120	14	0	0	0
cottonseed	1 cup	1927	218	0	0	0
cupu assu	1 tbsp	120	14	0	0	0
garlic oil	1 tbsp	150	17	0	0	0
grapeseed	1 tbsp	120	14	0	0	0
hazelnut	1 cup	1927	218	0	0	0
hazelnut	1 tbsp	120	14	0	0	0
mustard	1 cup	1927	218	0	0	0
mustard	1 tbsp	124	14	0	0	0
oat	1 tbsp	120	14	0	0	0
olive	1 cup	1909	216	0	0	0
olive	1 tbsp	119	14	0	0	0
palm	1 tbsp	120	14	0	0	0
palm	1 cup	1927	218	0	0	0
palm kernel	1 cup	1879	218	0	0	0
palm kernel	1 tbsp	117	14	0	0	0
peanut	1 cup	1909	216	0	0	0
peanut	1 tbsp	119	14	0	0	0
peppermint	1 tsp	42	4	0	0	0
poppyseed	1 tbsp	120	14	0	0	0
pumpkin seed	1 oz	217	29	0	0	0
rice bran	1 tbsp	120	14	0	0	0

FOOD	PORTION	CAL	FAT	CARB	SUGAR	FIBER
safflower	1 cup	1927	218	0	0	0
safflower	1 tbsp	120	14	0	0	0
sesame	1 tbsp	120	14	0	0	0
sheanut	1 tbsp	120	14	0	0	0
soybean	1 tbsp	120	14	0	0	0
soybean	1 cup	1927	218	0	0	0
sunflower	1 cup	1927	218	0	0	0
sunflower	1 tbsp	120	14	0	0	0
teaseed	1 tbsp	120	14	0	0	0
tomatoseed	1 tbsp	120	14	0	0	0
vegetable	1 cup	1927	218	0	0	0
vegetable	1 tbsp	120	14	0	0	0
walnut	1 cup	1927	218	0	0	0
walnut	1 tbsp	120	14	0	0	0
wheat germ	1 tbsp	120	14	0	0	0
Annie's Homegrown						
Basil Oil	1 tbsp (0.5 oz)	120	14	0	0	0
Dipping Oil	1 tbsp (0.5 oz)	100	11	0	0	0
Azukar Organics						
Virgin Coconut	1 tbsp (0.5 oz)	125	14	0	0	0
Bella Sun Luci						
Olive Extra Virgin Cold Pressed	1 tbsp (0.5 oz)	120	14	0	0	0
Carotino						
Palm Fruit Oil	1 tbsp (0.5 oz)	121	14	0	0	0
Red Palm & Canola	1 tbsp	120	14	0	0	0
Gaea						
Olive Carbon Neutral	1 tbsp (0.5 oz)	130	14	0	0	0

FOOD	PORTION	CAL	FAT	CARB	SUGAR	FIBER
LouAna						
Canola	1 tbsp (0.5 oz)	120	14	0	0	0
Pam						
All Varieties	¼ sec spray	0	0	0	0	0
Penny's PopSurprise						
Organic Extra Virgin Olive Spicy	1 tbsp (0.5 oz)	130	14	0	0	0
Pillsbury						
Baking Spray w/ Flour	⅙ sec spray	0	0	0	0	0
Planters						
100% Pure Peanut	1 tbsp (0.5 oz)	120	14	0	0	0
Sadaf						
Avocado Cold Pressed	1 tbsp (0.5 oz)	130	14	0	0	0
Grapeseed	1 tbsp (0.5 oz)	120	14	0	0	0
Light Olive	1 tbsp (0.5 oz)	120	14	0	0	0
Smart Balance						
Omega Oil	1 tbsp (0.5 oz)	120	14	0	0	0
Sonoma Gourmet						
Dip-N-Toss Olive Oil Basil Parmesan	1 tbsp (0.5 oz)	120	0	0	0	0
Spectrum						
Almond	1 tbsp (0.5 oz)	120	14	0	0	0
Apricot Kernel	1 tbsp (0.5 oz)	120	14	0	0	0
Avocado	1 tbsp (0.5 oz)	120	14	0	0	0

FOOD	PORTION	CAL	FAT	CARB	SUGAR	FIBER
Coconut Organic	1 tbsp (0.5 oz)	120	14	0	0	0
Grapeseed	1 tbsp (0.5 oz)	120	14	0	0	0
Olive Organic	1 tbsp (0.5 oz)	120	14	0	0	0
Sesame	1 tbsp (0.5 oz)	120	14	0	0	0
Walnut	1 tbsp (0.5 oz)	120	14	0	0	0
OKRA						
CANNED						
pickled	6 pods (2.3 oz)	18	tr	4	1	2
FRESH						
cooked w/ salt	8 pods	19	tr	4	2	2
luffa chinese okra cooked	1 cup	39	tr	8	4	4
sliced cooked w/ salt	½ cup	18	tr	4	2	2
TAKE-OUT						
batter dipped fried	10 pieces (2.6 oz)	142	10	12	3	2
OLIVES						
black	2 med (0.3 oz)	8	1	tr	0	tr
greek	1 (0.5 oz)	16	1	1	0	tr
green	1 sm (0.2 oz)	8	1	tr	tr	tr
green	2 med (0.2 oz)	10	1	tr	tr	tr
green	2 lg (0.3 oz)	11	1	tr	tr	tr
green	2 extra lg (0.5 oz)	19	2	1	tr	tr
green chopped	¼ cup (1.2 oz)	48	5	1	tr	1
green olive tapenade	1 tbsp	25	3	1	1	0
green stuffed	2 sm (0.2 oz)	9	1	tr	tr	tr

FOOD	PORTION	CAL	FAT	CARB	SUGAR	FIBER
green stuffed	2 med (0.3 oz)	10	1	tr	tr	tr
green stuffed	2 lg (0.3 oz)	12	1	tr	tr	tr
green stuffed	¼ cup (1.3 oz)	47	5	1	tr	1
ripe	2 sm (0.2 oz)	7	1	tr	0	tr
ripe	2 lg (0.3 oz)	10	1	1	0	tr
ripe	2 extra lg (0.4 oz)	12	1	1	0	tr
ripe sliced	¼ cup (1.2 oz)	35	3	2	0	1
spanish stuffed	5 (0.5 oz)	15	1	1	0	0
Martinis						
Kalamata Pitted	4 (0.5 oz)	40	4	tr	0	tr
Matiz						
Olivada Spread Sweet	2 tbsp	87	6	9	9	1
Olivada Spread Traditional & Hot	2 tbsp	114	12	3	tr	2
Priorat Natur						
Natural Olives	10	30	3	1	tr	1
Progresso						
Tapenade	1 tbsp (0.5 oz)	20	2	1	0	0
Sadaf						
Sun Dried Oil Cured	2 (0.5 oz)	15	2	1	–	–
Victoria						
Almond Stuffed	2 (0.5 oz)	25	3	tr	0	0
Calamata	2 (0.5 oz)	30	3	2	0	2
Gaeta	3 (0.5 oz)	45	3	3	0	0
Jalapeno Stuffed	2 (0.5 oz)	20	2	tr	0	0
Manzanilla Stuffed	5 (0.5 oz)	25	3	tr	0	0
Queen Stuffed	2 (0.5 oz)	20	2	tr	0	0
Zatarain's						
Cocktail	7 (0.5 oz)	25	3	0	0	0
Stuffed	6 (0.5 oz)	25	3	0	0	0

FOOD	PORTION	CAL	FAT	CARB	SUGAR	FIBER
ONION						
CANNED						
cocktail	½ cup	41	tr	9	4	2
Dietz & Watson						
Sweet Vidalia In Sauce	1 tbsp (0.5 oz)	12	0	3	0	0
McSweet						
Pickled Onions	4 (1 oz)	10	0	2	tr	0
DRIED						
flakes	1 tbsp	17	tr	4	2	1
powder	1 tsp	7	tr	2	1	tr
shallots	1 tbsp	3	0	1	–	–
Seneca						
Crisp Onions	1 tbsp (7 g)	40	3	4	1	0
FRESH						
cooked w/o salt	1 sm (2 oz)	26	tr	6	3	1
cooked w/o salt	1 med (3.3 oz)	41	tr	10	4	1
cooked w/o salt	1 lg (4.5 oz)	56	tr	13	6	2
cooked w/o salt chopped	1 tbsp	7	tr	2	1	tr
raw chopped	½ cup	32	tr	7	3	1
raw chopped	1 tbsp	4	tr	1	tr	tr
raw slice	1 (0.5 oz)	6	tr	1	1	tr
raw sliced	½ cup	23	tr	5	2	1
scallions raw	1 med (0.5 oz)	5	tr	1	tr	tr
scallions raw chopped	¼ cup	8	tr	2	1	1
shallots raw chopped	¼ cup	29	tr	7	–	–
sweet whole raw	1 (11.6 oz)	106	tr	25	17	3
whole raw	1 sm (2.5 oz)	28	tr	7	3	1
whole raw	1 med (4 oz)	44	tr	10	5	2
whole raw	1 lg (5.3 oz)	60	tr	14	6	3
Bland Farms						
Vidalia Sweet	1 (5 oz)	60	0	14	5	3

FOOD	PORTION	CAL	FAT	CARB	SUGAR	FIBER
RealSweet						
Vidalia	1 (5.2 oz)	45	0	11	9	3
TAKE-OUT						
creamed	1 cup	187	9	22	10	2
fried	½ cup	57	5	3	tr	1
rings breaded & fried	8 to 9 (3 oz)	276	16	31	–	–
OPOSSUM						
roasted	3 oz	188	9	0	0	0
ORANGE						
CANNED						
Del Monte						
Mandarin In Light Syrup	1 pkg (4 oz)	70	0	17	17	–
Mandarin No Sugar Added	½ cup (4.3 oz)	45	0	13	6	1
SunFresh Mandarin In Light Syrup	½ cup (4.5 oz)	70	0	17	15	0
Dole						
Mandarin In Fruit Juice	1 pkg (4 oz)	80	0	19	18	1
FRESH						
california valencia	1 (4.2 oz)	59	tr	14	–	3
california valencia sections	½ cup (3.2 oz)	44	tr	11	–	2
cara cara navel	1 (5.4 oz)	80	0	19	14	3
florida	1 (5.3 oz)	69	tr	17	14	4
florida sections	½ cup (3.2 oz)	43	tr	11	8	2
fresh	1 sm (3.4 oz)	45	tr	11	9	2
fresh	1 med (4.6 oz)	62	tr	15	12	3
fresh	1 lg (6.5 oz)	86	tr	22	17	4
navel	1 (4.9 oz)	69	tr	18	12	3
navel sections	1 cup (5.8 oz)	81	tr	21	14	4
peel	1 tbsp (0.2 oz)	3	tr	1	tr	1

FOOD	PORTION	CAL	FAT	CARB	SUGAR	FIBER
Dole						
Orange	1 med (4.2 oz)	60	0	14	13	3
Sunkist						
Cara Cara	1 med (5.4 oz)	80	0	19	14	3
Mandarin	1 (2.2 oz)	40	0	9	8	tr
Minneola Tangelo	1 (3.8 oz)	70	1	13	9	2
Moro	1 (5.4 oz)	70	1	15	14	3
Navel	1 med (5.4 oz)	80	0	19	14	3
Satsuma Mandarin	1 (3.8 oz)	50	0	11	10	2
ORANGE JUICE						
chilled bottled	1 cup (8.7 oz)	112	1	26	21	1
fresh	1 cup (8.7 oz)	112	1	26	21	1
mandarin orange	7 oz	94	tr	20	–	–
Dole						
100% Juice w/ Calcium	8 oz	120	0	27	–	0
Genesis Today						
Omega Orange 100% Juice	8 oz	90	0	23	13	3
Italian Volcano						
Organic Blood Orange	8 oz	101	0	25	23	–
Izze						
Esque Sparkling Mandarin	1 bottle (12 oz)	50	0	12	11	–
Minute Maid						
100% Juice Heart Wise	8 oz	110	0	27	24	–
100% Juice No Pulp	8 oz	110	0	26	22	–
100% Juice w/ Calcium & Vitamin D	8 oz	110	0	27	24	–
Orangeade	8 oz	110	0	31	30	–
Ocean Spray						
Juice	8 oz	100	0	31	31	–
Old Orchard						
100% Juice	8 oz	130	0	31	29	–

FOOD	PORTION	CAL	FAT	CARB	SUGAR	FIBER
Snapple						
Orangeade	8 oz	100	0	26	26	–
Tropicana						
100% Juice	8 oz	110	0	27	22	–
TAKE-OUT						
orange julius	1 cup (9.2 oz)	212	tr	39	35	tr
OREGANO						
crumbled	1 tsp	3	tr	1	tr	tr
ground	1 tsp	6	tr	1	tr	1

ORGAN MEATS (*see* BRAINS, GIBLETS, GIZZARDS, HEART, KIDNEY, LIVER, SWEETBREAD)

FOOD	PORTION	CAL	FAT	CARB	SUGAR	FIBER
OROBLANCO						
Sunkist						
Fresh	½ (5.4 oz)	100	1	22	11	4
OSTRICH						
cooked	4 oz	195	8	0	0	0
cooked diced	1 cup (4.7 oz)	215	9	0	0	0
OYSTERS						
canned eastern	1 cup	112	4	6	0	0
eastern baked	6 med	47	1	4	–	0
eastern raw	6 med	50	1	5	–	0
eastern sauteed	6 med	76	5	3	0	0
smoked	6	33	1	2	0	0
Chicken Of The Sea						
Smoked In Oil	1 can (3.75 oz)	170	8	8	0	0
Whole	¼ can (2 oz)	80	3	6	0	0
TAKE-OUT						
breaded & fried	6	368	18	40	–	–
fritter	1 (1.4 oz)	121	6	12	tr	tr
oysters rockefeller	1 cup	302	17	22	2	4
stew	1 cup	208	13	11	9	0

FOOD	PORTION	CAL	FAT	CARB	SUGAR	FIBER
PANCAKE/WAFFLE SYRUP						
light	¼ cup	98	0	27	20	0
pancake syrup	¼ cup	209	tr	55	50	0
pancake syrup	1 pkg (2 oz)	156	tr	41	38	0
Ali's All Natural						
All Flavors	¼ cup (2 oz)	5	0	1	0	tr
IHOP At Home						
Blueberry	¼ cup (2.1 oz)	200	0	50	21	–
Lite	¼ cup (2.1 oz)	110	0	27	26	–
Original	¼ cup (2.1 oz)	220	0	54	28	–
Strawberry	¼ cup (2.1 oz)	200	0	50	23	–
Sugar Free	¼ cup (2.1 oz)	20	0	7	0	–
Log Cabin						
Lite	¼ cup (2 oz)	100	0	25	22	–
Smucker's						
Breakfast Syrup Sugar Free	¼ cup (2.1 oz)	20	0	8	0	–
Wholesome Sweeteners						
Organic	¼ cup	240	0	60	60	0
PANCAKES						
FROZEN						
Aunt Jemima						
Blueberry	3 (3.7 oz)	260	6	44	13	1
Buttermilk	3 (3.7 oz)	250	6	41	9	1
Buttermilk Lowfat	3 (3.6 oz)	200	2	41	8	1
Oatmeal	3 (3.7 oz)	230	4	42	11	4
Whole Grain	3 (3.6 oz)	240	6	42	9	3
Dr. Praeger's						
Broccoli	1 (2 oz)	80	4	9	1	2

FOOD	PORTION	CAL	FAT	CARB	SUGAR	FIBER
Potato	1 (2.2 oz)	100	4	13	1	3
Sweet Potato Bites	1 (2 oz)	80	2	12	6	3
Golden						
Potato Latkes	1 (1.3 oz)	70	3	10	2	1
Jimmy Dean						
Griddle Sticks	1 (2.5 oz)	160	6	21	8	0
MIX						
Bisquick						
Shake 'N Pour Buttermilk as prep	3	220	3	42	7	1
Maple Grove Farms						
Buttermilk & Honey as prep	1	220	7	32	36	tr
Mix Gluten Free as prep	1	200	8	30	4	2
TAKE-OUT						
bu chu jun korean w/ vegetables	1 (4 oz)	83	4	11	–	1
buckwheat	1 (7 in)	142	5	19	4	2
norwegian lefse	1 (9 in) (2.7 oz)	163	5	27	2	2
pindaettok korean mung bean	1 (3.9 oz)	204	11	20	–	6
plain	1 (7 in)	183	3	35	10	1
potato	1 (1.3 oz)	70	4	8	tr	1
w/ butter & syrup	2 (8.1 oz)	520	14	91	–	–
whole wheat	1 (7 in)	183	8	23	5	3

PANCREAS (*see* SWEETBREAD)

PANINI (*see* SANDWICHES)

PAPAYA

canned in syrup	½ cup (2.3 oz)	50	tr	13	11	1
dried	1 strip (0.8 oz)	59	tr	15	9	3
fresh	1 sm (5.3 oz)	59	tr	15	9	3
fresh	1 lg (13.3 oz)	148	1	37	22	7

FOOD	PORTION	CAL	FAT	CARB	SUGAR	FIBER
fresh cubed	1 cup (4.9 oz)	55	tr	14	8	3
green cooked	½ cup (2.3 oz)	18	tr	5	3	1
Crunchy N'Yummy						
Organic Papaya	1 pkg (1 oz)	55	0	13	0	2
Dole						
Fresh	½ (4.9 oz)	60	0	15	9	3
PAPAYA JUICE						
nectar	1 cup (8.8 oz)	142	tr	36	35	2
Old Orchard						
Nectar Cocktail	8 oz	75	0	17	17	–
PAPRIKA						
dried	1 tsp	1	tr	tr	tr	tr
PARSLEY						
dried	1 tbsp	4	tr	1	tr	1
freeze dried	1 tbsp	1	tr	tr	–	tr
fresh chopped	¼ cup	5	tr	1	tr	1
fresh chopped	1 tbsp	1	tr	tr	tr	tr
fresh sprigs	5 (1.8 oz)	18	tr	3	tr	2
PARSNIPS						
fresh sliced cooked w/o salt	½ cup (2.7 oz)	55	tr	13	4	3
whole cooked	1 (5.6 oz)	114	tr	27	8	6
TAKE-OUT						
creamed	1 cup (8 oz)	237	11	31	10	5
PASSION FRUIT						
fresh	1 (0.6 oz)	17	tr	4	2	2
fresh cut up	½ cup (4.1 oz)	114	1	28	13	12
PASSION FRUIT JUICE						
nectar	1 cup (8.8 oz)	168	tr	44	43	tr
yellow lilikoi	1 cup (8.7 oz)	138	tr	35	34	1

FOOD	PORTION	CAL	FAT	CARB	SUGAR	FIBER
Welch's						
Passion Fruit Cocktail	8 oz	150	0	38	37	–
PASTA (*see also* NOODLES, PASTA DINNERS, PASTA SALAD)						
DRY						
corn cooked	1 cup (4.9 oz)	176	1	39	–	7
elbows not prep	1 cup	389	2	78	–	–
elbows cooked	1 cup (4.9 oz)	197	1	40	–	2
shells small cooked	1 cup (4 oz)	162	1	33	–	2
spaghetti cooked	1 cup (4.9 oz)	197	1	40	–	2
spinach spaghetti cooked	1 cup (4.9 oz)	182	1	37	–	–
spirals cooked	1 cup (4.7 oz)	189	tr	38	–	2
vegetable cooked	1 cup (4.7 oz)	172	tr	36	–	6
whole wheat all shapes cooked	1 cup	174	tr	37	–	4
Barilla						
Lasagne not prep	2 pieces (1.8 oz)	180	0	37	1	2
Piccolini Mini Penne not prep	2 oz	210	1	43	2	6
Plus Spaghetti not prep	2 oz	210	2	38	2	4
Rotini Tri-Color not prep	2 oz	200	1	42	2	2
Rotini Whole Grain not prep	2 oz	200	2	41	2	6
Spaghetti Whole Grain not prep	1/7 box (2 oz)	200	2	41	2	6
Tortellini Three Cheese not prep	3 cup (2 oz)	230	8	32	2	3
Heartland						
Gluten Free not prep	2 oz	200	1	45	0	1
Naturals Penne not prep	3/4 cup (2 oz)	210	1	41	2	2
Perfect Balance Elbow Macaroni not prep	1/2 cup (2 oz)	200	1	41	2	3

FOOD	PORTION	CAL	FAT	CARB	SUGAR	FIBER
Whole Wheat Rotini not prep	¾ cup (2 oz)	210	2	41	2	5
Jovial						
Organic Einkorn All Shapes	2 oz	200	2	35	1	4
Organic Einkorn White All Shapes	2 oz	200	2	40	1	2
Organic Gluten Free Brown Rice All Shapes	2 oz	210	2	43	0	2
Lundberg						
Organic Spaghetti Brown Rice not prep	2 oz	190	3	40	1	4
MagNoodles						
Organic Smart not prep	2 oz	204	1	41	–	5
Mara's Pasta						
100% Whole Wheat not prep	2 oz	190	1	40	0	7
Mueller's						
100% Whole Grain Spaghetti not prep	1/7 pkg (2 oz)	200	2	40	2	5
Racconto						
Essentials Heart Health Rigatoni not prep	1/6 pkg (2 oz)	190	1	41	0	7
Rienzi						
Catanisella Lunga	2 oz	200	1	43	2	1
Ronzoni						
Alphabets not prep	⅓ cup (2 oz)	210	1	42	2	2
Bow Ties not prep	1 cup (2 oz)	210	1	42	2	2
Elbows not prep	½ cup (2 oz)	210	1	42	2	2
Garden Delight Rotini not prep	2 oz	200	1	40	3	2
Quick Cook Penne Rigate not prep	¾ cup (2 oz)	210	1	42	2	2

FOOD	PORTION	CAL	FAT	CARB	SUGAR	FIBER
Smart Taste Angel Hair not prep	1/7 pkg (2 oz)	170	1	40	1	5
Wacky Mac						
Veggie Bows not prep	1/6 pkg (2 oz)	200	1	41	0	1
FRESH						
cooked	2 oz	75	1	14	–	–
spinach cooked	2 oz	74	1	14	–	–
Buitoni						
Angel Hair	1/3 pkg (2.8 oz)	230	2	44	1	2
Ravioli Four Cheese	1 serv (3.7 oz)	340	12	42	2	3
Reserva Quattro Formaggi Agnolotti	1 serv (4.4 oz)	360	17	35	2	2
Tortellini Spinach Cheese	1 serv (3.7 oz)	320	7	49	4	3
Tortelloni Whole Wheat Cheese	1 serv (3.7 oz)	330	10	45	3	6
Nasoya						
Pasta Zero Plus Shirataki Fettuccine or Spaghetti	2/3 cup (4 oz)	20	0	4	0	3
Pasta Prima						
Ravioli Butternut Squash	1/2 pkg (4 oz)	250	6	36	2	2
Ravioli Gluten Free Butternut Squash	1 cup (3.5 oz)	180	4	30	2	2
Ravioli Gluten Free Five Cheese	1 cup (3.5 oz)	230	10	24	1	2
Ravioli Italian Sausage	1/2 pkg (4 oz)	290	13	25	1	2
Ravioli Lobster	1/2 pkg (4 oz)	250	7	31	2	2
Ravioli Spinach & Cheese	1 cup (3.5 oz)	210	7	29	1	2

FOOD	PORTION	CAL	FAT	CARB	SUGAR	FIBER
FROZEN						
Pasta Prima						
Ravioli Spinach & Mozzarella	1 cup (4 oz)	200	5	29	0	4
Solterra						
Fettuccine Gluten Free	⅓ pkg (4 oz)	330	6	54	1	3
Tofutti						
Ravioli Dairy Free	4 (3.2 oz)	210	10	28	1	1

PASTA DINNERS (*see also* PASTA SALAD)

FOOD	PORTION	CAL	FAT	CARB	SUGAR	FIBER
CANNED						
Annie's Homegrown						
Organic Cheesy Ravioli	1 cup (8.5 oz)	180	4	31	9	3
Organic P'sghetti Loops	1 cup (8.4 oz)	190	4	29	9	2
Chef Boyardee						
Beef Ravioli	1 cup (8.6 oz)	230	8	31	5	3
Beefaroni	1 cup (8.7 oz)	240	10	30	5	3
Mini Ravioli	1 cup (8.8 oz)	250	9	35	5	3
Mini-Bites Spaghetti & Meatballs	1 cup (8.8 oz)	240	10	28	6	3
Spaghetti & Meat Balls	1 cup (9 oz)	260	11	30	7	4
Hormel						
Kid's Kitchen Microwave Meals Cheezy Mac 'N Beef	1 pkg (7.5 oz)	250	6	34	8	1
Kid's Kitchen Microwave Meals Cheezy Mac 'N Cheese	1 pkg (7.5 oz)	270	14	24	3	1
Kid's Kitchen Microwave Meals Mini Beef Ravioli	1 pkg (7.5 oz)	240	6	38	6	1
Kid's Kitchen Microwave Meals Spaghetti Rings & Franks	1 pkg (7.5 oz)	240	8	32	11	1

FOOD	PORTION	CAL	FAT	CARB	SUGAR	FIBER
Lasagna w/ Meat Sauce	1 pkg (7.5 oz)	210	5	31	14	3
Spaghetti w/ Meat Sauce	1 pkg (7.5 oz)	210	5	31	14	3
SpaghettiOs						
Sliced Franks	1 cup (8.8 oz)	220	6	32	9	4
FROZEN						
Buitoni						
Braised Beef & Sausage Ravioli w/ Creamy Marinara Sauce	½ pkg (11.9 oz)	590	19	72	9	5
Chicken & Mushroom Ravioli w/ Marsala Wine Sauce	½ pkg (10.9 oz)	530	20	59	7	5
Four Cheese & Spinach Ravioli w/ Tomato Basil Sauce	½ pkg (12.9 oz)	550	21	55	12	7
Grilled Chicken w/ Spinach Cannelloni w/ Alfredo Sauce	½ pkg (10.9 oz)	560	26	46	7	3
Candle Cafe						
Macaroni & Vegan Cheese	1 pkg (9 oz)	300	12	41	tr	5
Tofu Spinach Ravioli	1 pkg (9 oz)	320	10	48	4	4
Celentano						
Cheese Ravioli	4 (4.3 oz)	220	5	34	1	2
Healthy Choice						
Chicken Fettuccini Alfredo	1 pkg (11.4 oz)	300	7	39	16	7
Hearty Beef Stroganoff	1 pkg (10.9 oz)	280	7	33	17	6
Lobster Cheese Ravioli	1 pkg (8.9 oz)	270	6	41	9	4
Roasted Red Pepper Marinara	1 pkg (8.5 oz)	270	6	43	6	5

FOOD	PORTION	CAL	FAT	CARB	SUGAR	FIBER
Tortellini Primavera Parmesan	1 pkg (8.9 oz)	240	5	37	7	6
Lean Cuisine						
Cafe Cuisine Three Cheese Stuffed Rigatoni	1 pkg (9 oz)	230	6	32	6	4
Dinnertime Selects Chicken Fettuccini	1 pkg (12 oz)	330	6	42	3	4
Market Creations Tortelloni Mushroom	1 pkg (10 oz)	280	7	43	7	5
Simple Favorites Alfredo Pasta w/ Chicken & Broccoli	1 pkg (10 oz)	300	6	45	5	3
Simple Favorites Angel Hair Pomodoro	1 pkg (10 oz)	250	5	42	10	4
Simple Favorites Cheese Ravioli	1 pkg (8.5 oz)	220	5	33	8	3
Simple Favorites Chicken Fettuccini	1 pkg (9.25 oz)	270	6	32	6	0
Simple Favorites Fettuccini Alfredo	1 pkg (9.25 oz)	330	7	54	6	3
Simple Favorites Lasagna Chicken Florentine	1 pkg (10 oz)	280	6	36	6	3
Simple Favorites Lasagna Classic Five Cheese	1 pkg (11.5 oz)	350	7	51	11	4
Simple Favorites Lasagna w/ Meat Sauce	1 pkg (10.5 oz)	320	8	45	8	4
Simple Favorites Macaroni & Cheese	1 pkg (10 oz)	290	7	41	7	1

FOOD	PORTION	CAL	FAT	CARB	SUGAR	FIBER
Simple Favorites Spaghetti w/ Meat Sauce	1 pkg (11.5 oz)	300	4	49	9	4
Simple Favorites Spaghetti w/ Meatballs	1 pkg (9.5 oz)	270	6	38	6	3
Spa Cuisine Ravioli Butternut Squash	1 pkg (9.9 oz)	260	7	40	11	5
Mom Made						
Cheesy Mac	1 pkg (7 oz)	200	3	36	4	4
Spaghetti w/ Turkey Meatballs & Sauce	1 pkg (7 oz)	180	4	26	3	3
Tabatchnick						
Macaroni & Cheese	1 serv (7.5 oz)	250	8	34	4	tr
Weight Watchers						
Chicken & Broccoli Alfredo	1 pkg (11.8 oz)	300	4	39	3	4
Smart Ones Sesame Chicken	1 pkg (11.8 oz)	360	7	49	10	6
Smart Ones Ziti w/ Meatballs & Cheese	1 pkg (11.7 oz)	390	9	52	8	6
MIX						
Annie's Homegrown						
Gluten Free Rice Pasta & Cheddar as prep	1 cup	280	4	54	4	1
Mac & Cheese Lower Sodium as prep	1 cup	280	4	47	5	2
Organic 5-Grain Elbows & White Cheddar as prep	1 cup	270	4	48	5	3
Organic Classic Mac & Cheese as prep	1 cup	280	4	48	5	2
Organic Peace Pasta & Parmesan as prep	1 cup	270	4	47	4	2

FOOD	PORTION	CAL	FAT	CARB	SUGAR	FIBER
Organic Shells & Real Aged Wisconsin Cheddar as prep	1 cup	270	4	47	5	2
Organic Skillet Meals Beef Stroganoff as prep	1 cup	360	18	33	3	1
Organic Skillet Meals Cheesy Lasagna as prep	1 cup	440	18	32	6	1
Organic Skillet Meals Tuna Spirals as prep	1 cup	320	8	39	4	2
Shells & White Cheddar as prep	1 cup	270	5	47	5	2
Kraft						
Macaroni & Cheese White Cheddar as prep	⅓ pkg	380	15	48	7	0
Simply Shari's						
Mac & Cheese Gluten Free as prep	¼ pkg (4 oz)	280	6	17	1	2
REFRIGERATED						
NoOodle						
Mamma Mia! Marinara	1 pkg (10 oz)	70	3	13	3	4
Say Cheese Pleeeze!	1 pkg (10 oz)	100	10	6	2	4
Terri-Yaki Chicken	1 pkg (10 oz)	80	2	10	5	4
Simply Sensible						
Lasagna w/ Meat Sauce	½ pkg (8 oz)	200	5	28	8	2
Mediterranean Style Chicken	1½ cups (7.2 oz)	250	6	36	3	2
SHELF-STABLE						
Barilla						
Mezze Penne w/ Tomato & Basil Sauce	1 pkg (9 oz)	320	5	59	8	6
Healthy Choice						
Balsamic Vegetable Medley	1 pkg (6.9 oz)	290	3	56	6	7

FOOD	PORTION	CAL	FAT	CARB	SUGAR	FIBER
Fresh Mixers Rotini & Zesty Marinara Sauce	1 pkg (9.9 oz)	300	4	56	11	7
Fresh Mixers Ziti & Meat Sauce	1 pkg (6.9 oz)	340	6	56	10	8
Pasta Margherita	1 pkg (6.9 oz)	270	4	52	7	4
Hormel						
Compleats Microwave Meals Chicken & Noodles	1 pkg (9.9 oz)	240	8	27	3	2
TAKE-OUT						
lasagna meatless	1 piece (9 oz)	356	11	46	8	3
lasagna w/ meat	1 piece (8 oz)	362	14	37	6	3
lasagna w/ vegetables	1 serv (9 oz)	315	10	41	8	4
macaroni & cheese w/ ham	1 cup	542	33	41	7	3
manicotti cheese w/ marinara sauce	1 (5 oz)	229	10	22	3	1
manicotti cheese w/ meat sauce	1 (5 oz)	239	11	20	1	3
pasta w/ pesto sauce	1 cup	370	25	27	1	2
ravioli cheese & spinach w/ cream sauce	1 cup	362	17	38	5	2
ravioli cheese w/ tomato sauce	1 cup	335	14	38	4	2
ravioli meat w/ marinara sauce	1 cup	372	16	36	5	3
rigatoni w/ sausage sauce	¾ cup	260	12	28	–	3
spaghetti w/ red clam sauce	1 cup	285	8	41	3	3
spaghetti w/ sauce & meatballs	2 cups	670	26	80	15	12

FOOD	PORTION	CAL	FAT	CARB	SUGAR	FIBER
spaghetti w/ white clam sauce	1 cup	456	20	43	1	3
tortellini cheese w/ tomato sauce	1 cup	332	14	38	4	2
tortellini meat w/ marinara sauce	1 cup	281	10	33	3	2
tortellini spinach w/ marinara sauce	1 cup	238	8	32	3	2

PASTA SALAD

MIX

Suddenly Salad

FOOD	PORTION	CAL	FAT	CARB	SUGAR	FIBER
Caesar as prep	1 cup (1.8 oz)	310	14	38	3	1
Classic as prep	¾ cup	250	8	39	4	1
Creamy Italian as prep	¾ cup	350	20	36	4	2
Creamy Parmesan as prep	¾ cup	370	22	33	2	1

TAKE-OUT

FOOD	PORTION	CAL	FAT	CARB	SUGAR	FIBER
pasta salad w/ crab vegetables & mayonnaise	1 cup	317	16	33	2	2
pasta salad w/ shrimp vegetables & mayonnaise	1 cup (6.2 oz)	335	17	35	6	2
tortellini salad cheese filled w/ vinaigrette dressing	1 cup	333	18	30	1	1

PATE

FOOD	PORTION	CAL	FAT	CARB	SUGAR	FIBER
chicken liver canned	1 tbsp	26	2	1	0	0
duck pate	1 oz	96	8	1	tr	–
fish pate	1 oz	76	7	1	–	–
liver w/ truffle	1 serv (2 oz)	183	16	4	–	–
mushroom anchovy pate	1 (2.25 oz)	130	11	7	1	1

FOOD	PORTION	CAL	FAT	CARB	SUGAR	FIBER
pate de foie gras smoked canned	1 tbsp	60	6	1	–	0
pork pate	1 oz	107	10	1	1	0
pork pate en croute	1 oz	91	7	3	tr	tr
rabbit pate	1 oz	66	5	1	–	–
shrimp pate	1 can (2.25 oz)	140	10	7	1	0

PEACH

CANNED

FOOD	PORTION	CAL	FAT	CARB	SUGAR	FIBER
halves in heavy syrup	½ cup (2.6 oz)	85	tr	22	20	2
halves in light syrup	1 half (3.4 oz)	53	tr	14	13	1
halves juice pack	1 half (3.4 oz)	43	tr	11	10	1
peach sauce	½ cup	120	0	32	31	1
pickled	½ cup (4.2 oz)	143	tr	35	34	1
pickled whole	1 (3.1 oz)	104	tr	26	25	1
slices in light syrup	½ cup (4.4 oz)	68	tr	18	17	2
slices juice pack	½ cup (4.4 oz)	55	tr	14	13	2
slices water pack	½ cup (4.3 oz)	29	tr	7	6	2
spiced in heavy syrup	½ cup (4.2 oz)	91	tr	24	23	2
Del Monte						
Diced In Light Syrup	1 pkg (4 oz)	70	0	17	16	–
Freestone Slices Lite	½ cup (4.4 oz)	60	0	14	13	1
Peaches In Strawberry Banana Gel	1 pkg (4.5 oz)	60	0	14	12	–
Sliced 100% Juice	½ cup (4.4 oz)	60	0	15	14	1
Sliced In Heavy Syrup	½ cup (4.5 oz)	100	0	24	23	1

DRIED

FOOD	PORTION	CAL	FAT	CARB	SUGAR	FIBER
halves	1 (0.5 oz)	31	tr	8	5	1
halves	½ cup (2.8 oz)	191	1	49	33	7
halves cooked w/o sugar	½ cup (4.5 oz)	99	tr	25	22	4

FOOD	PORTION	CAL	FAT	CARB	SUGAR	FIBER
FRESH						
peach	1 med (5.3 oz)	58	tr	14	13	2
peach	1 lg (6.1 oz)	68	tr	17	15	3
sliced	½ cup (2.7 oz)	30	tr	8	6	1
Dole						
Peach	1 lg (5.2 oz)	60	0	14	12	2
FROZEN						
Dole						
Sliced	¾ cup (4.9 oz)	50	0	13	10	1
REFRIGERATED						
Dole						
Fruit Crisp Peach	1 pkg (4 oz)	150	4	28	20	2
Parfait Peaches & Creme	1 pkg (4.3 oz)	120	2	23	21	1

PEACH JUICE

FOOD	PORTION	CAL	FAT	CARB	SUGAR	FIBER
nectar	1 cup (8.7 oz)	134	tr	35	33	2
Froose						
Playful Peach	1 box (4.2 oz)	80	0	19	7	3
Minute Maid						
Fruit Drink	8 oz	120	0	31	30	–

PEANUT BUTTER (*see also* INDIVIDUAL NUT NAMES, NUT BUTTER)

FOOD	PORTION	CAL	FAT	CARB	SUGAR	FIBER
chunky	2 tbsp (1.1 oz)	188	16	7	3	3
no sugar added	2 tbsp (1.1 oz)	208	18	5	1	3
reduced sodium	2 tbsp (1.1 oz)	202	16	7	3	2
smooth	2 tbsp (1.1 oz)	188	16	7	3	2
Jake & Amos						
Schmier	1 tbsp (0.6 oz)	60	3	8	8	0
Jif						
Simply	2 tbsp (1.1 oz)	190	16	6	2	2
Kettle Brand						
Organic Unsalted	2 tbsp (1 oz)	160	14	5	3	2
Maple Grove Farms						
Crunchy No Salt Added	2 tbsp (1.1 oz)	190	15	6	2	2

FOOD	PORTION	CAL	FAT	CARB	SUGAR	FIBER
Peanut Butter & Co.						
Cinnamon Raisin Swirl	2 tbsp (1.1 oz)	160	11	13	9	2
Dark Chocolate Dreams	2 tbsp (1.1 oz)	170	13	12	7	2
Old Fashioned Crunchy	2 tbsp (1.1 oz)	190	16	6	1	2
The Bee's Knees	2 tbsp (1.1 oz)	180	14	12	8	1
Planters						
Creamy or Crunchy	2 tbsp (1.1 oz)	180	15	8	3	2
Natural Creamy	2 tbsp (1.1 oz)	190	17	6	3	3
Skippy						
Extra Chunky Super Chunk	2 tbsp (1.1 oz)	190	16	7	3	2
Reduced Fat Creamy	2 tbsp (1.3 oz)	180	12	15	4	2
Smart Balance						
Omega Creamy & Chunky	2 tbsp (1.1 oz)	200	17	8	1	2
Smucker's						
Chunky	2 tbsp (1.1 oz)	200	16	6	1	2
Creamy No Salt Addded	2 tbsp (1.1 oz)	210	16	6	1	2
Creamy Reduced Fat	2 tbsp (1.2 oz)	190	12	12	2	2
Creamy Honey	2 tbsp (1.2 oz)	200	16	9	4	2
Goober Grape	3 tbsp (1.9 oz)	240	13	24	21	2
Goober Peanut Butter & Chocolate Spread	3 tbsp (2 oz)	230	11	27	23	2
Wild Squirrel						
Chocolate Coconut	2 tbsp (1.1 oz)	200	17	3	2	3
Cinnamon Raisin	2 tbsp (1.1 oz)	180	15	9	3	3
Honey Pretzel	2 tbsp (1.1 oz)	190	16	8	2	2

PEANUTS

chocolate coated	¼ cup	193	12	18	14	2
chocolate coated	1	21	1	2	2	tr
cooked w/ salt	½ cup	286	20	19	2	8
dry roasted w/ salt	28 (1 oz)	164	14	6	2	1
dry roasted w/o salt	28 (1 oz)	164	14	6	1	2

FOOD	PORTION	CAL	FAT	CARB	SUGAR	FIBER
dry roasted w/o salt	¼ cup	214	18	8	2	3
honey roasted	¼ cup	191	16	8	5	3
sugar coated	¼ cup	203	13	18	16	2
yogurt coated	¼ cup	230	16	18	15	2
Frito Lay						
Salted In Shells	1 oz	160	14	6	1	2
Planters						
Bar Big Double	1 (1.6 oz)	220	13	21	12	3
Dry Roasted	1 oz	160	14	5	2	2
Dry Roasted Lightly Salted	1 oz	160	14	5	1	2
Dry Roasted Unsalted	1 oz	170	14	5	1	2
Five Alarm Chili Dry Roasted	39 (1 oz)	160	14	5	2	1
Honey & Dry Roasted	1 oz	160	13	7	4	2
Roasted In Milk Chocolate	¼ cup (1.4 oz)	210	15	18	15	2
Virginia Cocktail Peanuts						
Jalapeno	⅕ can (1 oz)	170	13	7	tr	5
Milk Chocolate	⅓ pkg (1.5 oz)	230	14	23	14	4
Sea Salt	⅕ can (1 oz)	170	13	7	tr	5
Toffee	⅕ can (1 oz)	210	7	16	14	2
Unsalted	⅕ can (1 oz)	170	13	7	tr	5

PEAR

CANNED

FOOD	PORTION	CAL	FAT	CARB	SUGAR	FIBER
halves in heavy syrup	1 (1.7 oz)	36	tr	9	8	1
halves in heavy syrup	½ cup (3.5 oz)	74	tr	19	17	3
halves in light syrup	1 (2.7 oz)	43	tr	12	9	1
halves in light syrup	½ cup (4.4 oz)	72	tr	19	15	2
halves juice pack	1 (2.7 oz)	38	tr	10	7	1
halves juice pack	½ cup (4.4 oz)	62	tr	16	12	2
halves water pack	1 (2.7 oz)	22	tr	6	5	1

FOOD	PORTION	CAL	FAT	CARB	SUGAR	FIBER
Del Monte						
Halves In Heavy Syrup	½ cup (4.6 oz)	100	0	24	23	1
Halves Lite	½ cup (4.4 oz)	60	0	15	14	1
Dole						
Diced In Fruit Juice	1 pkg (4 oz)	90	0	21	18	2
DRIED						
halves	1 (0.6 oz)	47	tr	13	11	1
halves	½ cup (3.2 oz)	236	1	63	56	7
halves	5 (3 oz)	229	1	61	54	7
halves cooked w/o sugar	½ cup (4.5 oz)	162	tr	43	35	8
Crispy Green						
Crispy Asian Pears	1 pkg (0.35 oz)	40	0	8	7	1
Crunchies						
Freeze Dried	¼ cup (6 g)	20	0	5	3	1
FRESH						
asian	1 med (4.3 oz)	51	tr	13	9	4
asian	1 lg (9.6 oz)	116	1	30	19	10
pear	1 sm (5.2 oz)	86	tr	23	15	5
pear	1 med (6.2 oz)	103	tr	28	17	6
pear	1 lg (8.1 oz)	133	tr	36	23	7
sliced w/ skin	1 cup (4.9 oz)	81	tr	22	14	4
Dole						
Pear	1 med (5.8 oz)	100	0	26	16	5
PEAR JUICE						
nectar canned	1 cup (8.8 oz)	150	tr	39	38	2
Smart Juice						
Organic 100% Juice	8 oz	110	0	31	25	2

FOOD	PORTION	CAL	FAT	CARB	SUGAR	FIBER
PEAS						
CANNED						
green	½ cup (4.4 oz)	66	tr	12	4	4
green low sodium	½ cup (4.4 oz)	66	tr	12	4	4
Bush's						
Crowder Peas	½ cup (4.6 oz)	80	0	18	0	5
Field Peas w/ Snaps	½ cup (4.6 oz)	80	0	16	0	2
Purple Hull	½ cup (4.6 oz)	90	0	19	0	5
Butter Kernel						
Sweet	½ cup (4.4 oz)	60	0	13	6	4
Del Monte						
Sweet	½ cup (4.4 oz)	60	0	13	6	3
Sweet No Salt Added	½ cup (4.4 oz)	60	0	13	6	3
Le Sueur						
Very Young Small	½ cup (4.2 oz)	60	0	12	4	3
DRIED						
split cooked w/o salt	1 cup (6.9 oz)	231	1	41	6	16
Crunchies						
Freeze Dried Organic	¼ cup (0.5 oz)	50	1	9	8	3
Goya						
Green Split Peas not prep	¼ cup (1.6 oz)	110	0	27	1	11
FRESH						
green cooked w/o salt	½ cup (2.8 oz)	67	tr	13	5	4
green raw	½ cup (2.5 oz)	59	tr	10	4	4
snap peas cooked w/o salt	1 cup (5.6 oz)	67	tr	11	6	5
snap peas raw	10 (1.2 oz)	14	tr	3	1	1
snap peas raw	1 cup (2.2 oz)	26	tr	5	3	2
Dole						
Sugar Snap Peas	1 cup (3 oz)	35	0	6	3	2
Eat Smart						
Sugar Snap	1 serv (3 oz)	40	0	7	3	2

FOOD	PORTION	CAL	FAT	CARB	SUGAR	FIBER
Mann's						
Snow Peas	1 serv (3 oz)	35	0	6	3	2
FROZEN						
creamed	1 cup (4.3 oz)	132	6	15	6	4
green cooked w/o salt	½ cup (2.8 oz)	62	tr	11	4	4
Birds Eye						
Baby Sweet Peas	⅔ cup (3 oz)	70	0	12	4	4
Lisa's Organics						
Sweet Peas In Parmesan Herb Sauce	½ pkg (4 oz)	80	1	13	0	3
PECANS						
candied	1 oz	190	17	10	4	5
chopped dried w/o salt	¼ cup (0.9 oz)	188	20	4	1	3
halves dried w/o salt	19 (1 oz)	196	20	4	1	3
halves dried w/o salt	¼ cup (0.9 oz)	171	18	3	1	2
halves oil roasted w/ salt	15 (1 oz)	203	21	4	1	3
oil roasted w/ salt	¼ cup (1 oz)	197	21	4	1	3
Planters						
Halves	1 oz	200	20	4	1	3
Sante						
Cinnamon Pecan	¼ cup (1 oz)	190	17	9	5	2
PECTIN						
liquid	1 oz	3	0	1	0	1
powder	1 pkg (1.75 oz)	162	tr	45	–	4
PEPEAO						
dried	¼ cup	18	tr	5	–	–
raw sliced	1 cup	25	tr	7	–	–

FOOD	PORTION	CAL	FAT	CARB	SUGAR	FIBER
PEPPER						
black	1 tsp	5	tr	1	tr	1
cayenne	1 tsp	6	tr	1	tr	1
white	1 tsp	7	tr	2	–	1
Badia						
Lemon Pepper	¼ tsp (0.9 g)	0	0	0	0	0
McCormick						
Lemon Pepper w/ Garlic & Onion California Style	¼ tsp (0.6 g)	0	0	0	0	0
PEPPERMINT						
fresh chopped	2 tbsp	2	tr	tr	–	tr
PEPPERS						
CANNED						
chili green hot	1 (2.6 oz)	15	tr	4	2	1
chili green hot chopped	½ cup (2.4 oz)	14	tr	3	2	1
chili pepper paste	1 tbsp	6	1	1	–	1
green halves	1 cup (4.9 oz)	25	tr	5	–	2
jalapeno	1 (0.8 oz)	6	tr	1	tr	1
jalapeno chopped	1 cup (4.8 oz)	37	1	6	3	4
Costa Peruana						
Organic Aji Paste All Flavors	1 tbsp (0.5 oz)	10	0	2	0	0
Dietz & Watson						
Sweet Roasted	1 oz	5	0	1	0	0
Gedney						
Hot Banana Pepper Rings	¼ cup (1 oz)	10	0	1	0	0
Jalapeno Sliced	¼ cup (1 oz)	10	0	2	2	0
Jake & Amos						
Mild Sweet Stuffed	2 tbsp	15	0	7	0	0
Matiz						
Organic Piquillo Peppers	2	20	0	4	3	tr
Piparras	½ jar (1 oz)	5	0	1	0	0

FOOD	PORTION	CAL	FAT	CARB	SUGAR	FIBER
Victoria						
Jalapeno Hot Roasted	1 oz	10	0	2	0	1
Red & Green Roasted	⅓ cup (4.6 oz)	24	0	5	2	1
DRIED						
ancho	1 tsp	3	tr	1	–	tr
ancho	1 (0.6 oz)	48	1	9	–	4
casabel	1 tsp	3	tr	1	–	tr
chili hot sun-dried	¼ cup (0.3 oz)	30	1	6	4	3
chili hot sun-dried	1 (0.5 g)	2	tr	tr	tr	tr
chipotle smoked	1 tsp	3	tr	1	–	tr
green freeze dried	1 tbsp (0.4 g)	1	tr	1	1	tr
guajillo	1 tsp	3	tr	1	–	tr
mulato	1 tsp	3	tr	1	–	tr
pasilla	1 tsp	3	tr	1	–	tr
pasilla	1 (7 g)	24	1	4	–	2
red sweet freeze-dried	1 tbsp (0.4 g)	1	tr	tr	tr	tr
FRESH						
banana	1 lg (2.6 oz)	20	tr	4	1	3
banana	1 (4 in) (1.2 oz)	9	tr	2	1	1
banana	1 cup (4.4 oz)	33	1	7	2	4
chili green hot	1 (1.6 oz)	18	tr	4	2	1
chili green hot chopped	½ cup (2.6 oz)	30	tr	7	4	1
chili red hot	1 (1.6 oz)	18	tr	4	2	1
chili red hot chopped	½ cup (2.6 oz)	30	tr	7	4	1
green chopped	1 cup (5.2 oz)	30	tr	7	4	3
green chopped fried	1 cup (4 oz)	146	14	5	3	2
green chopped or strips cooked w/o salt	1 cup (4.7 oz)	38	tr	9	4	2
green sweet	1 med (4.2 oz)	24	tr	6	3	2
habanero	1 tsp	9	tr	2	–	1
hungarian	1 (0.9 oz)	8	tr	2	1	tr
jalapeno	1 (0.5 oz)	4	tr	1	1	tr
jalapeno sliced	1 cup (3.2 oz)	26	tr	6	4	3
red	1 med (4.2 oz)	37	tr	7	5	3

FOOD	PORTION	CAL	FAT	CARB	SUGAR	FIBER
red	1 lg (5.6 oz)	51	tr	10	7	3
red chopped	1 cup (5.2 oz)	46	tr	9	6	3
red chopped cooked w/o salt	½ cup (2.4 oz)	19	tr	5	3	1
red sweet	1 lg (5.8 oz)	33	tr	8	4	3
red sweet ring	1 (0.4 oz)	2	tr	tr	tr	tr
serrano	1 (6 g)	2	tr	tr	tr	tr
serrano chopped	1 cup (3.7 oz)	34	tr	7	4	4
yellow	1 lg (6.5 oz)	50	tr	12	–	2
yellow strips	10 (1.8 oz)	14	tr	3	–	1
FROZEN						
Farm Rich						
Stuffed Jalapeno	2 (1.7 oz)	120	8	10	1	0

PERCH

FOOD	PORTION	CAL	FAT	CARB	SUGAR	FIBER
FRESH						
cooked	1 fillet (1.6 oz)	54	1	0	0	0
cooked	3 oz	99	1	0	0	0
ocean perch atlantic cooked	3 oz	103	2	0	0	0
ocean perch atlantic cooked	1 fillet (1.8 oz)	60	1	0	0	0
ocean perch atlantic raw	3 oz	80	1	0	0	0
raw	3 oz	77	1	0	0	0
red raw	3.5 oz	114	4	0	0	0
FROZEN						
Bell						
Cajun Nuggets	12 (4.5 oz)	170	3	16	0	1
Fillets Breaded	1 piece (4.5 oz)	170	3	16	0	tr
Fillets Unbreaded	1 piece (3.5 oz)	80	1	0	0	0

FOOD	PORTION	CAL	FAT	CARB	SUGAR	FIBER
PERSIMMONS						
dried japanese	1 (1.2 oz)	93	tr	25	–	5
fresh	1 (6 oz)	118	tr	31	21	6
PHEASANT						
breast boneless cooked	½ (4.4 oz)	312	15	0	0	0
cooked diced	1 cup	332	16	0	0	0
drumstick & thigh cooked	1 (2.6 oz)	184	9	0	0	0
PHYLLO						
sheet	1 (0.7 oz)	57	1	10	tr	tr
Athens						
Fillo Dough Sheets	5 (2 oz)	160	1	31	1	1
Kataifi Shredded Fillo Dough	⅛ pkg (2 oz)	120	2	22	0	tr
Mini Fillo Shells	2 (7 g)	25	1	4	0	0
Spanakopita Spinach & Cheese Appetizers	2 (2 oz)	160	8	17	1	1
Tyropita Three Cheese Appetizers	2 (2 oz)	180	11	14	1	0
Ekizian						
Sheets	2 (4 oz)	433	9	76	2	3
PICANTE (*see* SALSA)						
PICKLES						
bread & butter	6 slices	39	tr	9	4	1
dill	1 lg (4.7 oz)	24	tr	6	5	2
dill low sodium	1 med (2.3 oz)	12	tr	3	–	1
dill sliced	6 slices	7	tr	2	1	1
sweet gherkin	1 (1.2 oz)	41	tr	11	5	tr
tsukemono japanese pickles sliced	¼ cup	10	tr	2	1	1

FOOD	PORTION	CAL	FAT	CARB	SUGAR	FIBER
B&G						
Crunchy Kosher Dill Gherkins	1 (1 oz)	5	0	1	–	–
Claussen						
Sandwich Slices Hearty Garlic	2 (1.2 oz)	5	0	1	tr	–
Dietz & Watson						
New Half Sours	2 pieces (1 oz)	0	0	0	0	0
Gedney						
Dill	½ lg (1 oz)	5	0	1	0	0
Kosher Dill Babies	3 (1 oz)	5	0	1	0	0
State Fair Norwegian Dills	1 med (1 oz)	5	0	1	tr	0
Sweet Bread & Butter Chips	5 (1 oz)	30	0	8	7	0
Jake & Amos						
Bread & Butter Chips	2 tbsp	20	0	5	2	0
Mt. Olive						
Bread & Butter Spears	2–4 spears (1 oz)	20	0	6	4	–
Vlasic						
Farmer's Garden Deli Halves	½ (1 oz)	0	0	1	–	–
Kosher Dill Spears Reduced Sodium	⅔ spear (1 oz)	0	0	tr	0	0
Stackers Kosher Dill	1 (1 oz)	0	0	tr	0	–
Stackers Kosher Dill Reduced Sodium	1 (1 oz)	0	0	tr	0	0
PIE (*see also* PIE CRUST, PIE FILLING)						
FROZEN						
Edwards						
Pie Slices Key Lime	1 slice (3.25 oz)	330	16	42	33	tr

FOOD	PORTION	CAL	FAT	CARB	SUGAR	FIBER
Mom Made						
Munchie Apple	1 (2.5 oz)	220	10	30	8	1
MIX						
Jell-O						
No Bake Lemon Meringue as prep	⅛ pie	270	10	44	29	1
READY-TO-EAT						
Foods By George						
Gluten Free Pecan Tarts	1 (4 oz)	470	26	51	26	3
TAKE-OUT						
apple one crust	1 slice (5.3 oz)	363	14	59	36	2
apple tart	1 (4.2 oz)	370	19	48	20	1
apple two crust	1 slice (5.3 oz)	350	17	51	23	2
apricot tart	1 (4.2 oz)	356	17	48	20	2
apricot two crust	1 slice (5.3 oz)	417	19	59	28	3
banana cream	1 slice (5.1 oz)	387	20	47	17	1
blackberry one crust	1 slice (4.4 oz)	341	17	44	18	4
blackberry two crust	1 slice (5.3 oz)	394	19	54	24	5
blueberry one crust	1 slice (4.8 oz)	292	12	45	23	3
blueberry tart	1 (4.2 oz)	346	17	47	21	2
blueberry two crust	1 slice (5.3 oz)	348	15	52	15	2
cherry one crust	1 slice (4.8 oz)	312	12	50	30	2
cherry two crust	1 slice (5.3 oz)	390	17	60	21	1

FOOD	PORTION	CAL	FAT	CARB	SUGAR	FIBER
chess	1 slice (3 oz)	365	18	48	37	1
chocolate cream	1 slice (5 oz)	380	18	50	29	2
coconut creme	1 slice (5 oz)	429	24	54	52	2
custard	1 slice (4.8 oz)	286	16	28	16	2
grasshopper	1 slice (3.5 oz)	341	19	33	23	1
key lime	1 slice (5 oz)	420	14	71	28	tr
lemon meringue	1 slice (4.8 oz)	367	12	65	33	2
lemon meringue tart	1 (4.1 oz)	298	14	41	22	1
mince two crust	1 slice (5.3 oz)	434	16	72	42	4
peach two crust	1 slice (5.3 oz)	334	15	49	9	1
pear two crust	1 slice (5.3 oz)	400	18	57	27	3
pecan	1 slice (4 oz)	456	21	65	32	4
pineapple two crust	1 slice (5.3 oz)	394	18	55	23	2
plum two crust	1 slice (5.3 oz)	441	21	61	29	2
prune one crust	1 slice (5.3 oz)	450	14	77	55	2
pumpkin	1 slice (5.4 oz)	323	15	42	21	4
raisin tart	1 (4.2 oz)	348	16	49	21	2
raisin two crust	1 slice (5.3 oz)	376	16	55	26	2
raspberry one crust	1 slice (4.8 oz)	330	13	52	29	6
raspberry two crust	1 slice (5.3 oz)	422	20	58	25	5

FOOD	PORTION	CAL	FAT	CARB	SUGAR	FIBER
rhubarb two crust	1 slice (5.3 oz)	444	23	55	16	2
shoo-fly	1 slice (4 oz)	404	13	69	39	1
strawberry rhubarb two crust	1 slice (5.3 oz)	422	21	53	18	2
strawberry two crust	1 slice (6 oz)	386	16	58	29	3
sweet potato	1 piece (5.4 oz)	276	14	32	13	2
PIE CRUST						
baked	⅙ crust (1 oz)	147	9	14	1	tr
chocolate wafer	⅛ crust (1.2 oz)	177	11	19	8	1
chocolate wafer tart shell	1 (0.8 oz)	111	7	12	5	tr
deep dish frzn	⅛ crust (1.8 oz)	266	16	27	–	1
graham cracker	⅙ crust (1.2 oz)	172	9	23	13	1
graham cracker tart shell	1 (0.8 oz)	109	5	14	8	tr
puff pastry shell	1 (1.4 oz)	223	15	18	tr	1
tart shell	1 (1 oz)	149	10	14	1	tr
Jiffy						
Mix as prep	1/16 pkg	80	5	8	0	0
Pepperidge Farm						
Puff Pastry Sheets frzn	⅙ sheet	160	10	16	1	1
Puff Pastry Shell frzn	1	180	11	18	1	2
Pillsbury						
Pet Ritz Deep Dish frzn	⅛ (0.6 oz)	90	5	11	1	0
PIE FILLING						
apple	1 cup	155	tr	41	34	2
blueberry	1 cup	474	1	116	99	7
cherry	1 cup	317	2	76	66	2

FOOD	PORTION	CAL	FAT	CARB	SUGAR	FIBER
lemon	1 cup	923	18	185	166	1
pumpkin pie mix canned	1 cup (9.5 oz)	281	tr	71	–	22
Comstock						
Apple No Sugar Added	⅓ cup (3 oz)	35	0	8	5	1
Apple Caramel	⅓ cup (3 oz)	90	0	23	21	1
Berry Medley	⅓ cup	90	0	21	16	1
Blackberry	⅓ cup (3 oz)	100	0	22	13	1
Blueberry More Fruit	⅓ cup (3 oz)	90	0	22	18	2
Cherry Dark Sweet	⅓ cup (3 oz)	70	0	18	14	0
Cherry More Fruit Lite	⅓ cup (3 oz)	90	0	21	16	0
Cherry No Sugar Added	⅓ cup (3 oz)	35	0	8	4	0
Key Lime Crème	⅓ cup (3.2 oz)	170	3	36	28	0
Lemon Crème	⅓ cup (3.2 oz)	130	2	28	20	0
Peach Country	⅓ cup (3 oz)	100	0	26	17	1
Strawberry	⅓ cup (3 oz)	100	0	24	10	0
PIEROGI						
potato	1 (1.3 oz)	70	2	11	tr	1
PIGEON PEAS						
dried cooked	1 cup	204	1	39	–	–
dried cooked w/ salt	½ cup (2.9 oz)	102	tr	20	–	6
PIGNOLIA (*see* PINE NUTS)						
PIG'S FEET						
cooked	1	201	14	0	0	0
pickled	1	177	14	tr	tr	0
PIKE						
northern cooked	3 oz	96	1	0	0	0
northern cooked	½ fillet (5.4 oz)	176	1	0	0	0
northern raw	3 oz	75	1	0	0	0

FOOD	PORTION	CAL	FAT	CARB	SUGAR	FIBER
roe raw	1 oz	37	tr	tr	–	–
walleye baked	3 oz	101	1	0	0	0
walleye fillet baked	4.4 oz	147	2	0	0	0
PILLNUTS						
canarytree dried	1 oz	204	23	1	–	–
PIMIENTOS						
canned	1 slice	0	0	tr	–	–
canned	1 tbsp	3	tr	1	–	–
PINE NUTS						
pine nuts dried	¼ cup (1.2 oz)	277	23	4	1	1
pinyon dried	1 oz	178	17	5	–	3
pinyon dried	20 (2 g)	13	1	tr	–	tr
PINEAPPLE						
CANNED						
in heavy syrup crushed sliced or chunks	1 cup (8.9 oz)	198	tr	51	50	2
in heavy syrup slice	1 (1.7 oz)	38	tr	10	8	tr
in juice crushed sliced or chunks	1 cup (8.7 oz)	149	tr	39	36	2
in light syrup crushed sliced or chunks	1 cup (8.8 oz)	131	tr	34	32	2
in light syrup slice	1 (1.7 oz)	25	tr	6	6	tr
in water crushed sliced or chunks	1 cup (8.6 oz)	79	tr	20	18	2
juice pack slice	1 (1.6 oz)	28	tr	7	7	tr
water pack slice	1 (1.6 oz)	15	tr	4	4	tr
Del Monte						
Crushed In 100% Juice	½ cup (4.3 oz)	70	0	17	15	1
Slices in 100% Juice	2 (4 oz)	60	0	16	14	1
Slices In Heavy Syrup	2 (4 oz)	60	0	16	14	1

FOOD	PORTION	CAL	FAT	CARB	SUGAR	FIBER
Dole						
Crushed In Heavy Syrup	½ cups (4.3 oz)	90	0	24	22	1
Crushed Juice Pack	½ cup (4.3 oz)	70	0	18	16	1
Slices In Heavy Syrup	2 (4.1 oz)	90	0	24	22	1
Slices Juice Pack	2 (4 oz)	60	0	15	13	1
DRIED						
dried	1 piece (1 oz)	71	tr	19	14	2
Crispy Green						
Crispy Pineapple	1 pkg (0.35)	35	0	9	7	1
Crunchies						
Freeze Dried	1 pkg (9 g)	35	0	8	6	tr
Crunchy N'Yummy						
Organic Freeze Dried	1 pkg (1 oz)	100	0	23	0	2
FRESH						
chunks	1 cup (5.8 oz)	82	tr	22	16	2
slice	1 slice (3 oz)	42	tr	11	8	1
whole	1 (2 lbs)	452	1	119	89	13
Dole						
Pineapple	2 slices (3.9 oz)	60	0	15	12	2
FROZEN						
chunks sweetened	1 cup (8.6 oz)	211	tr	54	52	3
Dole						
Chunks	¾ cup (4.9 oz)	70	0	18	3	2
Tropical Gold	1 pkg (3 oz)	45	0	11	8	1

PINEAPPLE JUICE

FOOD	PORTION	CAL	FAT	CARB	SUGAR	FIBER
canned unsweetened w/ vitamin C	1 cup (8.8 oz)	132	tr	32	25	1
frzn unsweetened as prep w/ water	1 cup (8.8 oz)	130	tr	32	31	1
Del Monte						
Juice	8 oz	110	0	26	23	0

FOOD	PORTION	CAL	FAT	CARB	SUGAR	FIBER
Dole						
100% Juice	1 can (6 oz)	90	0	22	21	1
Fizzy Lizzy						
Pineapple	1 bottle (12 oz)	100	0	25	25	–
PINK BEANS						
dried cooked	1 cup	252	1	47	–	–
PINTO BEANS						
dried cooked	1 cup	245	1	45	1	15
TAKE-OUT						
stewed w/ viandas	1 cup	222	8	27	2	6
PISTACHIOS						
dry roasted w/ salt	49 nuts (1 oz)	161	13	8	2	3
dry roasted w/o salt	49 nuts (1 oz)	162	13	8	2	3
in shells	½ cup	165	13	8	2	3
Planters						
Dry Roasted In Shell	½ cup	160	13	8	2	3
Sante						
Candied	¼ cup (1 oz)	200	16	11	7	1
Wonderful						
Roasted & Salted In Shells	½ cup	160	14	8	2	3
PITANGA						
fresh	1 cup	57	1	13	–	–
fresh	1	2	tr	1	–	–
PIZZA (*see also* PIZZA CRUST)						
A.C.LaRocco						
Thin Crust Whole Grain Tomato & Feta	⅓ pie (4.8 oz)	250	8	40	3	9
Ultra Thin Sprouted Grain Bruschetta	½ pie (3.5 oz)	170	8	17	0	1

FOOD	PORTION	CAL	FAT	CARB	SUGAR	FIBER
Bellatoria						
Fire Grilled Flatbread Buffalo Chicken	⅓ pie (5.8 oz)	340	17	34	4	5
Fire Grilled Flatbread Chicken Ranch w/ Uncured Bacon	¼ pie (4.5 oz)	270	13	25	3	3
Ultra Thin Crust Margherita	⅓ pie (4.9 oz)	280	16	23	2	1
Ultra Thin Crust Ultimate Pepperoni	¼ pie (4.3 oz)	300	18	21	3	1
Bold Organics						
Deluxe	½ pie (6.7 oz)	460	24	56	12	5
Meat Lovers	½ pie (6 oz)	450	24	54	11	5
Vegan Cheese	½ pie (5.5 oz)	380	18	54	11	5
Veggie Lovers	½ pie (6.2 oz)	390	18	55	12	5
Farm Rich						
Pizza Slices Pepperoni	2 (3.5 oz)	280	14	22	6	1
Foods By George						
Gluten Free Cheese	1 pie (6.5 oz)	400	15	44	5	2
Lean Cuisine						
Casual Cuisine Deep Dish Roasted Vegetable	1 pkg (6 oz)	320	5	52	6	3
Casual Cuisine Deep Dish Spinach & Mushroom	1 pkg (6 oz)	340	7	52	5	2
Casual Cuisine Deep Dish Three Meat	1 pkg (6.4 oz)	390	9	55	7	3
Casual Cuisine Flatbread Melts Chicken Philly	1 pkg (6.5 oz)	350	9	46	5	5
Casual Cuisine Traditional Deluxe	1 pkg (6 oz)	340	8	49	6	4
Casual Cuisine Traditional Four Cheese	1 pkg (6 oz)	350	6	55	6	3

FOOD	PORTION	CAL	FAT	CARB	SUGAR	FIBER
Casual Cuisine Traditional Mushroom	1 pkg (6 oz)	300	5	50	5	4
Casual Cuisine Traditional Pepperoni	1 pkg (6 oz)	380	9	55	6	3
Casual Cuisine Wood Fire Bacon Alfredo	1 pkg (6 oz)	320	9	42	4	2
Casual Cuisine Wood Fire Margherita	1 pkg (6 oz)	310	7	46	7	3
Simple Favorites French Bread Cheese	1 pkg (6 oz)	340	7	53	7	5
Lunchables						
Extra Cheesy	1 pkg	280	9	31	6	3
Pizza w/ Pepperoni	1 pkg	310	13	31	6	3
Mom Made						
Munchie Cheese Pizza	1 (2.5 oz)	160	9	13	2	1
Pacific Foods						
BBQ Chicken	⅓ pie (4.5 oz)	270	9	30	3	1
Herb Garlic Chicken	⅓ pie (4.5 oz)	270	9	30	3	1
Supreme	⅓ pie (4.8 oz)	270	11	31	4	2
Simply Shari's						
Gluten Free Cheese	½ pie (5 oz)	290	11	35	3	2
Gluten Free Pepperoni	½ pie (5 oz)	320	13	35	3	2
Gluten Free Pesto Margherita	½ pie (5 oz)	340	15	36	3	3
Gluten Free Spinach Feta	¼ pkg (5 oz)	280	10	35	4	2
Gluten Free Vegetable Margherita	¼ pie (5 oz)	220	5	38	4	3
Solterra						
Cheese Margherita	½ pie (4.1 oz)	200	9	22	2	2
Vegan	½ pie (4.1 oz)	210	10	27	2	3
Tandoor Chef						
Naan Pizza Margherita	½ pie (4 oz)	220	3	38	6	2

FOOD	PORTION	CAL	FAT	CARB	SUGAR	FIBER
Naan Pizza Roasted Eggplant	½ pie (4.6 oz)	320	6	53	8	4
Naan Pizza Spinach & Paneer Cheese	½ pie (4.2 oz)	290	5	50	6	4
Tofutti						
Pan Crust Pizzaz Dairy Free	1 slice (2.7 oz)	180	7	24	6	1
Vitalicious						
VitaPizza Cheese & Tomato	1 (5.3 oz)	190	3	38	4	11
VitaPizza Meatless Pepperoni Supreme	1 (5.3 oz)	190	3	38	4	19
TAKE-OUT						
cheese	⅛ of 16 in pie	423	18	46	5	3
cheese	16 in pie	3384	144	372	44	23
cheese deep dish individual	1 (5.5 oz)	460	24	47	4	2
cheese & vegetables	⅛ of 16 in pie	428	16	55	5	3
ground beef	16 in pie	3753	172	392	25	20
ham & pineapple	⅛ of 16 in pie	439	16	55	7	3
no cheese	⅛ of 16 in pie	262	7	43	3	2
pepperoni	⅛ of 16 in pie	469	22	49	3	3
white pizza	⅛ of 16 in pie	484	17	61	1	2

PIZZA CRUST

Crust	1 slice (1.7 oz)	130	2	25	1	1
whole wheat	⅛ crust (2 oz)	120	2	24	0	4
Jiffy						
Crust Mix as prep	⅕ pie	140	3	26	1	tr
Stonefire						
Italian Thin w/ Sauce	1 serv (1.9 oz)	130	3	22	2	1
Stonebaked Original	⅙ (1.8 oz)	140	3	24	1	1

FOOD	PORTION	CAL	FAT	CARB	SUGAR	FIBER
Udi's						
Gluten Free	½ crust (4.2 oz)	300	9	47	5	2
PLANTAINS						
cooked mashed	1 cup	232	tr	62	28	5
sliced cooked	1 cup	179	tr	48	22	4
Dole						
Fresh cooked	½ med (3.2 oz)	100	0	28	13	2
Isleno						
Chips	1 oz	150	9	17	0	2
TAKE-OUT						
mofongo	1 serv	320	3	71	31	5
ripe fried	1 serv (2.8 oz)	214	7	38	–	4
sweet baked w/ ice cream	1 serv	285	8	57	35	3
PLUMS						
canned purple in heavy syrup	1 cup	163	tr	42	39	3
canned purple juice pack	1 cup	146	tr	38	35	2
canned purple water pack	1 cup	102	tr	27	25	2
dried japanese	1	9	tr	2	1	tr
fresh	1	30	tr	8	7	1
pickled	1	34	tr	9	9	tr
Dole						
Fresh	2 (5.3 oz)	70	0	17	15	2
Fruit Bliss						
Soft Dried	5 (1.5 oz)	100	0	28	17	3

FOOD	PORTION	CAL	FAT	CARB	SUGAR	FIBER
POI						
poi	1 cup	240	0	65	–	1
POKEBERRY SHOOTS						
cooked	½ cup	16	tr	3	–	–
fresh	½ cup	18	tr	3	–	–
POLLACK						
atlantic baked	3 oz	100	1	0	0	0
atlantic fillet baked	5.3 oz	178	2	0	0	0
POMEGRANATE						
fresh	1 (5.4 oz)	105	tr	26	26	1
Navitas Naturals						
Pomegranate Powder	1 tbsp (0.5 oz)	50	0	13	3	0
POM						
Poms Fresh Arils	1 pkg (4.3 oz)	100	1	20	9	6
POMEGRANATE JUICE						
KeVita						
Sparkling Probiotic Drink Organic	8 oz	20	0	4	4	–
POM						
100% Juice	8 oz	150	0	38	32	0
100% Juice Concentrate	3 tbsp (1.5 oz)	150	0	36	30	0
Lite Pomegranate Cocktail	8 oz	75	0	19	18	0
Lite Pomegranate Dragonfruit	8 oz	80	0	20	17	0
Pomegranate Blueberry	8 oz	150	0	36	31	0
Pomegranate Cherry	8 oz	150	0	36	29	0
Smart Juice						
Organic 100% Juice	8 oz	149	0	37	33	1
Ultra Lo-Gly						
Pomegranate	1 bottle (10 oz)	45	0	10	9	0

FOOD	PORTION	CAL	FAT	CARB	SUGAR	FIBER
Pomegranate Mojita	1 bottle (10 oz)	40	0	9	7	0
POMPANO						
smoked	2 oz	109	6	0	0	0
steamed or poached	4 oz	156	9	0	0	0
TAKE-OUT						
battered & fried	4 oz	304	21	8	tr	tr
breaded & fried	4 oz	242	15	10	1	1
POPCORN						
air popped	1 cup (0.3 oz)	31	tr	6	–	2
caramel coated	1 cup (1.2 oz)	152	5	28	14	2
caramel coated w/ peanuts	⅔ cup (1 oz)	114	2	23	11	1
cheese	1 cup (0.4 oz)	58	4	6	–	1
oil popped	1 cup (0.4 oz)	55	3	6	tr	1
Bachman						
Regular	2¾ cups (1 oz)	160	10	14	0	6
Chip'ins						
Chips Hot Buffalo Wing	18 (1 oz)	130	5	21	0	1
Chips Jalapeno Ranch	18 (1 oz)	130	4	21	0	1
Chips Sea Salt	8 (1 oz)	120	3	22	0	1
Chips White Cheddar	18 (1 oz)	130	4	21	1	1
Cracker Jack						
The Original	½ cup (1 oz)	120	2	23	15	1
G.H.Cretors						
Caramel Nut Crunch	½ cup (1 oz)	130	6	19	16	1
Chicago Mix	1¼ cup (1 oz)	140	8	17	10	1
Just The Caramel	¾ cup (1 oz)	120	5	21	17	1
Just The Cheese	2 cups (1 oz)	170	13	10	0	2
Kettle Corn	2 cups (1 oz)	130	7	18	6	2

FOOD	PORTION	CAL	FAT	CARB	SUGAR	FIBER
Orville Redenbacher's						
Microwave Smart Pop 94% Fat Free as prep	1 cup	15	0	3	–	1
Popcorn Indiana						
Kettlecorn Cinnamon Sugar	2½ cups (1 oz)	130	5	21	7	2
Kettlecorn Sweet & Tangy BBQ	2½ cups (1 oz)	130	5	21	7	2
Original Movie Theater	2 cups (1 oz)	160	12	13	0	3
Sea Salt	3 cups (1 oz)	130	6	18	0	3
Smartfood						
Kettle Corn	1¼ cups (1 oz)	140	6	20	11	2
Reduced Fat White Cheddar	3 cups (1 oz)	130	6	18	0	3
White Cheddar	1¾ cups (1 oz)	160	10	14	2	2
The Whole Earth						
Organic Kettle Corn Salty & Sweet	2 cups (1 oz)	120	5	20	9	2
POPOVER						
home recipe as prep w/ 2% milk	1 (1.4 oz)	87	3	11	–	–
home recipe as prep w/ whole milk	1 (1.4 oz)	90	3	11	–	–
mix as prep	1 (1.2 oz)	67	2	10	–	–
POPPY SEEDS						
poppy seeds	1 tbsp	47	4	2	1	1
PORGY						
fresh	3 oz	77	tr	0	0	0

FOOD	PORTION	CAL	FAT	CARB	SUGAR	FIBER
PORK (*see also* HAM, JERKY, PORK DISHES)						
CANNED						
Spam						
Classic	2 oz	180	16	1	0	0
Less Sodium	2 oz	180	16	1	0	0
Smoked	2 oz	180	16	1	0	0
Spread	2 oz	140	12	1	1	0
FRESH						
boneless loin lean & fat roasted	3.5 oz	195	9	0	0	0
center loin chop bone in broiled	1 (3 oz)	178	9	0	0	0
center rib chop lean & fat bone in broiled	1 (3 oz)	189	11	0	0	0
country style ribs bone in lean & fat braised	3.5 oz	288	19	0	0	0
dehydrated oriental style	1 cup (0.8 oz)	135	14	tr	0	0
fresh ham rump half lean & fat roasted	4 oz	278	16	0	0	0
fresh ham shank half lean & fat roasted	4 oz	319	22	0	0	0
fresh ham whole lean & fat roasted	4 oz	302	19	0	0	0
ground cooked	4 oz	328	23	0	0	0
ham hock cooked	1	167	12	0	0	0
shoulder chop bone in braised	1 (3 oz)	229	15	0	0	0
sirloin roast lean & fat bone in roasted	4 oz	231	13	0	0	0
spareribs bone in roasted	3 oz	304	26	0	0	0
tail simmered	3 oz	336	30	0	0	0

FOOD	PORTION	CAL	FAT	CARB	SUGAR	FIBER
tenderloin roast boneless lean & fat roasted	4 oz	145	4	0	0	0
top loin chop boneless lean & fat broiled	1 (3.5 oz)	195	9	0	0	0
Dietz & Watson						
Chops Boneless Smoked	3 oz	110	3	3	3	0
Shoulder Butt	3 oz	150	9	1	1	0
Spare Ribs Canadian Center Cut	1 serv (5 oz)	300	20	15	1	0
Hatfield						
Chop Center Cut Boneless	1 (4 oz)	130	4	2	0	0
Hormel						
Always Tender Loin Filet Honey Mustard	1 serv (4 oz)	140	5	4	4	0
Always Tender Loin Filet Lemon Garlic	1 serv (4 oz)	130	5	1	0	0
Always Tender Tenderloin Apple Bourbon	1 serv (4 oz)	140	4	5	4	0
Pork Chops Smoked Thin Cut Bone-In	3 oz	140	9	0	0	0
Organic Prairie						
Chop Bone In	1 (3.3 oz)	220	13	0	0	0
FROZEN						
Organic Prairie						
Ribs Boneless Country Style	1 (4 oz)	160	7	0	0	0
Tenderloin	4 oz	150	6	0	0	0
TAKE-OUT						
char siu chinese style	1 piece (4 oz)	28	2	2	–	0

FOOD	PORTION	CAL	FAT	CARB	SUGAR	FIBER
chicharrones pork cracklings fried	1 cup	492	38	1	0	0
chop breaded & fried	1 med (3.4 oz)	304	18	13	1	1
chop breaded & fried	1 lg (5 oz)	441	26	19	2	1
chop stewed	1 lg (4.6 oz)	315	18	0	0	0
PORK DISHES						
Lloyd's						
Babyback Pork Ribs w/ Original BBQ Sauce	1 serv (5 oz)	340	21	12	12	0
TAKE-OUT						
kalua pork	1 cup (7 oz)	497	34	1	–	0
pork satay w/ peanut sauce	5 sticks (3.5 oz)	214	13	14	–	3
pulled pork w/ barbecue sauce	1 serv (5 oz)	240	14	15	12	1
spareribs barbecue w/ sauce	2 med (2.8 oz)	248	18	3	1	tr
tourtiere	1 piece (4.9 oz)	451	34	21	–	–
POT PIE						
Bell & Evans						
Chicken	1 cup (7.9 oz)	520	29	48	3	2
Pacific Foods						
Organic Beef	1 cup (8 oz)	410	21	40	0	6
Organic Turkey	1 cup (8 oz)	400	19	46	1	7
TAKE-OUT						
beef	1 (14.6 oz)	938	57	72	4	5
chicken	1 (14.6 oz)	897	52	69	5	6
ham	1 serv (11 oz)	752	45	58	3	4
oyster	1 serv (11.5 oz)	817	53	67	6	3

FOOD	PORTION	CAL	FAT	CARB	SUGAR	FIBER
puerto rican pastelon de carne	1 piece (5 oz)	666	48	35	1	2
st. stephen's day pie	1 serv (16.7 oz)	549	29	38	5	6
tuna	1 (27 oz)	1715	102	126	10	10
vegetarian w/ meat substitute	1 (8 oz)	511	32	39	3	5

POTATO (*see also* CHIPS, KNISH, PANCAKES)

FOOD	PORTION	CAL	FAT	CARB	SUGAR	FIBER
CANNED						
potatoes	½ cup	54	tr	12	–	–
Butter Kernel						
Whole	⅔ cup (5.4 oz)	60	0	13	0	2
Del Monte						
New Whole	2 med (5.5 oz)	70	0	15	1	1
FRESH						
baked skin only	1 skin (2 oz)	115	tr	27	–	2
baked w/ skin	1 (6.5 oz)	220	tr	51	–	–
baked w/o skin	½ cup	57	tr	13	–	1
baked w/o skin	1 (5 oz)	145	tr	34	–	2
boiled	½ cup	68	tr	16	–	1
microwaved	1 (7 oz)	212	tr	49	–	–
microwaved w/o skin	½ cup	78	tr	18	–	–
raw w/o skin	1 (3.9 oz)	88	tr	20	–	–
red new boiled	5 sm (5 oz)	120	0	27	3	2
Dole						
Idaho	1 (5.3 oz)	110	0	26	1	2
Green Giant						
Klondike Gourmet	5 sm (5.3 oz)	110	0	26	1	2
Masser's						
Roasted Russet Triple Washed	1 (5.3 oz)	110	0	26	1	2

FOOD	PORTION	CAL	FAT	CARB	SUGAR	FIBER
Melissa's						
Dutch Yellow Baby diced	¾ cup (3.9 oz)	80	0	20	tr	2
FROZEN						
french fries	10 strips	111	4	17	–	2
french fries thick cut	10 strips	109	4	17	–	–
hash browns	½ cup	170	9	22	–	–
potato puffs	1	16	1	2	–	–
potato puffs	½ cup	138	7	19	–	–
Alexia						
Sweet Potato Puffs	⅔ cup (3 oz)	130	4	23	8	2
Birds Eye						
Steamfresh Roasted Red Potatoes w/ Garlic Butter Sauce	1¼ cups (5.1 oz)	190	7	30	0	3
Lean Cuisine						
Simple Favorites Cheddar Potato w/ Broccoli	1 pkg (10.25 oz)	210	4	34	6	4
McCain						
5 Minute Fries	1 serv (3 oz)	120	5	16	tr	1
Farmer's Kitchen Oven Baked Crinkles	12 pieces (2 oz)	50	1	11	0	1
Purely Potatoes Whole Baby Skin On	1 serv (3 oz)	100	0	16	0	tr
MIX						
au gratin as prep	½ cup	160	9	14	–	–
instant mashed flakes as prep w/ whole milk & butter	½ cup	118	6	16	–	–
instant mashed flakes not prep	½ cup	78	tr	18	–	–

FOOD	PORTION	CAL	FAT	CARB	SUGAR	FIBER
instant mashed granules as prep w/ whole milk & butter	½ cup	114	5	15	–	–
instant mashed granules not prep	½ cup	372	1	86	–	–
scalloped	½ cup	105	5	13	–	–
Betty Crocker						
Mashed Creamy Butter as prep	⅔ cup	80	1	17	1	3
Idahoan						
Mashed Buttery Homestyle as prep	½ cup	110	3	20	2	1
Mashed Buttery Yukon as prep	½ cup	110	3	21	2	2
Mashed Original as prep	½ cup	170	7	24	0	2
Mashed Roasted Garlic as prep	½ cup	110	3	20	2	1
REFRIGERATED						
Country Crock						
Homestyle Mashed	⅔ cup (5 oz)	160	9	18	1	1
TAKE-OUT						
au gratin w/ cheese	½ cup	178	10	17	–	–
baked topped w/ cheese sauce	1	475	29	47	–	–
baked topped w/ cheese sauce & bacon	1	451	26	44	–	–
baked topped w/ cheese sauce & broccoli	1 (12 oz)	403	21	47	–	–
baked topped w/ cheese sauce & chili	1	481	22	56	–	–
baked topped w/ sour cream & chives	1	394	22	50	–	–

FOOD	PORTION	CAL	FAT	CARB	SUGAR	FIBER
french fries	1 reg	235	12	29	–	–
hash browns	½ cup (2.5 oz)	151	9	16	–	–
indian yogurt potatoes	1 serv	315	9	52	–	0
mashed	½ cup	111	4	18	–	–
o'brien	1 cup	157	3	30	–	–
potato pancakes	1 (1.3 oz)	101	7	11	–	–
potato salad	½ cup	179	10	14	–	2
scalloped	½ cup	127	5	18	–	–
twice baked w/ cheese	1 half (10 oz)	392	18	48	–	4
POTATO STARCH						
potato starch	1 oz	96	tr	24	–	–
POUT						
ocean baked	3 oz	87	1	0	0	0
ocean fillet baked	1 (4.8 oz)	140	2	0	0	0
PRETZELS						
chocolate covered	1 (0.4 oz)	47	1	8	2	tr
soft	1 lg (5 oz)	483	4	99	tr	2
twists salted	10 (2.1 oz)	229	2	48	–	2
twists w/o salt	10 (2.1 oz)	229	2	48	1	2
whole wheat	2 sm (1 oz)	103	1	23	–	2
yogurt covered	1 cup (3 oz)	391	13	61	30	1
yogurt covered	1 (4 g)	19	1	3	1	tr
Annie's Homegrown						
Organic Bunnies	32 (1 oz)	100	1	19	1	1
Bachman						
Honey Wheat Splits	9 (1 oz)	110	1	23	3	1
Mini Low Sodium	17 (1 oz)	110	0	25	–	1
Original Twist	5 (1 oz)	100	1	22	1	1
Rolled Rods	2 (1 oz)	110	0	23	1	1
Thin N Rights	12 (1 oz)	120	1	23	1	1

FOOD	PORTION	CAL	FAT	CARB	SUGAR	FIBER
Better Balance						
Cinnamon Toast Gluten Free	1 oz	120	5	9	0	3
Golden Butter Twists Gluten Free	1 oz	110	5	12	1	2
Jalapeno Mustard Gluten Free	1 oz	120	5	9	2	3
Farm Rich						
Stuffed Bites frzn	3 (1.7 oz)	110	3	18	2	1
Mary's Gone Crackers						
Sticks & Twigs Sea Salt Organic	15 (1 oz)	150	5	21	0	4
Rold Gold						
Braided Twists Honey Wheat	8 (1 oz)	110	1	24	3	1
Rods	3 (1 oz)	110	1	22	1	1
Sourdough	1 (0.8 oz)	90	1	19	tr	2
Sticks	53 (1 oz)	100	0	23	1	1
Tiny Twists Fat Free	18 (1 oz)	110	0	23	tr	tr
PRUNE JUICE						
jarred	1 cup	182	tr	45	42	3
Del Monte						
100% Juice	8 oz	180	0	42	25	3
PRUNES						
cooked w/o sugar	½ cup	133	tr	35	31	4
dried	1	20	tr	5	3	1
Del Monte						
Dried	5 (1.4 oz)	100	0	26	15	3
Dried Pitted	5 (1.5 oz)	100	0	24	12	3
Sunsweet						
Ones	4 (1.4 oz)	100	0	24	12	3
Pitted	5 (1.4 oz)	100	0	24	12	3

FOOD	PORTION	CAL	FAT	CARB	SUGAR	FIBER
PUDDING						
MIX						
Jell-O						
Banana Cream Instant as prep w/ 2% milk	½ cup	150	3	30	18	0
Butterscotch Cook & Serve as prep w/ 2% milk	½ cup	160	3	30	19	0
Chocolate Cook & Serve Sugar Free Fat Free as prep w/ fat free milk	½ cup	70	0	15	0	0
Chocolate Cook & Serve as prep w/ 2% milk	½ cup	150	3	27	15	0
Coconut Cream Instant as prep w/ 2% milk	½ cup	160	5	27	16	0
Rice Fat Free as prep w/ fat free milk	½ cup	140	0	30	13	0
Tapioca Fat Free Cook & Serve as prep w/ fat free milk	½ cup	130	0	27	15	0
Vanilla Instant as prep	1 serv	90	0	23	19	0
READY-TO-EAT						
Cocon						
Mixed Mini Pudding w/ Nata De Coco	2 (1 oz)	15	0	3	3	0
Jell-O						
Boston Cream Pie Sugar Free Reduced Calorie	1 pkg (3.7 oz)	60	1	13	0	0
Chocolate	1 pkg (4 oz)	120	2	25	19	1
Chocolate Fat Free	1 pkg (4 oz)	100	0	23	17	1
Chocolate Vanilla Swirl	1 pkg (4 oz)	110	2	24	19	1
Creme Brulee Sugar Free Reduced Calorie	1 pkg (3.7 oz)	70	2	12	0	0

FOOD	PORTION	CAL	FAT	CARB	SUGAR	FIBER
Dulce De Leche Sugar Free Reduced Calorie	1 pkg (3.7 oz)	60	1	13	0	0
Orange Ice Cream Shop	1 pkg (3.9 oz)	120	3	23	18	0
Rice Sugar Free Reduced Calorie	1 pkg (3.7 oz)	70	2	12	0	0
Tapioca	1 pkg (4 oz)	110	2	25	19	0
Vanilla	1 serv (4 oz)	110	2	23	18	0
Vanilla Sugar Free Reduced Calorie	1 pkg (3.7 oz)	60	1	13	0	0
Kozy Shack						
Banana	1 pkg (4 oz)	130	5	19	15	0
Bread Pudding Apple Cinnamon	1 pkg (3.5 oz)	150	3	26	19	0
Butterscotch	1 pkg (4 oz)	120	2	23	19	0
Chocolate Lactose Free	1 pkg (4 oz)	130	4	22	17	1
Chocolate No Sugar Added	1 pkg (4 oz)	60	1	10	4	4
Old Fashioned Tapioca	1 pkg (4 oz)	130	3	23	17	0
Rice Lactose Free	1 pkg (4 oz)	120	3	20	13	0
Rice No Sugar Added	1 pkg (4 oz)	70	1	14	5	3
Rice Original	1 pkg (4 oz)	130	3	21	14	0
Soda Shoppe Orange Cream Pop	1 pkg (3.7 oz)	110	1	21	17	0
Soda Shoppe Root Beer Float	1 pkg (3.7 oz)	100	1	20	17	0
Tapioca Lactose Free	1 pkg (4 oz)	120	3	20	15	0
Tapioca No Sugar Added	1 pkg (4 oz)	70	1	14	6	3
Vanilla	1 pkg (4 oz)	130	3	21	18	0
Vanilla No Sugar Added	1 pkg (4 oz)	90	3	10	5	4
Snack Pack						
Banana Cream Pie	1 pkg (3.5 oz)	110	4	18	13	0
Butterscotch	1 pkg (3.5 oz)	110	3	21	16	0
Caramel Cream	1 pkg (3.5 oz)	120	3	21	17	0

FOOD	PORTION	CAL	FAT	CARB	SUGAR	FIBER
Chocolate	1 pkg (3.5 oz)	130	3	23	16	tr
Chocolate Daredevil Triples	1 pkg (3.5 oz)	130	4	23	18	tr
Chocolate Fat Free	1 pkg (3.5 oz)	80	0	20	15	tr
Chocolate No Sugar Added	1 pkg (3.5 oz)	70	4	15	0	1
Lemon	1 pkg (3.5 oz)	130	3	25	20	0
Tapioca	1 pkg (3.5 oz)	120	4	20	15	0
Tapioca Fat Free	1 serv (3.5 oz)	80	0	18	13	0
Vanilla	1 pkg (3.5 oz)	120	4	21	14	1
SoYummi						
Dark Chocolate	1 pkg (3.5 oz)	110	3	17	11	4
Key Lime	1 pkg (3.5 oz)	115	4	17	11	2
Rice	1 pkg (3.5 oz)	110	2	19	6	2
Tapioca	1 pkg (3.5 oz)	110	3	18	8	3
TAKE-OUT						
blancmange	1 serv (4.7 oz)	154	5	25	–	tr
bread w/ raisins	1 cup	306	9	47	29	2
coconut	1 cup	291	9	45	38	2
corn	1 cup	328	13	43	17	4
guinataan coconut milk pudding	1 cup (9 oz)	331	11	59	–	3
indian pudding	½ cup	156	4	25	16	1
noodle pudding kugel	1 cup	297	10	44	15	2
plum pudding	1 slice (1.5 oz)	125	5	20	12	1
pumpkin	½ cup (4.6 oz)	139	4	24	19	tr
queen of puddings	1 serv (4.4 oz)	266	10	41	–	tr
rice pudding	1 cup	302	4	60	37	1
sweet potato	½ cup	107	3	19	7	3

FOOD	PORTION	CAL	FAT	CARB	SUGAR	FIBER
tapioca	1 cup	236	7	35	31	0
yorkshire	1 serv (3 oz)	177	8	22	–	tr
PUFFERFISH						
raw	3 oz	72	0	0	0	0
PUMMELO						
fresh white	1 (21.4 oz)	231	tr	59	–	6
sections white	1 cup (6.7 oz)	72	tr	18	–	2
Sunkist						
Fresh	¼ (5.3 oz)	90	1	20	11	4
PUMPKIN						
butter	1 tbsp	32	0	8	8	–
canned w/o salt	1 cup (8.6 oz)	83	1	20	8	7
cooked mashed w/o salt	1 cup (8.6 oz)	49	tr	12	3	3
flowers cooked w/o salt	1 cup (4.7 oz)	20	tr	4	3	1
leaves cooked w/o salt	1 cup (2.5 oz)	15	tr	2	tr	2
Farmer's Market						
Organic Puree	½ cup (4.3 oz)	50	0	10	4	4
Libby's						
Pumpkin	½ cup (4.3 oz)	40	1	9	4	5
TAKE-OUT						
indian sago	1 serv (2.3 oz)	75	5	6	3	3
pumpkin fritters	1 (1.2 oz)	84	3	14	8	tr
PUMPKIN SEEDS						
kernels dried	¼ cup (1.1 oz)	180	16	3	tr	2
kernels roasted w/o salt	¼ cup (1 oz)	169	14	4	tr	2
whole roasted w/o salt	¼ cup (0.5 oz)	71	3	9	–	3
David						
Kernels	1 pkg (2.5 oz)	280	22	6	tr	2
Spitz						
Seasoned Hulled	¼ cup (1 oz)	180	15	4	0	4

FOOD	PORTION	CAL	FAT	CARB	SUGAR	FIBER
Sunrich Naturals						
Pepitas Lightly Salted	1 pkg (1 oz)	160	14	4	0	2
PURSLANE						
cooked	1 cup	21	tr	4	–	–
cresh	1 cup	7	tr	1	–	–
QUAIL						
cooked bone removed	1 (2.7 oz)	177	11	0	0	0
QUICHE						
La Terra Fina						
Cheddar & Broccoli	⅕ pie (4.6 oz)	300	18	24	3	2
Lorraine	⅕ pie (4.6 oz)	320	19	22	2	1
Spinach & Artichoke	⅕ pie (4.6 oz)	290	17	23	2	2
TAKE-OUT						
cheese pie	⅛ (9 in)	566	44	27	1	1
lorraine pie	⅛ (9 in)	568	44	27	1	1
mushroom	1 slice (3 oz)	256	18	17	–	1
spinach pie	⅛ (9 in)	342	26	17	1	1
QUINCE						
fresh	1	53	tr	14	–	–
Matiz						
Quince Paste	2 tbsp	83	0	20	13	1
QUINCE JUICE						
Smart Juice						
Organic 100% Juice	8 oz	110	0	31	21	0
QUINOA						
cooked	1 cup (6.5 oz)	222	4	39	–	5
quinoa not prep	¼ cup (1.5 oz)	156	3	27	–	3
Simply Shari's						
Quinoa + Marinara Gluten Free as prep	¼ pkg (4 oz)	175	2	35	4	5

FOOD	PORTION	CAL	FAT	CARB	SUGAR	FIBER
TruRoots						
Organic not prep	¼ cup (1.6 oz)	172	3	31	3	3
Village Harvest						
Whole Grain Medley Golden Quinoa	¾ cup (5 oz)	220	3	43	0	4
Whole Grain Medley Red Quinoa & Brown Rice	1 cup (5 oz)	300	4	58	0	3
RABBIT						
domestic w/o bone roasted	3 oz	167	7	0	0	0
wild w/o bone stewed	3 oz	147	3	0	0	0
RACCOON						
roasted	3 oz	217	12	0	0	0
RADICCHIO						
raw shredded	½ cup	5	tr	1	–	–
RADISHES						
chinese dried	½ cup	157	tr	37	–	–
chinese raw	1 (12 oz)	62	tr	14	–	–
chinese raw sliced	½ cup	8	tr	2	–	–
chinese sliced cooked	½ cup	13	tr	3	–	–
daikon dried	½ cup	157	tr	37	–	–
daikon raw	1 (12 oz)	62	tr	14	–	–
daikon raw sliced	½ cup	8	tr	2	–	–
daikon sliced cooked	½ cup	13	tr	3	–	–
red raw	10	7	tr	2	–	–
red sliced	½ cup	10	tr	2	–	–
white icicle raw	1 (0.5 oz)	2	tr	tr	–	–
white icicle raw sliced	½ cup	7	tr	1	–	–
TAKE-OUT						
korean kimchee	½ cup	31	1	6	–	–

FOOD	PORTION	CAL	FAT	CARB	SUGAR	FIBER
moo namul saengche korean salad	1 serv (3.7 oz)	34	tr	8	6	2
RAISINS						
cinnamon coated	¼ cup	108	tr	29	21	1
cooked	¼ cup	162	tr	42	35	1
golden seedless	¼ cup	109	tr	29	21	1
jumbo golden	¼ cup	130	0	31	29	2
milk chocolate coated	28 (1 oz)	109	4	19	17	1
milk chocolate coated	¼ cup	176	7	31	28	2
seedless	55 (1 oz)	86	tr	23	17	1
sultanas	1 oz	88	0	23	–	2
Dole						
Golden Seedless	¼ cup (1.4 oz)	120	0	32	24	1
Sun-Maid						
Chocolate Covered	30 (1.4 oz)	160	6	27	24	2
RAMBUTAN						
canned in syrup	1 cup (4.3 oz)	123	tr	31	–	1
canned in syrup	1 (0.3 oz)	7	tr	2	–	tr
puerto rican fresh	5 (1.6 oz)	34	tr	8	8	tr
RASPBERRIES						
black fresh	1 cup	70	1	16	6	9
canned in heavy syrup	½ cup	116	tr	30	26	4
canned water pack	1 cup	43	1	10	4	5
fresh	1 pt	162	2	37	14	20
fresh	1 cup	64	1	15	5	8
frzn sweetened	1 cup	129	tr	33	27	6
frzn unsweetened	1 cup	65	1	15	6	8
Dole						
Fresh	1 cup (4.3 oz)	60	1	15	5	8
Raspberries frzn	1 cup (4.9 oz)	70	1	17	7	9

FOOD	PORTION	CAL	FAT	CARB	SUGAR	FIBER
RASPBERRY JUICE						
Izze						
Esque Sparkling Black Raspberry	1 bottle (12 oz)	50	0	12	11	–
Old Orchard						
100% Juice	8 oz	130	0	31	29	–
RELISH						
hamburger	1 tbsp	19	tr	5	–	–
hamburger	½ cup	158	1	42	–	–
hot dog	1 tbsp	14	tr	4	–	–
hot dog	½ cup	111	1	28	–	–
piccalilli	1.4 oz	13	tr	2	–	1
sweet	½ cup	159	1	43	–	–
sweet	1 tbsp	19	tr	5	–	–
tomato	¼ cup (2.8 oz)	119	tr	28	26	1
Gedney						
Sweet	1 tbsp (0.5 oz)	15	0	4	3	0
Jake & Amos						
Chow Chow Sweet & Sour	1 serv (4 oz)	140	0	31	19	5
Corn	2 tbsp	40	0	8	6	0
Green Tomato	1 serv (1 oz)	25	0	7	6	–
RENNIN						
tablet	1 (0.9 g)	1	0	tr	–	–
RHUBARB						
fresh	½ cup	13	tr	3	–	–
frozen	½ cup	60	tr	3	–	–
frzn as prep w/ sugar	½ cup	139	tr	37	–	–
RICE (*see also* RICE CAKES)						
arborio	½ cup	100	0	22	–	–
brown long grain cooked	1 cup (6.8 oz)	216	2	45	–	4

FOOD	PORTION	CAL	FAT	CARB	SUGAR	FIBER
brown medium grain cooked	1 cup (6.8 oz)	218	2	46	–	4
glutinous cooked	1 cup (6.1 oz)	169	tr	37	–	2
starch	1 oz	98	0	24	–	–
white long grain cooked	1 cup (5.5 oz)	205	tr	45	–	1
white long grain instant cooked	1 cup (5.8 oz)	162	tr	35	–	1
white medium grain cooked	1 cup (6.5 oz)	242	tr	53	–	1
white short grain cooked	1 cup (6.5 oz)	242	tr	53	–	–
Birds Eye						
Steamfresh Whole Grain Brown Rice as prep	1 cup (4.8 oz)	150	1	31	0	2
Carolina						
White Medium Grain as prep	1 cup	160	0	35	0	1
Gourmet House						
Indian Basmati as prep	¾ cup	160	0	35	0	0
Italian Arborio as prep	¾ cup	160	0	37	0	tr
Organic Brown as prep	¾ pkg	150	1	32	0	1
Organic White as prep	¾ cup	150	0	35	0	0
Goya						
Yellow Rice not prep	¼ cup (1.6 oz)	160	0	35	0	tr
Lundberg						
Organic Heat & Eat Short Grain	1 pkg (7.4 oz)	290	3	65	1	5
Organic Risotto Florentine not prep	¼ pkg (1.4 oz)	140	0	31	2	1
Organic Risotto Tuscan not prep	¼ pkg (1.4 oz)	140	0	31	2	1
Risotto Butternut Squash not prep	¼ pkg (1.4 oz)	140	1	31	1	1

FOOD	PORTION	CAL	FAT	CARB	SUGAR	FIBER
Mahatma						
Jasmine as prep	¾ cup	160	0	36	0	0
White as prep	¾ cup	150	0	35	0	0
Whole Grain Brown as prep	¾ cup	150	1	32	0	1
Minute						
Brown as prep	⅔ cup	150	2	34	0	2
Ready To Serve Brown & Wild Rice	1 pkg (4.4 oz)	230	5	42	0	5
Ready To Serve Pilaf	1 pkg (4.4 oz)	220	4	41	3	2
Ready To Serve Spanish Rice	1 pkg (4.4 oz)	230	5	41	1	2
Ready To Serve Whole Grain Brown	1 pkg (4.4 oz)	230	4	40	0	2
Steamers Broccoli & Cheese	1 cup (6.4 oz)	200	4	37	2	1
Steamers Fried Rice	1 cup (6.5 oz)	280	6	50	0	2
White as prep	1 cup	200	0	45	0	0
River Rice						
Brown as prep	¾ cup	150	0	32	0	1
Stahlbush Island Farms						
Organic Brown Rice & Black Beans frzn	1 cup (6.2 oz)	200	2	39	0	7
Success						
Boil In Bag Whole Grain Brown as prep	1 cup	150	1	33	0	2
Boil-In-Bag Jasmine as prep	¾ cup	150	0	36	0	0
Boil-In-Bag White as prep	1 cup	190	0	43	0	0
Uncle Ben's						
Boil-In-Bag Whole Grain Brown Rice	1 cup	170	2	36	0	2

FOOD	PORTION	CAL	FAT	CARB	SUGAR	FIBER
Ready Rice Spanish	1 cup (5 oz)	200	3	40	3	2
Ready Rice Whole Grain Medley	1 cup (5 oz)	210	4	41	1	4
Ready Rice Whole Grain Medley Roasted Garlic	1 cup (4.9 oz)	200	3	38	0	3
Whole Grain White Broccoli Cheddar as prep	1 cup	200	2	41	1	4
Whole Grain White Creamy Chicken as prep	1 cup	200	2	44	1	5
Whole Grain White Garden Vegetable as prep	1 cup	180	1	40	2	4
Whole Grain White Long Grain as prep	1 cup	170	1	38	1	4
Whole Grain White Sweet Tomato as prep	1 cup	210	2	46	4	5
Whole Grain White Taco as prep	1 cup	160	2	35	1	4
Village Harvest						
Whole Grain Creations w/ Corn & Black Beans	¾ cup (4.3 oz)	140	2	27	4	4
Whole Grain Medley Brown Red & Wild Rice frzn	1 cup (5 oz)	250	3	52	0	3
Water Maid						
Medium Grain as prep	¾ cup	160	0	36	0	1
Zatarain's						
Black Eyed Peas & Rice as prep	1 cup	220	1	46	0	4
Caribbean Rice Mix as prep	1 cup	160	2	34	0	tr

FOOD	PORTION	CAL	FAT	CARB	SUGAR	FIBER
Cheddar Broccoli as prep	1 cup	220	2	45	3	tr
Yellow as prep	1 cup	190	0	43	tr	tr
TAKE-OUT						
coconut rice	1 serv	500	42	30	–	2
congee	½ cup (4.1 oz)	44	–	10	–	–
dirty rice w/ chicken giblets	1 cup (6.9 oz)	291	10	38	tr	1
nasi goreng indonesian rice & vegetables	1 cup (4.9 oz)	130	0	28	1	1
pea palau rice & peas fried in ghee	1 serv	144	5	21	1	2
pilaf	½ cup	84	3	11	–	3
rice & black beans	1 cup (5.1 oz)	220	6	36	1	5
risotto	1 serv (6.6 oz)	426	18	65	–	3
spanish	¾ cup	363	27	19	–	–
RICE CAKES						
Lundberg						
Eco-Farmed Apple Cinnamon	1 (0.7 oz)	80	1	16	2	1
Eco-Farmed Toasted Sesame	1 (0.7 oz)	70	0	16	0	1
Organic Caramel Corn	1 (0.7 oz)	80	1	18	2	1
Organic Flax w/ Tamari	1 (0.7 oz)	80	1	17	1	1
Organic Mochi Sweet	1 (0.7 oz)	60	1	14	0	1
Organic Popcorn Rice	1 (0.7 oz)	60	1	14	0	1
Organic Sesame Tamari	1 (0.7 oz)	60	1	14	0	1
Organic Wild Rice Lightly Salted	1 (0.6 oz)	70	0	15	0	1
Mother's						
Caramel	1 (0.5 oz)	45	0	10	3	–
Plain Salted	1 (0.3 oz)	35	0	7	–	–

FOOD	PORTION	CAL	FAT	CARB	SUGAR	FIBER
Plain Unsalted	1 (0.3 oz)	35	0	7	–	–
Salted Butter	1 (0.3 oz)	35	0	8	–	–
Quaker						
Apple Cinnamon	1 (0.5 oz)	50	0	11	3	–
Butter Popped Corn	1 (0.3 oz)	35	0	8	0	–
Lightly Salted	1 (0.3 oz)	35	0	7	–	–
Quakes Chocolate	13 (1 oz)	120	2	26	7	1
Quakes Vanilla Crème Brulee	13 (1 oz)	120	1	26	8	1
ROCKFISH						
pacific cooked	1 fillet (5.2 oz)	180	3	0	0	0
pacific cooked	3 oz	103	2	0	0	0
pacific raw	3 oz	80	1	0	0	0
ROE (*see also* INDIVIDUAL FISH NAMES)						
fresh baked	1 oz	58	2	1	–	0
ROLL						
READY-TO-EAT						
bialy	1 (2.2 oz)	138	0	32	–	1
brioche sweet roll	1 (3.5 oz)	410	23	41	5	3
cheese	1 (2.3 oz)	238	12	29	–	1
cinnamon raisin	1 (2.1 oz)	223	10	31	19	1
dinner	1 (1 oz)	78	1	14	2	1
egg	1 (1.2 oz)	107	2	18	2	1
french	1 (1.3 oz)	105	2	19	tr	1
garlic	1 (1.5 oz)	133	3	22	2	1
hamburger or hot dog	1 (1.5 oz)	120	2	21	3	1
hamburger or hot dog multi grain	1 (1.5 oz)	113	3	19	3	2
hamburger or hot dog reduced calorie	1 (1.5 oz)	84	1	18	2	3

FOOD	PORTION	CAL	FAT	CARB	SUGAR	FIBER
hamburger or hot dog whole wheat	1 (1.5 oz)	114	2	22	4	3
hard	1 (2 oz)	167	2	30	1	1
hoagie or submarine roll whole wheat	1 (4.7 oz)	359	6	69	11	10
hot cross bun	1	202	4	38	–	1
mexican bolillo	1 (4.1 oz)	305	2	60	tr	2
oat bran	1 (1.2 oz)	78	2	13	2	1
oatmeal	1 (1.3 oz)	103	2	17	2	1
pumpernickel	1 (1.3 oz)	100	1	19	tr	2
rye	1 med (1.3 oz)	103	1	19	tr	2
sourdough	1 (1.6 oz)	130	1	25	1	1
wheat	1 (1 oz)	76	2	13	tr	1
whole wheat	1 med (1.3 oz)	96	2	18	3	3
Arnold						
Wheat Hot Dog	1 (1.8 oz)	130	2	25	5	2
Calise						
Kaiser 100% Whole Wheat	1 (2.5 oz)	190	3	33	5	3
J.J. Cassone						
Sandwich	1 (2.5 oz)	190	2	38	2	2
Martin's						
Potato	1 (1.9 oz)	130	2	25	7	3
Pepperidge Farm						
Deli Flats Soft 100% Whole Wheat	1	100	2	19	3	5
Deli Flats Soft Honey Wheat	1	100	1	21	3	5
Dinner Classic	1	90	2	17	3	1
Hamburger 100% Whole Wheat	1	110	2	17	2	2
Hot Dog Top Sliced	1	150	3	24	4	<2

FOOD	PORTION	CAL	FAT	CARB	SUGAR	FIBER
Sandwich Mini	1	100	2	18	3	1
Soft Hoagie	1	210	6	35	3	2
Stone Baked Artisan Ciabatta Sourdough	1	140	1	27	1	3
Stone Baked Artisan French Dinner	1	120	0	25	tr	1
Stone Baked Artisan Multi-Grain Dinner	1	120	1	25	5	3
Udi's						
Gluten Free Cinnamon	1 (3 oz)	260	7	48	25	2
REFRIGERATED						
crescent	1 (1 oz)	78	1	14	2	1
ROSE APPLE						
fresh	3.5 oz	32	tr	7	–	–
ROSE HIP						
fresh	1 oz	26	0	5	–	–
ROSELLE						
fresh	1 cup	28	tr	6	–	–
ROSEMARY						
dried	1 tsp	4	tr	1	–	1
fresh	1 tbsp	1	tr	tr	–	tr
ROUGHY						
orange baked	3 oz	75	1	0	0	0
RUBS (*see* HERBS/SPICES)						
RUTABAGA						
cooked mashed	1 cup	94	1	21	14	4
cubed cooked	1 cup	66	tr	14	10	3
SABLEFISH						
baked	3 oz	213	17	0	0	0
fillet baked	5.3 oz	378	30	0	0	0

FOOD	PORTION	CAL	FAT	CARB	SUGAR	FIBER
smoked	3 oz	218	17	0	0	0
smoked	1 oz	72	6	0	0	0
SAFFLOWER						
seeds dried	1 oz	147	11	10	–	–
SAFFRON						
dried	1 tsp	2	tr	tr	–	tr
SAGE						
ground	1 tsp	2	tr	tr	tr	tr
SALAD (*see also* SALAD TOPPINGS)						
Dole						
American Blend	1½ cups (3 oz)	15	0	3	1	2
Butter Bliss	1½ cups (3 oz)	15	0	2	1	1
European Blend	1½ cups (3 oz)	15	0	3	1	1
Field Greens	1½ cups (3 oz)	20	0	4	1	2
Italian Blend	1½ cups (3 oz)	15	0	3	2	1
Kit Asian Island Crunch as prep	1½ cups (3.5 oz)	130	7	15	9	3
Seven Lettuces	1½ cups (3 oz)	20	0	4	1	1
Spring Mix	1½ cups (3 oz)	20	0	3	2	2
Very Veggie Blend	1½ cups (3 oz)	20	0	4	2	2
Eat Smart						
Asian Salad Kit as prep	1 serv (3 oz)	120	8	9	4	3
Broccoli Salad Kit as prep	1 serv (3 oz)	90	4	10	5	3
Chipotle Salad Kit as prep	1 serv (3 oz)	140	10	9	2	2
Mann's						
Rainbow	1 serv (3 oz)	25	0	5	2	2
Ready Pac						
All American	2 cups (3 oz)	15	0	3	2	1

FOOD	PORTION	CAL	FAT	CARB	SUGAR	FIBER
American Blue Cheese Mix as prep	1¾ cups (3.5 oz)	110	8	8	2	1
Baby Romaine Blend	4½ cups (3 oz)	20	0	3	0	2
Baby Spinach Mix as prep	2 cups (3.5 oz)	140	3	24	12	2
Chef	1 pkg (7.7 oz)	270	20	10	5	2
Cobb	1 pkg (7.2 oz)	300	23	7	4	2
Garden	2 cups (3 oz)	15	0	3	2	1
Grand Asian Mix as prep	1¼ cups (3.5 oz)	130	6	19	11	2
Spinach Bacon	1 pkg (4.7 oz)	240	12	19	8	3
Spring Mix	4½ cups	20	0	4	0	2
Spring Mix Spinach	5 cups (3 oz)	20	0	4	1	2
Veggie Medley	2 cups (3 oz)	15	0	4	2	1
River Ranch						
American Blend	2 cups (3 oz)	15	0	3	2	1
Classic Garden	2 cups (3 oz)	15	0	3	2	1
Complete Caesar Salad Kit as prep	2 cups (3.5 oz)	150	11	10	2	2
Heritage Blend	4 cups (3 oz)	25	0	4	1	3
TAKE-OUT						
7-layer salad	2 cups	557	51	15	8	3
caesar	4 cups	734	61	28	6	7
chef salad w/o dressing	3 cups	535	32	9	–	–
cobb w/ dressing	4 cups	645	49	23	9	11
greek w/ dressing	4 cups	424	29	14	8	4
mixed salad greens shredded	1 cup	9	tr	2	tr	1
somen w/ lettuce egg fish pork	2 cups	550	17	57	4	4
spinach w/o dressing	4 cups	429	19	45	5	6
tossed w/ avocado w/o dressing	2 cups	90	6	9	4	5

FOOD	PORTION	CAL	FAT	CARB	SUGAR	FIBER
tossed w/ chicken w/o dressing	3 cups	194	4	5	3	2
tossed w/ egg w/o dressing	2 cups	93	5	6	4	2
tossed w/ shrimp w/o dressing	1½ cups (8.3 oz)	106	2	7	–	–
tossed w/ shrimp & egg w/o dressing	3 cups	185	5	5	3	2
tossed w/o dressing	2 cups	22	tr	5	3	2
waldorf	1 cup	242	21	15	10	3
wilted lettuce w/ bacon dressing	1 cup	99	8	3	1	1
SALAD DRESSING (*see also* SALAD TOPPINGS)						
MIX						
Good Seasons						
Italian as prep	2 tbsp	130	13	3	tr	–
Italian not prep	⅛ pkg (3 g)	5	0	1	tr	–
READY-TO-EAT						
blue cheese	1 tbsp	77	8	1	–	–
french	1 tbsp	67	6	3	–	–
french reduced calorie	1 tbsp	22	1	4	–	–
italian	1 tbsp	69	7	2	–	–
italian reduced calorie	1 tbsp	16	2	1	–	–
russian	1 tbsp	76	8	2	–	–
russian reduced calorie	1 tbsp	23	1	5	–	–
sesame seed	1 tbsp	68	7	1	–	–
thousand island	1 tbsp	59	6	2	–	–
thousand island reduced calorie	1 tbsp	24	2	3	–	–
Annie's Homegrown						
Cowgirl Ranch	2 tbsp (1 oz)	90	11	3	2	–
Tuscany Italian	2 tbsp (1 oz)	100	9	3	2	–
Vinaigrette Lite Gingerly	2 tbsp (1.1 oz)	40	3	3	2	–

FOOD	PORTION	CAL	FAT	CARB	SUGAR	FIBER
Vinaigrette Lite Honey Mustard	1 tbsp (1.1 oz)	40	3	4	3	–
Vinaigrette Mango Fat Free	2 tbsp (1.1 oz)	20	0	5	5	–
Vinaigrette Roasted Red Pepper	2 tbsp (1.1 oz)	60	6	3	2	–
Cains						
Caesar Fat Free	2 tbsp (1 oz)	30	0	6	2	0
Creamy Dill Cucumber Fat Free	2 tbsp (1 oz)	35	0	8	3	0
French	2 tbsp (1 oz)	120	11	6	4	0
French Light	2 tbsp (1 oz)	80	5	10	6	0
Italian Bellissimo	2 tbsp (2 oz)	150	16	1	1	0
Italian Fat Free	2 tbsp (1 oz)	15	0	4	2	0
Italian Light	2 tbsp (1 oz)	50	4	4	2	0
Peppercorn Ranch Fat Free	2 tbsp (1 oz)	45	0	10	3	0
Ranch	2 tbsp (1 oz)	180	19	1	1	0
Ranch Light	2 tbsp (1 oz)	80	6	6	2	0
Ranch w/ Bacon	2 tbsp (1 oz)	170	17	3	1	0
Vinaigrette Chianti	2 tbsp (1 oz)	130	12	5	3	0
Vinaigrette Citrus	2 tbsp (1 oz)	120	12	4	3	0
Vinaigrette White Balsamic	2 tbsp (1 oz)	130	10	10	7	0
David's Unforgettables						
Balsamic Vinaigrette Low Fat	1 tbsp (0.5 oz)	40	3	3	3	0
Balsamic Vinaigrette Original	1 tbsp (0.5 oz)	70	7	3	3	0
Gazebo Room						
Lite Greek	1 tbsp (0.5 oz)	40	4	0	0	0
Jake & Amos						
Bacon	2 tbsp (1 oz)	90	5	10	10	1

FOOD	PORTION	CAL	FAT	CARB	SUGAR	FIBER
Ken's						
Light Vinaigrette Balsamic	2 tbsp (1 oz)	60	5	4	4	0
Maple Grove Farms						
Asiago & Garlic	2 tbsp (1 oz)	40	4	2	1	–
Caesar Lite	2 tbsp (1 oz)	50	5	4	3	–
Cranberry Balsamic Fat Free	2 tbsp (1 oz)	30	0	7	6	–
Creamy Ranch Sugar Free	2 tbsp (1 oz)	100	12	tr	–	–
Honey Dijon Fat Free	2 tbsp (1 oz)	35	0	9	8	tr
Poppyseed Fat Free	2 tbsp (1 oz)	35	0	7	7	–
Sesame Ginger	2 tbsp (1 oz)	45	2	6	5	–
Strawberry Balsamic	1 tbsp (1 oz)	30	0	6	6	–
Sweet'n Sour	2 tbsp (1 oz)	90	6	10	9	–
Vidalia Onion Fat Free	2 tbsp (1 oz)	20	0	5	4	–
Vinaigrette Balsamic Sugar Free	2 tbsp (1 oz)	5	0	1	–	–
Vinaigrette Champagne	2 tbsp (1 oz)	100	11	2	1	–
Newman's Own						
Lighten Up Light Balsamic Vinaigrette	2 tbsp (1 oz)	45	4	2	2	0
OrganicVille						
Coleslaw Non Dairy	2 tbsp (1 oz)	70	5	6	6	0
French	2 tbsp (1 oz)	130	7	9	8	0
Miso Ginger	2 tbsp (1 oz)	100	10	1	tr	0
Pomegranate	2 tbsp (1 oz)	100	10	2	2	0
Ranch Non Dairy	2 tbsp (1 oz)	90	9	1	1	0
Thousand Island Non Dairy	2 tbsp (1 oz)	80	7	4	3	0
Sonoma Gourmet						
Blue Cheese	2 tbsp (1 oz)	170	18	1	0	0
Caesar	2 tbsp (1 oz)	130	14	1	0	0

FOOD	PORTION	CAL	FAT	CARB	SUGAR	FIBER
Greek	2 tbsp (1 oz)	60	7	0	0	0
Raspberry	2 tbsp (1 oz)	60	6	0	0	0
Soy Vay						
Toasted Sesame	3 tbsp	190	15	11	9	0
Walden Farms						
Sesame Ginger Calorie Free	2 tbsp (1 oz)	0	0	0	0	0
Wishbone						
Buffalo Blue Cheese	2 tbsp (1 oz)	120	13	1	tr	0
Chunky Blue Cheese Fat Free	2 tbsp (1 oz)	30	0	7	2	tr
Guacamole Ranch	2 tbsp (1 oz)	130	13	2	1	0
Italian	2 tbsp (1 oz)	160	12	11	11	0
Ranch Light	2 tbsp (1 oz)	70	5	4	2	0
Robusto Italian	2 tbsp (1 oz)	80	7	4	3	0
TAKE-OUT						
vinegar & oil	1 tbsp	72	8	tr	–	–

SALAD TOPPINGS

FOOD	PORTION	CAL	FAT	CARB	SUGAR	FIBER
McCormick						
Salad Toppins	1.3 tbsp (7 g)	35	2	3	tr	0
Salad Toppins Garden Vegetable	1.3 tbsp (7 g)	35	2	3	tr	0

SALMON

FOOD	PORTION	CAL	FAT	CARB	SUGAR	FIBER
CANNED						
w/ bone	½ cup	106	5	0	0	0
Chicken Of The Sea						
Pink	¼ cup (2.2 oz)	90	5	0	0	0
Pink Skinless & Boneless	⅓ pkg (2 oz)	60	2	0	0	0
Pink Smoked Pacific	1 pkg (3 oz)	120	4	1	1	0
Red	¼ cup	110	7	0	0	0

FOOD	PORTION	CAL	FAT	CARB	SUGAR	FIBER
Sea Fare Pacific						
Smoked Alaskan Red Sockeye	½ pkg (1.5 oz)	70	4	0	0	0
Tonnino						
Wild Sockeye In Olive Oil	2 oz	220	17	tr	0	tr
Wild Planet						
Salmon Wild Alaskan Pink	2 oz	65	2	0	0	0
Salmon Wild Alaskan Sockeye	2 oz	85	4	0	0	0
FRESH						
atlantic farmed baked	4 oz	233	14	0	0	0
coho wild poached	4 oz	209	9	0	0	0
pink baked	4 oz	169	5	0	0	0
roe raw	1 oz	59	3	tr	–	–
sockeye baked	4 oz	245	12	0	0	0
FROZEN						
Gorton's						
Classic Grilled Fillets	1 (3 oz)	100	3	2	1	–
SMOKED						
lox	1 oz	33	1	0	0	0
TAKE-OUT						
guisado salmon stew	1 serv (7.4 oz)	320	16	18	3	3
roulette w/ spinach stuffing	1 serv (4 oz)	160	6	10	0	tr
salmon cake	1 (4.2 oz)	264	16	14	1	1
salmon loaf	1 slice (3.7 oz)	206	11	9	2	tr

SALSA

black bean & corn	2 tbsp	15	0	3	1	tr

FOOD	PORTION	CAL	FAT	CARB	SUGAR	FIBER
citrus	2 tbsp (1 oz)	10	0	2	2	0
peach	2 tbsp	15	0	4	4	0
tomatoless corn & chile	2 tbsp	45	0	10	6	tr
Frontera						
Chipotle Hot	2 tbsp (1 oz)	10	0	2	2	0
Corn & Poblano Medium	2 tbsp (1 oz)	10	0	2	tr	0
Guajillo Medium	2 tbsp (1 oz)	10	1	2	1	1
Spanish Olive Mild	2 tbsp (1 oz)	10	1	1	tr	0
Jake & Amos						
Black Bean	2 tbsp (1 oz)	15	0	3	3	0
Peach	2 tbsp (1 oz)	20	0	6	5	0
Margaritaville						
Medium	2 tbsp	10	0	2	2	tr
Peppadew Chipotle Garlic	1 oz	10	0	2	2	0
Peppadew Mild	1 oz	10	0	2	2	0
Newman's Own						
Mild	2 tbsp (1.1 oz)	10	0	2	1	tr
OrganicVille						
Medium	2 tbsp (1 oz)	15	0	3	1	0
Pineapple	2 tbsp (1 oz)	15	0	4	3	0
Ready Pac						
Pico De Gallo	2 tbsp (1 oz)	5	0	2	1	0
Tostitos						
All Natural Chunky Mild	2 tbsp (1 oz)	10	0	2	2	tr
Con Queso	2 tbsp	40	3	5	tr	tr
SALSIFY						
fresh sliced cooked	½ cup	46	tr	10	–	–
SALT SUBSTITUTES						
gomasio sesame salt	2 tsp	34	3	2	–	1
SALT/SEASONED SALT						
kosher	¼ tsp	0	0	0	0	0

FOOD	PORTION	CAL	FAT	CARB	SUGAR	FIBER
salt	1 tsp (6 g)	0	0	0	0	0
salt	1 tbsp (0.6 oz)	0	0	0	0	0
sea salt coarse	1 tsp	0	0	0	0	0
sea salt fine	¼ tsp	0	0	0	0	0
BaconSalt						
Original	¼ tsp (1 g)	0	0	0	0	0
Peppered	¼ tsp (1 g)	0	0	0	0	0
David's						
Kosher Salt	¼ tsp (1.5 g)	0	0	0	0	0
Lawry's						
Original Seasoned Salt	¼ tsp	0	0	0	0	0
Manischewitz						
Kosher	¼ tsp (1.5 g)	0	0	0	0	0
McCormick						
Grinder Garlic Sea Salt	¼ tsp	0	0	0	0	0
Grinder Sea Salt	¼ tsp	0	0	0	0	0
NutraSalt						
African Medley	1 serv (1g)	0	0	0	0	0
Sea Salt	1 serv (1g)	0	0	0	0	0
Seasoned Salt	1 serv (1g)	0	0	0	0	0
SANDWICHES						
Aunt Jemima						
Biscuit Sausage Egg & Cheese	1 (4 oz)	340	21	27	2	tr
Griddlecake Sausage Egg & Cheese	1 (4.4 oz)	350	20	30	11	tr
Sausage Egg & Cheese On French Toast	1 (4.7 oz)	310	18	23	6	tr
Farm Rich						
Philly Cheese	2 (3 oz)	220	11	18	3	1
Steak Sandwich Melts	2 (4.2 oz)	290	14	22	1	1

FOOD	PORTION	CAL	FAT	CARB	SUGAR	FIBER
IHOP At Home						
Breakfast Sandwich Flatbread Apple Bacon	1 (3.1 oz)	250	13	22	2	2
Wrap Griddle 'N Sausage Blueberry	1 (1.5 oz)	150	10	11	2	0
Wrap Griddle 'N Sausage Original	1 (1.6 oz)	140	11	11	2	0
Lean Cuisine						
Casual Cuisine Panini Chicken Club	1 pkg (6 oz)	360	9	45	6	4
Casual Cuisine Panini Spinach Artichoke Chicken	1 pkg (6 oz)	320	9	40	5	5
Casual Cuisine Panini Steak Cheddar & Mushroom	1 pkg (6 oz)	340	9	43	5	5
Lifestyle Chefs						
Meal-In-A-Bun Channa Masala	1 (4.5 oz)	250	10	37	4	7
Meal-In-A-Bun Creamy Vegetable Medley	1 (4.5 oz)	260	12	32	3	5
Meal-In-A-Bun Herb Vegetable Melange	1 (4.5 oz)	270	14	34	4	6
Meal-In-A-Bun Peas Paneer	1 (4.5 oz)	260	13	32	3	6
Meal-In-A-Bun Thai Satay	1 (4.5 oz)	270	14	33	3	5
Lunchables						
Cracker Stackers Bologna & American	1 pkg	390	22	33	11	2
Cracker Stackers Ham & Cheddar	1 pkg	410	21	39	14	1

FOOD	PORTION	CAL	FAT	CARB	SUGAR	FIBER
Sub Sandwich Ham + American	1 pkg	240	7	33	7	1
Sub Sandwich Turkey & Cheddar	1 pkg	230	6	34	8	1
Mom Made						
Munchie Turkey Sausage	1 (2.5 oz)	220	11	24	1	1
Munchies Chicken	1 (2.5 oz)	220	11	24	1	2
Saffron Road						
Crispy Samosas w/ Saag Paneer	⅓ pkg (2.75 oz)	160	7	21	3	2
Crispy Samosas w/ Vegetables	⅓ pkg (2.75 oz)	180	8	25	2	2
Smucker's						
Uncrustables Peanut Butter & Grape Jelly On Whole Wheat	1 (2 oz)	210	9	26	9	3
Uncrustables Peanut Butter & Strawberry Jam	1 (2 oz)	210	9	28	9	2
Uncrustables Peanut Butter On Wheat Bread	1 (2 oz)	210	9	26	9	3
Soul						
Wrap Butter Chicken	1 (7 oz)	390	15	51	5	1
Wrap Chicken Tikka Masala	1 (7 oz)	370	11	53	3	1
Wrap Chicken Vandaloo	1 (7 oz)	400	11	58	3	1
Wrap Vegetable Curry	1 (7 oz)	410	16	61	5	2
Vegetarian Plus						
Vegan Tuna Roll	1 serv (2.5 oz)	160	8	14	0	0
TAKE-OUT						
bacon & egg	1 (6.2 oz)	388	21	28	4	1

FOOD	PORTION	CAL	FAT	CARB	SUGAR	FIBER
bacon lettuce & tomato w/ mayo	1 (5.8 oz)	344	17	35	5	3
beef barbecue w/ bun	1 (6.7 oz)	417	12	42	6	2
calzone beef & cheese	1 (14 oz)	1476	76	131	1	6
calzone cheese	1 (15 oz)	1632	93	117	2	5
chicken fillet	1 (6.4 oz)	515	29	39	–	–
chicken fillet w/ cheese	1 (8 oz)	632	39	42	–	–
chicken salad	1 (5 oz)	333	16	28	3	2
crab cake w/ bun	1	308	8	36	4	2
crispy chicken fillet w/ lettuce tomato & mayo	1 (7.7 oz)	537	26	49	tr	3
croque monsieur	1 (12.4 oz)	765	46	43	9	2
egg salad	1 (5.6 oz)	485	35	28	3	1
french dip w/ roll	1 (6.8 oz)	357	13	34	4	1
fried egg	1 (3.4 oz)	226	9	26	3	1
grilled cheese	1 (2.9 oz)	290	16	28	4	1
gyro	1 (13.7 oz)	593	12	74	8	4
ham & egg	1 (4.4 oz)	272	11	27	3	2
ham w/ cheese lettuce & mayo	1 (5.4 oz)	369	18	32	4	2
hot turkey w/ gravy	1	389	10	32	2	2
peanut butter	1 (3.3 oz)	342	17	38	5	3
peanut butter & banana	1	617	14	43	11	4
peanut butter & jelly	1 (3.3 oz)	327	14	42	12	3
reuben w/ sauerkraut & cheese	1 (6.4 oz)	463	29	30	7	4
roast beef w/ gravy	1 (7.8 oz)	386	16	30	2	2
sloppy joe pork on bun	1 (6.5 oz)	318	9	34	6	2
tuna melt	1 (5.3 oz)	350	16	30	6	1
tuna salad w/ lettuce	1 (5.9 oz)	289	7	37	6	2
turkey w/ mayo	1 (5 oz)	329	11	26	2	1

FOOD	PORTION	CAL	FAT	CARB	SUGAR	FIBER
SAPODILLA						
fresh	1	140	2	34	–	–
fresh cut up	1 cup	199	3	48	–	–
SAPOTES						
fresh	1	301	1	76	–	–
SARDINES						
CANNED						
atlantic in oil w/ bone	2	50	3	0	0	0
atlantic in oil w/ bone	1 can (3.2 oz)	192	11	0	0	0
pacific in tomato sauce w/ bone	1 (1.3 oz)	68	5	0	0	0
pacific in tomato sauce w/ bone	1 can (13 oz)	658	44	0	0	0
Chicken Of The Sea						
In Hot Sauce	1 can (3.75 oz)	120	3	3	0	1
In Oil Lightly Smoked	1 can (3.75 oz)	150	10	0	0	0
In Tomato Sauce	1 can (3.75 oz)	90	2	4	2	1
In Water	1 can (3.75 oz)	90	2	0	0	0
King Oscar						
In Dijon Mustard	1 can (3.5 oz)	160	11	0	0	0
In Pure Spring Water Low Sodium	1 can (3.5 oz)	140	10	0	0	0
In Tomato Sauce	1 can (3.5 oz)	170	12	0	0	0
Skinless Boneless In Olive Oil drained	1 serv (3 oz)	210	15	0	0	0
Matiz						
In Olive Oil	½ pkg (2 oz)	120	7	0	0	0

FOOD	PORTION	CAL	FAT	CARB	SUGAR	FIBER
Wild Planet						
Sardines Wild In Extra Virgin Olive Oil	2 oz	110	8	0	0	0
Sardines Wild In Marinara Sauce	2 oz	60	2	0	0	0
Sardines Wild In Oil w/ Lemon	2 oz	110	8	0	0	0
Sardines Wild In Spring Water	2 oz	73	2	0	0	0
FRESH						
raw	3.5 oz	135	5	0	0	0

SAUCE (*see also* BARBECUE SAUCE, CURRY, GRAVY, SPAGHETTI SAUCE)

FOOD	PORTION	CAL	FAT	CARB	SUGAR	FIBER
adobo fresco	2 tbsp	81	8	7	tr	1
bearnaise	1 oz	177	19	1	–	tr
cheese mix as prep w/ milk	1 cup	307	17	23	–	–
enchilada sauce green	¼ cup	46	4	3	2	1
enchilada sauce red	¼ cup	79	8	2	1	1
fish sauce chinese	1 tbsp	9	0	tr	–	0
fish sauce Vietnamese nuoc mam	1 tbsp	6	0	1	–	0
hoisin	1 tbsp	35	1	7	–	tr
moroccan tagine	½ cup (4 oz)	70	3	10	10	1
mushroom mix as prep w/ milk	1 cup	228	10	24	–	–
oyster	1 tbsp	8	0	2	–	0
plum sauce	0.5 oz	42	0	10	10	0
satay peanut sauce	1 oz	77	6	3	3	1
sour cream mix as prep w/ milk	1 cup	509	30	45	–	–
stroganoff mix as prep	1 cup	271	11	34	–	–
sweet & sour mix as prep	1 cup	294	tr	73	–	–

FOOD	PORTION	CAL	FAT	CARB	SUGAR	FIBER
teriyaki	1 tbsp	15	0	3	–	–
teriyaki mix as prep	1 cup	131	1	28	–	–
white sauce mix as prep w/ milk	1 cup	241	13	21	–	–
Annie's Homegrown						
Organic Worcestershire	1 tsp (5 g)	5	0	1	1	–
Cains						
Tartar	2 tbsp (1 oz)	160	16	2	1	0
Chef Hymie Grande						
New Mexico Sweet Basting Sauce	2 tbsp (1.2 oz)	35	0	8	6	–
Chun's						
Sweet N' Sour	2 tbsp (1.2 oz)	45	0	12	9	0
Del Monte						
Chili Sauce	1 tbsp (0.6 oz)	20	0	5	4	–
Seafood Cocktail	¼ cup	100	0	24	22	0
Fischer & Wieser						
Bourbon Charred Pineapple	1 tbsp (0.7 oz)	35	0	8	8	0
Chipotle Original Roasted Raspberry	1 tbsp (0.7 oz)	40	0	10	9	1
Grilling Chipotle Plum	1 tbsp (0.7 oz)	40	0	10	10	–
Grilling Spicy Garlic Steak	1 tbsp (0.7 oz)	20	1	2	2	0
Habanero Mango Ginger	1 tbsp (0.7 oz)	40	0	11	9	–
Marinade All Purpose Vegetable & Meat	1 tbsp (0.7 oz)	35	3	3	2	0
Onion Glaze Sweet & Savory	1 tbsp (0.7 oz)	45	0	11	11	–
Roasted Blackberry Chipotle	1 tbsp (0.7 oz)	35	0	9	9	–
Soppin' Big Bold Red	1 tbsp (0.7 oz)	35	0	7	6	–

FOOD	PORTION	CAL	FAT	CARB	SUGAR	FIBER
Frontera						
Hot Sauce Habanero	1 tsp	5	0	1	0	0
Hot Squeeze						
Original	2 tbsp (1 oz)	110	0	27	25	–
Kikkoman						
Marinade Quick & Easy Honey & Mustard	1 tbsp (0.6 oz)	30	0	6	5	–
Peanut Sauce Thai Style	2 tbsp (1.2 oz)	80	4	10	8	tr
Teriyaki Less Sodium	1 tbsp (0.5 oz)	15	0	3	3	–
Teriyaki Sauce & Marinade	1 tbsp (0.5 oz)	15	0	2	2	–
Teriyaki Takumi Original	1 tbsp (0.6 oz)	30	0	6	6	–
Lawry's						
Marinade Szechuan Sweet & Sour BBQ	1 tbsp (0.5 oz)	35	0	8	7	–
Marinade Tuscan Sun-Dried Tomato	1 tbsp (0.5 oz)	15	0	2	1	–
Lea & Perrins						
Worcestershire	1 tsp (0.2 oz)	5	0	1	1	–
Loney's						
Bar-B-Q Chicken as prep	¼ cup (2.1 oz)	15	0	3	0	0
Manwich						
Sloppy Joe Original	¼ cup (2.2 oz)	40	0	9	6	2
Margaritaville						
ConQueso In Paradise	1 oz	45	3	2	1	0
Matiz						
Paella Sofrito	¼ cup	137	12	6	5	1
McCormick						
Cocktail For Seafood Original	¼ cup (2.1 oz)	90	1	19	16	1
Seafood Sauce Asian	2 tbsp (1.2 oz)	50	2	7	4	0
Seafood Sauce Cajun Style	1 tbsp (1.1 oz)	15	0	3	3	0

FOOD	PORTION	CAL	FAT	CARB	SUGAR	FIBER
Seafood Sauce Scampi	1 tbsp (1 oz)	160	17	2	1	0
Tartar Fat Free	2 tbsp (1.1 oz)	30	0	7	5	1
Tartar Original	2 tbsp (1 oz)	140	14	3	3	0
More Than Gourmet						
Bearnaise	1 pkg (1.8 oz)	120	12	tr	0	tr
Demi-Glace Classic French	2 tsp (0.4 oz)	30	1	3	1	0
Hollandaise	1 pkg (1.8 oz)	120	12	2	tr	0
Red Wine Shallot	1 pkg (1.8 oz)	70	6	3	tr	0
White Wine	¼ cup (2.1 oz)	45	3	2	0	0
Mrs. Dash						
10 Minute Marinade Zesty Garlic Herb	1 tbsp (0.5 oz)	25	2	3	1	–
Old Bay						
Tartar Sauce	2 tbsp (1.1 oz)	130	12	3	–	0
OrganicVille						
Sesame Teriyaki	1 tbsp (0.5 oz)	25	1	4	3	0
Progresso						
Bruschetta	2 tbsp (1 oz)	10	1	1	1	0
Recipe Starters Cooking Sauce Creamy Parmesan Basil	½ cup	90	7	4	0	0
Recipe Starters Cooking Sauce Creamy Portabella Mushroom	½ cup	90	6	6	1	0
Recipe Starters Cooking Sauce Creamy Three Cheese	½ cup	90	7	5	tr	0
Saffron Road						
Simmer Sauce Moroccan Tagine	1 oz	50	2	8	6	tr
Simmer Sauce Rogan Josh	1 oz	25	1	3	2	0

FOOD	PORTION	CAL	FAT	CARB	SUGAR	FIBER
Simmer Sauce Tikka Masala	1 oz	35	2	4	3	0
Saucy Susan						
Peach Apricot	2 tbsp (1.3 oz)	80	0	19	11	2
Soy Vay						
Hoisin Garlic Asian Glaze & Marinade	1 tbsp	40	1	7	7	0
Island Teriyaki	1 tbsp	30	1	5	4	0
Veri Veri Teriyaki	1 tbsp	35	1	6	5	0
Steel's						
Cocktail w/ Dill & Lemon No Sugar Added Gluten Free	¼ cup (2.4 oz)	35	0	9	6	2
Hoisin No Sugar Added Gluten Free	2 tbsp (1 oz)	30	0	6	4	1
Thai Kitchen						
Pineapple & Chili	2 tbsp (1 oz)	25	0	7	6	0
Premium Fish Sauce	1 tbsp (0.5 oz)	10	0	0	0	0
Sweet Red Chili	2 tbsp (1 oz)	70	0	18	14	0
Thai Chili & Ginger	2 tbsp (1 oz)	40	0	10	8	0
Walden Farms						
Calorie Free Scampi Sauce	2 tbsp (1 oz)	0	0	0	0	0
TAKE-OUT						
cucumber yogurt sauce	1½ tbsp	20	0	3	–	0

SAUERKRAUT

FOOD	PORTION	CAL	FAT	CARB	SUGAR	FIBER
canned	½ cup	22	tr	5	–	–
Del Monte						
Sweet Bavarian	2 tbsp (1 oz)	15	0	4	3	0
Gedney						
Sauerkraut	½ cup (4 oz)	15	0	3	0	0
Hebrew National						
Sauerkraut	2 tbsp (1.1 oz)	5	0	1	–	–

FOOD	PORTION	CAL	FAT	CARB	SUGAR	FIBER
SAUSAGE						
beef & pork	1 link (2.3 oz)	196	17	1	0	0
beef & pork w/ cheddar cheese	1 link (2.7 oz)	228	20	2	tr	0
bierschinken	3.5 oz	174	11	tr	–	–
bierwurst	3.5 oz	258	21	0	0	0
blutwurst uncooked	3.5 oz	424	39	0	0	0
bockwurst	3.5 oz	276	25	0	0	0
bratwurst chicken cooked	1 (3 oz)	148	9	0	0	0
bratwurst pork cooked	1 link (2.5 oz)	226	19	2	2	0
brotwurst pork & beef	1 link (2.5 oz)	226	19	2	2	0
chipolata	3.5 oz	342	32	1	1	0
chorizo	1 link (2.1 oz)	273	23	1	0	0
fleischwurst	3.5 oz	305	29	0	0	0
free range chicken breakfast	2 links (2.7 oz)	110	6	1	1	0
gelbwurst uncooked	3.5 oz	363	33	0	0	0
italian pork cooked	1 (2.4 oz)	230	18	3	1	1
italian turkey smoked	1 (2 oz)	88	5	3	2	1
jagdwurst	3.5 oz	211	16	0	0	0
knockwurst pork & beef	1 (2.5 oz)	221	20	2	0	0
mettwurst uncooked	3.5 oz	483	45	0	0	0
plockwurst uncooked	3.5 oz	312	45	0	0	0
polish kielbasa	2 oz	127	10	2	0	0
pork cooked	2 links (1.7 oz)	163	14	0	0	0
regensburger uncooked	3.5 oz	354	31	0	0	0
venison patty	1 (1 oz)	84	8	1	0	0
vienna canned	1 link (0.5 oz)	37	3	tr	0	0
vienna canned	1 can (4 oz)	260	22	3	0	0
weisswurst uncooked	3.5 oz	305	27	0	0	0
zungenwurst (tongue)	3.5 oz	285	24	0	0	0

FOOD	PORTION	CAL	FAT	CARB	SUGAR	FIBER
Al Fresco						
Chicken Buffalo	1 (3 oz)	130	6	4	2	0
Chicken Hot Italian	1 (2.7 oz)	120	7	2	1	0
Chicken Roasted Garlic	1 (3 oz)	140	7	3	1	0
Chicken Smoked Andouille	1 (3 oz)	140	7	3	1	1
Chicken Spicy Chipotle	1 (2.7 oz)	120	6	1	1	0
Chicken Spinach & Feta	1 (3 oz)	130	7	1	0	–
Chicken Sweet Apple	1 (3 oz)	160	7	10	9	0
Chicken Wild Blueberry	1 (1.2 oz)	70	3	5	4	0
Banquet						
Brown'N Serve Turkey	3 (2.1 oz)	110	7	2	1	0
Coleman						
Bratwurst	1 (3 oz)	240	21	tr	0	0
Chicken Spicy Chorizo	1 (3 oz)	150	8	1	0	0
Dietz & Watson						
Italian	1 (2 oz)	160	14	1	0	0
Italian Chicken	1 (3.4 oz)	130	8	0	0	0
Jerk Chicken	1 (3.4 oz)	130	8	0	0	0
Polska Kielbasa	1 (2 oz)	150	13	1	0	0
Scrapple Philadelphia	2 oz	120	8	7	0	1
Foster Farms						
Turkey Breakfast Links	2 (2 oz)	120	10	0	0	0
Hans All Natural						
Breakfast Links Skinless Chicken	2 (1.7 oz)	60	4	0	0	0
Chicken Spinach & Feta	1 (2.7 oz)	130	8	1	0	0
Hebrew National						
Knockwurst Beef	1 (3 oz)	270	25	2	0	0
High Plains Bison						
Wild Rice & Asiago	1 (3.2 oz)	260	21	6	0	0
Jones						
All Natural Light	3 (2.1 oz)	130	9	3	–	–

FOOD	PORTION	CAL	FAT	CARB	SUGAR	FIBER
Murray's						
Chicken Cheese & Parsley	3 oz	130	7	0	0	0
Chicken Spinach & Garlic	3 oz	130	7	1	–	–

SAUSAGE DISHES

FOOD	PORTION	CAL	FAT	CARB	SUGAR	FIBER
TAKE-OUT						
italian sausage w/ peppers & onions	1 cup	210	11	14	–	–
sausage roll	1 (2.3 oz)	311	24	22	–	1

SAUSAGE SUBSTITUTES

FOOD	PORTION	CAL	FAT	CARB	SUGAR	FIBER
meatless	1 patty (1.3 oz)	98	7	4	0	1
meatless	1 link (0.9 oz)	64	5	2	0	1
Harmony Valley						
Vegetarian Breakfast Sausage Mix as prep	1 (2 oz)	90	4	6	1	3

SAVORY

FOOD	PORTION	CAL	FAT	CARB	SUGAR	FIBER
ground	1 tsp	4	tr	1	–	tr

SCALLOP

FOOD	PORTION	CAL	FAT	CARB	SUGAR	FIBER
raw	3 oz	75	1	2	–	–
TAKE-OUT						
breaded & fried	2 lg	67	3	3	–	–

SCONE

FOOD	PORTION	CAL	FAT	CARB	SUGAR	FIBER
TAKE-OUT						
apricot	1	232	7	39	–	–
blueberry	1 (3 oz)	270	9	41	7	2
cheese	1 (3.5 oz)	364	18	44	–	2
orange poppy	1 (3 oz)	260	6	47	12	2
plain	1 (3.5 oz)	362	14	54	–	2
raisin	1 (3 oz)	270	8	43	12	2

FOOD	PORTION	CAL	FAT	CARB	SUGAR	FIBER
SCUP						
fresh baked	3 oz	115	3	0	0	0
SEA BASS (*see* BASS)						
SEA CUCUMBER						
dried	1 oz	74	1	1	–	0
fresh	1 oz	20	tr	tr	–	0
SEA TROUT (*see* TROUT)						
SEA URCHIN						
canned	1 oz	39	1	3	–	0
fresh	1 oz	36	1	3	–	tr
roe paste	1 tbsp	19	tr	3	–	0
SEAWEED						
agar dried	1 oz	92	tr	24	1	2
agar fresh	⅛ cup (0.4 oz)	3	0	1	tr	0
furikake	1 tbsp (5 g)	15	1	2	–	0
hijiki rehydrated	1 tbsp (3 g)	1	0	0	0	0
hijiki dried	1 tbsp	9	0	2	–	1
irishmoss fresh	⅛ cup (0.4 oz)	5	tr	1	tr	tr
kelp dried	¼ cup (4 g)	11	tr	2	tr	tr
kelp fresh	⅛ cup (0.4 oz)	4	tr	1	tr	tr
kelp strip	1 (0.5 g)	1	tr	tr	tr	0
konbu dried	1 piece (5 g)	11	0	2	–	1
konbu fresh	1 oz	12	tr	3	–	–
laver fresh	⅛ cup (0.4 oz)	4	tr	1	tr	0
nori fresh	1 oz	10	tr	1	–	–
nori sheet dried	1 (8 x 8 in)	5	0	1	–	1
ogo fresh	1 cup (2.8 oz)	24	0	5	–	0
pickled	¼ cup (1.3 oz)	58	tr	14	13	tr
seahair dried	1 tbsp	13	0	3	–	tr
seaweed w/ soy sauce	½ cup (1.7 oz)	21	tr	4	tr	tr
spirulina dried	¼ cup (1 oz)	81	2	7	1	1

FOOD	PORTION	CAL	FAT	CARB	SUGAR	FIBER
spirulina fresh	1 oz	8	tr	1	–	–
steamed	½ cup (1.4 oz)	15	tr	3	tr	tr
tangle fresh	1 oz	12	tr	3	–	–
wakame rehydrated	1 tbsp (3 g)	1	0	0	0	0
wakame fresh	⅛ cup (0.4 oz)	4	tr	1	tr	0
Annie Chun's						
Roasted Snacks Sesame	1 pkg (1.5 g)	5	0	0	0	0
Roasted Snacks Wasabi	1 pkg (1.5 g)	10	tr	0	0	0
Sea's Gift						
Roasted	1 pkg (5 g)	30	2	1	0	1
Roasted Snack Organic	1 pkg (5 g)	30	2	1	0	1
Roasted Snack Wasabi	1 pkg (5 g)	30	2	1	0	1
Sweet Snack	1 pkg (6 g)	35	3	2	tr	1

SEEDS

FOOD	PORTION	CAL	FAT	CARB	SUGAR	FIBER
SaviSeed						
Cocoa Kissed	⅕ pkg (1 oz)	170	13	10	5	4
Karmalized	⅕ pkg (1 oz)	160	11	11	8	3
Oh Natural	⅕ pkg (1 oz)	190	15	5	0	5

SEITAN (*see* WHEAT)

SEMOLINA

FOOD	PORTION	CAL	FAT	CARB	SUGAR	FIBER
dry	1 cup (5.9 oz)	601	2	122	–	7

SESAME

FOOD	PORTION	CAL	FAT	CARB	SUGAR	FIBER
seeds	1 tsp	16	2	tr	–	–
sesame butter	1 tbsp	95	8	4	–	1
sesame crunch candy	1 oz	146	9	14	–	–
sesame crunch candy	20 pieces (1.2 oz)	181	12	18	–	–
tahini from roasted & toasted kernels	1 tbsp	89	8	3	–	–
tahini from stone ground kernels	1 tbsp	86	7	4	–	–

FOOD	PORTION	CAL	FAT	CARB	SUGAR	FIBER
tahini from unroasted kernels	1 tbsp	85	8	3	–	–
Oskri						
Organic Sesame Bars	1 (1.9 oz)	217	6	35	20	1
SESBANIA						
flower	1 (3 g)	1	0	tr	–	–
flowers	1 cup (0.7 oz)	5	tr	1	–	–
flowers cooked	1 cup	23	tr	5	–	–
SHAD						
american baked	3 oz	214	15	0	0	0
cooked	1 oz	55	3	1	tr	0
roe baked w/ butter & lemon	1 oz	36	1	tr	–	–
SHALLOTS (*see* ONION)						
SHARK						
raw	3 oz	111	4	0	0	0
TAKE-OUT						
batter-dipped & fried	3 oz	194	12	5	–	–
SHEEPSHEAD FISH						
cooked	3 oz	107	1	0	0	0
cooked	1 fillet (6.5 oz)	234	3	0	0	0
raw	3 oz	92	2	0	0	0
SHELLFISH (*see individual fish names,* SHELLFISH SUBSTITUTES)						
SHELLFISH SUBSTITUTES						
crab imitation	1 cup (4.4 oz)	144	1	16	0	tr
scallop imitation	3 oz	84	tr	9	–	–
shrimp imitation	3 oz	86	1	8	–	0
surimi	3 oz	84	1	6	–	–

FOOD	PORTION	CAL	FAT	CARB	SUGAR	FIBER
Louis Kemp						
Crab Delights Flake Style	½ cup (3 oz)	90	0	15	3	0
Crab Delights Leg Style	½ cup (3 oz)	90	0	15	3	0
Crab Delights Snack Delights	1 stick (1.5 oz)	35	0	5	2	0
Lobster Delights Chunk Style	½ cup (3 oz)	90	0	15	3	0
TAKE-OUT						
crab salad	1 cup	395	26	21	1	1
SHELLIE BEANS						
canned	½ cup	37	tr	8	–	–
SHERBET						
orange	1 bar (2.75 fl oz)	91	1	20	–	–
orange	½ gal	2158	31	469	–	–
orange	½ cup (4 fl oz)	132	2	29	–	–
SHRIMP (*see also* ASIAN FOOD, EGG ROLLS)						
CANNED						
canned drained	10 (1.1 oz)	32	tr	0	0	0
canned drained	1 cup (4.5 oz)	128	2	0	0	0
chinese shrimp paste	1 tbsp	46	0	10	8	tr
Chicken Of The Sea						
Tiny	½ can (2 oz)	45	1	1	1	0
Small	½ can (2 oz)	45	1	1	1	0
Medium	½ can (2 oz)	45	1	1	1	0
Wild Planet						
Shrimp Wild Pink	2 oz	50	1	0	0	0
DRIED						
dried	1 oz	72	1	0	0	0
dried	10 (5 g)	13	tr	0	0	0

FOOD	PORTION	CAL	FAT	CARB	SUGAR	FIBER
FRESH						
broiled jumbo	3 (1 oz)	44	1	tr	0	0
broiled small	3 (0.4 oz)	18	1	tr	0	0
broiled tiny popcorn	3 (3 g)	4	tr	tr	0	0
prawn broiled	3 (0.6 oz)	27	1	tr	0	0
steamed jumbo	3 (1 oz)	41	1	tr	0	0
steamed large	3 (0.6 oz)	25	tr	tr	0	0
steamed medium	3 (0.5 oz)	21	tr	tr	0	0
Chicken Of The Sea						
Ring w/ Cocktail Sauce	⅓ pkg (3 oz)	100	1	6	3	0
FROZEN						
Chicken Of The Sea						
Tempura w/ Soy Dipping Sauce	3	200	13	14	1	0
Margaritaville						
Island Lime	6 (4 oz)	240	11	5	2	0
Jammin' Jerk	7 (4 oz)	210	10	4	–	1
Plum Crazy + Sauce	7 + 2 oz sauce	270	12	33	13	1
SeaPak						
Butterfly	7 (3 oz)	210	10	20	2	tr
Popcorn	15 (3 oz)	210	10	20	2	1
Scampi	8 (4 oz)	350	29	2	0	0
Shrimp Burgers						
Cajun	1 (4 oz)	160	3	8	0	0
Original	1 (4 oz)	160	3	8	0	0
Teriyaki	1 (4 oz)	150	3	8	2	0
TAKE-OUT						
battered jumbo	3 (3 oz)	268	17	16	1	1
battered large	3 (1.8 oz)	152	9	9	tr	1
battered medium	3 (1.2 oz)	98	5	6	tr	tr
battered small	3 (0.6 oz)	54	3	3	tr	tr
battered tiny popcorn	3 (6 g)	18	1	1	tr	tr

FOOD	PORTION	CAL	FAT	CARB	SUGAR	FIBER
breaded & fried	1 lg (0.6 oz)	44	3	2	–	0
cocktail w/ cocktail sauce	4 shrimp (3.2 oz)	78	1	7	3	2
creole w/o rice	1 cup (8.6 oz)	335	13	11	3	2
jambalaya w/ rice	1 cup (8.5 oz)	294	9	28	2	2
scampi	1 cup	310	22	1	tr	0
shish kabob w/ vegetables	1 (7.1 oz)	184	5	9	5	2
shrimp cake	1 (4.2 oz)	238	13	14	1	1
shrimp egg patty torta de cameron seco	2 (1.3 oz)	152	11	3	1	tr
shrimp in garlic sauce	1 cup (7.4 oz)	649	54	6	1	tr
shrimp newburg	1 cup (8.6 oz)	605	50	11	tr	tr
shrimp salad	1 cup (6.4 oz)	258	16	4	2	1
shrimp w/ crab stuffing	3 (1.7 oz)	94	5	3	tr	tr
tempura	1 (0.9 oz)	65	4	3	–	0
toast fried	3 pieces (2.5 oz)	219	14	16	2	2
SMELT						
rainbow cooked	3 oz	106	3	0	0	0
rainbow raw	3 oz	83	2	0	0	0
SMOOTHIES (*see also* FRUIT DRINKS, YOGURT DRINKS)						
Arizona						
Smoothie Mix Orchard Peach as prep	8 oz	150	0	39	38	0
Chia|Vie						
Acerola-Pina	1 bottle (10.4 oz)	160	3	32	27	4
Banapple-Berry	1 bottle (10.4 oz)	170	4	32	26	5
Cogo						
Coconut Milk Cappuccino	1 bottle (7.5 oz)	130	3	24	14	4

FOOD	PORTION	CAL	FAT	CARB	SUGAR	FIBER
Coconut Milk Mango	1 bottle (7.5 oz)	120	3	23	16	4
Coconut Milk Strawberry	1 bottle (7.5 oz)	130	3	24	15	4
Coconut Milk Vanilla	1 bottle (7.5 oz)	110	4	18	9	4
Del Monte						
Ready-To-Blend Mango Pineapple	1 serv (6 oz)	115	0	29	26	3
Ready-To-Blend Pomegranate Peach Pear	1 serv (6 oz)	125	0	31	22	4
Ready-To-Blend Strawberry Peach	1 serv (6 oz)	120	0	30	21	4
Ready-To-Blend Strawberry Peach Lite	1 serv (6 oz)	80	0	20	15	4
Dole						
Shakers Mixed Berry not prep	1 pkg (4 oz)	100	2	17	13	3
Jamba Juice						
Mango-A-Go-Go not prep	½ pkg (4 oz)	70	0	17	15	1
Razzmatazz not prep	½ pkg (4 oz)	60	0	14	10	2
Strawberries Wild not prep	½ pkg (4 oz)	60	0	15	11	1
Main St Cafe						
Protein Smoothie Mixed Berry	1 bottle (11 oz)	270	2	33	42	1
Protein Smoothie Peach	1 bottle (11 oz)	260	2	54	43	1
Protein Smoothie Strawberry	1 bottle (11 oz)	280	2	58	48	1

FOOD	PORTION	CAL	FAT	CARB	SUGAR	FIBER
Oatworks						
Oat & Fruit Mango & Peach	1 bottle (10.8 oz)	150	0	38	31	2
Oat & Fruit Pomegranate & Blueberry	1 bottle (10.8 oz)	160	0	40	32	2
Simpli						
OatShake Tropical Fruits	1 (8.4 oz)	160	2	30	23	8
Vega						
Energizing Choc-a-lot	1 pkg (1 oz)	105	3	9	1	7
Energizing Natural	1 pkg (0.8 oz)	90	2	8	1	5
Energizing Tropical Tango	1 pkg (0.8 oz)	95	2	9	1	5
Yasso						
Greek Yogurt Mango Pineapple as prep	8 oz	120	0	24	13	4
Greek Yogurt Mixed Berry as prep	8 oz	110	0	21	9	4
Yoplait						
Mixed Berry as prep	1 serv (12 oz)	160	2	27	14	1
Strawberry Banana Orange as prep	1 serv (12 oz)	170	2	27	14	1

SNACKS

FOOD	PORTION	CAL	FAT	CARB	SUGAR	FIBER
cheese puffs	1 oz	122	3	21	2	3
oriental mix	1 oz	155	12	9	–	–
pork skins	1 oz	154	9	0	0	0
pork skins barbecue	1 oz	152	9	1	–	–
Annie's Homegrown						
Organic Cheddar Snack Mix	40 pieces (1 oz)	140	5	20	1	0
Organic Pizza Snack Mix	½ cup (1 oz)	140	5	18	1	0

FOOD	PORTION	CAL	FAT	CARB	SUGAR	FIBER
Bachman						
Baked Cheese	23 (1 oz)	140	7	17	2	0
Curls Onion Rings	½ pkg (1 oz)	130	6	19	1	1
Baken-ets						
Pork Skins Hot 'N Spicy	9 (0.5 oz)	80	5	0	0	0
Pork Skins Traditional	9 (0.5 oz)	80	5	0	0	0
Better Balance						
Kruncheeze White Cheddar Gluten Free	1 oz	130	6	10	0	2
Cheetos						
Baked Crunchy	34 (1 oz)	130	5	20	tr	tr
Corn BBQ	29 (1 oz)	150	10	16	tr	1
Natural White Cheddar	1 oz	150	9	16	1	tr
Puffs	13 (1 oz)	160	10	13	1	0
Chester's						
Puffcorn Butter	1 oz	160	11	14	0	tr
Snack Mix Crazy Cheddar	1¼ cups (1 oz)	140	7	17	tr	1
DrSears						
Popumz BBQ	1 pkg (0.74 oz)	70	2	11	1	2
Popumz Caramel Drizzle	1 pkg (0.75 oz)	90	3	13	5	2
Popumz Cheddar	1 pkg (0.74 oz)	80	3	11	1	2
Popumz Cool Ranch	1 pkg (0.74 oz)	80	2	12	2	2
Popumz Vanilla Drizzle	1 pkg (0.74 oz)	90	3	13	5	2
Funyuns						
Onion Rings	13 (1 oz)	140	7	18	tr	tr
Garden Of Eatin'						
Puffs Baked Cheddar	32 (1 oz)	150	10	15	1	1
Hawaiian Snacks						
Sweet Maui Onion Rings	27 (1 oz)	130	6	19	3	tr
Hi I'm Skinny Sticks						
Multi Grain Cheddar	34 (1 oz)	130	6	16	2	1
Multi Grain Sea Salt	34 (1 oz)	130	6	17	1	1

FOOD	PORTION	CAL	FAT	CARB	SUGAR	FIBER
Multi Grain Sweet Onion	34 (1 oz)	120	6	17	2	1
Multi Grain Sweet Potato	34 (1 oz)	120	7	18	5	1
Multi Grain Tangy BBQ	34 (1 oz)	130	6	17	2	1
Multi Grain Veggie Tortilla	34 (1 oz)	130	7	16	0	2
I Heart Keenwah						
Quinoa Cluster Almond	7 to 8 (1 oz)	130	5	18	7	tr
Quinoa Cluster Chocolate Sea Salt	7 (1 oz)	130	5	18	8	1
Quinoa Cluster Cranberry Cashew	¼ pkg (1 oz)	120	4	20	9	tr
Quinoa Cluster Ginger Peanut	7 to 8 (1 oz)	120	4	20	10	tr
Kay's Naturals						
Snack Mix Sweet BBQ Gluten Free	1 oz	120	5	11	5	2
Munchies						
Snack Mix Totally Ranch	¾ cup (1 oz)	140	7	18	1	2
Quaker						
Fiber Crisps Wild Blueberry	13 (1 oz)	110	2	23	6	3
Sabritones						
Puffed Wheat Chili & Lime	23 pieces (1 oz)	150	10	13	0	1
Sweet Emotions						
Chocolate Passion	1 pkg (0.5 oz)	60	3	10	2	2
Cinnamon Joy	1 pkg (0.5 oz)	60	3	10	2	2
SNAIL						
cooked	3 oz	233	1	13	–	–
raw	3 oz	117	tr	7	–	–

FOOD	PORTION	CAL	FAT	CARB	SUGAR	FIBER
TAKE-OUT						
escargot cooked	5	25	0	1	–	0
SNAKE						
fresh	3 oz	78	tr	3	–	0
SNAPPER						
cooked	1 fillet (6 oz)	217	3	0	0	0
cooked	3 oz	109	1	0	0	0
raw	3 oz	85	1	0	0	0
SODA						
club	12 oz	0	0	0	0	0
cola	12 oz	151	tr	39	–	–
cream	12 oz	191	0	49	–	–
diet cola	12 oz	2	0	tr	–	–
ginger ale	12 oz	124	0	32	–	–
grape	12 oz	161	0	42	–	–
lemon lime	12 oz	149	0	38	–	–
orange	12 oz	177	0	46	–	–
pepper type	12 oz	151	tr	38	–	–
quinine	12 oz	125	0	32	–	–
root beer	12 oz	152	0	39	–	–
shirley temple	1 serv	159	0	41	–	0
tonic water	12 oz	125	0	32	–	–
CasCal						
Crisp White	1 can (12 oz)	70	0	18	11	–
Ripe Rouge	1 can (12 oz)	60	0	15	10	–
Fresh Ginger						
Ginger Ale Jasmine Green Tea	1 bottle (12 oz)	160	0	40	37	0
Ginger Ale Original	1 bottle (12 oz)	160	0	40	37	0
Ginger Ale Pomegranate w/ Hibiscus	1 bottle (12 oz)	160	0	41	37	0

FOOD	PORTION	CAL	FAT	CARB	SUGAR	FIBER
Gus						
Dry Valencia Orange	1 bottle (12 oz)	95	0	24	24	–
In The Raw						
Cola	1 bottle (12 oz)	150	0	39	37	–
Joia						
Grapefruit Chamomile & Cardamon	1 bottle (12 oz)	110	0	31	28	–
Lime Hibiscus & Clove	1 bottle (12 oz)	120	0	35	28	–
Pineapple Coconut & Nutmeg	1 bottle (12 oz)	110	0	38	26	–
Minta						
Diet	1 bottle (12 oz)	5	0	6	0	–
Original	1 bottle (12 oz)	120	0	30	30	–
OrganicVille						
Carbonate Beverage	1 bottle (12 oz)	140	0	35	34	0
Pepsi						
Cola	8 oz	100	0	28	28	–
Diet	8 oz	0	0	0	0	0
Diet Vanilla	8 oz	0	0	0	0	0
One	8 oz	1	0	0	0	–
Wild Cherry	8 oz	100	0	28	28	–
Spindrift						
Sparkling Blackberry	8 oz	70	0	18	17	0
Sparkling Cranberry Raspberry	8 oz	60	0	16	16	0
Sparkling Grapefruit	8 oz	80	0	21	21	0

FOOD	PORTION	CAL	FAT	CARB	SUGAR	FIBER
Sparkling Mango Orange	8 oz	80	0	21	21	0
Stewart's						
Birch Beer	1 bottle (12 oz)	170	0	42	42	–
Sunkist						
Grape	8 oz	120	0	31	30	–
Orange	8 oz	110	0	30	29	–
Pineapple	8 oz	130	0	35	34	–
Taylor's Tonics						
Chai Cola	1 bottle (12 oz)	135	0	32	32	–
Cola Azteca	1 bottle (12 oz)	95	0	28	28	–
Mate Majito Mint & Lime	1 bottle (12 oz)	98	0	28	28	–
The Pop Shoppe						
Cola	1 bottle (12 oz)	180	0	46	45	–
Cream	1 bottle (12 oz)	190	0	47	46	–
Lime Ricky	1 bottle (12 oz)	150	0	38	37	–
Pineapple	1 bottle (12 oz)	240	0	60	58	–
Welch's						
Sparkling Grape	1 bottle (20 oz)	330	0	81	78	–
Sparkling Strawberry	1 can (8 oz)	120	0	34	34	–
Zevia						
All Flavors	1 can (12 oz)	0	0	7	0	0

FOOD	PORTION	CAL	FAT	CARB	SUGAR	FIBER
SOLE						
cooked	1 fillet (4.5 oz)	148	2	0	0	0
cooked	3 oz	99	1	0	0	0
lemon raw	3.5 oz	85	1	0	0	0
TAKE-OUT						
breaded & fried	3.2 oz	211	11	15	–	–
SORGHUM						
sorghum	1 cup (6.7 oz)	651	6	143	–	–
SOUFFLE						
Garden Lites						
Butternut Squash Souffle	1 pkg (7 oz)	180	5	35	18	3
Pizza Souffle	1 pkg (7 oz)	200	4	31	6	3
Roasted Vegetable	1 pkg (7 oz)	140	2	28	8	4
Southwestern Souffle	1 pkg (7 oz)	180	3	30	4	4
Spinach Souffle	1 pkg (7 oz)	140	2	26	6	4
Zucchini Souffle	1 pkg (7 oz)	140	2	30	6	3
TAKE-OUT						
cheese	1 cup	194	15	6	3	tr
chicken	1 cup (5.6 oz)	278	18	9	4	tr
corn	1 cup	257	11	34	11	3
lime chilled	1 cup	388	18	48	45	2
seafood	1 cup	245	15	9	4	tr
spinach	1 cup	124	8	7	3	1
SOUP						
CANNED						
Campbell's						
100% Natural Caramelized French Onion	1 cup (8.4 oz)	80	3	12	4	1

FOOD	PORTION	CAL	FAT	CARB	SUGAR	FIBER
100% Natural Creole Chicken w/ Red Beans & Rice	1 cup (8.4 oz)	130	3	18	4	2
100% Natural Harvest Tomato w/ Basil	1 cup (8.4 oz)	100	0	22	15	2
100% Natural Light Vegetable & Pasta	1 cup (8.4 oz)	60	0	13	3	4
100% Natural Southwest White Chicken Chili	1 cup (8.4 oz)	140	2	21	3	5
98% Fat Free Cream Of Chicken as prep	1 cup (8.4 oz)	70	3	10	0	1
Chunky Creamy Chicken & Dumplings	1 cup (8.4 oz)	170	8	17	3	3
Chunky Italian Wedding	1 cup (8.4 oz)	130	3	21	6	3
Chunky Split Pea & Ham	1 cup (8.4 oz)	170	3	24	4	5
Go Soup Creamy Red Pepper w/ Smoked Gouda	1 cup	220	15	15	8	2
Go Soup Moroccan Style Chicken w/ Chickpeas	1 cup	160	2	23	11	6
Gourmet Bisques Thai Tomato Coconut	1 cup	200	9	28	17	3
Gourmet Bisques Tomato Roasted Garlic Bacon	1 cup	240	10	33	25	3
Healthy Kids Goldfish Pasta as prep	1 cup	80	2	12	1	1
Italian Wedding Light as prep	1 cup (8.4 oz)	80	2	12	2	2
Light Chicken Gumbo as prep	1 cup (8.4 oz)	70	1	12	2	1

FOOD	PORTION	CAL	FAT	CARB	SUGAR	FIBER
Minestrone as prep	1 cup (8.4 oz)	90	1	17	3	3
Slow Kettle Burgundy Beef Stew w/ Baby Bella Mushrooms & Roasted Garlic	1 cup (8.4 oz)	160	4	19	5	4
Slow Kettle Portobello Mushroom & Madeira Bisque w/ Shallots	1 cup (8.4 oz)	230	17	14	7	4
Slow Kettle Southwest Chicken Chile w/ Black Beans & Sweet Corn	1 cup (8.4 oz)	190	2	27	6	7
Slow Kettle Tuscan Chicken & White Bean w/ Asiago Cheese Thyme & Rosemary	1 cup (8.4 oz)	140	3	17	4	4
Sun-Ripened Yellow Tomato as prep	1 cup	100	1	22	13	1
V8 Garden Broccoli	1 cup (8.4 oz)	90	2	15	6	3
College Inn						
Beef Broth 99% Fat Free	1 cup (8.4 oz)	25	1	0	0	0
Beef Broth Fat Free Lower Sodium	1 cup (8.4 oz)	15	0	0	0	0
Bold Stock Rotisserie Chicken	1 cup (8.4 oz)	30	0	4	1	0
Bold Stock Tender Beef	1 cup (8.4 oz)	45	0	4	2	0
Chicken Broth 99% Fat Free	1 cup (8.5 oz)	15	1	3	1	0
Chicken Broth Light & Fat Free 50% Less Sodium	1 cup (8.4 oz)	5	0	0	0	0
Chicken Broth w/ Roasted Garlic	1 cup (8.5 oz)	20	0	3	1	0

FOOD	PORTION	CAL	FAT	CARB	SUGAR	FIBER
Chicken Broth w/ Roasted Vegetables & Herbs	1 cup (8.5 oz)	20	0	3	1	0
Culinary Broth Thai Coconut Curry	1 cup (8.4 oz)	20	1	5	4	0
Culinary Broth Wine & Herbs	1 cup (8.4 oz)	5	1	1	1	1
Garden Vegetable Broth	1 cup (8.4 oz)	25	1	6	4	0
Turkey Broth	1 cup (8.4 oz)	20	1	0	0	0
Dr. McDougall's						
Chunky Tomato Gluten Free	1 cup (8.6 oz)	90	0	20	8	3
Lentil	1 cup (8.6 oz)	115	1	21	1	8
Organic Black Bean Lower Sodium	1 cup (8.6 oz)	150	1	28	3	6
Organic Tortilla	1 cup (8.6 oz)	100	1	20	2	4
Split Pea	1 cup (8.6 oz)	110	0	20	1	8
Frontera						
Gourmet Mexican Classic Tortilla	1 cup (8.6 oz)	80	2	15	5	3
Gourmet Mexican Roasted Vegetable	1 cup (8.6 oz)	80	2	14	5	2
Healthy Choice						
Bean & Ham	1 cup (8.7 oz)	180	3	28	3	6
Chicken & Dumplings	1 cup (8.8 oz)	150	3	22	2	3
Chicken w/ Rice	1 cup (8.4 oz)	110	2	17	tr	2
Garden Vegetable	1 cup (8.6 oz)	130	1	25	4	5
Italian Wedding	1 cup (8.6 oz)	120	3	16	1	3
New England Clam Chowder	1 cup (8.4 oz)	110	2	20	3	3
Split Pea & Ham	1 cup (8.8 oz)	160	3	27	3	6
Tomato Basil	1 cup (8.8 oz)	100	0	22	10	3

FOOD	PORTION	CAL	FAT	CARB	SUGAR	FIBER
Hormel						
Bean & Ham	1 pkg (7.5 oz)	190	4	29	2	7
Chicken Noodle	1 pkg (7.5 oz)	100	3	12	0	0
Chicken w/ Rice	1 pkg (7.5 oz)	110	3	18	3	1
Manischewitz						
Borscht Low Calorie	¾ cup (6.2 oz)	15	0	4	2	tr
Borscht Reduced Sodium	¾ cup (6.2 oz)	50	0	13	11	tr
Borscht w/ Shredded Beets	¾ cup (6.2 oz)	50	0	13	11	tr
Matzo Ball Chicken	1 cup (8.4 oz)	120	5	12	2	1
Matzo Ball Chicken Reduced Sodium	1 cup (8.4 oz)	120	5	12	2	1
Marie Callender's						
Classic Chicken & Rice	1 cup (7.8 oz)	80	3	9	tr	1
Homestyle Vegetable	1 cup (7.8 oz)	80	1	16	4	3
More Than Gourmet						
Roasted Duck & Chicken Stock	2 tsp (0.4 oz)	40	3	tr	0	0
Seafood & Shrimp Stock	2 tsp (0.4 oz)	15	0	1	1	0
Venison Stock	2 tsp (0.4 oz)	25	0	2	0	0
New England Country Soup						
Caribbean Black Bean	1 cup (8.8 oz)	210	3	38	4	8
Chicken Pomodoro	1 cup (8.6 oz)	140	6	16	3	2
Nana's Chicken	1 cup (8.6 oz)	120	4	2	2	4
Sweet Chicken Curry	1 cup (8.8 oz)	160	4	27	9	3
Yankee White Bean	1 cup (9.3 oz)	380	9	52	41	12
Pacific Foods						
Beef Broth Organic	1 cup (8 oz)	20	1	1	1	0
Butternut Squash Organic	1 cup (8 oz)	90	2	17	4	3
Cashew Carrot Ginger Bisque	1 cup (8.4 oz)	130	5	20	8	4

FOOD	PORTION	CAL	FAT	CARB	SUGAR	FIBER
Chicken Broth Free Range	1 cup (8 oz)	10	0	1	1	0
Chicken Broth Free Range Low Sodium Organic	1 cup (8 oz)	15	0	1	0	0
Cream Of Celery	1 cup (8.6 oz)	70	3	11	1	0
Curried Red Lentil	1 cup (8 oz)	140	5	19	8	5
French Onion Organic	1 cup (8 oz)	30	1	5	3	0
Minestone w/ Chicken Meatballs	1 cup (8.8 oz)	130	4	19	3	3
Mushroom Broth Organic	1 cup (8 oz)	5	0	1	0	0
Pho Beef Broth Organic	1 cup (8 oz)	35	0	5	5	0
Pho Vegetarian Soup Base Organic	1 cup (8 oz)	25	0	5	5	0
Poblano Pepper & Corn Chowder	1 cup (8.7 oz)	190	10	22	2	1
Red Pepper & Tomato Light Sodium Organic	1 cup (8 oz)	110	2	16	12	1
Rosemary Potato Chowder	1 cup (8.7 oz)	230	8	36	0	2
Thai Sweet Potato	1 cup (8.6 oz)	160	6	25	3	3
Tomato Light Sodium Organic	1 cup (8 oz)	100	2	16	12	1
Vegetable Broth Organic	1 cup (8 oz)	15	0	3	2	1
Progresso						
High Fiber Chicken Tuscany	1 cup (8.7 oz)	130	3	20	2	7
High Fiber Creamy Tomato Basil	1 cup (8.8 oz)	130	4	26	13	7
Light Chicken Noodle	1 cup (8.3 oz)	70	2	10	1	1
Light Vegetable & Noodle	1 cup (8.7 oz)	60	1	13	2	4

FOOD	PORTION	CAL	FAT	CARB	SUGAR	FIBER
Reduced Sodium Chicken Gumbo	1 cup (8.7 oz)	110	2	18	3	4
Reduced Sodium Chicken Noodle	1 cup (8.4 oz)	90	2	13	1	1
Rich & Hearty Chicken & Homestyle Noodles	1 cup (8.6 oz)	100	3	14	2	1
Traditional Chicken Noodle	1 cup (8.3 oz)	100	3	12	1	1
Vegetable Classics Lentil	1 cup (8.5 oz)	160	2	30	2	5
Saffron Road						
Chicken Broth Artisan Roasted	1 cup (8.4 oz)	20	1	0	0	0
Spoonful Of Comfort						
Chicken Soup	1 serv (8 oz)	80	2	11	1	1
Swanson						
50% Low Sodium Beef Broth	1 cup	15	0	1	1	0
Beef Stock	1 cup	30	0	3	3	0
Chicken Broth	1 cup	10	0	1	1	0
Chicken Stock	1 cup	20	0	1	1	0
Tabatchnick						
Garden Fresh Vegetable Broth	⅔ cup (5.5 oz)	10	0	2	1	0
Wisconsin Cheddar Cheese	⅔ cup (5.5 oz)	150	11	10	2	0
FROZEN						
Kettle Cuisine						
Chicken w/ Rice Noodles Gluten Free	1 pkg (10 oz)	140	3	15	1	2
Thai Curry Chicken Gluten Free Dairy Free	1 pkg (10 oz)	330	11	44	2	4
Three Bean Chili Gluten Free	1 pkg (10 oz)	220	4	36	11	13

FOOD	PORTION	CAL	FAT	CARB	SUGAR	FIBER
Tabatchnick						
Cabbage	1 serv (7.5 oz)	90	1	21	11	1
Chicken Broth w/ Noodles & Dumplings	1 serv (7.25 oz)	150	6	19	1	tr
Corn Chowder	1 serv (7.5 oz)	130	5	21	4	2
Organic Vegetarian Chili	1 serv (7.5 oz)	180	4	28	3	8
Soup Singles Split Pea	1 bowl (10.9 oz)	210	1	50	1	20
Split Pea	1 serv (7.5 oz)	140	0	34	0	13
Vegetable	1 serv (7.5 oz)	90	2	17	3	4
Vegetable Low Sodium	1 serv (7.5 oz)	90	2	17	3	4
Wilderness Wild Rice	1 serv (7.5 oz)	80	1	16	1	1
Yankee Bean	1 serv (7.5 oz)	180	2	33	2	10
MIX						
beef broth cube	1 cube	6	tr	1	–	–
chicken broth cube	1 cube (4.8 g)	9	tr	1	–	–
Annie Chun's						
Ramen Soy Ginger as prep	1 pkg (4.9 oz)	230	1	45	tr	1
Ramen Spring Vegetable as prep	1 pkg (4.9 oz)	230	1	48	2	2
Dr. McDougall's						
Black Bean & Lime not prep	1 pkg (3.3 oz)	340	2	60	4	28
Chicken Noodle Light Sodium not prep	1 pkg (1.4 oz)	140	1	28	2	2
Chinese Chicken Noodle Light Sodium not prep	1 pkg (1.4 oz)	140	1	28	2	2
Minestrone & Pasta not prep	1 pkg (2.3 oz)	200	1	40	2	8
Tamale w/ Baked Chips not prep	1 pkg (2.4 oz)	200	2	36	2	6

FOOD	PORTION	CAL	FAT	CARB	SUGAR	FIBER
Tortilla w/ Baked Chips not prep	1 pkg (2 oz)	200	2	34	2	6
White Bean & Pasta Light Sodium not prep	1 pkg (1.8 oz)	170	1	34	2	8
Herb Ox						
Beef Cubes	1 (3.5 g)	5	0	1	0	0
Beef Instant	1 pkg (4 g)	5	0	1	0	0
Chicken Cubes	1 (4 g)	5	0	1	0	0
Chicken Instant	1 pkg (3.5 g)	5	0	1	0	0
Chicken Instant Sodium Free	1 pkg (4 g)	10	0	2	1	0
Kikkoman						
Instant Tofu Miso	1 pkg (6 g)	15	0	3	0	0
Instant Wakame Seaweed	1 pkg (10 g)	35	1	3	0	0
Knorr						
Chicken Reduced Sodium Concentrated Stock as prep	1 cup	20	1	2	–	–
TAKE-OUT						
ban mien fish head	1 serv (10 oz)	277	10	27	2	4
beef stew soup	1 cup (8.8 oz)	221	5	20	–	–
bird's nest	1 cup (8.6 oz)	112	3	8	1	0
black bean turtle soup	1 cup (6.5 oz)	240	1	45	1	10
broccoli cheese	1 cup	165	9	15	7	2
brunswick stew soup	1 cup (8.5 oz)	232	6	17	–	–
caldo de res beef soup	1 cup	143	5	12	3	2
corn & cheese chowder	¾ cup	215	12	21	–	3
duck soup	1 cup (8.6 oz)	412	37	2	tr	tr
egg drop	1 cup	73	4	1	tr	0
gazpacho	1 cup	46	tr	5	–	–
greek lemon	¾ cup	63	2	7	–	2
hot & sour	1 serv (14 oz)	173	9	9	3	3

FOOD	PORTION	CAL	FAT	CARB	SUGAR	FIBER
matzo ball soup	1 cup	118	5	10	tr	1
minestrone	1 cup	233	13	22	4	4
miso w/ tofu	1 cup	84	3	8	2	2
onion soup gratinee	1 serv	492	27	38	6	4
oxtail	1 cup	68	2	9	2	1
pasta e fagioli	1 cup (8.8 oz)	194	5	30	–	–
ratatouille	1 cup (7.5 oz)	266	25	12	–	–
seaweed	1 cup (8 oz)	80	3	6	1	1
shark fin	1 bowl (10 oz)	164	9	9	–	0
shrimp bisque	1 cup	263	14	13	10	tr
shrimp gumbo	1 cup (8.6 oz)	163	7	18	5	3
sopa de albondigas	1 cup	171	11	9	3	1
thai lemon grass	1 bowl	100	4	5	–	–
vietnamese pho beef noodle	1 serv (7.8 oz)	480	12	78	2	1
wonton soup	1 cup	183	7	14	tr	1
yookgaejang korean beef	1 cup (8.4 oz)	94	6	4	–	1
zupa koprowa polish dill soup	1 bowl	54	2	6	–	–
SOUR CREAM						
fat free	1 tbsp	12	0	3	tr	0
fat free	½ cup (4.5 oz)	95	0	20	1	0
reduced fat	1 tbsp (0.5 oz)	29	2	1	tr	0
reduced fat	½ cup (4.4 oz)	224	17	9	tr	0
sour cream	1 tbsp (0.4 oz)	23	2	tr	tr	0
sour cream	½ cup (4 oz)	222	23	3	3	0
Friendship						
Light	2 tbsp (1 oz)	40	3	2	2	0
Green Valley						
Sour Cream	2 tbsp	100	10	1	1	0

FOOD	PORTION	CAL	FAT	CARB	SUGAR	FIBER
SOUR CREAM SUBSTITUTES						
imitation	½ cup (4 oz)	239	22	8	8	0
Tofutti						
Better Than Sour Cream	2 tbsp (1 oz)	85	5	9	2	0
SOURSOP						
fresh	1	416	2	105	–	–
fresh cut up	1 cup	150	1	38	–	–
SOY (*see also* CHEESE SUBSTITUTES, ICE CREAM AND FROZEN DESSERTS, MILK SUBSTITUTES, MISO, SMOOTHIES, SOY SAUCE, SOYBEANS, TEMPEH, TOFU, YOGURT FROZEN)						
natto	½ cup (3.1 oz)	187	10	13	4	5
SOY DRINKS (*see* MILK SUBSTITUTES, SMOOTHIES)						
SOY SAUCE						
shoyu	1 tbsp	9	tr	2	–	–
soy sauce	1 tbsp	7	tr	1	–	–
tamari	1 tbsp	11	tr	1	–	–
Kikkoman						
Less Sodium	1 tbsp (0.5 oz)	10	0	1	–	–
Ponzu	1 tbsp (0.5 oz)	10	0	2	2	–
Soy Sauce	1 tbsp (0.5 oz)	10	0	0	0	0
Sushi Sashimi	1 tbsp (0.5 oz)	15	0	2	2	–
Lee Kum Kee						
Less Sodium	1 tbsp (0.5 oz)	10	0	2	1	–
San-J						
Tamari Organic Gluten Free	2 pkg (0.5 oz)	10	0	tr	–	–
Soy Vay						
Wasabi Teriyaki	1 tbsp	35	1	6	5	0
SOYBEANS						
dried cooked	1 cup	298	15	17	–	–
dry roasted	½ cup	387	19	28	–	–

FOOD	PORTION	CAL	FAT	CARB	SUGAR	FIBER
green cooked	½ cup	127	6	10	–	4
roasted	½ cup	405	22	29	–	–
roasted & toasted	1 cup	490	26	33	–	–
roasted & toasted salted	1 cup	490	26	33	–	–
sprouts raw	½ cup	43	2	3	–	–
sprouts steamed	½ cup	38	2	3	–	–
sprouts stir fried	1 cup	125	7	9	–	–
Crunchies						
Freeze Dried Edamame	⅜ cup (1 oz)	124	6	9	2	3
Freeze Dried Edamame Grilled	⅜ cup (0.9 oz)	84	1	13	1	1
Freeze Dried Edamame Salted	¼ cup (0.9 oz)	90	4	7	0	3
KooLoos						
Soy Nuts & Flaxseed BBQ	1 pkg (1 oz)	130	4	16	1	3
Soy Nuts & Flaxseed Original	1 pkg (1 oz)	140	5	15	1	3
South Beach						
Dark Chocolate Covered	1 pkg (0.71 oz)	100	6	13	6	2
Sunrich Naturals						
Edamame Fiesta Blend frzn	½ cup (3 oz)	90	3	12	1	3
Edamame In The Shell frzn	½ cup (3 oz)	120	5	9	3	4
Soy Honey Nutz	1 pkg (1 oz)	130	6	12	3	4

SPAGHETTI (*see* PASTA, PASTA DINNERS, PASTA SALAD, SPAGHETTI SAUCE)

SPAGHETTI SAUCE

JARRED

FOOD	PORTION	CAL	FAT	CARB	SUGAR	FIBER
marinara sauce	1 cup	171	8	25	–	–
spaghetti sauce	1 cup	272	12	40	–	–

FOOD	PORTION	CAL	FAT	CARB	SUGAR	FIBER
Barilla						
Toscana Tuscan Herb	½ cup (4.4 oz)	70	2	10	6	3
Bella Sun Luci						
Sun Dried Tomato Pesto w/ Whole Pine Nuts	¼ cup (1.9 oz)	270	27	8	5	1
Del Monte						
Garlic & Onion	½ cup (4.4 oz)	70	1	14	6	2
Hunt's						
Pasta Sauce Four Cheese	½ cup (4.4 oz)	60	1	10	5	3
Pasta Sauce Garlic & Herb	½ cup (4.4 oz)	40	1	8	4	3
Pasta Sauce Meat	½ cup (4.4 oz)	60	1	10	6	3
Pasta Sauce Mushroom	½ cup (4.4 oz)	50	1	10	6	3
Tomato Sauce	¼ cup (2.2 oz)	20	0	4	2	1
Tomato Sauce No Salt Added	¼ cup (2.2 oz)	20	0	5	3	1
Traditional Pasta Sauce	½ cup (4.4 oz)	50	1	11	5	3
Lucini						
Tuscan Marinara w/ Roasted Garlic	½ cup (4.4 oz)	60	3	8	5	1
Manischewitz						
Tomato & Mushroom	¼ cup (2.2 oz)	40	2	6	3	1
Mom's						
Artichoke Heart & Asiago Cheese	½ cup (4.2 oz)	90	6	7	3	3
Fresh Garlic Basil	½ cup (4.2 oz)	30	3	7	4	2
Martini	½ cup (4.2 oz)	120	4	6	3	1
Puttanesca	½ cup (4.2 oz)	90	6	8	5	2
OrganicVille						
Marinara	½ cup (4 oz)	50	1	9	3	2
Mushroom	½ cup (4 oz)	45	1	8	3	2
Pizza Sauce	½ cup (2 oz)	25	1	3	2	1

FOOD	PORTION	CAL	FAT	CARB	SUGAR	FIBER
Pomi						
Strained	½ cup (4.4 oz)	30	0	5	5	3
Prego						
Veggie Smart	½ cup (4.2 oz)	90	2	16	10	3
Progresso						
Lobster Sauce	½ cup (4.3 oz)	100	7	6	3	2
Pesto Arrabiata	2 tbsp (1 oz)	140	11	7	2	2
Pesto Basil & Roasted Garlic	2 tbsp (1 oz)	130	13	3	0	0
Red Clam w/ Tomato & Basil	½ cup (4.4 oz)	60	1	8	4	1
White Clam w/ Garlic & Herb	½ cup (4.4 oz)	120	10	4	1	1
Racconto						
Essentials Heart Health Roasted Garlic	½ cup (4.4 oz)	90	5	10	5	2
Ragu						
Light Tomato & Basil No Sugar Added	½ cup (4.4 oz)	50	1	9	6	3
Old World Style Meat	½ cup (4.4 oz)	70	3	9	6	2
Randazzo's						
Alfredo	¼ cup (2.2 oz)	200	20	3	1	0
Fra Diavolo	½ cup (4.4 oz)	90	4	9	4	4
Puttanesca	½ cup (4.4 oz)	100	6	9	4	4
Vodka	½ cup (4.4 oz)	230	20	7	3	3
Sonoma Gourmet						
Fennel Romano	½ cup (4.4 oz)	70	4	7	4	2
Puttanesca	½ cup (4.4 oz)	70	5	7	4	2
Red Clam	½ cup (4.4 oz)	60	4	7	3	2

FOOD	PORTION	CAL	FAT	CARB	SUGAR	FIBER
Vodka Cream	½ cup (4.4 oz)	100	6	8	3	1
Victoria						
Bolognese	½ cup (4 oz)	120	8	7	4	tr
Italian w/ Imported Cheeses	½ cup (4 oz)	150	12	4	3	2
Marinara	½ cup (4 oz)	70	4	4	3	2
Pesto	¼ cup (2 oz)	380	37	4	1	2
Sicilian Caponata	½ cup (4 oz)	70	4	4	3	2
Eggplant Tomato Basil	½ cup (4 oz)	70	4	4	3	2
White Clam Sauce	½ cup (4.4 oz)	140	9	5	0	0
Walden Farms						
Alfredo Sauce Calorie Free	3 tbsp (1.6 oz)	0	0	0	0	0
MIX						
Loney's						
Carbonara as prep	¼ cup (2.1 oz)	33	3	3	0	0
Rose as prep	¼ cup (2.1 oz)	29	3	6	1	0
REFRIGERATED						
Buitoni						
Alfredo	¼ cup (2.1 oz)	140	12	4	2	0
Alfredo Light	¼ cup (2.1 oz)	90	6	5	1	0
Marinara	½ cup (4.4 oz)	70	3	10	6	2
Pesto	¼ cup (2.2 oz)	270	23	6	4	1
Pesto Basil Reduced Fat	¼ cup (2.2 oz)	230	17	8	6	2
Vodka Sauce	½ cup (4.2 oz)	90	6	5	3	1
TAKE-OUT						
bolognese	5 oz	195	15	4	–	tr

FOOD	PORTION	CAL	FAT	CARB	SUGAR	FIBER
SPANISH FOOD						
FRESH						
Texas Tamale Company						
Tamales Beef	2 (3 oz)	160	12	8	0	2
Tamales Chicken	2 (3 oz)	130	7	8	1	1
Tamales Spinach	2 (3 oz)	140	8	12	0	0
FROZEN						
Dr. Praeger's						
Burrito Bites	2 (2 oz)	130	3	20	1	4
Farm Rich						
Quesadillas	2 (3.1 oz)	200	10	19	1	1
Glutenfreeda						
Burrito Breakfast Beef	1 (3.9 oz)	199	8	23	1	2
Burrito Vegetarian Bean & Cheese	1 (3.9 oz)	196	7	29	0	3
Jose Ole						
Burrito Steak & Jalapeno	1 (5 oz)	300	9	43	tr	3
Lean Cuisine						
Simple Favorites Chicken Enchilada Suiza	1 pkg (9 oz)	290	5	51	8	3
Mom Made						
Fiesta Rice	1 pkg (7 oz)	200	1	38	2	5
Munchie Bean Burrito	1 (2.5 oz)	140	9	10	1	1
Pjs Organics						
Burrito Breakfast	1 (6 oz)	310	7	46	1	2
Burrito Five Layer	1 (6 oz)	390	11	55	1	4
Burrito Skinny	1 (6 oz)	310	2	55	0	4
Burrito Traditional Chicken	1 (6 oz)	380	8	58	1	4
READY-TO-EAT						
taco shell corn	1 (6.5 inch)	98	5	13	tr	2
taco shell flour	1 (7 inch)	173	9	19	tr	1

FOOD	PORTION	CAL	FAT	CARB	SUGAR	FIBER
Garden Of Eatin'						
Taco Shells Yellow Corn	2 (0.9 oz)	140	7	17	0	1
TAKE-OUT						
arroz con coco	1 cup	532	38	46	5	4
burrito w/ beans	1 med (5 oz)	295	8	45	1	7
burrito w/ beans & rice	1 (3.5 oz)	221	5	37	tr	4
burrito w/ beef	1 sm (3.4 oz)	297	13	25	tr	1
burrito w/ beef & beans	1 med (5 oz)	331	13	36	1	6
burrito w/ beef beans & cheese	1 med (5 oz)	379	19	30	1	5
burrito w/ chicken & beans	1 med (5 oz)	295	9	34	1	5
burrito w/ pork & beans	1 med (5 oz)	320	12	35	1	6
chiles rellenos meat & cheese filled	1 (5 oz)	213	16	9	3	2
chimichanga w/ bean cheese lettuce & tomato	1 (4.1 oz)	271	18	22	2	3
chimichanga w/ beef & rice	1 (10 oz)	634	36	58	5	5
chimichanga w/ beef beans lettuce & tomato	1 (4.1 oz)	254	15	22	2	3
chimichanga w/ beef cheese lettuce & tomato	1 (4.1 oz)	337	24	19	1	1
chimichanga w/ chicken sour cream lettuce & tomato	1 (4 oz)	277	20	17	1	1
empanada fruit filled	1 (3.8 oz)	452	25	55	25	2
empanada meat & vegetable	1 (7.8 oz)	881	61	66	1	3
empanada sweet potato	1 (7.8 oz)	546	23	76	22	4
enchilada w/ beans	1 (4.1 oz)	179	6	27	2	6
enchilada w/ beans & cheese	1 (4.6 oz)	233	11	25	2	5

FOOD	PORTION	CAL	FAT	CARB	SUGAR	FIBER
enchilada w/ beef	1 (4 oz)	214	10	21	2	3
enchilada w/ beef & beans	1 (4 oz)	195	8	25	2	4
frijoles	1 cup	278	2	49	6	9
frijoles w/ cheese	1 cup	225	8	29	–	–
nachos w/ beans & cheese	1 serv (9.4 oz)	616	33	57	2	13
nachos w/ beef beans cheese & sour cream	1 serv (19 oz)	1620	97	133	4	19
paella	1 serv (7 oz)	308	16	17	–	3
pupusa meat filled	1 (3.6 oz)	187	6	26	1	3
quesadilla w/ cheese	1 (5 oz)	498	28	40	1	3
quesadilla w/ meat & cheese	1 (6.5 oz)	605	35	40	1	2
taco de jueye w/ crab meat	1 (4.2 oz)	266	14	18	1	2
taco w/ beans lettuce tomato & salsa	1 (2.8 oz)	117	5	16	1	4
taco w/ chicken lettuce tomato & salsa	1 (2.5 oz)	114	5	10	1	1
taco w/ fish lettuce tomato & salsa	1 (2.7 oz)	101	4	10	1	1
tostada w/ beef lettuce tomato & salsa	1 (2.7 oz)	143	8	11	1	2

SPICES (*see* INDIVIDUAL NAMES, HERBS/SPICES)

SPINACH

CANNED

FOOD	PORTION	CAL	FAT	CARB	SUGAR	FIBER
drained	1 cup	49	1	7	1	5
Del Monte						
Leaf No Salt Added	½ cup (4 oz)	30	0	4	0	2
Whole Leaf	½ cup (4 oz)	30	0	4	0	2

FOOD	PORTION	CAL	FAT	CARB	SUGAR	FIBER
FRESH						
baby raw	2 cups	20	0	5	0	3
cooked	1 cup	41	tr	7	1	4
malabar cooked	1 cup	10	tr	1	–	1
mustard cooked	1 cup	29	tr	5	–	4
new zealand cooked	1 cup	22	tr	4	–	–
raw	1 cup	7	tr	1	tr	1
Dole						
Baby Spinach	1½ cups (3 oz)	20	0	3	0	2
Ready Pac						
Microwave Spinach as prep	½ cup (3 oz)	20	0	3	0	1
River Ranch						
Baby Spinach	3 cups (3 oz)	20	0	3	0	2
FROZEN						
chopped cooked	1 cup	30	tr	5	tr	4
Birds Eye						
Creamed	½ cup (4.4 oz)	90	4	9	3	4
Seabrook Farms						
Chopped	⅓ cup (2.9 oz)	20	0	2	1	2
Creamed	½ cup (4.4 oz)	100	5	10	3	2
Tabatchnick						
Creamed	1 serv (3.7 oz)	40	1	7	1	1
Tandoor Chef						
Palak Paneer	½ pkg (5 oz)	170	14	6	1	2
TAKE-OUT						
indian saag	1 serv	28	2	2	–	1
spanakopita spinach pie	1 serv (3 oz)	148	11	8	1	1

SPINACH JUICE

juice	7 oz	14	0	2	–	–

SPORTS DRINKS (*see* ENERGY DRINKS)

FOOD	PORTION	CAL	FAT	CARB	SUGAR	FIBER
SPOT						
baked	3 oz	134	5	0	0	0
SPROUTS						
kidney bean	½ cup	27	tr	4	–	–
lentil sprouts	½ cup	40	tr	8	–	–
mung bean	½ cup	16	tr	3	–	–
mung bean canned	½ cup	8	tr	1	–	–
mung bean cooked	½ cup	13	tr	3	–	–
pea	½ cup (2.1 oz)	74	tr	16	–	–
radish	½ cup	8	tr	1	–	–
Brassica						
BroccoSprouts	½ cup (1 oz)	16	0	2	–	1
TAKE-OUT						
mung bean stir fried	½ cup	31	tr	7	–	–
SQUAB						
boneless baked	1 (4 oz)	242	14	0	0	0
SQUASH (*see also* SQUASH SEEDS, ZUCCHINI)						
CANNED						
crookneck sliced	½ cup	14	tr	3	–	–
FRESH						
acorn cooked mashed	½ cup	41	tr	11	–	3
acorn cubed baked	½ cup	57	tr	15	–	2
butternut baked	½ cup	41	tr	11	–	2
crookneck sliced cooked	½ cup	18	tr	4	–	1
hubbard baked	½ cup	51	tr	11	–	3
hubbard cooked mashed	½ cup	35	tr	8	–	3
scallop sliced cooked	½ cup	14	tr	3	–	1
spaghetti cooked	½ cup	23	tr	5	–	2
Mann's						
Butternut Cubes	1 serv (3 oz)	40	0	10	2	2

FOOD	PORTION	CAL	FAT	CARB	SUGAR	FIBER
Plainville Farm						
Butternut Peeled	½ cup (3 oz)	40	0	10	5	1
FROZEN						
butternut cooked mashed	½ cup	47	tr	12	–	3
crookneck sliced cooked	½ cup	24	tr	5	–	–
TAKE-OUT						
fritter	1 (0.8 oz)	81	5	8	1	1
squash pie	1 slice (5.4 oz)	291	12	40	24	2

SQUASH SEEDS

FOOD	PORTION	CAL	FAT	CARB	SUGAR	FIBER
kernels dried	¼ cup (1.1 oz)	180	16	3	tr	2
kernels roasted	¼ cup (1 oz)	169	14	4	tr	2
kernels roasted w/ salt	¼ cup (1 oz)	169	14	4	tr	2
whole roasted w/ salt	¼ cup (0.5 oz)	71	3	9	–	3
whole roasted w/o salt	¼ cup (0.5 oz)	71	3	9	–	3

SQUID

FOOD	PORTION	CAL	FAT	CARB	SUGAR	FIBER
baked	1 cup	192	6	5	0	0
canned in its own ink	1 can (4 oz)	122	2	4	0	0
dried	1 sm (1.5 oz)	147	2	5	0	0
pickled	1 oz	26	tr	1	tr	0
steamed	1 cup	147	2	5	0	0
Margaritaville						
Captain's Calamari Rings + Sauce	3 + 2 tbsp sauce	320	21	25	3	1
TAKE-OUT						
arroz con calamares	1 cup	400	17	47	2	1
calamari breaded & fried	1 cup	296	12	17	1	1

SQUIRREL

FOOD	PORTION	CAL	FAT	CARB	SUGAR	FIBER
roasted	3 oz	147	4	0	0	0

FOOD	PORTION	CAL	FAT	CARB	SUGAR	FIBER
STARFRUIT						
fresh	1	42	tr	10	–	–
STRAWBERRIES						
canned in heavy syrup	½ cup	117	tr	30	28	2
fresh halves	1 cup	49	tr	12	7	3
fresh whole	1 pint	114	1	27	17	7
fresh whole	1 cup	46	tr	11	7	3
frzn sweetened sliced	½ cup	122	tr	33	31	2
frzn sweetened whole	1 cup	199	tr	54	48	5
frzn whole unsweetened	1 cup	77	tr	20	10	5
organic fresh whole	8 med	45	0	12	8	4
Crunchies						
Freeze Dried	¼ cup (6 g)	20	0	5	3	1
Crunchy N'Yummy						
Organic Freeze Dried	1 pkg (1 oz)	60	0	11	0	3
Dole						
Sliced frzn	1 pkg (3 oz)	35	0	8	4	2
Squish'ems	1 pkg	70	0	16	15	1
Whole Fresh	1 cup (5.2 oz)	45	0	11	7	3
Whole frzn	1 cup (4.9 oz)	50	0	13	61	3
STUFFING/DRESSING						
Mrs. Cubbison's						
Corn Bread not prep	½ cup (1.2 oz)	130	1	25	2	2
Focaccia not prep	½ cup (1 oz)	110	2	11	3	4
Multi-Grain Cranberry not prep	⅓ cup (1 oz)	110	3	18	3	1
Pepperidge Farm						
Cornbread	¾ cup	170	2	33	2	2
Country Style	¾ cup	140	1	27	2	2
Herb Seasoned	¾ cup	170	2	33	2	3

FOOD	PORTION	CAL	FAT	CARB	SUGAR	FIBER
TAKE-OUT						
bread	1 cup	352	17	44	5	2
cornbread	½ cup	179	9	22	0	3
kishke stuffed derma	1 piece (1.3 oz)	166	12	13	tr	1
oyster	1 cup	304	18	29	3	2
sausage	½ cup	292	11	40	–	1
STURGEON						
broiled	3 oz	115	4	0	0	0
roe raw	1 oz	59	3	tr	–	–
smoked	1 oz	49	1	0	0	0
TAKE-OUT						
breaded & fried	4 oz	252	15	9	1	1
SUCKER						
white baked	3 oz	101	3	0	0	0
SUGAR (*see also* FRUCTOSE, SYRUP)						
brown organic	1 tsp	17	0	4	4	0
brown packed	1 cup (7.7 oz)	828	0	214	214	–
brown unpacked	1 cup (5.1 oz)	547	0	141	140	0
cinnamon sugar	1 tsp	16	tr	4	4	tr
cube	1 (2 g)	9	0	2	2	0
maple	1 piece (1 oz)	99	tr	25	24	0
powdered	1 tbsp (0.3 oz)	31	0	8	8	–
powdered unsifted	1 cup (4.2 oz)	467	tr	119	115	–
raw	1 pkg (5 g)	19	0	5	5	0
sugarcane stem	3 oz	54	0	14	–	3
white	1 pkg (3 g)	12	0	3	3	0
white	1 cup (7 oz)	773	0	200	200	–
white	1 tbsp (0.4 oz)	49	0	13	13	0
white	1 tsp (4 g)	15	0	4	4	–
Coconut World						
Coconut Sugar	1 tsp (3 g)	10	0	3	3	0

FOOD	PORTION	CAL	FAT	CARB	SUGAR	FIBER
Domino						
White	1 tsp	15	0	4	–	–
In The Raw						
Granulated	1 pkg (5 g)	20	0	5	5	–
Liquid Cane	1 tsp (6 g)	20	0	5	5	0
Maple Grove Farms						
Granulated Maple	1 tsp (4 g)	15	0	4	3	–
Wholesome Sweeteners						
Organic	1 tsp (4 g)	15	0	4	4	0
Organic Fair Trade Dark Brown Sugar	1 tsp (4 g)	15	0	4	4	0
Organic Fair Trade Powdered	¼ cup (1 oz)	120	0	30	30	0
SUGAR SUBSTITUTES						
Domino						
Light	½ tsp (1.7 g)	5	0	2	2	–
Emerald City						
Erythritol	1 tsp (4 g)	0	0	4	0	0
Emerald Forest						
Xylitol	1 tsp (4 g)	10	0	4	0	0
Fibrelle						
Fiber-Rich Sweetener	1 tsp (4 g)	5	0	4	0	2
Fruit-Sweetness						
Sugar Substitute	1 serv (0.9 oz)	0	0	0	0	0
Ideal						
Brown	1 tsp (1.5 g)	0	0	2	0	0
Confectionary	¼ cup (1 oz)	86	0	30	0	0
Packets	1 (1.5 g)	0	0	2	0	0
White Granulated	1 tsp (1.5 g)	0	0	2	0	0
In The Raw						
Monk Fruit	1 pkg (0.8 g)	0	0	tr	0	–
Stevia	1 pkg (1 g)	0	0	tr	0	–

FOOD	PORTION	CAL	FAT	CARB	SUGAR	FIBER
Nevella						
No Calorie Sweetener	1 tsp (0.5 g)	0	0	tr	0	0
Pyure						
Organic Stevia	1 pkg (1 g)	0	0	1	0	1
Splenda						
Nectresse	1 pkg (2.4 g)	0	0	2	tr	–
No Calorie Sweetener w/ Antioxidants	1 pkg	0	0	tr	0	–
No Calorie Sweetener w/ B Vitamins	1 pkg	0	0	tr	0	0
No Calorie Sweetener w/ Fiber	1 pkg	0	0	2	0	1
Steel's						
Nature Sweet Brown Crystals	1 tsp (3 g)	6	0	3	0	0
Nature Sweet Crystals	1 tsp (4 g)	8	0	4	0	0
Sugar Free Vanilla Flavor	1 tbsp (0.5 oz)	23	0	11	0	0
Sugar Twin						
Granulated Brown	1 tsp (0.4 g)	0	0	tr	0	0
Packets	1 (0.8 g)	0	0	1	–	–
Sun Crystals						
Natural Sweetener	1 pkg (5 g)	5	0	1	1	–
Suzanne						
Somersweet Baking Blend	1 tsp (4 g)	5	0	4	0	2
Swerve						
Sweetener	1 tsp (5 g)	0	0	5	0	–
Whey Low						
Gold	1 tsp (4 g)	4	0	4	4	0
Granular	1 tsp (4 g)	4	0	4	4	0
Maple	¼ cup (2 oz)	57	0	57	57	0
Powder	1 tsp (4 g)	4	0	4	4	0

FOOD	PORTION	CAL	FAT	CARB	SUGAR	FIBER
SUGAR-APPLE						
fresh	1	146	tr	37	–	–
fresh cut up	1 cup	236	1	59	–	–
SUNCHOKE						
fresh raw sliced	½ cup	57	tr	13	–	–
SUNFISH						
pumpkinseed baked	3 oz	97	1	0	0	0
SUNFLOWER						
seeds dry roasted w/ salt	¼ cup	186	16	8	1	3
seeds dry roasted w/o salt	¼ cup	186	16	8	1	4
seeds w/ hulls dried	¼ cup	66	6	2	tr	1
David						
Kernels	¼ cup (1.1 oz)	190	15	4	tr	3
Seeds Reduced Sodium w/o Shell	¼ cup (1.1 oz)	190	14	7	tr	3
Seeds w/o Shell	¼ cup (1.1 oz)	190	15	5	tr	4
Frito Lay						
Seeds	1 oz	190	16	5	tr	3
Kaia Foods						
Seeds Sprouted Cocoa Mole	⅙ pkg (1 oz)	80	6	5	3	2
Sprouted Seeds Sweet Curry	⅙ pkg (1 oz)	80	6	4	2	2
Planters						
Kernels	1 oz	160	14	5	1	3
Seeds Roasted & Salted	¾ cup (1 oz)	160	14	7	0	3
Somersaults						
Snacks Pacific Sea Salt	14 (1.1 oz)	150	8	14	1	3

FOOD	PORTION	CAL	FAT	CARB	SUGAR	FIBER
South Beach						
Dark Chocolate Covered	1 pkg (0.67 oz)	100	8	8	6	1
Spitz						
Seeds Salted	⅓ pkg (1 oz)	180	15	5	tr	3
Sunrich Naturals						
Kernels Cocoa Sunnies	1 pkg (2 oz)	280	16	30	13	4
Kernels Honey Roasted	1 pkg (1 oz)	170	14	6	3	2
Kernels Lightly Salted	1 pkg (1 oz)	170	16	4	1	2

SUSHI

TAKE-OUT

FOOD	PORTION	CAL	FAT	CARB	SUGAR	FIBER
california roll	1 (1.2 oz)	48	1	8	1	tr
crabmeat mayonnaise	1 (1.2 oz)	60	2	10	–	tr
futomaki roll	1 (1.8 oz)	73	1	14	3	1
ikura salmon roe & cucumber	1 (1.1 oz)	50	1	7	1	1
inari	1 sm (1.2 oz)	46	1	9	–	0
kappa cucumber roll	1 (1.1 oz)	43	0	9	2	tr
kim bap	1 (1.2 oz)	56	2	8	–	0
nigiri	1 (0.7 oz)	27	0	5	–	0
prawn cooked	1 (1.1 oz)	36	0	8	–	1
preserved radish roll	1 (0.3 oz)	9	0	2	0	tr
saba raw mackerel	1 (0.8 oz)	33	1	5	1	tr
salmon slice	1 (1.2 oz)	59	1	10	1	tr
sashimi ahi	1 slice (0.3 oz)	10	0	0	0	0
scallop cooked	1 (1.1 oz)	43	tr	8	–	tr
seasoned baby octopus	1 (1.2 oz)	55	tr	10	1	tr
seasoned jellyfish	1 (1.2 oz)	58	1	11	2	tr
seaweed roll	1 (1.1 oz)	43	1	9	1	1
sweet beancurd	1 (1.2 oz)	64	2	10	3	1
tekka tuna maki	1 (0.6 oz)	25	0	5	–	0
torigai cockle	1 piece (1.1 oz)	41	0	7	–	tr
tuna roll	1 (0.6 oz)	19	0	4	0	tr

FOOD	PORTION	CAL	FAT	CARB	SUGAR	FIBER
unagi grilled eel	1 (1 oz)	54	2	8	1	1
vegetable roll	1 (1.2 oz)	27	1	5	tr	–
vinegared ginger	⅓ cup (1.6 oz)	48	tr	12	4	–
wasabi	2 tsp (0.3 oz)	5	tr	1	–	–
yellowtail roll	1 (0.6 oz)	25	1	3	tr	–
SWAMP CABBAGE						
chopped cooked w/o salt	1 cup	20	tr	4	–	2
SWEET POTATO (*see also* YAM)						
baked w/ skin w/o salt	1 med (4 oz)	103	tr	24	7	4
baked w/ skin w/o salt	1 lg (6.3 oz)	162	tr	37	12	6
canned in syrup	½ cup	106	tr	25	6	3
canned mashed	½ cup	129	tr	30	7	2
leaves cooked w/o salt	1 cup	22	tr	5	3	1
paste dulce de calabaza	1 oz	82	tr	21	20	tr
Jake & Amos						
Sweet Potato Butter	1 tbsp (0.5 oz)	25	0	6	3	0
Mann's						
Fresh Cubes	1 serv (3 oz)	60	0	15	3	3
Fries Fresh	1 serv (3 oz)	60	0	15	3	3
TAKE-OUT						
candied	1 serv (3.7 oz)	151	3	29	–	3
white fried batata blanca frita	1 serv (8 oz)	792	29	129	2	19
SWEETBREAD (PANCREAS)						
beef braised	3 oz	230	15	0	0	0
lamb braised	3 oz	199	13	0	0	0
pork braised	3 oz	186	9	0	0	0
veal braised	3 oz	218	12	0	0	0
SWISS CHARD						
cooked	½ cup	18	tr	4	–	–
raw chopped	½ cup	3	tr	1	–	–

FOOD	PORTION	CAL	FAT	CARB	SUGAR	FIBER
SWORDFISH						
cooked	3 oz	132	4	0	0	0
raw	3 oz	103	3	0	0	0
SYRUP						
corn dark & light	¼ cup	240	tr	65	65	0
date syrup	1 tbsp	63	tr	15	–	0
maple	1 cup (11.1 oz)	824	1	212	191	–
maple	1 tbsp	52	0	13	12	–
raspberry	1 oz	76	0	19	–	–
rose hip	1 oz	9	0	2	2	0
sorghum	1 tbsp (0.7 oz)	61	0	16	16	–
sorghum	1 cup (11.6 oz)	957	0	247	247	–
sugar syrup	¼ cup	76	0	20	20	0
Domino						
Agave Nectar Organic Light or Amber	1 tbsp (0.7 oz)	60	0	16	16	–
In The Raw						
Agave	1 tbsp (0.7 oz)	60	0	16	15	–
Karo						
Corn Syrup Light	2 tbsp (1 oz)	120	0	30	10	–
Lundberg						
Organic Sweet Dreams Brown Rice	2 tbsp (1.5 oz)	150	0	36	22	0
Maple Grove Farms						
Apricot	¼ cup (2.1 oz)	170	0	42	40	–
Butter Flavor Sugar Free	¼ cup (2.1 oz)	30	0	11	0	–
Red Raspberry	¼ cup (2.1 oz)	230	0	46	45	–

FOOD	PORTION	CAL	FAT	CARB	SUGAR	FIBER
Nature's Agave						
Agave Nectar Organic Amber Clear or Raw	1 tbsp (0.7 oz)	60	0	16	16	–
Smucker's						
Blackberry	¼ cup (2.1 oz)	200	0	51	44	–
Blueberry Sugar Free	¼ cup (2.1 oz)	25	0	8	0	1
Plate Scrapers Caramel	2 tbsp (1.4 oz)	100	0	25	20	0
Plate Scrapers Raspberry	2 tbsp (1.3 oz)	100	0	25	17	0
Plate Scrapers Vanilla	2 tbsp (1.4 oz)	110	1	24	19	0
Pure Maple	¼ cup (2.1 oz)	210	0	53	47	–
Red Raspberry	¼ cup (2.1 oz)	200	0	51	44	–
Steel's						
Maple Flavor No Sugar Added	3 tbsp (1.6 oz)	64	0	16	0	0
Wholesome Sweeteners						
Organic Blue Agave Maple	2 tbsp (1 oz)	120	0	16	16	0
Organic Corn Syrup	2 tbsp (1 oz)	120	0	30	30	0

TAHINI (*see* SESAME)

TAMARIND

FOOD	PORTION	CAL	FAT	CARB	SUGAR	FIBER
dried sweetened pulpitas	1 piece (0.8 oz)	56	tr	15	14	1
dried sweetened pulpitas	½ cup	279	1	73	68	5
fresh	1 (2 g)	5	tr	1	0	tr
fresh cut up	1 cup	143	tr	38	34	3

TAMARIND JUICE

FOOD	PORTION	CAL	FAT	CARB	SUGAR	FIBER
nectar	1 cup	143	tr	37	32	1

FOOD	PORTION	CAL	FAT	CARB	SUGAR	FIBER
TANGERINE						
CANNED						
in light syrup	1 cup	154	tr	41	39	2
juice pack	1 cup	92	tr	24	22	2
FRESH						
fresh	1 sm (2.7 oz)	40	tr	10	8	1
fresh	1 med (3.1 oz)	47	tr	12	9	2
fresh	1 lg (4.2 oz)	64	tr	16	13	2
sections	1 cup	103	1	26	21	4
Sunkist						
Fresh	1 med (3.8 oz)	50	0	13	9	2
TANGERINE JUICE						
canned sweetened	1 cup	124	1	30	29	1
fresh	1 cup	106	tr	25	24	1
Italian Volcano						
Organic	8 oz	113	1	24	23	–
TAPIOCA						
pearl dry	¼ cup (1.3 oz)	136	tr	34	1	tr
starch	1 oz	98	tr	24	–	–
TARO						
chips	10 (0.8 oz)	115	6	16	–	–
leaves cooked	½ cup	18	tr	3	–	–
raw sliced	½ cup	56	tr	14	–	–
shoots sliced cooked	½ cup	10	tr	2	–	–
sliced cooked	½ cup (2.3 oz)	94	tr	23	–	–
tahitian sliced cooked	½ cup	30	tr	5	–	–
TARPON						
fresh	3 oz	87	2	0	0	0
TARRAGON						
dried crumbled	1 tsp	2	tr	tr	–	0
ground	1 tsp	5	tr	1	–	tr

FOOD	PORTION	CAL	FAT	CARB	SUGAR	FIBER
TEA/HERBAL TEA (*see also* ICED TEA)						
HERBAL						
chamomile brewed	1 cup	2	tr	tr	0	0
Bambusland						
Bamboo Tea Blueberry as prep	1 tea bag	0	0	1	0	0
Bamboo Tea Organic	1 tea bag	0	0	1	0	0
Bigelow						
Cozy Chamomile	1 tea bag	0	0	0	0	0
Celestial Seasonings						
Chamomile Honey Vanilla as prep	1 cup (8 oz)	0	0	0	0	0
Nature's Guru						
Cardamon Chai Sweetened Instant	1 pkg (0.9 oz)	35	1	8	7	0
Lemongrass Sweetened Instant	1 pkg	65	0	13	7	0
REGULAR						
brewed tea	1 cup (6 oz)	2	0	1	–	0
Hansen's						
Tea Stix Blackberry	½ pkg (2 g)	5	0	1	0	–
Lipton						
Black Tea as prep	8 oz	0	0	0	0	0
Green Tea as prep	1 cup (8 oz)	0	0	0	0	0
Green Tea Cranberry Pomegranate	1 tea bag	0	0	0	0	0
Green Tea Decaffeinated as prep	1 tea bag	0	0	0	0	0
Tastefully Simple						
Oh My! Itty Bitty Chai Mix as prep w/ water	1 pkg (1.2 oz)	140	3	25	22	0
Tetley						
Classic Black as prep	1 tea bag	0	0	0	0	0

FOOD	PORTION	CAL	FAT	CARB	SUGAR	FIBER
TAKE-OUT						
chai spiced latte	1 cup	130	3	23	18	0
TEMPEH						
tempeh	½ cup (2.9 oz)	160	9	8	–	–
TESTICLES						
prairie oysters cooked	1 pair (6.8 oz)	241	6	0	0	0
THYME						
dried crumbled	1 tsp	3	tr	1	tr	tr
fresh	1 tsp	1	tr	tr	–	tr
ground	1 tsp	4	tr	1	tr	1
TILAPIA						
Beacon Light						
Boneless Fillet Farm Raised	1 (3 oz)	85	1	1	0	0
Dr. Praeger's						
Fillets Lightly Breaded	1 (4.5 oz)	220	9	20	3	3
Gorton's						
Grilled Fillets Roasted Garlic & Butter	1 (3 oz)	80	3	tr	–	–
TAKE-OUT						
battered & fried	1 fillet (4 oz)	206	9	8	tr	tr
breaded & fried	1 fillet (4 oz)	300	14	16	2	1
broiled w/o fat	1 fillet (3.5 oz)	128	3	0	0	0
TILEFISH						
cooked	½ fillet (5.3 oz)	220	7	0	0	0
cooked	3 oz	125	4	0	0	0
raw	3 oz	81	2	0	0	0

FOOD	PORTION	CAL	FAT	CARB	SUGAR	FIBER
TOFU						
firm	¼ block (3 oz)	118	7	3	–	1
firm	½ cup	183	11	5	–	2
fresh fried	1 piece (0.5 oz)	35	3	1	–	tr
fuyu salted & fermented	1 block (⅓ oz)	13	1	1	–	tr
koyadofu dried frozen	1 piece (½ oz)	82	5	2	–	tr
okara	½ cup	47	1	8	–	1
regular	½ cup	94	6	2	–	1
regular	¼ block (4 oz)	88	6	2	–	1
Azumaya						
Extra Firm	3 oz	70	4	2	0	1
Lite Extra Firm	⅕ pkg (2.8 oz)	60	2	3	0	1
Silken	⅕ pkg (3.2 oz)	40	2	1	0	tr
Nasoya						
Extra Firm	⅕ pkg (2.8 oz)	80	4	2	0	1
Silken	⅕ pkg (3.2 oz)	160	1	1	0	0
Sprouted	3 oz	160	6	3	1	1
TofuTown						
Tofu Tenders Havana Black Bean	½ pkg (5 oz)	210	8	18	13	2
Tofu Tenders Mediterranean Tahini	½ pkg (5 oz)	240	13	16	9	3
White Wave						
Baked Garlic Herb Italian	1 piece (2 oz)	90	5	2	0	1
Baked Zesty Lemon Pepper	1 piece (2 oz)	90	5	3	1	1
Organic Extra Firm	⅕ block (3.2 oz)	110	6	3	0	1

FOOD	PORTION	CAL	FAT	CARB	SUGAR	FIBER
Organic Soft	⅕ block (3.2 oz)	110	6	3	0	1
TAKE-OUT						
breaded deep fried w/ soy sauce japanese style	1 piece (0.4 oz)	15	1	1	0	tr
soy sauce marinated & grilled	1 serv (4 oz)	181	11	6	–	1
stir-fried w/ vegetables	1 cup (7.6 oz)	186	10	21	–	3
TOMATILLO						
fresh	1 (1.2 oz)	11	tr	2	1	1
fresh chopped	½ cup (2.3 oz)	21	1	4	3	1
TOMATO						
CANNED						
green pickled	½ cup (2.5 oz)	26	tr	6	5	1
green whole pickled	1 (2.6 oz)	27	tr	6	5	1
paste	¼ cup (2.3 oz)	54	tr	12	8	3
paste	1 can (6 oz)	139	1	32	21	7
paste no salt added	1 can (6 oz)	139	1	32	21	7
puree	1 cup (8.8 oz)	95	1	22	12	5
puree	1 can (28 oz)	312	2	74	40	16
puree w/o salt	1 can (28 oz)	312	2	74	40	16
sauce	1 cup (8.6 oz)	59	tr	13	10	4
stewed	1 cup (8.9 oz)	66	tr	16	9	3
Bella Sun Luci						
Bruschetta w/ Italian Basil	¼ cup (1.9 oz)	190	17	6	4	2
Sun Dried Halves w/ Italian Herbs	1 tbsp (0.7 oz)	70	5	6	3	1
Sun Dried Julienne Cut w/ Italian Herbs	1 tbsp (0.7 oz)	70	5	6	3	1

FOOD	PORTION	CAL	FAT	CARB	SUGAR	FIBER
Del Monte						
Diced Organic	½ cup (4.4 oz)	20	0	3	2	1
Diced w/ Mushrooms & Garlic	½ cup (4.4 oz)	45	0	10	6	1
Diced Zesty Chili	½ cup (4.5 oz)	30	0	18	6	2
Organic Diced w/ Basil Garlic & Oregano	½ cup (4.4 oz)	45	0	10	5	1
Peeled Diced	½ cup (4.2 oz)	25	0	4	3	1
Peeled Diced No Salt Added	½ cup (4.4 oz)	25	0	6	4	2
Petite Cut Garlic & Olive Oil	½ cup (4.4 oz)	40	1	9	6	1
Petite Diced No Salt Added	½ cup (4.4 oz)	25	0	6	4	2
Wedges	½ cup (4.4 oz)	35	0	7	4	1
Hunt's						
Crushed	½ cup (4.2 oz)	45	0	9	4	3
Diced	½ cup (4.2 oz)	30	0	6	3	2
Diced Fire Roasted	½ cup (4.3 oz)	30	0	6	3	2
Diced In Sauce	½ cup (4.3 oz)	35	0	7	3	2
Diced No Salt Added	½ cup (4.2 oz)	30	0	6	3	2
Diced Petite	½ cup (4.2 oz)	30	0	6	2	2
Diced w/ Roasted Garlic	½ cup (4.2 oz)	35	0	8	4	2
Stewed	½ cup (4.2 oz)	45	0	10	6	2
Stewed No Salt Added	½ cup (4.2 oz)	40	0	8	5	2
Whole	½ cup (4.2 oz)	25	0	5	3	2
Whole No Salt Added	½ cup (4.2 oz)	30	0	6	3	2
Redpack						
Crushed w/ Basil Garlic & Oregano	¼ cup (2.1 oz)	20	0	4	1	1
Rienzi						
Italian Cherry Tomatoes No Salt Added	⅓ can (4.5 oz)	30	0	6	4	1

FOOD	PORTION	CAL	FAT	CARB	SUGAR	FIBER
DRIED						
sun dried	1 piece (2 g)	5	tr	1	1	tr
sun dried	¼ cup (0.5 oz)	35	tr	8	5	2
sun dried in oil drained	¼ cup (1 oz)	59	4	6	–	2
sun dried in oil drained	1 piece (3 g)	6	tr	1	–	tr
tomato powder	1 oz	85	tr	21	12	5
Bella Sun Luci						
Sun Dried w/ Italian Basil	⅐ pkg (0.5 oz)	35	0	6	4	1
Sun Dried w/ Zesty Peppers	⅐ pkg (0.5 oz)	35	0	6	4	1
FRESH						
bruschetta	¼ cup	50	3	6	4	tr
cherry	1 (0.6 oz)	3	tr	1	tr	tr
cherry	½ cup (2.6 oz)	13	tr	3	2	1
grape tomatoes	20	30	0	6	4	1
green	1 sm (3.2 oz)	21	tr	5	4	1
green	1 med (4.3 oz)	28	tr	6	5	1
green	1 lg (6.4 oz)	42	tr	9	7	2
green chopped	1 cup (6.3 oz)	41	tr	9	7	2
orange	1 (4 oz)	18	tr	4	–	1
orange chopped	1 cup (5.5 oz)	25	tr	5	–	1
plum	1 (2.2 oz)	11	tr	2	2	1
red	1 sm (3.2 oz)	16	tr	4	2	1
red	1 med (4.3 oz)	22	tr	5	3	2
red	1 lg (6.4 oz)	33	tr	7	5	2
red chopped	½ cup (3.2 oz)	16	tr	4	2	1
red slice	1 lg (0.9 oz)	5	tr	1	1	tr
roma	1 (2.2 oz)	11	tr	2	2	1
yellow	1 (7.4 oz)	32	1	6	–	2
yellow chopped	½ cup (2.4 oz)	10	tr	2	–	1
Ready Pac						
Bruschetta	2 tbsp (1.6 oz)	70	7	3	1	1

FOOD	PORTION	CAL	FAT	CARB	SUGAR	FIBER
TAKE-OUT						
aspic	½ cup (4 oz)	32	tr	6	5	tr
broiled slices	2 (2.9 oz)	18	tr	4	3	1
broiled whole	1 med (3.7 oz)	23	tr	5	3	2
bruschetta on toasted Italian bread	1 slice	106	3	18	2	tr
fried slices	2 (2.5 oz)	122	9	8	2	1
scalloped	½ cup (4 oz)	99	5	12	5	1
stewed	½ cup (1.8 oz)	40	1	7	–	1
stuffed w/ rice	1 (5.2 oz)	110	3	20	3	2
stuffed w/ rice & meat	1 (5.2 oz)	142	6	15	3	2
TOMATO JUICE						
tomato juice	1 cup (8.5 oz)	41	tr	10	9	1
tomato juice w/o added salt	1 cup (8.5 oz)	41	tr	10	9	1
TONGUE						
beef simmered	3 oz	241	19	0	0	0
lamb braised	3 oz	234	17	0	0	0
pork braised	3 oz	230	16	0	0	0
veal braised	3 oz	172	9	0	0	0
TORTILLA						
corn	1 (6 in diam)	56	1	12	–	1
corn w/o salt	1 (6 in diam)	56	1	12	–	1
flour w/o salt	1 (8 in diam)	114	3	20	–	1
Garden Of Eatin'						
Organic Whole Wheat	1 (1.6 oz)	110	1	22	0	3
Shells Blue Corn	2 (0.9 oz)	140	7	17	0	1
La Tortilla Factory						
Corn Chipotle	1 (1.4 oz)	90	1	14	0	1
Smart & Delicious 100 Calorie 100% Whole Wheat	1 (2 oz)	100	2	24	3	8

FOOD	PORTION	CAL	FAT	CARB	SUGAR	FIBER
Smart & Delicious 100 Calorie Traditional	1 (2 oz)	100	2	24	0	8
Smart & Delicious Low Carb Whole Wheat	1 (2.2 oz)	80	3	18	1	12
White Corn	1 (1.4 oz)	90	1	14	0	1

TORTILLA CHIPS (*see* CHIPS)

TRAIL MIX

FOOD	PORTION	CAL	FAT	CARB	SUGAR	FIBER
Bear Naked						
Peak Chocolate Cherry	½ cup (1.1 oz)	120	5	21	11	2
Peak Pecan Apple Flax	½ cup (1.1 oz)	140	8	16	6	2
Craisins						
Cranberry & Chocolate	1 pkg (1.75 oz)	230	28	26	18	–
Fruit & Nuts	1 pkg (1.4 oz)	230	10	31	18	–
Emerald						
Breakfast On The Go Berry Nut Blend	1 pkg (1.5 oz)	180	9	24	16	3
Breakfast On The Go Breakfast Nut Blend	1 pkg (1.5 oz)	180	7	27	20	3
Breakfast On The Go Smores Nut Blend	1 pkg (1.5 oz)	200	10	24	14	2
Frito Lay						
Nut & Fruit	1 oz	150	9	12	7	2
Original	3 tbsp	160	9	14	11	2
Planters						
Daybreak Blend Berry & Almond	⅕ pkg (1.5 oz)	180	7	27	19	3
Energy Go-Paks	1 (1.5 oz)	250	20	14	6	3
Fruit & Nut	⅙ pkg (1 oz)	140	9	14	10	2
Nut & Chocolate	1 oz	150	9	14	12	2

FOOD	PORTION	CAL	FAT	CARB	SUGAR	FIBER
Sweet & Nutty	⅕ pkg (1.1 oz)	160	10	15	11	2
SunRidge Farms						
Mountain Rainbow Mix	¼ cup (1 oz)	150	9	16	12	2
TREE FERN						
chopped cooked	½ cup	28	tr	8	–	–
TRIPE						
beef simmered	3 oz	80	3	2	0	0
TAKE-OUT						
mondongo w/ potatoes	1 cup	300	11	26	5	6
TRITICALE						
dry	½ cup (3.4 oz)	323	2	69	–	–
TROUT						
baked	3 oz	162	7	0	0	0
rainbow cooked	3 oz	129	4	0	0	0
seatrout baked	3 oz	113	4	0	0	0
TRUFFLES						
fresh	0.5 oz	4	tr	9	–	2
Aux Delices Des Bois						
Black Truffle Butter	0.5 oz	90	10	0	0	0
TUNA						
CANNED						
light in oil	1 can (6 oz)	399	14	0	0	0
light in oil	3 oz	169	7	0	0	0
light in water	1 can (5.8 oz)	192	1	0	0	0
light in water	3 oz	99	1	0	0	0
white in oil	3 oz	158	7	0	0	0
white in oil	1 can (6.2 oz)	331	14	0	0	0
white in water	3 oz	116	2	0	0	0
white in water	1 can (6 oz)	234	4	0	0	0

FOOD	PORTION	CAL	FAT	CARB	SUGAR	FIBER
Arroyabe						
Bonito In Olive Oil	2 oz	109	5	0	0	0
Chicken Of The Sea						
Albacore Chunk White In Water	½ can (2.5 oz)	50	1	0	0	0
Albacore Solid White In Oil	2 oz	90	4	0	0	0
Albacore Solid White In Water	2 oz	80	4	0	0	0
Chunk Light 50% Less Sodium	2 oz	180	1	0	0	0
Chunk Light In Oil	2 oz	100	6	0	0	0
Chunk Light In Water	2 oz	50	1	0	0	0
Chunk White In Water Very Low Sodium	2 oz	50	1	0	0	0
Genova						
Tonno In Olive Oil	2 oz	110	6	0	0	0
Progresso						
Light Olive Oil drained	¼ cup (2 oz)	120	6	0	0	0
Wild Planet						
Albacore Wild	2 oz	120	6	0	0	0
Albacore Wild Fillet	2 oz	120	6	0	0	0
Albacore Wild No Salt	2 oz	120	6	0	0	0
Albacore Wild Smoked Troll Caught	2 oz	90	5	0	0	0
Skipjack Wild Light	2 oz	69	2	0	0	0
FRESH						
bluefin cooked	3 oz	157	5	0	0	0
bluefin raw	3 oz	122	4	0	0	0
skipjack baked	3 oz	112	1	0	0	0
yellowfin baked	3 oz	118	1	0	0	0

FOOD	PORTION	CAL	FAT	CARB	SUGAR	FIBER
SHELF-STABLE						
Sea Fare Pacific						
Albacore Wild Caught Jalapeno	⅓ pkg (2 oz)	160	13	0	0	0
Albacore Wild Caught Salt Free	⅓ pkg (2 oz)	100	6	0	0	0
Albacore Wild Caught Sea Salt	⅓ pkg (2 oz)	100	6	0	0	0
Albacore Wild Caught Smoked	⅓ pkg (2 oz)	100	6	0	0	0
TAKE-OUT						
tuna salad	1 cup	383	19	19	–	–
TURBOT						
european baked	3 oz	104	3	0	0	0
TURKEY (*see also* JERKY, TURKEY DISHES, TURKEY SUBSTITUTES)						
CANNED						
w/ broth	1 cup	220	9	0	0	0
Hormel						
Chunk White & Dark	2 oz	70	3	0	0	0
Premium Chunk White	2 oz	60	2	0	0	0
Spam						
Oven Roasted	2 oz	80	5	1	0	0
FRESH						
breast roasted pre-basted w/ skin	3.5 oz	126	3	0	0	0
breast roasted w/ skin	4 oz	212	8	0	0	0
breast roasted w/o skin	4 oz	212	4	0	0	0
dark meat w/o skin roasted	1 cup (5 oz)	262	10	0	0	0
dark meat w/o skin roasted	3 oz	170	7	0	0	0
ground cooked	3 oz	193	11	0	0	0

FOOD	PORTION	CAL	FAT	CARB	SUGAR	FIBER
leg w/ skin roasted	1 (19 oz)	1136	54	0	0	0
light meat w/ skin roasted half turkey	2.3 lbs	2069	87	0	0	0
light meat w/o skin roasted	4 oz	183	4	0	0	0
neck simmered	1 (5.3 oz)	274	11	0	0	0
skin roasted	1 oz	141	13	0	0	0
skin roasted from half turkey	8.7 oz	1096	98	0	0	0
tail cooked	1 (2 oz)	197	16	0	0	0
w/ skin roasted	½ turkey (4 lbs)	3857	181	0	0	0
w/ skin roasted	1 serv (4.2 oz)	249	12	0	0	0
w/o skin roasted	1 cup (5 oz)	238	7	0	0	0
w/o skin roasted	1 serv (3.7 oz)	177	5	0	0	0
wing w/ skin roasted	1 (6.5 oz)	426	23	0	0	0
wing w/o skin roasted	1 (5.2 oz)	237	5	0	0	0
Empire						
Ground	4 oz	220	16	0	0	0
Foster Farms						
Breast Cutlets	4 oz	120	1	0	0	0
Necks	4 oz	150	6	0	0	0
Tails	4 oz	380	36	0	0	0
Perdue						
Whole Breast Bone-In Seasoned	4 oz	140	7	1	0	0
Shady Brook						
Breast Tenderloin Lemon Garlic	4 oz	130	4	4	1	0
Breast Tenderloin Rotisserie	4 oz	130	4	4	1	0

FOOD	PORTION	CAL	FAT	CARB	SUGAR	FIBER
FROZEN						
roast boneless seasoned light & dark meat roasted	3.5 oz	155	6	3	0	0
sticks breaded fried	1 (2.2 oz)	179	11	11	–	–
Organic Prairie						
Whole Young	4 oz	90	10	0	0	0
READY-TO-EAT						
bologna	1 slice (1 oz)	59	4	1	1	tr
breast	1 slice (0.7 oz)	22	tr	1	1	tr
ham	1 slice (1 oz)	35	1	1	tr	tr
pastrami	2 oz	70	2	2	2	tr
salami	1 slice (1 oz)	48	3	tr	tr	0
Foster Farms						
Breast Honey Roasted	1 slice (1 oz)	25	0	1	1	0
Breast Oven Roasted	1 slice (1 oz)	30	0	0	0	0

TURKEY DISHES

FOOD	PORTION	CAL	FAT	CARB	SUGAR	FIBER
CANNED						
Dinty Moore						
Turkey Stew	½ can	140	3	19	3	2
FROZEN						
gravy & turkey	1 cup (8.4 oz)	160	6	11	–	–
TAKE-OUT						
boneless breast w/ cranberry apple stuffing	1 serv (5 oz)	260	9	10	2	1
turkey a la king	1 cup (8.5 oz)	465	34	16	4	1
turkey creole w/o rice	1 cup	189	4	9	5	2
turkey croquette	1 (2 oz)	158	9	8	2	tr
turkey divan	1 cup	321	14	9	2	3
turkey fricassee	1 cup	322	18	8	tr	tr

FOOD	PORTION	CAL	FAT	CARB	SUGAR	FIBER
turkey meatloaf	1 lg slice (5 oz)	243	9	11	3	1
turkey salad	1 cup	417	32	3	1	1
turkey tetrazzini	1 cup	369	18	29	2	2
TURKEY SUBSTITUTES						
Quorn						
Turk'y Burger	1 (2.5 oz)	90	4	6	0	2
TURMERIC						
ground	1 tsp	8	tr	1	tr	tr
TURNIPS						
canned greens	½ cup	17	tr	3	–	–
cooked mashed	½ cup (4.2 oz)	47	tr	10	–	–
cubed cooked	½ cup (3 oz)	33	tr	7	–	–
fresh greens chopped cooked	½ cup	15	tr	3	–	2
frzn greens cooked	½ cup	24	tr	4	–	2
greens raw chopped	½ cup	7	tr	2	–	1
raw cubed	½ cup (2.4 oz)	25	tr	6	–	–
TURTLE						
raw	3.5 oz	85	1	0	0	0
TUSK FISH						
raw	3.5 oz	79	tr	0	0	0
VANILLA						
vanilla extract	1 tbsp (0.5 oz)	37	tr	2	2	0
vanilla extract	1 tsp (4.2 g)	12	0	1	1	0
vanilla extract alcohol free	1 tsp (4.2 g)	2	0	1	1	0
Nielsen-Massey						
Madagascar Bourbon Extract	1 tsp	11	tr	tr	tr	tr

FOOD	PORTION	CAL	FAT	CARB	SUGAR	FIBER
VEAL (*see also* VEAL DISHES)						
breast braised	3 oz	226	14	0	0	0
chop breaded fried	1 med (6.5 oz)	290	12	13	0	tr
chop cooked	1 med (6.5 oz)	230	13	0	0	0
cubed braised	3 oz	160	4	0	0	0
cutlet cooked	3 oz	141	4	0	0	0
ground broiled	3 oz	146	6	0	0	0
leg roasted	3 oz	136	4	0	0	0
loin roasted	3 oz	184	10	0	0	0
patty breaded fried	1 (2.8 oz)	211	13	7	1	tr
shank braised	3 oz	162	5	0	0	0
VEAL DISHES						
TAKE-OUT						
cordon bleu	1 serv (8 oz)	490	35	4	2	1
marengo	1 serv (8.8 oz)	274	9	7	3	1
marsala	1 slice + sauce (3.4 oz)	268	19	6	2	tr
paprikash	1 serv (8.6 oz)	280	12	5	1	1
parmigiana	1 serv (6.4 oz)	362	21	15	3	2
picatta	1 piece + sauce (3.5 oz)	154	9	2	tr	tr
scallopini	1 slice + sauce (3.4 oz)	238	17	2	1	tr
stew	1 serv (8.8 oz)	192	6	18	4	3

FOOD	PORTION	CAL	FAT	CARB	SUGAR	FIBER
VEGETABLE JUICE (*see also* INDIVIDUAL VEGETABLE NAMES, FRUIT DRINKS)						
low sodium tomato & vegetable juice	1 cup	53	tr	11	9	2
vegetable juice cocktail	8 oz	46	tr	11	8	2
V8						
100% Juice Low Sodium	8 oz	50	0	10	7	2
Low Sodium Spicy Hot	8 oz	50	0	11	8	2
Original Hint Of Black Pepper	8 oz	50	0	10	7	2
Vegetable Juice Original	8 oz	50	0	10	8	2
VEGETABLES MIXED						
CANNED						
mixed vegetables	½ cup	39	tr	8	–	–
peas & carrots	½ cup (4.5 oz)	48	tr	11	–	3
peas & onions	½ cup (2.1 oz)	31	tr	5	–	1
succotash	½ cup	102	1	23	–	–
Butter Kernel						
Mixed	½ cup (4.4 oz)	45	0	10	3	2
Del Monte						
Mixed Vegetables w/ Potatoes	½ cup (4.3 oz)	45	0	10	3	2
Peas And Carrots	½ cup (4.5 oz)	60	0	13	4	4
Victoria						
Fancy Giardiniera	¼ cup (1 oz)	5	0	1	0	0
Italian Antipasto	¼ jar (2 oz)	130	12	3	0	1
DRIED						
Crunchies						
Freeze Dried Power Veggies Buttered	½ cup (0.7 oz)	110	3	17	6	4
Freeze Dried Power Veggies Herb Spiced	½ cup (0.7 oz)	110	3	17	6	5
Freeze Dried Roasted Veggies	⅝ cup (1 oz)	100	1	21	10	2

FOOD	PORTION	CAL	FAT	CARB	SUGAR	FIBER
Freeze Dried Roasted Veggies BBQ	½ cup (0.8 oz)	100	2	20	7	4
FRESH						
Dole						
Stir Fry Medley	1 cup (3 oz)	30	0	7	3	2
Vegetable Medley	3 oz	30	0	6	2	2
Eat Smart						
Broccoli & Carrots	1 serv (3 oz)	30	0	6	2	2
Harvest Blend	1 serv (3 oz)	30	0	6	1	2
Vegetable Medley	1 serv (3 oz)	25	0	5	3	2
Mann's						
Broccoli & Carrots	1 serv (3 oz)	25	0	5	3	2
Broccoli & Cauliflower	1 serv (3 oz)	25	0	4	2	2
California Stir Fry	1 serv (3 oz)	30	0	6	3	2
Low Mein Stir Fry	1 serv (3 oz)	80	1	14	5	2
Medley	1 serv (3 oz)	25	0	5	3	2
Ready Pac						
Carrots & Celery w/ Ranch Dressing	1 pkg (7 oz)	250	21	14	8	3
Ready Fixin's Chop Suey	1½ cups (3 oz)	15	0	2	1	1
FROZEN						
mixed vegetables cooked	½ cup	54	tr	12	–	2
peas & carrots cooked	½ cup (2.8 oz)	38	tr	8	3	3
peas & carrots creamed	½ cup (4.3 oz)	111	6	12	5	2
succotash cooked	½ cup	79	1	17	–	–
Green Giant						
Steamers Basil Vegetable Medley as prep	¾ cup	45	1	10	5	2
Lisa's Organics						
California In Balsamic Glaze	½ pkg (4 oz)	35	0	8	4	2

FOOD	PORTION	CAL	FAT	CARB	SUGAR	FIBER
Southwest In Ranchero Sauce	½ pkg (4 oz)	60	1	14	4	2
TAKE-OUT						
buddha's delight	1 serv (16 oz)	174	5	17	8	3
fukujinzuke japanese pickled vegetables	1 tbsp (6 g)	8	0	2	–	0
pakoras	4 (1.7 oz)	57	2	7	1	2
ratatouille	1 serv (3.5 oz)	96	7	7	7	4
samosa	1 (2.4 oz)	206	11	22	1	2
stir fry mixed vegetables	1 serv (4 oz)	66	5	3	2	2
succotash	½ cup	111	1	23	–	–

VENISON (*see also* JERKY)

FOOD	PORTION	CAL	FAT	CARB	SUGAR	FIBER
cubed stewed	1 cup (5 oz)	266	6	0	0	0
hamburger grilled	1 (3.3 oz)	174	8	0	0	0
loin steak lean only broiled	1 (2 oz)	81	1	0	0	0
shoulder lean only braised	3 oz	162	3	0	0	0
tenderloin roasted	3 oz	127	2	0	0	0
top round lean only broiled	3 oz	129	2	0	0	0
TAKE-OUT						
meatloaf	1 lg slice (5 oz)	238	10	9	2	1
stew w/ potatoes & vegetables	1 cup (8.8 oz)	179	2	22	5	4

VINEGAR

FOOD	PORTION	CAL	FAT	CARB	SUGAR	FIBER
balsamic	1 tbsp	14	0	3	2	–
cider	1 tbsp	3	0	tr	tr	0
coconut	1 tbsp (0.5 oz)	1	tr	tr	–	–
red wine	1 tbsp	3	0	tr	0	0
white	1 tbsp	3	0	tr	tr	0

FOOD	PORTION	CAL	FAT	CARB	SUGAR	FIBER
Gedney						
Apple Cider	1 tbsp (0.5 oz)	3	0	0	0	0
Distilled White	1 tbsp (0.5 oz)	3	0	0	0	0
Heinz						
Apple Cider	1 tbsp (0.5 oz)	0	0	0	0	0
Malt	1 tbsp (0.5 oz)	0	0	0	0	0
Red Wine	1 tbsp (1 oz)	0	0	0	0	0
Tarragon	1 tbsp (0.5 oz)	0	0	0	0	0
White	1 tbsp (0.5 oz)	0	0	0	0	0
Spectrum						
Apple Cider Organic	1 tbsp (0.5 oz)	7	0	2	0	0
Brown Rice Organic	1 tbsp (0.5 oz)	10	0	0	0	0
Golden Balsamic Organic	1 tbsp (0.5 oz)	6	0	2	2	0
Red Wine Organic	1 tbsp (0.5 oz)	0	0	0	0	0
Victoria						
Balsamic	1 tbsp (0.5 oz)	5	0	2	0	0

WAFFLES

FROZEN

FOOD	PORTION	CAL	FAT	CARB	SUGAR	FIBER
Aunt Jemima						
Blueberry	2 (2.5 oz)	170	5	27	5	tr
Buttermilk	2 (2.5 oz)	190	5	29	3	tr
Homestyle	2 (2.5 oz)	160	5	25	2	tr
Low Fat	2 (2.5 oz)	160	3	27	2	tr
Eggo						
Blueberry	2 (2.5 oz)	190	6	29	6	tr
Cinnamon Toast	3 sets (3.3 oz)	300	11	46	17	1
FiberPlus Calcium Buttermilk	2 (2.5 oz)	160	6	29	3	9
Homestyle Low Fat	2 (2.5 oz)	160	3	31	4	tr
Nutri-Grain Honey Oat	2 (2.5 oz)	190	6	31	7	3

FOOD	PORTION	CAL	FAT	CARB	SUGAR	FIBER
Nutri-Grain Whole Wheat	2 (2.5 oz)	170	6	26	3	3
Original	2 (2.5 oz)	210	8	30	4	tr
Thick & Fluffy Original	1 (2 oz)	160	7	21	3	tr
Frozen Guru						
Flour-Free Coconut Chia	2 (2.3 oz)	125	4	14	2	6
Flour-Free Sweet Banana	2 (2.3 oz)	115	3	15	4	5
Nature's Path						
Buckwheat Wild Blueberry Organic	2 (2.5 oz)	190	7	33	5	1
Hemp Plus Organic	2 (2.5 oz)	200	8	30	5	5
Maple Cinn Organic	2 (2.5 oz)	180	6	28	6	4
Pomegran Plus Organic	2 (2.5 oz)	160	4	27	5	4
Smucker's						
Snack'n Waffles Blueberry	1 (2 oz)	230	8	33	16	2
Snack'n Waffles Maple	1 (2 oz)	220	8	32	15	2
Van's						
Belgian	2 (2.7 oz)	210	9	29	5	1
Lite	2 (2.7 oz)	140	2	33	4	2
Minis	8 (1.9 oz)	140	4	25	4	tr
Organic w/ Vitamin Boost	2 (2.7 oz)	200	8	27	3	6
Wheat Gluten Free	2 (3 oz)	230	7	37	4	2
Whole Grain	2 (2.8 oz)	190	7	23	5	6
MIX						
plain as prep 7 in diam	1 (2.6 oz)	218	11	25	–	–
READY-TO-EAT						
Mrs. Huber						
Fresh Egg Waffles	1 (1 oz)	100	5	11	7	0
Unique Belgique						
Imported From Belgium	2 (2.3 oz)	230	12	27	15	1

FOOD	PORTION	CAL	FAT	CARB	SUGAR	FIBER
TAKE-OUT						
belgian	1 (4.7 oz)	412	13	65	6	3
blueberry 9 in sq	1 (7 oz)	556	16	90	12	5
round 10 in diam	1 (6.8 oz)	598	18	94	9	5
square 9 in	1 (7 oz)	620	19	98	9	5
whole wheat 9 in sq	1 (7 oz)	534	22	67	15	5
WALNUTS						
black chopped	¼ cup	193	18	3	tr	2
english chopped	¼ cup	191	19	4	1	2
english ground	¼ cup	131	13	3	1	1
english halves	14 (1 oz)	185	18	4	1	2
english in shell	7 (1 oz)	183	18	4	1	2
honey roasted	¼ cup	172	16	7	4	2
Planters						
Halves	1 oz	190	18	4	1	2
NUT-rition Omega-3 Mix	¼ cup (1.1 oz)	160	10	15	12	2
Recipe Ready Pieces	½ pkg (1 oz)	210	19	4	1	2
Sante						
Candied	¼ cup (1 oz)	200	17	10	8	2
WASABI (*see* HORSERADISH)						
WATER						
ice cubes	3	0	0	0	0	0
tap water	8 oz	0	0	0	0	0
Aquafina						
Pure Water	8 oz	0	0	0	0	0
Arizona						
Rescue Relax	8 oz	25	0	7	6	–
Vapor	8 oz	0	0	0	0	0
EX						
Aqua Vitamins Raspberry	1 bottle (16.9 oz)	110	0	27	27	–

FOOD	PORTION	CAL	FAT	CARB	SUGAR	FIBER
Mash						
Water Drink Grapefruit Citrus Zing	8 oz	40	0	10	10	–
Water Drink Ripe Mango Blood Orange	8 oz	40	0	10	10	–
Pellegrino						
Mineral Water	8 oz	0	0	0	0	0
Propel						
Fitness Water All Flavors	1 bottle (24 oz)	30	0	6	6	–
R.W. Knudsen						
Organic Sparkling Essence Lemon	1 can (10.5 oz)	0	0	0	0	0
Snapple						
Antioxidant Water Awaken Dragonfruit	8 oz	50	0	12	12	–
Antioxidant Water Restore Agave Melon	8 oz	60	0	13	13	–
Lyte Water	8 oz	0	0	0	0	–
SoBe						
Lifewater Blood Orange Mango	1 bottle (20 oz)	0	0	7	0	–
Lifewater w/ Coconut Water	1 bottle (20 oz)	80	0	21	20	5
SoNu						
Organic 10 Calories All Flavors	8 oz	10	0	4	3	0
Organic All Flavors	8 oz	45	0	13	13	0
Sparkling Ice						
All Flavors	1 bottle (16 oz)	0	0	0	0	0
Victoria's Kitchen						
Almond Water	8 oz	55	0	15	15	0

FOOD	PORTION	CAL	FAT	CARB	SUGAR	FIBER
WATER CHESTNUTS						
chinese sliced	½ cup	35	tr	9	–	–
canned fresh sliced	½ cup	66	tr	15	–	–
WATERCRESS						
cooked w/o fat	1 cup	15	tr	2	tr	1
raw chopped	1 cup	4	tr	tr	tr	tr
WATERMELON						
cut up	1 cup	46	tr	12	10	1
seeds dried	¼ cup	150	13	4	–	–
wedge	1 sm (2.5 oz)	21	tr	5	4	tr
wedge	1 med (10 oz)	86	tr	22	18	1
wedge	1 lg (20 oz)	172	1	43	35	2
whole melon	1 (9 lb)	1227	6	309	254	16
Jake & Amos						
Pickled Sweet Rind	2 tbsp (1 oz)	70	0	17	12	0
WATERMELON JUICE						
juice	8 oz	71	tr	18	15	1
Arizona						
Fruit Juice Cocktail	8 oz	100	0	25	24	0
Izze						
Esque Sparkling Watermelon	1 bottle (12 oz)	50	0	14	14	–
Minute Maid						
Flavored Drink	8 oz	100	0	27	26	–
WHALE						
beluga dried	1 oz	93	2	0	0	0
beluga raw	3.5 oz	111	1	0	0	0
WHEAT						
sprouted	1 cup (3.8 oz)	214	1	46	–	1
starch	3.5 oz	348	tr	86	–	–

FOOD	PORTION	CAL	FAT	CARB	SUGAR	FIBER
WHEAT GERM						
plain	¼ cup	108	3	14	2	4
Mother's						
Wheat Germ	2 tbsp (0.5 oz)	50	1	6	1	2
WHEY						
acid dry	1 tbsp	10	tr	2	2	0
sweet dry	1 tbsp	26	tr	6	6	0
sweet fluid	½ cup	33	tr	6	6	0
whey cheese	1 oz	126	8	9	0	0
Action Whey						
Dream Shake All Flavors	1 scoop (0.8 oz)	90	3	3	2	1
Premier						
100% Whey Isolate	2 scoops (1.5 oz)	160	2	8	1	2
WHIPPED TOPPINGS						
dairy fat free pressurized	¼ cup (0.6 oz)	24	1	4	3	tr
nondairy fat free frzn	¼ cup (0.7 oz)	28	1	5	3	tr
nondairy frzn	¼ cup (0.7 oz)	60	5	4	4	0
nondairy lowfat frzn	¼ cup (0.7 oz)	42	2	4	4	0
nondairy pressurized	¼ cup (0.6 oz)	46	4	3	3	0
Reddiwip						
Chocolate	2 tbsp (5 g)	15	1	1	tr	0
Fat Free	2 tbsp (5 g)	5	0	1	tr	0
Soyatoo						
Rice Whip	2 tbsp (6 g)	10	1	1	1	0
Soy Whip	2 tbsp (6 g)	10	1	1	1	0
Truwhip						
Whipped Topping	2 tbsp (0.4 oz)	30	2	3	2	0
WHITE BEANS						
canned	1 cup (9.2 oz)	299	1	56	1	13

FOOD	PORTION	CAL	FAT	CARB	SUGAR	FIBER
dried small cooked w/o salt	1 cup (6.3 oz)	254	1	46	–	19
Bush's						
White Beans	½ cup (4.6 oz)	80	0	17	0	7
WHITEFISH						
baked	3 oz	146	6	0	0	0
fillet grilled no added fat	1 (5.4 oz)	265	12	0	0	0
smoked boneless	1 oz	31	tr	0	0	0
WHITING						
broiled w/o fat	3 oz	99	1	0	0	0
fillet broiled w/o fat	1 (2.5 oz)	84	1	0	0	0
fillet steamed w/o fat	1 (2.6 oz)	84	1	0	0	0
hake raw	3.5 oz	84	1	0	0	0
TAKE-OUT						
fillet battered & fried	1 (3.1 oz)	157	7	6	tr	tr
fillet breaded & fried	1 (3.1 oz)	191	10	7	1	tr
WILD RICE						
cooked	1 cup (5.8 oz)	166	1	35	1	3
Gourmet House						
Cracked as prep	1 cup	170	0	35	0	2
Quick Cooking not prep	½ cup	170	0	25	0	2
Thai Jasmine as prep	¾ cup	160	0	36	0	0
WINE						
chianti	1 serv (5 oz)	125	0	4	1	0
chinese cooking	1 bottle (15 oz)	559	0	3	0	0
cooking	¼ cup (2 oz)	29	0	4	1	0
haiku	1 serv	93	0	3	–	0
japanese plum	3 oz	139	tr	16	–	0
japanese sake	2 oz	78	0	3	0	0
kir	1 serv	78	0	3	–	0

FOOD	PORTION	CAL	FAT	CARB	SUGAR	FIBER
madeira	3.5 oz	169	0	10	10	0
nonalcoholic	1 serv (5 oz)	9	0	2	2	0
port	1 serv (3.5 oz)	165	0	14	8	0
red barbera	1 serv (5 oz)	125	0	4	–	–
red burgundy	1 serv (5 oz)	127	0	5	–	–
red cabernet franc	1 serv (5 oz)	122	0	4	–	–
red claret	1 serv (5 oz)	122	0	4	–	–
red gamay	1 serv (5 oz)	115	0	4	–	–
red lemberger	1 serv (5 oz)	118	0	4	–	–
red mourvedre	1 serv (5 oz)	129	0	4	–	–
red pinot noir	1 serv (5 oz)	121	0	3	–	–
red sangiovese	1 serv (5 oz)	126	0	4	–	–
red sauvignon cabernet	1 serv (5 oz)	122	0	4	–	–
red syrah	1 serv (5 oz)	122	0	4	–	–
red zinfandel	1 serv (5 oz)	129	0	4	–	–
sake screwdriver	1 serv	175	tr	23	–	tr
sangria	1 serv	88	tr	6	–	tr
sangria blanco	1 serv	155	tr	24	–	3
sherry	2 oz	84	0	5	–	–
vermouth dry	3.5 oz	105	0	1	–	–
vermouth sweet	3.5 oz	167	0	12	–	–
wassail wine	1 serv	142	tr	22	–	2
white	1 serv (5 oz)	121	0	4	1	0
white chardonnay	1 serv (5 oz)	123	0	3	1	0
white chenin blanc	1 serv (5 oz)	118	0	5	–	–
white fume blanc	1 serv (5 oz)	121	0	3	–	–
white gewurztaminer	1 serv (5 oz)	119	0	4	–	–
white muller thurgau	1 serv (5 oz)	112	0	5	–	–
white muscat	1 serv (5 oz)	123	0	8	–	–
white pinot blanc	1 serv (5 oz)	119	0	3	–	–
white pinot grigio	1 serv (5 oz)	122	0	3	–	–
white riesling	1 serv (5 oz)	128	0	6	–	–

FOOD	PORTION	CAL	FAT	CARB	SUGAR	FIBER
white riesling	1 serv (5 oz)	118	0	6	–	–
white sauvignon blanc	1 serv (5 oz)	119	0	3	–	–
white semillon	1 serv (5 oz)	121	0	5	–	–
wine cooler	1 (7 oz)	116	tr	14	11	0
wine spritzer	1 serv (7 oz)	73	0	2	1	0
Kedem						
Cooking Red	2 tbsp (1 oz)	30	0	1	–	–
Cooking Sherry	2 tbsp (1 oz)	40	0	1	1	–
Cooking Wine Marsala	2 tbsp (1 oz)	40	0	1	1	–
WINGED BEANS						
dried cooked w/o salt	1 cup	253	10	26	–	3
WRAPS (*see* BREAD, SANDWICHES)						
YAM (*see also* SWEET POTATO)						
FRESH						
mountain yam hawaii cooked w/o salt	1 cup	119	tr	29	–	–
yam cooked w/o salt	1 cup	158	tr	38	1	5
YARDLONG BEANS						
sliced cooked w/o salt	1 cup	49	tr	10	–	–
YAUTIA (*see* MALANGA)						
YEAST						
baker's compressed	1 cake (0.6 oz)	18	tr	3	0	1
baker's dry	1 tbsp	35	1	5	0	3
baker's dry	1 pkg (7 g)	21	tr	3	0	2
brewer's dry	1 tbsp	35	1	5	0	3
YELLOW BEANS						
fresh cooked w/o salt	1 cup	44	tr	10	2	4
fresh raw	1 cup	34	tr	8	–	4
Del Monte						
Cut Golden Wax Beans	½ cup (4.2 oz)	20	0	5	1	2

FOOD	PORTION	CAL	FAT	CARB	SUGAR	FIBER
YELLOWTAIL						
baked	4 oz	199	7	0	0	0
YOGURT (*see also* YOGURT DRINKS, YOGURT FROZEN)						
plain lowfat	8 oz	143	4	16	16	0
plain nonfat	8 oz	127	tr	17	17	0
plain whole milk	8 oz	138	7	11	11	0
tofu yogurt	1 cup	246	5	42	3	1
Activia						
Breakfast Blends Apple Cinnamon	1 pkg (6 oz)	190	3	30	25	–
Breakfast Blends Banana Bread	1 pkg (6 oz)	190	3	30	26	–
Breakfast Blends Maple Brown Sugar	1 pkg (6 oz)	190	3	30	26	–
Breakfast Blends Vanilla	1 pkg (6 oz)	190	3	30	26	–
Harvest Picks Strawberry	1 pkg (4 oz)	110	4	16	15	–
Strawberry	1 pkg (4 oz)	120	2	22	19	0
Strawberry Light	1 pkg (4 oz)	70	0	13	8	2
Alpina						
Restart All Fruit Flavors	1 pkg (6 oz)	180	3	27	19	1
Breyers						
Creme Savers All Flavors	1 pkg (6 oz)	160	2	31	26	0
Fruit On The Bottom Black Cherry	1 pkg (6 oz)	160	1	32	28	tr
Fruit On The Bottom Chocolate Raspberry	1 pkg (6 oz)	170	1	34	27	tr
Fruit On The Bottom Mixed Berry	1 pkg (6 oz)	160	1	31	26	tr
Fruit On The Bottom Peach Mango Orange	1 pkg (6 oz)	160	1	31	27	tr

FOOD	PORTION	CAL	FAT	CARB	SUGAR	FIBER
Fruit On The Bottom Pineapple	1 pkg (6 oz)	150	1	31	27	tr
Fruit On The Bottom Strawberry	1 pkg (6 oz)	150	1	31	26	tr
Inspirations Cherry Chocolate Chip	1 pkg (4 oz)	140	3	23	20	0
Inspirations Mint Chocolate Chip	1 pkg (4 oz)	140	4	23	19	0
Inspirations Vanilla Bean	1 pkg (4 oz)	110	1	21	17	0
Light Blueberry	1 pkg (4 oz)	50	0	8	5	tr
Smooth & Creamy Peaches 'N Cream	1 pkg (4 oz)	120	1	24	19	0
Smooth & Creamy Strawberry	1 pkg (4 oz)	110	1	23	18	0
Chobani						
0% Blueberry	1 pkg (6 oz)	140	0	20	20	tr
0% Honey	1 pkg (6 oz)	150	0	20	20	0
0% Peach	1 pkg (6 oz)	140	0	20	19	tr
0% Plain	1 pkg (6 oz)	100	0	7	7	0
0% Pomegranate	1 pkg (6 oz)	140	0	21	19	0
0% Raspberry	1 pkg (6 oz)	140	0	22	19	1
0% Strawberry	1 pkg (6 oz)	140	0	20	19	tr
0% Vanilla	1 pkg (6 oz)	120	0	13	13	0
2% Mango	1 pkg (6 oz)	160	3	21	20	0
2% Plain	1 pkg (6 oz)	130	4	7	7	0
Bite Fig w/ Orange Zest	1 pkg (3.5 oz)	100	2	13	12	tr
Champions Honey-nana	1 pkg (3.5 oz)	100	2	14	13	0
Champions VeryBerry	1 pkg (3.5 oz)	100	2	12	11	0
Champions Tube All Flavors	1 (2.25 oz)	70	1	9	8	0
Ehrmann						
Bavarian Lowfat Cherry	1 pkg	140	2	25	24	0
Bavarian Lowfat Peach	1 pkg	140	2	25	24	0

FOOD	PORTION	CAL	FAT	CARB	SUGAR	FIBER
Bavarian Lowfat Strawberry	1 pkg	140	2	25	24	0
Emmi						
Apricot Low-fat	1 pkg (6 oz)	170	3	27	25	0
Green Apple Low-fat	1 pkg (6 oz)	170	3	27	26	0
Pink Grapefruit Low-fat	1 pkg (6 oz)	170	3	27	26	0
Plain Low-fat	1 pkg (6 oz)	170	3	10	10	0
Fage						
Total Cherry	1 pkg (5.3 oz)	170	6	17	16	0
Total Peach	1 pkg (5.3 oz)	170	6	17	16	0
Total Plain	1 pkg (5.3 oz)	190	10	8	8	0
Total Strawberry	1 pkg (5.3 oz)	170	6	17	16	0
Total 0% Cherry	1 pkg (5.3 oz)	130	0	19	16	0
Total 0% Cherry Pomegranate	1 pkg (5.3 oz)	130	0	19	16	0
Total 0% Honey	1 pkg (5.3 oz)	120	0	17	16	0
Total 0% Mango Guanabana	1 pkg (5.3 oz)	120	0	18	17	0
Total 0% Peach	1 pkg (5.3 oz)	120	0	17	16	0
Total 0% Plain	1 pkg (5.3 oz)	100	0	7	7	0
Total 2% Cherry	1 pkg (5.3 oz)	140	3	17	16	0
Total 2% Plain	1 pkg (5.3 oz)	150	4	8	8	0
Total 2% Strawberry	1 pkg (5.3 oz)	140	3	17	16	0
Green Valley						
Organic Lactose Free Blueberry	1 pkg (6 oz)	140	2	23	16	0
Organic Lactose Free Honey	1 pkg (6 oz)	140	2	24	14	0
Organic Lactose Free Plain	1 pkg (6 oz)	100	3	11	4	0
Organic Lactose Free Vanilla	1 pkg (6 oz)	120	3	17	9	0

FOOD	PORTION	CAL	FAT	CARB	SUGAR	FIBER
Karoun						
Plain Lowfat	1 cup (8 oz)	180	5	16	15	0
Plain Whole Milk	1 cup (8 oz)	210	12	15	14	0
Liberte						
Plain Lowfat	1 pkg (6 oz)	110	4	10	7	0
Six Grains Peach	1 pkg (6 oz)	150	3	23	18	1
Six Grains Pear	1 pkg (6 oz)	160	3	23	18	1
Mountain High						
Black Cherry Classic Lowfat	1 pkg (6 oz)	140	2	24	23	0
Blueberry Classic Lowfat	1 pkg (6 oz)	140	2	24	23	0
Lemon Lowfat	1 pkg (8 oz)	190	2	34	33	0
Mountain Berry Classic Lowfat	1 pkg (6 oz)	150	2	26	25	0
Plain Fat Free	1 pkg (8 oz)	120	0	18	17	0
Plain Lowfat	1 pkg (8 oz)	140	3	18	16	0
Plain Original	1 pkg (8 oz)	180	8	17	15	0
Strawberry Classic Lowfat	1 pkg (6 oz)	140	2	24	23	0
Vanilla Fat Free	1 pkg (8 oz)	160	0	30	28	0
Vanilla Lowfat	1 pkg (8 oz)	180	3	29	28	0
Vanilla Original	1 pkg (8 oz)	210	7	28	27	0
Muller						
Corner Choco Balls	1 pkg (5.3 oz)	210	5	32	26	0
Corner Crispy Crunch	1 pkg (5.3 oz)	200	4	33	24	0
Corner Strawberry	1 pkg (5.3 oz)	140	2	25	23	0
FruitUp Luscious Lemon	1 pkg (5.3 oz)	150	2	28	24	0
FruitUp Peach Passion Fruit	1 pkg (5.3 oz)	140	2	26	23	0
FruitUp Radiant Raspberry	1 pkg (5.3 oz)	150	2	28	23	0

FOOD	PORTION	CAL	FAT	CARB	SUGAR	FIBER
Greek Corner Caramelized Almonds	1 pkg (5.3 oz)	220	9	21	18	1
Greek Corner Honeyed Apricots	1 pkg (5.3 oz)	130	2	20	17	0
Nancy's						
Lowfat Lemon	1 pkg (8 oz)	150	3	16	16	0
Lowfat Maple	1 pkg (8 oz)	180	3	26	26	0
Lowfat Peach	1 pkg (8 oz)	170	3	26	26	0
Lowfat Plain	1 pkg (8 oz)	150	3	16	16	0
Lowfat Vanilla	1 pkg (8 oz)	140	3	15	15	0
Organic Whole Milk Fruit On The Top Cherry	1 pkg (8 oz)	220	6	36	32	1
Organic Whole Milk Fruit On The Top Peach	1 pkg (8 oz)	220	5	38	38	tr
Organic Whole Milk Honey	1 pkg (8 oz)	170	8	17	17	0
Organic Soy Kiwi Lime	1 pkg (6 oz)	160	3	31	21	4
Organic Soy Plain	1 pkg (6 oz)	150	3	25	15	2
Organic Soy Vanilla	1 pkg (6 oz)	120	3	19	10	3
Oikos						
Caramel	1 pkg (4 oz)	110	0	17	16	0
Chocolate	1 pkg (4 oz)	110	0	17	16	tr
Strawberry	1 pkg (5.3 oz)	110	0	16	7	0
Super Fruits	1 pkg (5.3 oz)	130	0	18	16	0
Olympus						
Greek Strained Strawberry 1% Lowfat	1 pkg (6 oz)	155	2	23	22	tr
Silk						
Live! Blueberry	1 pkg (6 oz)	150	2	29	21	1
Stonyfield Farm						
0% Fat Chocolate Underground	1 pkg (6 oz)	150	0	30	29	1

FOOD	PORTION	CAL	FAT	CARB	SUGAR	FIBER
0% Fat Fruit On The Bottom Blueberry	1 pkg (6 oz)	120	0	22	20	0
0% Fat Fruit On The Bottom Pomegranate Raspberry	1 pkg (6 oz)	120	0	22	22	0
0% Fat Fruit On The Bottom Strawberry	1 pkg (6 oz)	110	0	22	21	0
0% Fat Smooth & Creamy Black Cherry	1 pkg (6 oz)	100	0	18	17	0
0% Fat Smooth & Creamy French Vanilla	1 pkg (6 oz)	100	0	17	17	0
0% Fat Smooth & Creamy Key Lime	1 pkg (6 oz)	100	0	17	16	0
0% Fat Smooth & Creamy Lemon	1 pkg (6 oz)	100	0	18	17	0
0% Fat Smooth & Creamy Peach	1 pkg (6 oz)	100	0	18	17	0
0% Fat Smooth & Creamy Plain	1 pkg (6 oz)	80	0	11	11	0
0% Fat Smooth & Creamy Pomegranate Berry	1 pkg (6 oz)	100	0	17	16	0
0% Fat Smooth & Creamy Strawberry	1 pkg (6 oz)	100	0	18	17	0
Whole Milk Cream Top White Chocolate Raspberry	1 pkg (6 oz)	170	6	23	23	0
Straus						
Organic Blueberry Pomegranate	1 cup (8 oz)	220	6	31	25	0
Organic Cinnamon Nonfat	1 cup (8 oz)	190	0	33	26	1

FOOD	PORTION	CAL	FAT	CARB	SUGAR	FIBER
Organic Maple Whole Milk	1 cup (8 oz)	210	6	28	23	0
Organic Plain Lowfat	1 cup (8 oz)	150	2	21	10	0
Organic Plain Nonfat	1 cup (8 oz)	120	0	17	10	1
Organic Vanilla Nonfat	1 cup (8 oz)	190	0	34	25	0
Voskos						
Greek Yogurt Plain Non Fat	1 pkg (8 oz)	140	0	9	8	0
Greek Yogurt Plain Original	1 pkg (8 oz)	280	20	15	10	0
Organic Vanilla Bean	1 pkg (5.3 oz)	130	0	20	17	0
Wallaby						
Lowfat Lemon	1 pkg (6 oz)	140	3	23	19	0
Lowfat Plain	1 pkg (8 oz)	140	4	15	9	0
Lowfat Vanilla	1 pkg (6 oz)	140	3	24	20	0
WholeSoy & Co.						
Apricot Mango	1 pkg (6 oz)	160	4	30	19	2
Cherry	1 pkg (6 oz)	170	4	31	19	2
Lemon	1 pkg (6 oz)	160	4	29	18	2
Plain	1 pkg (6 oz)	150	5	19	13	1
Strawberry	1 pkg (6 oz)	160	4	30	21	2
Vanilla	1 pkg (6 oz)	160	4	23	18	1
Yoplait						
Delights Chocolate Raspberry	1 pkg (4 oz)	100	2	18	13	0
Delights Triple Berry Creme	1 pkg (4 oz)	100	2	16	12	0
GoGurt Stawberry Ripetide & Sponge Berry	1 pkg (2.2 oz)	70	1	13	10	0
Original Lemon Burst	1 pkg (6 oz)	180	2	36	31	0
Original Pina Colada	1 pkg (6 oz)	170	2	33	28	0
Simplait Blackberry	1 pkg (6 oz)	200	7	28	24	–

FOOD	PORTION	CAL	FAT	CARB	SUGAR	FIBER
Simplait Vanilla	1 pkg (6 oz)	200	7	28	24	–
Yo Plus All Flavors	1 pkg (4 oz)	110	2	21	16	3
YOGURT DRINKS (*see also* KEFIR, SMOOTHIES)						
lassi	7 oz	78	5	8	8	0
Gopi						
Lassi	8 oz	126	10	4	4	0
Karoun						
Yogurt Drink	8 oz	126	10	4	4	0
Lifeway						
Lassi Mango	8 oz	160	2	25	21	3
Lassi Strawberry	8 oz	160	2	25	21	3
Yo-Goat						
All Flavors	8 oz	160	8	11	12	0
Plain	8 oz	150	9	11	40	0
Yoplait						
Kids All Flavors	1 bottle (3.1 oz)	70	2	11	10	–
YOGURT FROZEN						
chocolate soft serve	1 cup	230	9	36	–	3
vanilla soft serve	1 cup	236	8	35	35	0
Ben & Jerry's						
Greek Banana Peanut Butter	½ cup (3.5 oz)	210	8	30	26	tr
Greek Blueberry Vanilla Graham	½ cup (3.5 oz)	200	7	29	23	0
Greek Raspberry Fudge Chunk	½ cup (3.4 oz)	200	7	29	25	tr
Greek Strawberry Shortcake	½ cup (3.5 oz)	180	5	28	23	0
Haagen-Dazs						
Lowfat Coffee	½ cup (3.7 oz)	200	5	31	20	0

FOOD	PORTION	CAL	FAT	CARB	SUGAR	FIBER
Healthy Choice						
Blueberry	1 pkg (4 oz)	100	2	19	13	1
Raspberry	1 pkg (4 oz)	100	2	19	13	1
Strawberry	1 pkg (4 oz)	100	2	18	12	tr
Vanilla Bean	1 pkg (4 oz)	100	2	17	12	1
Julie's						
Organic Blackberry	½ cup	190	12	20	15	1
Organic Peanut Butter Fudge	½ cup	260	17	24	22	tr
Organic Strawberry	½ cup	200	12	22	20	0
Organic Vanilla	½ cup	220	15	20	18	0
Stonyfield Farm						
Fat Free After Dark Chocolate	1 serv (4 oz)	100	0	21	18	1
Low Fat Cookies 'N Cream	1 serv (4 oz)	130	2	25	20	0
Low Fat Creme Caramel	1 serv (4 oz)	130	2	26	25	0
Yasso						
Greek Yogurt Bar Raspberry	1 (2.6 oz)	70	0	13	12	0
Greek Yogurt Bar Strawberry	1 (2.6 oz)	70	0	12	11	0
ZUCCHINI						
baby raw	1 (0.5 oz)	3	tr	1	–	tr
canned italian style	1 cup	66	tr	16	–	–
fresh	1 sm (4.1 oz)	19	tr	4	2	1
pickled	¼ cup	16	tr	4	3	1
raw sliced	1 cup	19	tr	4	2	1
sliced cooked w/o salt	1 cup	29	tr	7	3	3
Del Monte						
Zucchini w/ Italian Tomato Sauce	½ cup (4.2 oz)	30	0	7	1	1

FOOD	PORTION	CAL	FAT	CARB	SUGAR	FIBER
Garden Lites						
Zucchini Marinara frzn	1 pkg (7 oz)	110	4	19	6	4
TAKE-OUT						
breaded & fried	6 slices (3 oz)	141	11	10	3	1
indian pakora	1 serv	46	2	7	–	2
sticks breaded & fried	6 (2 oz)	90	7	6	2	1

PART TWO

Restaurant Chains

A Cup of Joe to Go?

Drinking coffee lowers the risk for type 2 diabetes.
Research has shown that those who drank 3 to 4 cups of regular coffee a day had up to a 50% lower risk of developing type 2 diabetes.
Decaf didn't provide the same protection.

FOOD	PORTION	CAL	FAT	CARB	SUGAR	FIBER
BASKIN-ROBBINS						
BEVERAGES						
Cappuccino Blast w/ Whipped Cream	1 sm (16 oz)	330	14	48	42	0
Shake Chocolate Chip	1 sm (16 oz)	660	32	78	74	1
Shake Chocolate Chip Cookie Dough	1 sm (16 oz)	750	31	99	88	1
Shake Mint Chocolate Chip	1 sm (16 oz)	680	33	83	79	1
Shake Vanilla	1 sm (16 oz)	670	33	80	73	0
FROZEN YOGURT						
Cherries Jubilee	1 scoop (4 oz)	240	12	30	26	1
Vanilla Fat Free	1 scoop (4 oz)	150	0	32	31	0
ICE CREAM						
Butter Almond Crunch Reduced Fat No Sugar Added	1 scoop (4 oz)	220	11	31	7	4
Butter Pecan	1 scoop (4 oz)	280	18	24	24	1
Cabana Berry Banana Reduced Fat No Sugar Added	1 scoop (4 oz)	150	6	27	7	3
Chocolate	1 scoop (4 oz)	260	14	33	31	0
Chocolate Chip	1 scoop (4 oz)	270	16	28	26	1
Chocolate Chip Cookie Dough	1 scoop (4 oz)	310	15	36	30	0
Chocolate Overload Reduced Fat No Sugar Added	1 scoop (4 oz)	190	8	37	7	5

FOOD	PORTION	CAL	FAT	CARB	SUGAR	FIBER
Gold Medal Ribbon	1 scoop (4 oz)	260	13	34	33	0
Mint Chocolate Chip	1 scoop (4 oz)	270	16	28	26	1
Nutty Coconut	1 scoop (4 oz)	300	20	28	27	1
Oreo Cookies 'N Cream	1 scoop (4 oz)	280	15	32	27	1
Peanut Butter 'N Chocolate	1 scoop (4 oz)	320	20	31	28	1
Pistachio Almond	1 scoop (4 oz)	290	19	25	23	1
Pralines 'N Cream	1 scoop (4 oz)	280	14	35	31	1
Reese's Peanut Butter Cup	1 scoop (4 oz)	300	18	31	29	1
Rocky Road	1 scoop (4 oz)	290	15	36	32	5
Sundae Caramel Soft Serve	1 (10 oz)	580	21	89	78	1
Sundae Hot Fudge Soft Serve	1 (10 oz)	610	25	86	75	1
Sundae Strawberry Soft Serve	1 (10 oz)	450	18	59	57	1
Tax Crunch	1 scoop (4 oz)	330	20	32	28	1
Vanilla	1 scoop (4 oz)	260	16	26	26	0
Vanilla Soft Serve	1 serv (6 oz)	280	11	37	36	0
Very Berry Strawberry	1 scoop (4 oz)	320	11	28	27	0
ICES						
Sherbet Rainbow	1 scoop (4 oz)	160	2	34	34	0

FOOD	PORTION	CAL	FAT	CARB	SUGAR	FIBER
Sorbet Lemon	1 scoop (4 oz)	130	0	33	33	0
Sorbet Mango	1 scoop (4 oz)	120	0	32	30	0
Sorbet Strawberry	1 scoop (4 oz)	130	0	34	34	0
BILLY'S BURGER HUT						
BEVERAGES						
Shake Chocolate	1 (20 oz)	420	10	63	50	0
Shake Vanilla	1 (20 oz)	320	10	49	44	0
MAIN MENU SELECTIONS						
Big Billy's Roast Beef Sub	1	843	54	62	12	3
Billyburger	1	426	22	35	6	3
Billyburger w/ Cheese	1	498	35	35	8	4
Billy's Best Red Potato Salad	1 serv	190	9	12	4	3
Billy's Biggest Burger ½ Pounder w/ Everything	1	852	58	61	15	4
Billy's Famous 7 Layer Salad	1 serv	558	49	18	9	2
Billy's Seafood Sandwich	1	399	18	43	9	3
Caesar Side Salad	1 serv	360	28	12	1	4
Chili w/ Cheese & Onion	1 serv	380	12	35	8	7
Cowboy Cobb Salad	1 serv	735	45	25	10	9
Cowboy Coleslaw	1 serv	180	9	11	4	3
French Fries	1 reg	230	12	25	7	1
Onion Rings	1 serv	250	10	37	6	1
Super Billy Burger w/ Bacon	1	663	41	39	9	4

FOOD	PORTION	CAL	FAT	CARB	SUGAR	FIBER
BLIMPIE						
DESSERTS						
Cookie Chocolate Chunk	1 (1.5 oz)	200	10	25	16	0
Cookie Oatmeal Raisin	1 (1.5 oz)	180	7	27	16	tr
Cookie Peanut Butter	1 (1.5 oz)	210	13	21	13	tr
Cookie Sugar	1 (2.5 oz)	320	16	42	23	0
Cookie White Chocolate Macadamia Nut	1 (1.5 oz)	200	11	25	16	0
SALAD DRESSINGS AND SAUCES						
Dressing Blue Cheese	1 serv (1.5 oz)	230	24	2	2	–
Dressing Buttermilk Ranch	1 serv (1.5 oz)	230	24	2	1	–
Dressing Buttermilk Ranch Light	1 serv (1.5 oz)	70	4	8	3	–
Dressing Creamy Caesar	1 serv (1.5 oz)	210	21	2	1	–
Dressing Creamy Italian	1 serv (1.5 oz)	180	18	4	3	0
Dressing Dijon Honey Mustard	1 serv (1.5 oz)	180	17	8	7	–
Dressing Italian Fat Free	1 serv (1.5 oz)	25	0	5	3	0
Dressing Italian Light	1 serv (1.5 oz)	20	1	2	2	–
Dressing Peppercorn	1 serv (1.5 oz)	240	26	1	1	0
Dressing Thousand Island	1 serv (1.5 oz)	210	20	6	6	0
Guacamole	1 serv (1 oz)	45	4	2	0	1
Mayonnaise	1 serv (1 oz)	200	22	0	0	0
Mustard Yellow Deli	1 serv (0.5 oz)	15	0	0	0	0
Oil Blend	1 serv (0.5 oz)	130	14	0	0	0

FOOD	PORTION	CAL	FAT	CARB	SUGAR	FIBER
Sauce Blimpie Special	1 serv (0.5 oz)	40	5	0	–	–
Sauce Red Hot Original	1 serv (1 oz)	10	0	2	0	0
SALADS						
Antipasto	1 serv (11.6 oz)	254	14	12	6	4
Buffalo Chicken	1 serv (7.7 oz)	220	9	10	5	4
Chicken Caesar	1 serv (9.4 oz)	190	8	6	3	3
Cole Slaw	1 side (4 oz)	160	9	20	17	2
Garden	1 serv (6.5 oz)	30	0	6	3	3
Macaroni	1 side (5 oz)	330	22	28	8	2
Northwest Potato	1 side (5 oz)	260	17	22	3	3
Potato	1 side (4.7 oz)	230	12	28	8	3
Tuna	1 serv (9.4 oz)	270	19	6	3	3
Ultimate Club	1 serv (10.1 oz)	280	14	10	5	3
SANDWICHES						
6 Inch Sub Blimpie Best	1 (10.4 oz)	450	17	49	10	3
6 Inch Sub Blimpie Best Super Stacked	1 (12.8 oz)	550	22	52	12	3
6 Inch Sub Blimpie Trio Super Stacked	1 (13.5 oz)	510	15	51	11	3
6 Inch Sub BLT	1 (7.2 oz)	430	22	43	6	2
6 Inch Sub BLT Super Stacked	1 (8.4 oz)	640	41	43	6	2
6 Inch Sub Chicken Cheddar Bacon Ranch	1 (12.1 oz)	600	29	48	8	3
6 Inch Sub Chicken Teriyaki	1 (8.7 oz)	450	12	52	13	2
6 Inch Sub Club	1 (10.2 oz)	410	13	49	9	3

FOOD	PORTION	CAL	FAT	CARB	SUGAR	FIBER
6 Inch Sub Cuban	1 (8.2 oz)	410	11	43	6	1
6 Inch Sub French Dip	1 (13.4 oz)	410	11	46	3	1
6 Inch Sub Ham & Swiss	1 (10 oz)	420	14	49	10	3
6 Inch Sub Hot Pastrami	1 (7.2 oz)	430	16	42	5	1
6 Inch Sub Hot Pastrami Super Stacked	1 (10.1 oz)	570	23	43	7	1
6 Inch Sub Meatball	1 (10 oz)	580	31	50	6	4
6 Inch Sub Reuben	1 (9.2 oz)	530	20	52	7	3
6 Inch Sub Roast Beef & Provolone	1 (10.8 oz)	430	14	46	7	3
6 Inch Sub Roast Beef & Provolone On Wheat	1 (11.3 oz)	430	16	44	6	6
6 Inch Sub Tuna	1 (8.9 oz)	470	21	43	5	2
6 Inch Sub Turkey & Provolone	1 (10.8 oz)	410	13	49	8	3
6 Inch Sub Turkey & Provolone On Wheat	1 (11.3 oz)	420	14	47	8	6
6 Inch Sub VegiMax	1 (10.2 oz)	520	20	56	8	5
Blimpie Burger	1 (6 oz)	460	24	42	4	1
Blimpie Dog	1 (6.3 oz)	510	29	45	7	1
Ciabatta Buffalo Chicken	1 (11.3 oz)	540	23	49	5	3
Ciabatta French Dip	1 (13.8 oz)	430	11	49	2	2
Ciabatta Grilled Chicken Caesar	1 (10.1 oz)	580	20	62	4	3
Ciabatta Mediterranean	1 (10.1 oz)	450	8	65	6	3
Ciabatta Roast Beef Turkey & Cheddar	1 (10 oz)	520	24	51	6	3
Ciabatta Sicilian	1 (10 oz)	590	22	66	9	3
Ciabatta Spicy Chicken & Pepperoni	1 (10.1 oz)	710	34	65	4	3
Ciabatta Tuscan	1 (9.9 oz)	570	20	65	6	3
Ciabatta Ultimate Club	1 (7.4 oz)	520	24	47	5	2

FOOD	PORTION	CAL	FAT	CARB	SUGAR	FIBER
Wrap Chicken Caesar	1 (9.7 oz)	220	8	56	5	4
Wrap Southwestern	1 (10 oz)	530	22	61	10	4
SOUPS						
Bean w/ Ham	1 serv (8.6 oz)	140	1	23	2	11
Chicken Noodle	1 serv (8.6 oz)	130	4	18	5	2
Chicken w/ White & Wild Rice	1 serv (8.6 oz)	250	10	15	4	4
Cream Of Broccoli w/ Cheese	1 serv (8.6 oz)	250	19	13	2	tr
Cream Of Potato	1 serv (8.6 oz)	190	9	24	3	3
Garden Vegetable	1 serv (8.6 oz)	80	1	14	5	3
Grande Chili w/ Bean & Beef	1 serv (8.6 oz)	310	9	31	9	9
Tomato Basil w/ Raviolini	1 serv (8.6 oz)	110	1	22	5	0
Vegetable Beef	1 serv (8.6 oz)	80	2	13	3	2

BURGER KING

FOOD	PORTION	CAL	FAT	CARB	SUGAR	FIBER
BEVERAGES						
Apple Juice Minute Maid	1 (6.67 oz)	100	0	23	21	0
Barq's Root Beer	1 sm (16 oz)	160	0	46	46	0
Cherry Coke	1 sm (16 oz)	150	0	42	42	0
Chocolate Milk 1% Low Fat	1 (8 oz)	160	3	26	25	0
Coca-Cola Classic	1 sm (16 oz)	140	0	39	39	–
Coffee Iced Seattle's Best	1 sm	80	2	14	12	0
Coffee Iced Seattle's Best Caramel	1 sm	170	4	32	23	0
Coffee Iced Seattle's Best Mocha	1 sm	180	3	37	33	1

FOOD	PORTION	CAL	FAT	CARB	SUGAR	FIBER
Coffee Iced Seattle's Best Vanilla	1 sm	160	2	34	32	0
Coffee Seattle's Best Decaf Black	16 oz	0	0	0	0	0
Coffee Seattle's Best Regular Black	1 (16 oz)	0	0	0	0	0
Diet Coke	1 sm (16 oz)	0	0	0	0	0
Dr Pepper	1 sm (16 oz)	140	0	39	39	0
Fanta Orange	1 sm (16 oz)	160	0	42	42	0
Frappe Caramel	1 (12 oz)	410	19	58	39	0
Frappe Mocha	1 (12 oz)	410	19	58	39	0
Frozen Coke	1 sm (16 oz)	90	0	25	25	0
Hi-C Fruit Punch	1 sm (16 oz)	150	0	42	42	0
Iced Tea Southern Style Nestea	1 sm (16 oz)	180	0	50	50	0
Iced Tea Sweetened Nestea	1 sm (16 oz)	90	0	24	24	0
Iced Tea Unsweetened Nestea	1 sm (16 oz)	0	0	0	0	0
Lemonade Light Minute Maid	1 sm (16 oz)	5	0	1	0	0
Milk Fat Free	8 oz	90	0	13	12	0
Orange Juice Minute Maid	10 oz	140	0	33	30	0
Shake Chocolate	1 sm (12 oz)	580	17	97	83	0
Shake Strawberry	1 sm (12 oz)	500	16	79	67	0
Shake Vanilla	1 sm (12 oz)	550	16	91	81	0
Smoothie Strawberry Banana	1 (12 oz)	200	0	48	40	2
Smoothie Tropical Mango	1 (12 oz)	210	1	51	41	1
Sprite	1 sm (16 oz)	140	0	39	39	0
Sweet Tea Gold Peak	1 sm (16 oz)	120	0	31	31	0
Vault	1 sm (16 oz)	160	0	42	42	0

FOOD	PORTION	CAL	FAT	CARB	SUGAR	FIBER
BREAKFAST SELECTIONS						
Biscuit Bacon Egg & Cheese	1 (5.6 oz)	420	25	32	4	1
Biscuit Ham Egg & Cheese	1 (6.4 oz)	390	19	33	4	1
Biscuit Sausage	1 (4.4 oz)	420	27	32	3	1
Biscuit Sausage Egg & Cheese	1 (6.7 oz)	520	34	33	3	1
Biscuit Country Ham & Egg	1 (6.4 oz)	420	23	32	3	1
BK Breakfast Muffin Bacon Egg & Cheese	1 (4.6 oz)	250	11	22	2	1
BK Breakfast Muffin Egg & Cheese	1 (4.4 oz)	220	9	22	2	1
BK Breakfast Muffin Ham Egg & Cheese	1 (5.6 oz)	250	9	23	3	1
BK Breakfast Muffin Sausage & Cheese	1 (3.9 oz)	330	20	23	1	1
BK Breakfast Muffin Sausage Egg & Cheese	1 (5.9 oz)	390	23	23	2	1
BK Breakfast Platter Ultimate	1 (17.9 oz)	1450	84	134	41	5
Breakfast Burrito Sausage	1 (4.3 oz)	290	17	21	2	1
Breakfast Burrito Southwestern	1 (7.8 oz)	580	35	42	3	4
Breakfast Syrup	1 serv (1 oz)	120	0	30	18	0
Cinnabon Roll	1 (3.4 oz)	300	11	45	20	2
Croissan'wich Bacon Egg & Cheese	1 (4.6 oz)	320	18	25	4	1
Croissan'wich Double w/ Bacon Egg & Cheese	1 (5.2 oz)	390	24	25	4	1

FOOD	PORTION	CAL	FAT	CARB	SUGAR	FIBER
Croissan'wich Double w/ Ham Bacon Egg & Cheese	1 (6.2 oz)	390	22	26	5	1
Croissan'wich Double w/ Ham Egg & Cheese	1 (7 oz)	390	19	27	6	1
Croissan'wich Double w/ Ham Sausage Egg & Cheese	1 (7.5 oz)	530	34	27	5	1
Croissan'wich Double w/ Sausage Bacon Egg & Cheese	1 (6.6 oz)	530	36	26	4	1
Croissan'wich Double w/ Sausage Egg & Cheese	1 (8 oz)	660	48	27	4	1
Croissan'wich Egg & Cheese	1 (4.4 oz)	280	15	25	4	1
Croissan'wich Ham Egg & Cheese	1 (5.9 oz)	450	30	26	4	1
Croissan'wich Sausage & Cheese	1 (4 oz)	390	26	25	3	1
French Toast Sticks	3 (2.3 oz)	230	11	29	8	1
Hash Browns	1 sm (2.9 oz)	250	16	24	0	3
Jam Strawberry or Grape	1 pkg (0.4 oz)	30	0	7	6	0
Pancakes + Syrup	3 (6.6 oz)	500	19	77	36	1
Platter Pancake & Sausage	1 (13.7 oz)	670	34	78	36	1
Quaker Oatmeal Maple Brown Sugar	1 serv (6.1 oz)	270	4	55	29	5
Quaker Oatmeal Original	1 serv (4.4 oz)	140	4	23	1	3
DESSERTS						
Cookies Chocolate Chip	2 (2.7 oz)	330	15	47	29	1

FOOD	PORTION	CAL	FAT	CARB	SUGAR	FIBER
Cookies Oatmeal Raisin	2 (2.7 oz)	310	13	46	26	3
Cookies White Chocolate Macadamia Nut	2 (2.7 oz)	340	18	44	28	0
Dutch Apple Pie	1 (3.8 oz)	320	14	46	23	1
Hershey Sundae Pie	1 serv (2.8 oz)	310	19	32	22	1
Soft Serve Cone	1 (3.5 oz)	160	4	27	20	0
Soft Serve Cup	1 (3.3 oz)	140	4	23	19	0
Sundae Brownie	1 (8 oz)	530	17	89	70	2
Sundae Caramel	1 (4.9 oz)	280	6	52	37	0
Sundae Chocolate Fudge	1 (4.9 oz)	280	7	50	43	1
Sundae Mini M&M	1 (7.2 oz)	450	13	76	62	0
Sundae Oreo	1 (7.2 oz)	440	12	77	57	1
Sundae Strawberry	1 (4.9 oz)	190	4	35	31	0
MAIN MENU SELECTIONS						
Apple Slices	1 pkg (2 oz)	30	0	7	6	1
BK Stacker Double	1 (5.3 oz)	490	30	31	7	1
BK Stacker Quad	1 (8.4 oz)	760	51	33	8	1
BK Stacker Single	1 (4 oz)	370	21	32	7	1
BK Stacker Triple	1 (6.9 oz)	630	41	32	7	1
BK Veggie Burger	1 (7.3 oz)	410	16	44	8	7
Burger BK Bacon	1 (3.7 oz)	320	17	31	7	1
Cheeseburger	1 (4 oz)	280	12	32	7	1
Cheeseburger Bacon	1 (4.2 oz)	310	14	32	7	1
Cheeseburger Double	1 (5.2 oz)	370	18	32	7	1
Cheeseburger Double Bacon	1 (5.6 oz)	440	24	32	7	1
Chicken Nuggets	4 (2.2 oz)	190	11	10	0	1
Chicken Strips	2 (3.2 oz)	240	13	23	0	0
French Fries Salted	1 sm (4.5 oz)	340	15	49	0	4
Hamburger	1 (3.5 oz)	240	8	31	7	1
Mozzarella Sticks	4 (3.1 oz)	280	15	24	2	2

FOOD	PORTION	CAL	FAT	CARB	SUGAR	FIBER
Onion Rings	1 sm (3.2 oz)	320	16	41	4	3
Pickles	2 (0.4 oz)	10	0	0	0	0
Sandwich Chicken Crispy	1 (9.3 oz)	750	45	58	8	3
Sandwich Chicken Crispy Spicy	1 (5.2 oz)	480	27	40	6	2
Sandwich Chicken Grilled	1 (8.4 oz)	510	22	43	6	2
Sandwich Chicken Original	1 (7.6 oz)	630	39	46	4	3
Sandwich Country Pork	1 (10.5 oz)	810	42	78	10	4
Sandwich Premium Alaskan Fish	1 (8 oz)	590	31	57	8	3
Tacos	2 (6.1 oz)	390	16	18	4	5
Whopper	1 (9.7 oz)	630	35	57	13	3
Whopper Texas	1 (10.8 oz)	760	48	55	10	3
Whopper Texas Double	1 (13.7 oz)	1000	66	55	11	3
Whopper w/ Cheese	1 (10.5 oz)	710	42	59	14	3
Whopper Double	1 (12.2 oz)	830	50	57	13	3
Whopper Double w/ Cheese	1 (14 oz)	990	65	53	11	3
Whopper Jr.	1 (5.2 oz)	340	19	28	6	2
Whopper Jr. w/ Cheese	1 (5.6 oz)	380	23	29	6	2
Whopper Triple	1 (14.6 oz)	1020	65	57	13	3
Wrap Chicken Apple & Cranberry Garden Fresh Salad Crispy	1 (7.5 oz)	500	24	54	19	5
Wrap Chicken Apple & Cranberry Garden Fresh Salad Grilled	1 (7.3 oz)	430	18	47	17	4
Wrap Chicken BLT Garden Fresh Salad Crispy	1 (7.2 oz)	490	27	43	4	4

FOOD	PORTION	CAL	FAT	CARB	SUGAR	FIBER
Wrap Chicken BLT Garden Fresh Salad Grilled	1 (7.2 oz)	420	22	36	3	4
Wrap Chicken Caesar Garden Fresh Salad Crispy	1 (8.2 oz)	460	23	44	4	5
Wrap Chicken Caesar Garden Fresh Salad Grilled	1 (8 oz)	380	18	37	3	5
Wrap Honey Mustard Crispy Chicken	1 (5 oz)	390	23	34	6	2
Wrap Honey Mustard Grilled Chicken	1 (5.2 oz)	370	19	29	6	1
Wrap Ranch Crispy Chicken	1 (5 oz)	370	23	29	1	2
Wrap Ranch Grilled Chicken	1 (5.2 oz)	350	18	24	1	1
SALAD DRESSINGS AND SAUCES						
Dipping Sauce Barbecue	1 serv (1 oz)	40	0	11	10	0
Dipping Sauce BBQ Roasted Jalapeno	1 serv (1 oz)	50	0	13	11	0
Dipping Sauce Honey Mustard	1 serv (1 oz)	90	6	8	7	0
Dipping Sauce King Kung Pao	1 serv (1 oz)	60	0	13	12	0
Dipping Sauce Ranch	1 serv (1 oz)	140	15	1	1	0
Dipping Sauce Sweet And Sour	1 serv (1 oz)	45	0	11	10	0
Dipping Sauce Zesty Onion Ring	1 serv (1 oz)	150	15	3	2	1
Dressing Ken's Apple Cider Vinaigrette	1 pkg (1.75 oz)	210	18	10	7	0

FOOD	PORTION	CAL	FAT	CARB	SUGAR	FIBER
Dressing Ken's Avocado Ranch	1 pkg (1.8 oz)	170	17	4	3	0
Dressing Ken's Citrus Caesar	1 pkg (1.8 oz)	180	18	4	2	0
Dressing Ken's Honey Mustard	1 pkg (1.8 oz)	221	23	13	12	1
Dressing Ken's Lite Honey Balsamic	1 pkg (1.75 oz)	120	7	14	11	0
Ketchup	1 pkg (0.4 oz)	10	0	3	2	0
Mayonnaise	1 pkg (0.4 oz)	80	9	1	0	0
Sauce French Fry	1 serv (1 oz)	90	7	5	3	0
Sauce Marinara	1 serv (1 oz)	15	0	4	3	1
Sauce Picante/Taco	1 serv (1 oz)	10	0	2	1	0
SALADS						
Chicken Apple & Cranberry Garden Fresh w/ Tendercrisp & Dressing	1 (14 oz)	700	41	54	37	5
Chicken Apple & Cranberry Garden Fresh w/ Tendergrill & Dressing	1 (13.6 oz)	560	30	40	34	4
Chicken BLT Garden Fresh w/ Tendercrisp & Dressing	1 (14 oz)	690	48	31	8	4
Chicken BLT Garden Fresh w/ Tendergrill & Dressing	1 (13.6 oz)	550	37	17	5	3
Chicken Caesar Garden Fresh w/ Tendercrisp & Dressing	1 (13.5 oz)	670	43	40	8	5

FOOD	PORTION	CAL	FAT	CARB	SUGAR	FIBER
Chicken Caesar Garden Fresh w/ Tendergrill & Dressing	1 (13.1 oz)	530	32	26	6	3
Croutons Homestyle Caesar	1 pkg (0.5 oz)	60	2	9	1	0
Side Caesar w/ Dressing	1 (5 oz)	220	20	7	3	2
Side Garden w/ Avocado Ranch Dressing	1 (5.2 oz)	230	21	7	3	2

CARIBOU COFFEE

BEVERAGES

FOOD	PORTION	CAL	FAT	CARB	SUGAR	FIBER
Americano No Whip	1 sm (11 oz)	0	0	0	0	0
Apple Blast Cooler No Whip	1 sm (17 oz)	300	11	51	48	0
Apple Blast w/ Whip	1 med (17 oz)	400	11	76	71	0
Berry Black Tea Growlers	1 sm (9 oz)	110	0	28	26	0
Berry Mocha 2% Milk w/ Whip	1 sm (14 oz)	570	31	67	63	1
Berry Mocha Cooler Northern Lite No Whip	1 sm (17 oz)	170	3	52	27	8
Berry Mocha Cooler w/ Whip	1 sm (18 oz)	560	20	91	83	0
Berry Mocha Northern Lite Skim Milk No Whip	1 sm (11 oz)	185	6	23	22	0
Black Forest Caribou Cooler w/ Whip	1 sm (19 oz)	650	28	98	85	4
Black Tea	1 sm (12 oz)	0	0	0	0	0
Black Tea Peach Growlers	1 sm (9 oz)	90	0	23	22	0
Black Tea Peach No Whip	1 med (24 oz)	104	0	34	33	0
Breve No Whip	1 sm (12 oz)	350	31	12	0	0

FOOD	PORTION	CAL	FAT	CARB	SUGAR	FIBER
Campfire Mocha 2% Milk w/ Whip	1 med (14 oz)	560	31	65	62	1
Campfire Mocha Cooler w/ Whip	1 sm (18 oz)	510	20	89	81	0
Cappuccino 2% Milk No Whip	1 sm (6 oz)	45	2	4	4	0
Caramel Caribou Cooler Northern Lite No Whip	1 sm (16 oz)	90	2	30	11	6
Caramel Caribou Cooler w/ Whip	1 sm (17 oz)	420	16	71	63	0
Caramel High Rise 2% Milk w/ Whip	1 med (17 oz)	360	18	41	40	0
Caramel High Rise Northern Lite Skim Milk Nonfat Whip	1 sm (12 oz)	115	1	15	15	0
Chai 2% Milk No Whip	1 sm (13 oz)	250	6	38	38	0
Chai Blended 2% Milk No Whip	1 sm (16 oz)	210	4	40	39	0
Chai Iced 2% Milk No Whip	1 sm (13 oz)	210	4	40	39	0
Coffee Caribou Cooler Northern Lite No Whip	1 sm (16 oz)	100	2	34	13	7
Coffee Of The Day w/o Milk & Whip	1 sm (12 oz)	5	0	0	0	0
Cold Press Growlers	1 sm (8 oz)	0	0	0	0	0
Cold Press Iced Coffee No Whip	1 sm (14 oz)	5	0	0	0	0
Cookies & Cream Snowdrift 2% Milk w/ Whip	1 sm (19 oz)	590	25	82	71	1
Depth Charge	1 sm (12 oz)	5	0	0	0	0
Espresso	1 sm (3 oz)	0	0	0	0	0

FOOD	PORTION	CAL	FAT	CARB	SUGAR	FIBER
Espresso Caribou Cooler No Whip	1 sm (16 oz)	210	35	42	36	0
Espresso Caribou Cooler Northern Lite No Whip	1 sm (16 oz)	80	2	28	11	6
Green Tea	1 sm (12 oz)	0	0	0	0	0
Green Tea Lemonade Growlers	1 sm (9 oz)	140	0	36	35	0
Green Tea Lemonade No Whip	1 med (24 oz)	210	0	54	52	0
Herbal Tea	1 sm (12 oz)	0	0	0	0	0
Hot Chocolate 2% Milk w/ Whip	1 sm (10 oz)	410	26	35	33	1
Hot Chocolate Lite Skim Milk Nonfat Whip	1 sm (11 oz)	215	6	28	27	0
Juice Lemon Ginger Pomegranate	1 med (24 oz)	260	0	64	57	0
Juice Lemon Ginger Pomegranate Growlers	1 sm (9 oz)	170	0	43	38	0
Juice Very Berry	1 med (24 oz)	160	0	38	34	0
Juice Very Berry Growlers	1 sm (9 oz)	110	0	25	23	0
Latte 2% Milk No Whip	1 sm (12 oz)	140	6	13	13	0
Latte Iced 2% Milk No Whip	1 sm (12 oz)	80	3	7	7	0
Latte Iced Northern Lite Skim Milk No Whip	1 sm (12 oz)	45	0	6	6	0
Latte Northern Lite Skim Milk No Whip	1 sm (12 oz)	90	5	12	12	0
Macchiato 2% Milk No Whip	1 sm (4 oz)	15	1	1	1	0
Mint Condition 2% Milk w/ Whip	1 sm (14 oz)	520	31	68	65	1

FOOD	PORTION	CAL	FAT	CARB	SUGAR	FIBER
Mint Condition Cooler w/ Whip	1 sm (18 oz)	570	20	92	84	0
Mint Snowdrift 2% Milk w/ Whip	1 sm (18 oz)	490	21	67	64	0
Mocha 2% Milk w/ Whip	1 sm (10 oz)	360	24	31	28	1
Mocha Cooler Northern Lite No Whip	1 sm (17 oz)	190	3	56	29	9
Mocha Cooler w/ Whip	1 sm (18 oz)	530	21	79	70	0
Mocha Iced 2% Milk No Whip	1 sm (13 oz)	250	8	36	35	0
Mocha Iced Northern Lite Skim Milk No Whip	1 sm (12 oz)	140	3	21	20	0
Mocha Northern Lite Skim Milk Nonfat Whip	1 sm (10 oz)	185	6	23	22	0
Oolong Tea Iced Pomegranate 2% Milk No Whip	1 sm (13 oz)	140	3	27	26	0
Oolong Tea Pomegranate 2% Milk No Whip	1 sm (13 oz)	200	6	29	29	0
Rooibos Tea Iced Vanilla	1 sm (13 oz)	140	3	26	26	0
Rooibos Tea Vanilla 2% Milk No Whip	1 sm (13 oz)	200	6	28	28	0
Smoothie Mango Orange Key Lime No Whip	1 sm (19 oz)	360	0	90	82	0
Smoothie Strawberry Banana No Whip	1 sm (18 oz)	300	0	70	66	0
Smoothie White Peach Berry No Whip	1 sm (19 oz)	260	0	64	56	0
Tea Berry Black No Whip	1 med (24 oz)	170	0	42	39	0
Turtle Mocha 2% Milk w/ Whip	1 med (14 oz)	580	31	69	66	1

FOOD	PORTION	CAL	FAT	CARB	SUGAR	FIBER
Turtle Mocha Cooler Northern Lite No Whip	1 sm (17 oz)	488	3	53	27	8
Turtle Mocha Cooler w/ Whip	1 sm (18 oz)	570	20	93	85	0
Turtle Mocha Northen Lite Skim Milk Nonfat Whip	1 sm (11 oz)	185	6	24	22	0
Vanilla Caribou Cooler	1 sm (17 oz)	410	16	68	60	0
Vanilla Caribou Cooler Northern Lite No Whip	1 sm (16 oz)	90	2	30	11	6
Vanilla White Chocolate Mocha 2% Milk w/ Whip	1 sm (14 oz)	570	31	66	63	1
Vanilla White Chocolate Mocha Cooler Northern Lite No Whip	1 sm (17 oz)	170	3	52	27	8
Vanilla White Chocolate Mocha Cooler w/ Whip	1 sm (18 oz)	560	20	91	82	0
Vanilla White Chocolate Mocha Northern Lite Skim Milk Nonfat Whip	1 sm (11 oz)	185	6	23	22	0
White Tea Mint Lime Growlers	1 sm (9 oz)	160	0	40	39	0
White Tea Mint Lime No Whip	1 med (24 oz)	240	0	60	58	0
FOOD						
Croissant Butter	1 (2.5 oz)	280	13	35	5	1
Daybreaker Chicken Apple Sausage	1 (6.4 oz)	410	20	34	9	1
Daybreaker Egg White & Turkey Bacon	1 (5 oz)	320	13	36	7	3
Daybreaker Veggie	1 (5.5 oz)	370	16	40	7	4

FOOD	PORTION	CAL	FAT	CARB	SUGAR	FIBER
Mini Turkey Bacon	1 (2.4 oz)	190	10	17	1	1
Mini Turkey Sausage	1 (4 oz)	310	16	25	4	1
Muffin Carrot Cake	1 (5 oz)	510	24	71	47	2
Muffin Maine Blueberry	1 (5 oz)	620	38	65	33	1
Muffin Triple Berry	1 (5 oz)	600	34	69	42	1
Oatmeal Apple Cinnamon	1 serv (8 oz)	330	3	63	22	8
Oatmeal Blueberry Almond	1 serv (8 oz)	370	8	61	17	9
Oatmeal Classic	1 serv (6.6 oz)	260	3	47	8	7
Oatmeal Maple Brown Sugar Crunch	1 serv (7.2 oz)	206	4	57	16	7
Oatmeal Very Berry	1 serv (9 oz)	400	8	78	34	10
Sandwich Aged Cheddar Roast	1 (6.5 oz)	480	22	46	8	2
Sandwich Gouda Turkey Pesto	1 (7.2 oz)	510	24	46	7	2
Sandwich Italian Chicken Melt	1 (7 oz)	470	21	41	6	7
Sandwich Three Cheese	1 (5.2 oz)	500	25	46	9	1

CHICKEN OUT ROTISSERIE

MAIN MENU SELECTIONS

1/4 Dark Chicken w/ Skin	1 serv	337	18	5	4	1
1/4 Dark Chicken w/o Skin	1 serv	223	10	1	1	0
Apple Cornbread Stuffing	1 serv (7 oz)	453	21	58	7	2
Baked Potato Wedges	1 serv (8 oz)	220	6	39	12	6
Chunky Cinnamon Applesauce	1 serv (7 oz)	241	4	52	13	5
Cranberry Relish	1 serv (7 oz)	285	2	69	66	3
Creamed Spinach	1 serv (6 oz)	320	25	16	7	3

FOOD	PORTION	CAL	FAT	CARB	SUGAR	FIBER
Edamame Beans In Sweet Pepper Sauce	1 serv (7 oz)	200	8	18	6	8
Farm Fresh Cole Slaw	1 serv (7 oz)	226	17	18	13	3
Fresh Fruit Salad	1 serv (7 oz)	110	0	29	25	3
Grilled Chicken Filet Skinless	1 (6 oz)	290	6	3	3	0
Half Sandwich BBQ & Cole Slaw	1	340	7	41	16	2
Half Sandwich Classic Grilled Chicken	1	405	33	55	4	1
Half Sandwich Signature Chicken Salad	1	305	22	10	7	1
Just The Turkey Burger	1 (7 oz)	360	27	65	16	5
Macaroni & Cheese	1 serv (7 oz)	290	72	46	6	6
Mashed Sweet Potatoes	1 serv (7 oz)	423	1	102	54	4
Pulled BBQ Chicken	1 serv (6 oz)	380	7	27	22	0
Pulled Rotisserie Chicken Breast	1 serv (6 oz)	290	6	3	2	0
Red Skin Mashed Potatoes	1 serv (7 oz)	334	16	44	3	4
Sandwich Hot Openfaced Pulled Chicken On Biscuit	1	1180	47	113	10	7
Steamed Vegetable Medley	1 serv (7 oz)	30	0	6	2	2
Wrap Apricot Chicken Salad	½	412	19	37	9	3
Wrap Asian Chicken Salad	½	341	12	35	6	2
Wrap BBQ Chicken w/ Cole Slaw	½	395	9	43	14	2
Wrap Chopped Veggie	½	315	7	40	13	4
Wrap Cobb Salad	½	430	21	32	5	3

FOOD	PORTION	CAL	FAT	CARB	SUGAR	FIBER
Wrap Freshly Roasted Turkey w/ Cucumber Sauce	½	325	14	27	3	3
Wrap Garden Veggie & Cheese	½	352	18	32	4	3
Wrap Grilled Chicken	½	359	15	32	3	2
Wrap Grilled Chicken Caesar	½	386	18	31	2	2
Wrap Santa Fe	½	371	16	34	4	3
Wrap Spinach & Milan Cutlet	½	315	7	43	14	4
SALAD DRESSINGS						
Buttermilk Ranch	1 oz	110	11	1	0	0
Creamy Caesar	1 oz	181	20	0	0	0
Creamy Cole Slaw	1 oz	125	11	6	5	0
Honey Balsamic Vinaigrette	1 oz	161	16	4	3	0
Honey Mustard Fat Free	1 oz	50	0	11	9	0
Southwest	1 oz	146	16	2	0	1
SALADS						
Apricot Chicken Salad	1 serv (6 oz)	610	36	23	17	3
Asian Chicken w/o Dressing or Wontons	1 serv	325	9	21	12	7
Caesar Grilled Chicken w/o Dressing or Croutons	1 serv	310	10	10	5	5
Caesar w/o Dressing Croutons or Roll	1 serv	90	4	8	3	5
Chicken Cobb	1 serv	720	29	48	8	7
Chopped Veggie & Chicken w/o Dressing or Croutons	1 serv	300	5	25	12	9

FOOD	PORTION	CAL	FAT	CARB	SUGAR	FIBER
Freshly Roasted Turkey Breast	1 serv	320	10	13	5	7
Garden Grilled Chicken w/o Dressing or Croutons	1 serv	269	5	17	8	6
Green Leaf Fruit & Granola	1 serv	380	11	67	38	11
Milan Chicken Cutlet	1 serv	348	7	17	3	4
Santa Fe Chicken w/o Dressing or Tortilla Strips	1 serv	399	15	22	8	8
Signature Chicken Salad	1 serv (6 oz)	790	58	22	15	2
Spinach w/ Milan Cutlet	1 serv	550	22	46	26	8
SOUPS						
Chicken Noodle	1 serv (13 oz)	211	6	9	3	1
Vegetable Primavera	1 serv (13 oz)	330	7	45	20	10

CHICK-FIL-A

FOOD	PORTION	CAL	FAT	CARB	SUGAR	FIBER
BEVERAGES						
Coca-Cola	1 med	170	0	47	47	0
Coffee 100% Colombian	1 med	5	0	0	0	0
Diet Coke	1 med	0	0	0	0	0
Dr Pepper	1 med	180	0	48	48	0
Iced Tea Sweetened	1 med	130	0	32	32	0
Iced Tea Unsweetened	1 med	0	0	0	0	0
Lemonade	1 med	240	0	36	58	0
Lemonade Diet	1 med	20	0	7	2	0
Milkshake Chocolate	1 sm	600	23	90	86	1
Milkshake Peach	1 sm	780	19	139	118	1
Milkshake Strawberry	1 sm	610	23	88	85	1
BREAKFAST SELECTIONS						
Bagel Multigrain Chicken Egg & Cheese	1	490	20	49	8	3

FOOD	PORTION	CAL	FAT	CARB	SUGAR	FIBER
Biscuit Bacon Egg & Cheese	1	500	27	44	6	2
Biscuit Chicken	1	440	20	47	6	3
Biscuit Plain	1	310	14	41	5	2
Biscuit Sausage	1	590	39	43	5	2
Biscuit Spicy Chicken	1	450	20	50	5	2
Breakfast Burrito Chicken	1	450	20	43	3	2
Breakfast Burrito Sausage	1	510	28	40	3	2
Chick-N-Minis	3	280	10	30	5	1
Cinnamon Cluster	1 serv	430	17	63	29	2
Hashbrowns	1 serv	270	18	25	0	2
Yogurt Parfait	1	230	3	44	35	0
Yogurt Parfait w/ Chocolate Cookie Crumbs	1	240	5	47	36	0
Yogurt Parfait w/ Granola	1	290	6	53	39	1
DESSERTS						
Cheesecake	1 slice	310	23	22	14	1
Fudge Nut Brownie	1	370	19	45	28	3
Icedream	1 cup	290	7	50	49	0
Icedream Cone	1	170	4	31	25	0
Lemon Pie	1 slice	360	13	58	21	1
MAIN MENU SELECTIONS						
Chick-N-Strips	3	360	17	17	2	1
Cool Wrap Chargrilled Chicken	1	410	12	50	8	9
Cool Wrap Chicken Caesar	1	460	15	47	6	8
Cool Wrap Spicy Chicken	1	410	12	48	5	8

FOOD	PORTION	CAL	FAT	CARB	SUGAR	FIBER
Hearty Breast of Chicken Soup	1 med	140	4	19	3	2
Nuggets	8	260	12	11	1	1
Sandwich Chargrilled Chicken	1	290	5	36	9	3
Sandwich Chargrilled Chicken Club	1	410	12	37	10	3
Sandwich Chicken	1	430	17	38	6	3
Sandwich Chicken Deluxe	1	490	22	41	8	3
Sandwich Chicken Salad On Wheat Bread	1	490	19	55	12	5
Sandwich Spicy Chicken	1	480	20	44	6	3
Sandwich Spicy Chicken Deluxe	1	570	27	46	8	4
Waffle Potato Fries	1 med	360	19	43	0	5
SALAD DRESSINGS AND SAUCES						
Dressing Berry Balsamic Vinaigrette Reduced Fat	½ pkg (1.25 oz)	70	2	12	9	0
Dressing Blue Cheese	½ pkg (1.25 oz)	160	16	1	1	0
Dressing Buttermilk Ranch	½ pkg (1.25 oz)	160	17	1	1	0
Dressing Caesar	½ pkg (1.25 oz)	160	17	1	0	0
Dressing Honey Mustard Fat Free	½ pkg (1.25 oz)	60	0	14	12	0
Dressing Italian Light	½ pkg (1.25 oz)	15	1	2	2	0
Dressing Spicy	½ pkg (1.25 oz)	140	14	2	1	0

FOOD	PORTION	CAL	FAT	CARB	SUGAR	FIBER
Dressing Thousand Island	½ pkg (1.25 oz)	150	14	5	4	0
Sauce Barbecue	½ pkg (0.5 oz)	45	0	11	9	0
Sauce Buffalo	½ pkg (0.4 oz)	10	0	1	0	0
Sauce Buttermilk Ranch	½ pkg (0.4 oz)	110	12	1	1	0
Sauce Chick-fil-A	½ pkg (0.5 oz)	140	13	6	6	0
Sauce Honey Mustard	½ pkg (1.25 oz)	45	0	11	10	0
Sauce Honey Roasted BBQ	½ pkg	60	5	2	2	0
Sauce Polynesian	½ pkg (0.5 oz)	110	6	14	5	0
SALADS						
Carrot & Raisin Salad	1 med	260	12	40	32	4
Chargrilled Chicken Garden Salad	1 serv	180	6	11	6	4
Chargrilled & Fruit	1 serv	220	6	22	17	4
Chicken Salad Bacon & Egg	1 cup	350	22	9	6	1
Chick-N-Strips Salad	1 serv	460	22	26	6	5
Cole Slaw	1 med	360	31	19	16	3
Croutons Garlic & Butter	1 pkg	60	2	9	1	0
Fruit Cup	1 serv	70	0	17	14	2
Harvest Nut Granola	1 pkg	60	3	8	3	1
Honey Roasted Sunflower Kernels	1 pkg	90	7	4	1	1
Side Salad	1 serv	70	5	5	2	2
Southwest Chargrilled Salad	1 serv	240	9	18	6	5
Tortilla Strips	1 pkg	80	4	8	1	1

FOOD	PORTION	CAL	FAT	CARB	SUGAR	FIBER
CHILI'S						
CHILDREN'S MENU SELECTIONS						
Pepper Pals Cheese Pizza w/o Sides	1	570	24	67	–	3
Pepper Pals Chicken Crispers Crispy w/o Sides	1 serv	380	22	19	–	2
Pepper Pals Corn Dog w/o Sides	1	270	14	31	–	0
Pepper Pals Grilled Cheese w/o Sides	1 serv	530	42	30	–	1
Pepper Pals Grilled Chicken Platter w/o Sides	1 serv	160	4	2	–	0
Pepper Pals Little Chicken Crispers w/o Sides	1 serv	340	15	21	–	1
Pepper Pals Little Mouth Burger w/o Sides	1 serv	330	18	23	–	1
Pepper Pals Little Mouth Cheeseburger w/o Sides	1 serv	400	24	24	–	1
Pepper Pals Macaroni & Cheese w/o Sides	1 serv	500	18	69	–	3
Pepper Pals Quesadilla Cheese w/o Sides	1 serv	380	22	29	–	1
Pepper Pals Sandwich Grilled Chicken w/o Sides	1 serv	230	5	22	–	1
Pepper Pals Sides Celery Sticks w/ Ranch	1 serv	80	5	10	–	0
Pepper Pals Sides Corn Cob w/ Butter	1 serv	150	2	32	–	3

FOOD	PORTION	CAL	FAT	CARB	SUGAR	FIBER
DESSERTS						
Brownie Sundae	1	1290	61	195	–	8
Cheesecake	1 serv	710	42	68	–	0
Chocolate Chip Paradise Pie	1 serv	1250	64	163	–	4
Frosty Chocolate Shake	1 serv	690	33	92	–	0
Molten Chocolate Cake	1 serv	1020	46	144	–	5
MAIN MENU SELECTIONS						
Baby Back Ribs Half Rack	1 serv	760	49	14	–	2
Big Mouth Bites w/ Ranch w/ Fries	1 serv	2120	133	163	–	7
Black Beans	1 serv	100	1	18	–	5
Boneless Buffalo Wings w/ Bleu Cheese	1 serv	1490	88	94	–	2
Bottomless Tostada Chips w/ Salsa	1 serv	1020	51	125	–	11
Broccoli Steamed	1 serv	80	6	6	–	3
Burger Classic Bacon	1 serv	1570	91	125	–	9
Burger Ground Avocado On Wheat Bun w/ Fries	1 serv	1570	90	138	–	15
Burger Mushroom Swiss	1 serv	1540	88	126	–	10
Burger Oldtimer	1 serv	1310	65	128	–	10
Burger Shiner Bock BBQ	1 serv	1680	87	166	–	10
Cajun Pasta w/ Grilled Shrimp	1 serv	1460	78	125	–	6
Chicken Crispers Honey Chipotle w/ Ranch	1 serv	1660	70	196	–	13
Chicken Crispers w/ Honey Mustard	1 serv	1350	68	129	–	11
Chicken Crispers w/o Dressing	1 serv	1210	57	125	–	13
Cinnamon Apples	1 serv	280	11	48	–	9

FOOD	PORTION	CAL	FAT	CARB	SUGAR	FIBER
Classic Nachos	8	960	66	53	–	8
Classic Nachos Beef	8	1110	69	56	–	8
Classic Nachos Chicken	8	1120	69	55	–	8
Classic Ribeye	1 serv	1270	82	53	–	7
Classic Sirloin	1 (6 oz)	870	51	53	–	7
Cole Slaw	1 serv	240	20	15	–	2
Country Fried Steak	1 serv	1270	71	120	–	9
Crispy Onion String & Jalapeno Stack w/ Ranch	1 serv	1050	81	71	–	4
Fajitas Beef w/o Tortillas & Condiments	1 serv	510	29	23	–	8
Fajitas Chicken w/o Tortillas & Condiments	1 serv	360	10	24	–	7
Fajitas Trio w/o Tortillas & Condiments	1 serv	560	25	29	–	8
Fire Grilled Corn Guacamole w/ Chips	1 serv	1400	84	151	–	25
Fried Cheese w/ Marinara Sauce	1 serv	660	35	54	–	1
Fried Shrimp w/ Cocktail Sauce	1 serv	240	12	20	–	1
Grilled Salmon w/ Garlic & Herbs	1 serv	560	25	37	–	5
Homestyle Fries	1 serv	380	13	61	–	6
Hot Spinach & Artichoke Dip w/ Chips	1 serv	1610	103	139	–	14
Loaded Mashed Potatoes	1 serv	390	25	28	–	3
Loaded Potato Skins	1 serv	1050	84	36	–	3
Margarita Grilled Chicken	1 serv	550	14	62	–	8

FOOD	PORTION	CAL	FAT	CARB	SUGAR	FIBER
Mashed Potatoes w/ Black Pepper Gravy	1 serv	280	15	31	–	3
Monterey Chicken	1 serv	890	48	51	–	8
Pasta Cajun w/ Grilled Chicken	1 serv	1500	76	124	–	6
Quesadillas Bacon Ranch Chicken	1 serv	1480	103	70	–	4
Quesadillas Bacon Ranch Steak	1 serv	1470	103	72	–	4
Quesadillas Chicken Club	1 serv	1240	88	63	–	9
Ribs Memphis Dry Rub	½ rack	1080	57	82	–	8
Ribs Memphis Dry Rub	1 serv	1990	111	137	–	17
Ribs Original	1 serv	2170	123	137	–	20
Ribs Shiner Bock BBQ	1 serv	2310	123	168	–	20
Rice	1 serv	190	7	30	–	1
Sandwich Buffalo Chicken Ranch On White Bun w/ Fries	1 serv	1410	68	143	–	12
Sandwich California Club w/ Fries	1 serv	1490	76	147	–	15
Sandwich Cheesesteak w/ Fries	1 serv	1300	61	133	–	11
Sandwich Classic Turkey w/ Fries	1 serv	1340	64	138	–	11
Sandwich Fajita Chicken w/ Fries	1 serv	730	38	70	–	6
Sandwich Grilled Chicken On White Bun w/ Fries	1 serv	1290	63	121	–	9
Sandwich Grilled Ham & Swiss w/ Fries	1 serv	1360	71	137	–	9

FOOD	PORTION	CAL	FAT	CARB	SUGAR	FIBER
Sandwich Southwestern BLT w/ Fries	1 serv	630	33	68	–	5
Skillet Queso w/ Chips	1 serv	1710	101	147	–	13
Southwestern Eggrolls w/ Avocado Ranch	1 serv	780	41	81	–	7
Spicy Garlic & Lime Grilled Shrimp	1 serv	130	5	5	–	0
Sweet Corn On The Cob w/ Butter	1 serv	200	7	32	–	3
Tacos Chicken Club	1 serv	1130	56	100	–	10
Tacos Crispy Chicken	1 serv	1500	74	151	–	12
Tacos Grilled Shrimp	1 serv	1120	52	126	–	14
Texas Cheese Fries w/ Ranch	1 serv	1960	136	109	–	12
Wings Over Buffalo w/ Bleu Cheese	1 serv	690	53	7	–	1
Wrap Sante Fe Chicken w/ Ancho Chile Ranch w/ Fries	1 serv	1320	73	126	–	11
SALAD DRESSINGS AND SAUCES						
Dressing Ancho Chile	1 serv	190	19	3	–	0
Dressing Avocado Ranch	1 serv	140	14	3	–	1
Dressing Citrus Balsamic Vinaigrette	1 serv	250	25	6	–	0
Dressing Honey Lime	1 serv	200	17	13	–	0
Dressing Honey Mustard	1 serv	200	22	1	–	0
Dressing Honey Mustard No Fat	1 serv	70	0	11	–	0
Dressing Ranch	1 serv	180	19	2	–	0
Dressing Ranch Low Fat	1 serv	80	5	9	–	0
Gravy Black Pepper	1 serv	30	2	4	–	1
Guacamole	1 serv	45	4	3	–	2
Sauce BBQ	1 serv	50	0	12	–	1
Sauce Honey Chipotle	1 serv	140	0	34	–	0

FOOD	PORTION	CAL	FAT	CARB	SUGAR	FIBER
SALADS						
Boneless Buffalo Chicken	1 serv	990	68	48	–	8
Caribbean w/ Grilled Chicken w/ Dressing	1 serv	610	25	65	–	6
Caribbean w/ Grilled Shrimp w/ Dressing	1 serv	590	28	66	–	6
Chicken Caesar	1 serv	680	44	31	–	6
House w/o Dressing	1 serv	150	6	18	–	3
Quesadilla Explosion	1 serv	1300	86	75	–	9
Santa Fe Chicken w/ Dressing	1 serv	670	48	30	–	7
SOUPS						
Chicken Enchilada	1 cup	190	12	11	–	1
Loaded Baked Potato	1 cup	210	15	11	–	1
Southwest Chicken & Sausage	1 cup	160	10	13	–	2
Terlinger Chili w/ Toppings	1 cup	180	10	9	–	3

DAIRY QUEEN

FOOD	PORTION	CAL	FAT	CARB	SUGAR	FIBER
BEVERAGES						
Arctic Rush All Flavors	1 sm (13.6 oz)	210	0	41	41	0
Arctic Rush Float All Flavors	1 sm (13.2 oz)	330	6	65	61	0
Arctic Rush Freeze All Flavors	1 sm (11.8 oz)	380	10	65	58	0
Barq's	1 sm (17 oz)	180	0	48	48	0
Coca-Cola	1 sm (16.8 oz)	160	0	43	43	0
Coffee Black	1 (12 oz)	0	0	0	0	0
Diet Coca-Cola	1 sm (16.5 oz)	0	0	0	0	0
Diet Pepsi	1 sm (17 oz)	0	0	0	0	0

FOOD	PORTION	CAL	FAT	CARB	SUGAR	FIBER
Dr Pepper	1 sm (16.8 oz)	160	0	43	43	0
Lemonade Chiller Classic	1 sm (12.4 oz)	250	0	55	54	0
Lemonade Chiller Strawberry	1 sm (13.8 oz)	280	0	64	61	0
Malt Banana	1 sm (13 oz)	540	19	80	65	1
Malt Caramel	1 sm (13.3 oz)	610	20	95	72	0
Malt Cherry	1 sm (13.3 oz)	560	19	83	71	0
Malt Chocolate	1 sm (13.3 oz)	590	21	92	79	1
Malt Hot Fudge	1 sm (13.3 oz)	620	22	90	73	1
Malt Peanut Butter	1 sm (13.3 oz)	700	34	83	65	1
Malt Strawberry	1 sm (13.3 oz)	550	19	81	68	0
Malt Vanilla	1 sm (13.3 oz)	580	19	89	73	0
Milk 2%	8 oz	110	5	11	11	0
MooLatte Cappuccino	1 sm (13 oz)	450	16	65	58	0
MooLatte Caramel	1 sm (13.5 oz)	520	16	82	64	0
MooLatte French Vanilla	1 sm (13.6 oz)	500	15	80	67	0
MooLatte Mocha	1 sm (13.2 oz)	500	19	74	65	0
Mountan Dew	1 sm (17 oz)	190	0	51	51	0
Mug	1 sm (17 oz)	160	0	47	47	0
Pepsi	1 sm (16.5 oz)	160	0	44	44	0

FOOD	PORTION	CAL	FAT	CARB	SUGAR	FIBER
Shake Banana	1 sm (12.6 oz)	480	18	68	56	1
Shake Caramel	1 sm (12.8 oz)	560	20	83	63	0
Shake Cherry	1 sm (12.8 oz)	500	18	72	61	0
Shake Chocolate	1 sm (12.8 oz)	540	20	81	69	1
Shake Hot Fudge	1 sm (12.8 oz)	560	22	79	64	1
Shake Peanut Butter	1 sm (12.8 oz)	640	33	71	56	1
Shake Strawberry	1 sm (12.8 oz)	490	18	70	59	0
Shake Vanilla	1 sm (12.8 oz)	520	19	77	63	0
Sierra Mist	1 sm (17 oz)	170	0	43	43	0
Sprite	1 sm (17 oz)	150	0	42	42	0
BREAKFAST MENU SELECTIONS						
Biscuit Sandwich Bacon	1 (4.8 oz)	380	24	26	1	1
Biscuit Sandwich Ham	1 (5.4 oz)	360	21	26	2	1
Biscuit Sandwich Sausage	1 (5.4 oz)	440	30	25	1	1
Biscuit Twin Pack Sausage	1 (6.3 oz)	600	36	48	2	2
Biscuits & Gravy	1 serv (12.8 oz)	730	47	64	4	2
Hashbrowns	1 serv (2.5 oz)	190	12	18	0	2
Platter Country	1 (11 oz)	780	46	69	3	4
Platter Pancake	1 (5.6 oz)	310	6	57	9	3
Platter Ultimate Hashbrown	1 (12.4 oz)	660	43	45	1	5

FOOD	PORTION	CAL	FAT	CARB	SUGAR	FIBER
Ultimate Breakfast Burrito Ultimate	1 (10 oz)	640	37	55	2	4
CHILDREN'S MENU SELECTIONS						
Applesauce	1 serv (4 oz)	90	0	23	22	1
Banana	1 (4.4 oz)	110	0	29	15	3
Cheeseburger	1 (5.5 oz)	400	18	34	8	1
Chicken Strips	2 (2.8 oz)	220	12	15	0	2
Fries	1 serv (2.5 oz)	190	8	27	0	2
Grilled Cheese	1 (3.6 oz)	320	13	30	2	1
Hot Dog	1 (3.9 oz)	290	17	22	4	1
ICE CREAM						
Banana Split	1 (13 oz)	520	14	94	73	4
Blizzard Banana Cream Pie	1 sm (10.8 oz)	570	21	85	64	1
Blizzard Banana Split	1 sm (10.4 oz)	440	14	71	58	1
Blizzard Butterfinger	1 sm (9.2 oz)	460	17	69	58	1
Blizzard Chocolate Xtreme	1 sm (10 oz)	650	29	88	69	2
Blizzard Cookie Dough	1 sm (11.2 oz)	710	28	104	75	1
Blizzard French Silk Pie	1 sm (10.1 oz)	670	30	90	69	1
Blizzard Georgia Mud Fudge	1 sm (10 oz)	680	35	82	63	3
Blizzard Hawaiian	1 sm (9.9 oz)	440	15	67	55	1
Blizzard Heath	1 sm (10 oz)	600	26	83	73	1
Blizzard Midnight Truffle	1 sm (12 oz)	750	37	99	80	3
Blizzard Mint Oreo	1 sm (10 oz)	560	18	87	69	1
Blizzard Oreo CheeseQuake	1 sm (9.7 oz)	580	25	78	58	1
Blizzard Oreo Cookies	1 sm (9.9 oz)	550	20	81	61	1

FOOD	PORTION	CAL	FAT	CARB	SUGAR	FIBER
Blizzard Reese's Peanut Butter Cups	1 sm (10 oz)	530	21	74	62	1
Blizzard Snickers	1 sm (11.4 oz)	670	26	99	83	1
Blizzard Strawberry CheeseQuake	1 sm (9.8 oz)	510	20	69	54	0
Buster Bar Treat	1 (5.2 oz)	460	28	44	36	2
Cake 8 In Round	⅛ (7.3 oz)	410	15	59	46	1
Cake Blizzard Chocolate Xtreme 8 In	⅛ cake (8.7 oz)	620	29	83	64	2
Cake Blizzard Oreo 8 In	⅛ (8 oz)	550	24	75	58	1
Cake Blizzard Reese's Peanut Butter Cups 8 In	⅛ (8.4 oz)	580	27	76	62	2
Cone Chocolate	1 sm (5 oz)	240	7	37	25	0
Cone Vanilla	1 sm (5 oz)	230	7	36	26	0
Cone Dipped Chocolate	1 sm (5.5 oz)	330	15	42	31	0
Cone Kids' Chocolate	1 (3.5 oz)	180	5	28	17	0
Cone Kids' Dipped Chocolate	1 (3.7 oz)	220	9	30	30	0
Cone Kids' Vanilla	1 (3.5 oz)	170	5	27	18	0
Dilly Bar Butterscotch	1 (3 oz)	210	11	24	20	0
Dilly Bar Cherry	1 (3 oz)	210	12	24	20	0
Dilly Bar Chocolate	1 (3 oz)	240	15	24	20	1
Dilly Bar Chocolate Mint	1 (3 oz)	240	15	24	20	1
Dilly Bar Heath	1 (3 oz)	220	13	25	22	0
Dilly Bar No Sugar Added	1 (3 oz)	190	13	24	5	5
DQ Heart Cake	1/10 cake (5 oz)	290	11	42	32	1
DQ Log Cake	⅛ cake (5 oz)	310	12	44	33	1
DQ Sandwich	1 (3 oz)	190	5	31	18	1
DQ Sheet Cake	1/24 cake (5.4 oz)	320	13	47	35	1

FOOD	PORTION	CAL	FAT	CARB	SUGAR	FIBER
Fudge Bar	1 (2.3 oz)	50	0	13	4	6
Oreo Brownie Earthquake Treat	1 (10.7 oz)	740	27	149	86	2
Parfait Peanut Buster	1 (10.6 oz)	710	31	96	71	3
Peanut Butter Bash	1 (9 oz)	580	27	73	55	2
Pecan Mudslide Treat	1 (9.6 oz)	640	30	83	58	2
Starkiss Bar Cherry	1 (3 oz)	80	0	21	17	0
Starkiss Bar Stars & Stripes	1 (3 oz)	80	0	21	17	0
Strawberry Shortcake	1 (8.9 oz)	480	17	75	62	1
Sundae Banana	1 sm (5.7 oz)	230	7	37	29	1
Sundae Caramel	1 sm (5.7 oz)	300	8	50	35	0
Sundae Cherry	1 sm (5.7 oz)	240	7	39	33	0
Sundae Chocolate	1 sm (5.7 oz)	280	8	48	41	1
Sundae Hot Fudge	1 sm (5.7 oz)	300	10	46	36	0
Sundae Marshmallow	1 sm (5.7 oz)	290	7	50	42	0
Sundae Peanut Butter	1 sm (5.7 oz)	390	22	39	28	1
Sundae Pineapple	1 sm (5.7 oz)	230	7	38	32	0
Sundae Strawberry	1 sm (6.7 oz)	260	7	44	36	0
Sundae Waffle Bowl Chocolate Covered Strawberry	1 (11.2 oz)	760	38	96	74	2
Sundae Waffle Bowl Fudge Brownie Temptation	1 (11.2 oz)	940	48	121	89	2
Sundae Waffle Bowl Turtle	1 (10.7 oz)	810	35	115	72	2
Vanilla Orange Bar	1 (2.3 oz)	60	0	18	4	6
Waffle Cone Chocolate Coated w/ Soft Serve	1 (8.6 oz)	540	21	77	57	1
Waffle Cone w/ Soft Serve	1 (7.9 oz)	420	13	67	47	0

FOOD	PORTION	CAL	FAT	CARB	SUGAR	FIBER
MAIN MENU SELECTIONS						
Breaded Mushrooms	1 serv (4 oz)	250	9	36	1	2
Burger DQ Ultimate	1 (9 oz)	780	48	34	7	1
Cheese Curds	1 serv (4.9 oz)	550	45	0	0	0
Cheeseburger Deluxe	1 (6.2 oz)	400	19	35	9	1
Cheeseburger Deluxe Double	1 (8.7 oz)	640	34	35	9	1
Cheeseburger Original	1 (5.5 oz)	400	18	34	8	1
Cheeseburger Original Double	1 (7.9 oz)	630	34	34	9	1
Chick Strip Basket w/ Country Gravy	4 pieces (15.2 oz)	1030	53	105	4	9
Chili	1 cup (8 oz)	470	16	54	2	2
Chili Cheese Dog	1 (4.8 oz)	380	24	23	3	1
Chili Cheese Dog Foot-Long	1 (8.2 oz)	670	43	40	5	2
Chili Dog	1 (4.8 oz)	330	20	24	5	1
Corn Dog	1 (2.6 oz)	260	15	26	7	1
French Fries	1 reg (4 oz)	310	13	43	0	3
Fries Chili Cheese	1 serv (15 oz)	1020	51	116	4	10
GrillBurger ½ Lb FlameThrower	1 (11.3 oz)	1000	74	40	9	2
GrillBurger ½ Lb w/ Cheese	1 (11.3 oz)	800	51	44	13	3
GrillBurger ¼ Lb Bacon Cheese	1 (8.5 oz)	630	37	44	13	2
GrillBurger ¼ Lb Mushroom Swiss	1 (6.9 oz)	570	35	39	8	5
GrillBurger ¼ Lb w/ Cheese	1 (8.1 oz)	540	30	44	13	3
Hamburger Deluxe	1 (5.7 oz)	350	14	34	9	1

FOOD	PORTION	CAL	FAT	CARB	SUGAR	FIBER
Hamburger Deluxe Double	1 (7.7 oz)	540	26	34	9	1
Hot Dog	1 (4 oz)	290	17	22	4	1
Hot Dog Foot-Long	1 (7 oz)	560	35	39	6	2
Onion Rings	1 serv (4 oz)	360	16	47	3	2
Popcorn Shrimp Basket	1 (15 oz)	1000	49	116	3	7
Quesadilla Basket Chicken	1 (18 oz)	1160	60	110	7	6
Quesadilla Basket Veggie	1 (16.2 oz)	1100	59	110	6	7
Sandwich Barbecue Beef	1 (5 oz)	350	14	40	8	2
Sandwich Barbecue Pork	1 (5 oz)	310	9	41	9	2
Sandwich Crispy Chicken	1 (7.4 oz)	600	30	59	8	7
Sandwich Crispy Fish	1 (6.5 oz)	470	22	53	7	2
Sandwich Crispy Flame Thrower Chicken	1 (9.4 oz)	830	51	63	9	8
Sandwich Grilled Chicken	1 (6.3 oz)	360	15	32	5	1
Sandwich Iron Grilled Cheese	1 (5 oz)	420	14	52	3	2
Sandwich Iron Grilled Classic Club	1 (9.4 oz)	600	24	55	4	3
Sandwich Iron Grilled Supreme BLT	1 (6 oz)	600	34	40	2	2
Sandwich Iron Grilled Turkey	1 (8.2 oz)	550	23	43	2	2
Wrap Crispy Chicken	1 (4 oz)	350	21	30	1	2
Wrap Crispy Flame Thrower Chicken	1 (4 oz)	360	22	30	1	2
Wrap Grilled Chicken	1 (4 oz)	280	15	22	1	1

FOOD	PORTION	CAL	FAT	CARB	SUGAR	FIBER
SALAD DRESSINGS AND SAUCES						
Country Gravy	1 serv (4 oz)	90	6	8	1	0
Dipping Sauce Bleu Cheese	1 serv (2 oz)	210	21	5	4	0
Dipping Sauce Honey Mustard	1 serv (2 oz)	250	21	16	9	0
Dipping Sauce Ranch	1 serv (2 oz)	320	35	2	2	0
Dipping Sauce Sweet & Sour	1 serv (2 oz)	90	0	24	22	0
Dipping Sauce Wild Buffalo	1 serv (1.3 oz)	110	12	1	0	0
Dressing Italian Fat Free	1 serv (1.5 oz)	15	0	4	2	0
Dressing Ranch Fat Free	1 serv (1.5 oz)	35	0	5	4	0
Dressing Red French Fat Free	1 serv (1.5 oz)	40	0	10	7	0
Dressing Thousand Island Fat Free	1 serv (1.5 oz)	60	0	16	10	0
SALADS						
Crispy Chicken	1 (14.9 oz)	470	26	29	8	7
Grilled Chicken	1 (14.9 oz)	330	15	13	8	4
Side Salad	1 (4 oz)	20	0	5	3	2

DENNY'S

FOOD	PORTION	CAL	FAT	CARB	SUGAR	FIBER
BEVERAGES						
Apple Juice	1 sm (10 oz)	141	0	52	11	0
Cappuccino	1 (8 oz)	100	2	28	24	1
Chocolate Milk	1 sm (10 oz)	160	3	26	25	1
Hot Chocolate	1 (8 oz)	100	2	28	24	1
Iced Tea Raspberry	1 serv (16 oz)	78	0	21	–	0
Lemonade	1 serv (15 oz)	150	0	35	31	0
Milk	1 sm (10 oz)	130	5	12	12	0
Orange Juice	1 sm (10 oz)	140	0	34	30	0
Ruby Red Grapefruit	1 sm (10 oz)	164	0	40	36	0
Tomato Juice	1 sm (10 oz)	56	0	11	–	2

FOOD	PORTION	CAL	FAT	CARB	SUGAR	FIBER
BREAKFAST SELECTIONS						
All American Slam w/o Choices	1 serv (10 oz)	800	68	5	1	1
Bacon Turkey	4 slices	150	8	1	0	0
Bacon Strips	4	140	11	1	1	0
Banana	1	110	0	29	14	4
Egg	1 (2 oz)	120	11	0	0	0
Egg Whites	1 serv (4 oz)	50	1	1	0	0
English Muffin w/o Margarine	1	130	1	25	1	1
Grand Slam Slugger w/o Choices	1 serv (13 oz)	780	42	71	13	3
Grapes	1 serv (3 oz)	55	0	29	13	4
Grits w/ Margarine	1 serv (12 oz)	220	3	44	0	3
Ham Slice Grilled Honey	1 (3 oz)	120	5	8	6	0
Hash Browns	1 serv	210	12	26	1	2
Hashed Browns Cheddar Cheese	1 serv (5 oz)	300	19	26	2	2
Hashed Browns Everything	1 serv (8 oz)	340	21	33	3	2
Lumberjack Slam w/o Choices	1 serv (15 oz)	940	47	80	19	4
Moon Over My Hammy Omelette w/ Hash Browns w/o Choices	1 serv (16 oz)	770	53	31	5	2
Oatmeal w/ Milk	1 serv (16 oz)	290	8	39	20	4
Omelette Southern w/ Hash Browns w/o Bread	1 serv (18 oz)	1070	80	47	3	4
Omelette Veggie Cheese w/o Choices	1 serv (13 oz)	460	33	9	4	2
Omelette w/ Hash Browns w/o Choices	1 serv (16 oz)	700	46	32	5	2

FOOD	PORTION	CAL	FAT	CARB	SUGAR	FIBER
Pancakes Buttermilk	2	330	4	67	12	2
Platter Chocolate Chip Pancakes w/o Meat	1 serv (13 oz)	640	22	87	28	4
Sausage Links	4 (3 oz)	370	34	4	0	3
Senior Omelette w/o Choices	1 serv (9 oz)	470	37	7	3	1
Senior Scrambled Eggs & Cheddar	1 serv (13 oz)	870	48	72	12	4
Senior Slam Belgian Waffle w/ Egg w/o Choices	1 serv (8 oz)	450	31	29	1	0
Skillet Bananas Foster French Toast w/o Meat	1 serv (15 oz)	860	33	107	44	3
Slam Belgian Waffle w/ Margarine w/o Syrup	1 serv (13 oz)	1030	77	50	2	2
Slam Everyday Value w/ Bacon	1 serv (12 oz)	650	30	69	13	2
Slam Everyday Value w/ Sausage	1 serv (13 oz)	760	42	70	12	3
Slam French Toast	1 serv (15 oz)	940	55	66	13	3
Ultimate Omelette w/o Choices	1 serv (12 oz)	620	48	8	3	2
CHILDREN'S MENU SELECTIONS						
Jr Grand Slam	1 serv (5 oz)	380	19	39	7	2
Oreo Blender Blaster	1 serv (12 oz)	680	33	88	65	3
Pancake Softball w/ Meat	1 serv (4 oz)	250	11	30	5	1
Pancakes Chocolate Chip-In	1 serv (7 oz)	450	18	61	17	3
Pit Stop Pizza w/o Side	1 serv (8 oz)	590	26	70	4	5
Slam Dribblers	1 serv (6 oz)	410	11	74	41	2

FOOD	PORTION	CAL	FAT	CARB	SUGAR	FIBER
Slap Shot Slider w/o Side	1 (4 oz)	310	15	22	3	1
Spaghetti Set Go w/o Side	1 serv (6 oz)	260	7	40	4	7
Track & Cheese w/o Side	1 serv (7 oz)	340	11	48	11	2
DESSERTS						
Apple Crisp A La Mode	1 serv (13 oz)	740	21	134	89	5
Blender Blaster Oreo	1 serv (14 oz)	890	44	113	77	3
Cake Carrot	1 serv (8 oz)	820	45	100	77	2
Cake Hershey's Chocolate	1 serv (5 oz)	580	28	75	55	2
Cheesecake New York Style	1 serv (7 oz)	640	41	58	44	0
Float Rootbeer or Cola	1 (16 oz)	430	17	69	63	0
Hot Fudge Brownie A La Mode	1 serv (9 oz)	830	37	122	95	4
Milkshake	1 (12 oz)	560	26	76	65	tr
Pie Apple	1 serv (7 oz)	480	22	67	35	3
Pie Chocolate Peanut Butter Silk	1 serv (6 oz)	680	47	59	39	4
Pie Coconut Cream	1 serv (7 oz)	630	39	65	43	1
Pie Cookies & Cream	1 serv (7 oz)	630	39	67	44	3
Pie French Silk	1 serv (5 oz)	770	57	59	38	2
Pie Key Lime	1 serv (7 oz)	560	20	87	68	0
Pie Lemon Meringue	1 serv (7 oz)	500	19	82	56	1
Pie Pecan	1 serv (7 oz)	730	36	98	36	2
Pie Pumpkin	1 serv (7 oz)	500	18	77	34	3
Sundae Oreo	1 (9 oz)	760	37	103	76	3
Sundae Single Scoop	1 (4 oz)	300	16	36	16	1
Topping Cherry	1 serv (2 oz)	57	0	14	12	0
Topping Chocolate	1 serv (2 oz)	133	1	34	32	1
Topping Fudge	1 serv (2 oz)	201	10	30	29	1
Topping Strawberry	1 serv (2 oz)	77	1	17	–	1

FOOD	PORTION	CAL	FAT	CARB	SUGAR	FIBER
MAIN MENU SELECTIONS						
Basket Of Puppies w/o Syrup	10 pieces	520	11	94	16	3
Burger Bacon Cheddar w/o Choices	1 (15 oz)	900	50	50	10	3
Burger Classic & Fries	1 serv (19 oz)	1190	62	101	11	8
Burger Fit Fare Veggie w/o Choice	1 (10 oz)	460	10	65	13	8
Burger Mushroom Swiss w/o Choices	1 (18 oz)	880	49	56	13	4
Burger Veggie w/ Dressing w/o Choices	1 (11 oz)	520	12	75	23	9
Burger Western w/o Choice	1 (17 oz)	1120	61	73	17	6
Cheeseburger Double w/o Choices	1 serv (23 oz)	1420	87	53	12	4
Chicken Strips Sweet & Tangy BBQ w/o Dipping Sauce	1 serv (13 oz)	820	30	83	29	5
Chicken Wings Sweet & Tangy BBQ	1 serv (8 oz)	450	18	40	38	1
Chicken Wings w/ Buffalo Sauce	1 serv (8 oz)	330	20	3	2	1
Chopped Steak Mushroom Swiss w/o Choices	1 serv (13 oz)	900	66	13	4	1
Chopped Steak Spicy Cowboy w/o Choices	1 serv (15 oz)	1050	63	57	41	3
Club Sandwich w/o Choices	1 (10 oz)	550	32	39	7	3
Coleslaw	1 serv (5 oz)	260	22	15	12	3
Corn	1 serv (4 oz)	130	3	26	3	1

FOOD	PORTION	CAL	FAT	CARB	SUGAR	FIBER
Cottage Cheese	1 serv (3 oz)	70	2	5	3	0
Country Fried Steak w/ Gravy	1 serv (13 oz)	990	65	54	0	6
Dippable Veggies w/o Dressing	1 serv (2.5 oz)	30	0	5	3	1
Fiesta Corn	1 serv (4 oz)	100	0	21	4	3
Fit Fare Grilled Tilapia	1 serv (17 oz)	600	11	66	7	3
Fit Fare Sweet & Tangy BBQ Chicken w/ Vegetables & Tomatoes	1 serv (13 oz)	640	14	56	32	2
French Fries Salted	1 serv (5 oz)	430	23	50	0	5
Fried Shrimp Platter w/ Fries	1 serv (18 oz)	1050	59	109	24	13
Garlic Dinner Bread	2 pieces	170	9	21	0	1
Green Beans	1 serv (3 oz)	25	0	4	2	2
Haddock Fillet w/o Bread	1 serv (20 oz)	1330	81	116	18	8
Homestyle Meatloaf w/ Gravy	1 serv (7 oz)	600	46	14	33	0
Lemon Pepper Tilapia w/o Choices	1 serv (13 oz)	640	27	39	3	2
Mashed Potatoes Plain	1 serv (5 oz)	170	7	76	1	1
Mashed Potatoes Smoked Cheddar	1 serv (4 oz)	120	5	49	1	1
Mozzarella Sticks w/o Sauce	1 serv (8 oz)	560	20	58	4	2
Onion Rings	1 serv (5 oz)	520	36	48	6	3
Quesadilla Cheese	1 (8 oz)	690	42	48	5	6
Ranchero Tilapia w/o Bread	1 serv (19 oz)	450	15	56	4	4
Sampler w/o Sauce	1 serv (17 oz)	1380	71	139	11	6

FOOD	PORTION	CAL	FAT	CARB	SUGAR	FIBER
Sandwich Bacon Lettuce & Tomato w/o Choices	1 (7 oz)	520	35	35	7	2
Sandwich Chicken Ranch Melt w/o Choices	1 serv (12 oz)	790	38	74	3	3
Sandwich Fried Cheese Melt w/ Marinara Sauce w/o Choices	1 (12 oz)	830	40	82	8	3
Sandwich Hickory Grilled Chicken w/o Choices	1 (15 oz)	1020	60	72	15	4
Sandwich Patty Melt w/o Choices	1 (13 oz)	1040	73	41	10	4
Sandwich Philly Melt Prime Rib w/o Choices	1 serv (13 oz)	670	36	52	5	3
Sandwich Pulled BBQ Chicken w/ Coleslaw	1 serv (14 oz)	670	23	96	53	4
Sandwich Smoked Chicken Melt w/o Choices	1 (12 oz)	840	45	72	11	3
Sandwich Spicy Buffalo Chicken Melt w/o Choices	1 (15 oz)	860	48	76	3	3
Sandwich The Super Bird w/o Choices	1 (11 oz)	620	31	52	6	4
Seasoned Fries	1 serv (5 oz)	510	33	48	0	5
Senior Country Fried Steak w/o Choices	1 serv (8 oz)	520	34	30	0	3
Senior Grilled Chicken w/o Choices	1 serv (5 oz)	200	6	0	0	0
Senior Grilled Shrimp Skewer w/o Choices	1 serv (8 oz)	280	6	36	2	2

FOOD	PORTION	CAL	FAT	CARB	SUGAR	FIBER
Senior Homestyle Meatloaf w/o Choices	1 serv (4 oz)	290	23	5	2	0
Senior Mini Burgers Bacon Cheddar w/o Choice	1 (11 oz)	720	39	46	7	2
Senior Sandwich Club w/o Choices	1 (10 oz)	570	34	37	7	4
Senior Sandwich Grilled Cheese Deluxe w/o Choices	1 (7 oz)	520	28	49	5	2
Senior Slam French Toast w/ Egg	1 serv (5 oz)	300	14	29	5	1
Senior Starter w/o Choice	1 serv (3 oz)	210	19	1	0	1
Shrimp Breaded	6	190	8	20	5	2
Shrimp Grilled Skewer	1	90	4	1	0	0
Skillet Bacon Chipotle Chicken w/o Sides	1 serv (7 oz)	360	18	4	3	0
Skillet Prime Rib Premium	1 serv (21 oz)	850	46	64	9	7
Skillet Santa Fe	1 serv (14 oz)	710	52	30	5	5
Skillet Ultimate	1 serv (15 oz)	740	56	34	5	6
Slamburger Bacon w/ Fries	1 serv (15 oz)	1030	59	61	9	2
Smothered Cheese Fries	1 serv (10 oz)	860	53	75	3	7
Spinach Sauteed	1 serv (2 oz)	70	6	5	0	2
Spinach w/ Pico De Gallo	1 serv (3 oz)	110	8	6	1	2
T-Bone Steak w/o Choices	1 serv (12 oz)	640	42	6	0	0
T-Bone Steak & Breaded Shrimp	1 serv (13 oz)	830	50	25	5	2

FOOD	PORTION	CAL	FAT	CARB	SUGAR	FIBER
T-Bone Steak & Shrimp Skewer	1 serv (12 oz)	730	46	6	0	0
The Big Dipper w/ Salsa w/o Dipping Sauce	10 pieces	1230	50	145	13	14
Three Dip & Chips	1 serv (12 oz)	560	25	72	5	7
Tomatoes Slices	2	10	0	2	2	1
Tsing Tsing Chicken	1 serv (14 oz)	900	26	114	28	4
Vegetable Rice Pilaf	1 serv (5 oz)	190	3	35	2	2
Wrap Buffalo Chicken	1 (14 oz)	830	28	108	5	8
Zesty Nachos	1 serv (22 oz)	1340	61	140	10	12
SALAD DRESSINGS AND TOPPINGS						
BBQ Sweet & Spicy	1 serv (1.5 oz)	110	0	30	0	1
Cherry Topping	1 serv (3 oz)	86	0	21	12	0
Croutons	1 serv (0.25 oz)	90	3	15	0	0
Dressing Bleu Cheese	1 serv (1 oz)	110	11	1	1	0
Dressing Caesar	1 serv (1 oz)	100	10	0	0	0
Dressing French	1 serv (1 oz)	74	5	8	4	0
Dressing Honey Mustard	1 serv (1 oz)	160	15	5	4	0
Dressing Italian Fat Free	1 serv (1 oz)	9	0	3	2	0
Dressing Ranch	1 serv (1 oz)	130	14	0	0	0
Dressing Ranch Fat Free	1 serv (1 oz)	25	0	5	1	1
Dressing Thousand Island	1 serv (1 oz)	107	10	5	4	0
Pico De Gallo	1 serv (3 oz)	21	0	5	3	1
Sour Cream	1 serv (1.5 oz)	91	9	2	0	0
Syrup Maple Flavored	3 tbsp (1.5 oz)	143	0	36	28	0
Syrup Sugar Free Maple	1 serv (1.5 oz)	23	0	9	1	0
Vinaigrette Balsamic Low Fat	1 serv (1 oz)	35	1	7	7	0
Whipped Margarine	1 tbsp	50	6	0	0	0

FOOD	PORTION	CAL	FAT	CARB	SUGAR	FIBER
SALADS						
Cranberry Apple w/ Chicken w/o Dressing	1 serv (11 oz)	320	10	22	17	3
Deluxe Salad w/ Chicken Strips w/o Choices	1 serv (18 oz)	590	29	43	7	4
Deluxe Salad w/ Grilled Chicken Breast w/o Choices	1 serv (17 oz)	340	13	13	7	4
Nacho	1 serv (20 oz)	850	52	48	19	9
SOUPS						
Broccoli & Cheddar	1 serv (12 oz)	370	16	48	14	7
Chicken Noodle	1 serv (12 oz)	140	4	35	6	2
Clam Chowder	1 serv (12 oz)	270	17	24	12	1
Loaded Baked Potato	1 serv (12 oz)	310	23	22	5	2
Vegetable Beef	1 serv (12 oz)	140	5	17	3	3

DOMINO'S PIZZA

FOOD	PORTION	CAL	FAT	CARB	SUGAR	FIBER
OTHER MENU SELECTIONS						
Breadsticks	8	870	50	89	4	3
Buffalo Chicken Kickers	1 serv	510	21	36	0	7
Cheesy Bread	1 serv	930	51	91	5	3
Chocolate Lava Crunch Cakes	2	690	34	93	62	3
Cinna Stix	8	940	49	109	24	4
PIZZA MEDIUM						
Deep Dish Marinara Cheese	⅛ pie	219	9	27	2	3
Hand Tossed Marinara Cheese	⅛ pie	190	7	25	2	1
Thin Crust Marinara Cheese	¼ pie	141	12	14	2	1
TOPPINGS FOR 1 MEDIUM PIZZA						
Anchovies	1 serv	110	8	63	0	0
Bacon	1 serv	340	26	6	3	0

FOOD	PORTION	CAL	FAT	CARB	SUGAR	FIBER
Banana Peppers	1 serv	15	0	3	3	2
Beef	1 serv	300	26	0	0	–
Cheddar Cheese	1 serv	230	19	1	0	0
Cheese American	1 serv	310	26	3	2	0
Cheese Provolone	1 serv	200	16	1	0	0
Chicken	1 serv	140	5	3	0	0
Chorizo	1 serv	90	4	1	1	0
Feta Cheese	1 serv	90	6	1	0	0
Garlic	1 serv	40	0	9	0	1
Green Chile Pepper	1 serv	10	0	3	1	2
Green Pepper	1 serv	10	0	3	2	1
Ham	1 serv	90	5	0	0	0
Jalapenos	1 serv	15	0	3	3	2
Mushroom	1 serv	20	0	2	0	1
Olives Black	1 serv	100	10	2	0	2
Olives Green	1 serv	100	10	2	0	2
Onion	1 serv	15	0	4	0	1
Parmesan Shredded	1 serv	170	12	1	0	0
Pepperoni	1 serv	240	21	0	–	0
Philly Steak	1 serv	90	3	2	1	0
Pineapple	1 serv	60	0	16	14	1
Red Pepper Roasted	1 serv	10	0	2	1	1
Salami	1 serv	220	18	1	1	0
Sausage Italian	1 serv	350	30	9	4	0
Spinach	1 serv	10	0	2	0	1
Tomato	1 serv	20	0	5	3	2
Wing Sauce	1 serv	10	0	2	1	1

DONATOS PIZZA

PIZZA

FOOD	PORTION	CAL	FAT	CARB	SUGAR	FIBER
Hand Tossed Chicken Bacon Club	2 slices	780	46	61	–	5
Hand Tossed Chicken Spinach Mozzarella	2 slices	587	25	61	–	4

FOOD	PORTION	CAL	FAT	CARB	SUGAR	FIBER
Hand Tossed Chicken Vegy Medley	2 slices	517	17	63	–	5
Hand Tossed Classic Trio	2 slices	640	30	66	–	6
Hand Tossed Founder's Favorite	2 slices	678	31	66	–	5
Hand Tossed Fresh Mozzarella Trio	2 slices	690	34	66	–	6
Hand Tossed Hawaiian	2 slices	578	22	69	–	6
Hand Tossed Margherita	2 slices	583	27	60	–	4
Hand Tossed Mariachi Beef	2 slices	591	24	68	–	5
Hand Tossed Mariachi Chicken	2 slices	617	24	68	–	5
Hand Tossed Pepperoni	2 slices	499	27	65	–	5
Hand Tossed Pepperoni Zinger	2 slices	645	30	65	–	5
Hand Tossed Serious Cheese	2 slices	597	25	65	–	5
Hand Tossed Serious Meat	2 slices	735	37	66	–	5
Hand Tossed Vegy	2 slices	550	19	70	–	6
Hand Tossed The Works	2 slices	669	31	68	–	6
Thicker Crust Chicken Vegy Medley Large	¼ pie	580	20	66	–	5
Thicker Crust Founder's Favorite Large	¼ pie	780	36	70	–	5
Thicker Crust Hawaiian Large	¼ pie	680	26	76	–	6
Thicker Crust Mariachi Beef Large	¼ pie	710	31	73	–	6
Thicker Crust Mariachi Chicken Large	¼ pie	710	28	74	–	5
Thicker Crust Serious Meat Large	¼ pie	850	42	71	–	5

FOOD	PORTION	CAL	FAT	CARB	SUGAR	FIBER
Thicker Crust The Works Large	¼ pie	770	35	74	–	6
Thicker Crust Vegy Large	¼ pie	630	23	75	–	7
Thin Crust Chicken Medley Vegy Large	¼ pie	497	20	51	–	3
Thin Crust Classic Trio Large	¼ pie	674	37	52	–	3
Thin Crust Founder's Favorite Large	¼ pie	702	38	52	–	2
Thin Crust Hawaiian Large	¼ pie	588	27	56	–	4
Thin Crust Mariachi Beef Large	¼ pie	630	32	55	–	3
Thin Crust Mariachi Chicken Large	¼ pie	639	30	56	–	3
Thin Crust Pepperoni Large	¼ pie	627	34	50	–	2
Thin Crust Serious Cheese Large	¼ pie	710	31	69	–	5
Thin Crust Serious Meat Large	¼ pie	736	42	52	–	3
Thin Crust The Works	¼ pie	689	37	56	–	4
Thin Crust Vegy Large	¼ pie	544	24	57	–	4
SALAD DRESSINGS						
House Italian	1 serv (1.5 oz)	230	24	1	–	0
Italian Light	1 serv (1.5 oz)	20	1	2	–	0
Pizza Dip Chicken Bacon Ranch	1 serv (3 oz)	450	47	4	–	0
SALADS						
Chicken Harvest w/o Dressing Entree	1	540	32	32	–	6
Harvest Side	1 serv	81	3	13	–	2

FOOD	PORTION	CAL	FAT	CARB	SUGAR	FIBER
Italian Chef w/o Dressing Entree	1	290	20	8	–	1
Italian Side w/o Dressing	1	110	7	3	–	1
SIDES AND SUBS						
3 Cheese Garlic Bread	2 pieces	174	9	16	–	1
Big Don White Italian	1	717	34	68	–	3
Breadsticks w/ Pizza Sauce	2	261	9	38	–	3
Buffalo Wings Hot	5	597	48	11	–	0
Buffalo Wings Mild	5	618	48	13	–	0
Fresh Vegy Wheat	1	532	19	71	–	8
Stromboli 3 Meat	1	689	31	67	–	5
Stromboli Cheese	1	693	31	66	–	5
Stromboli Deluxe	1	613	25	68	–	5
Stromboli Pepperoni	1	716	34	67	–	5
Stromboli Vegy	1	606	24	69	–	5

DUNKIN' DONUTS

FOOD	PORTION	CAL	FAT	CARB	SUGAR	FIBER
BAGELS						
Blueberry	1	330	3	65	10	5
Cinnamon Raisin	1	330	4	65	13	5
Everything	1	350	5	66	5	5
Garlic	1	340	3	68	5	6
Multigrain	1	390	8	65	7	9
Onion	1	310	2	63	3	3
Plain	1	320	3	63	5	5
Poppy Seed	1	350	6	64	5	5
Salt	1	320	3	63	5	5
Sesame	1	360	6	63	5	5
Wheat	1	320	4	61	4	5
BAKED SELECTIONS						
Apple Fritter	1	400	15	63	22	2
Biscuit	1	280	14	32	2	1

FOOD	PORTION	CAL	FAT	CARB	SUGAR	FIBER
Bismark Chocolate Iced	1	350	14	53	22	1
Brownie	1	430	23	56	47	1
Coffee Roll	1	370	18	49	17	2
Coffee Roll Chocolate Frosted	1	380	19	50	18	2
Coffee Roll Maple Frosted	1	380	18	50	19	2
Coffee Roll Vanilla Frosted	1	380	18	50	19	2
Cookie Chocolate Chunk	1	540	23	80	48	3
Cookie Oatmeal Raisin	1	480	14	83	51	5
Croissant Plain	1	310	16	35	4	1
Danish Apple Cheese	1	330	16	41	18	1
Danish Cheese	1	330	17	39	17	1
Danish Strawberry Cheese	1	320	16	40	18	1
Donut Apple Crumb	1	460	14	80	49	2
Donut Apple N' Spice	1	240	11	32	8	1
Donut Bavarian Kreme	1	250	12	31	9	1
Donut Blueberry Cake	1	330	18	38	19	1
Donut Blueberry Crumb	1	470	14	84	52	2
Donut Boston Kreme	1	280	12	38	16	1
Donut Bow Tie	1	310	15	39	15	1
Donut Chocolate Coconut	1	340	18	42	24	2
Donut Chocolate Frosted	1	340	19	38	19	1
Donut Chocolate Glazed Cake	1	280	15	33	16	1
Donut Chocolate Kreme Filled	1	310	16	37	17	1
Donut Cinnamon	1	290	18	30	12	1
Donut Double Chocolate Cake	1	290	16	34	17	1

FOOD	PORTION	CAL	FAT	CARB	SUGAR	FIBER
Donut Glazed	1	220	9	31	12	1
Donut Glazed Cake	1	320	18	37	18	1
Donut Jelly Filled	1	260	11	36	6	1
Donut Maple Frosted	1	230	10	33	14	1
Donut Marble Frosted	1	230	10	32	13	1
Donut Old Fashioned	1	280	18	27	9	1
Donut Powdered	1	300	18	30	12	1
Donut Strawberry Frosted	1	230	10	33	14	1
Donut Sugar Raised	1	190	9	22	4	1
Donut Triple Chocolate	1	420	27	41	22	2
Donut Vanilla Kreme Filled	1	320	17	37	18	1
Éclair	1	350	14	53	22	1
English Muffin	1	160	2	31	2	2
French Cruller	1	250	20	18	10	0
Fritter Glazed	1	400	15	63	22	2
Muffin Blueberry	1	510	16	87	51	2
Muffin Blueberry Reduced Fat	1	450	10	86	45	2
Muffin Chocolate Chip	1	630	23	98	59	3
Muffin Coffee Cake	1	660	26	98	57	1
Muffin Corn	1	510	17	84	36	1
Muffin Cranberry Orange Low Fat	1	390	3	83	42	4
Muffin Honey Bran Raisin	1	500	14	86	48	5
Muffin Triple Chocolate	1	660	33	84	47	4
Munchkin Glazed Cake	1	60	3	8	4	0
Munchkins Cinnamon Cake	1	60	3	6	2	0
Munchkins Glazed	1	50	3	7	3	0
Munchkins Glazed Chocolate Cake	1	60	3	8	4	0

FOOD	PORTION	CAL	FAT	CARB	SUGAR	FIBER
Munchkins Jelly Filled	1	60	3	8	1	0
Munchkins Plain Cake	1	50	3	5	2	0
Munchkins Powdered Cake	1	60	4	6	3	0
Munchkins Sugar Raised	1	40	3	5	1	0
Stick Cinnamon Cake	1	310	20	30	12	1
Stick Glazed Cake	1	340	20	38	20	1
Stick Glazed Chocolate Cake	1	390	25	40	17	2
Stick Jelly	1	400	20	54	20	1
Stick Plain Cake	1	300	20	26	9	1
Stick Powdered Cake	1	320	20	31	13	1
BEVERAGES						
Cappuccino	1 sm (10 oz)	80	4	7	7	0
Cappuccino Frozen w/ Skim Milk	1 sm (16 oz)	280	0	62	53	0
Cappuccino Frozen w/ Whole Milk	1 sm (16 oz)	300	4	61	53	0
Cappuccino w/ Sugar	1 sm (10 oz)	140	4	24	24	0
Coffee Blueberry	1 sm (10 oz)	15	0	2	0	0
Coffee Caramel	1 sm (10 oz)	10	0	2	0	0
Coffee Cinnamon	1 sm (10 oz)	15	0	2	0	0
Coffee Coconut	1 sm (10 oz)	10	0	1	0	0
Coffee French Vanilla	1 sm (10 oz)	10	0	1	0	0
Coffee Hazelnut	1 sm (10 oz)	10	0	1	0	0
Coffee Mocha	1 sm (10 oz)	110	0	26	23	1
Coffee Mocha w/ Cream	1 sm (10 oz)	170	6	27	23	1
Coffee Raspberry	1 sm (10 oz)	15	0	2	0	0
Coffee Regular	1 med (14 oz)	10	0	1	0	0
Coffee Regular	1 lg (20 oz)	10	0	2	0	0
Coffee Regular	1 extra lg	15	0	2	0	0
Coffee Regular	1 sm (10 oz)	5	0	1	0	0
Coffee Toasted Almond	1 sm (10 oz)	10	0	1	0	0
Coffee White Chocolate	1 sm (10 oz)	110	0	25	19	0

FOOD	PORTION	CAL	FAT	CARB	SUGAR	FIBER
Coffee White Chocolate w/ Cream	1 sm (10 oz)	160	6	26	19	0
Coffee w/ Cream	1 sm (10 oz)	60	6	2	0	0
Coffee w/ Milk	1 sm (10 oz)	25	1	2	1	0
Coffee w/ Milk & Sugar	1 sm (10 oz)	80	1	20	19	0
Coffee w/ Skim Milk	1 sm (10 oz)	15	0	3	2	0
Coffee w/ Skim Milk & Splenda	1 sm (10 oz)	25	0	5	2	0
Coffee w/ Skim Milk & Sugar	1 sm (10 oz)	70	0	20	19	0
Coffee w/ Splenda	1 sm (10 oz)	15	0	3	0	0
Coffee w/ Sugar	1 sm (10 oz)	60	0	18	17	0
Coolatta Coffee w/ Cream	1 sm (16 oz)	400	23	49	43	0
Coolatta Coffee w/ Milk	1 sm (16 oz)	240	4	50	49	0
Coolatta Coffee w/ Skim Milk	1 sm (16 oz)	210	0	51	49	0
Coolatta Strawberry Fruit	1 sm (16 oz)	300	0	72	65	0
Coolatta Tropicana Orange	1 sm (16 oz)	220	0	52	50	0
Coolatta Vanilla Bean	1 sm (16 oz)	430	6	90	86	0
Dunkaccino	1 sm (10 oz)	230	11	35	24	1
Espresso	1 (1.75 oz)	0	0	0	0	0
Espresso w/ Sugar	1 (1.75 oz)	30	0	7	7	0
Hot Chocolate	1 sm (10 oz)	210	7	39	30	2
Iced Coffee	1 sm (16 oz)	10	0	2	0	0
Iced Coffee Mocha w/ Cream	1 sm (16 oz)	180	6	28	23	1
Iced Coffee White Chocolate w/ Cream	1 sm (16 oz)	170	6	27	19	1
Iced Coffee w/ Cream	1 sm (16 oz)	70	6	3	0	0
Iced Coffee w/ Cream & Sugar	1 sm (16 oz)	120	6	20	17	0

FOOD	PORTION	CAL	FAT	CARB	SUGAR	FIBER
Iced Coffee w/ Milk	1 sm (16 oz)	30	1	3	1	0
Iced Coffee w/ Milk & Sugar	1 sm (16 oz)	90	1	21	19	0
Iced Coffee w/ Skim Milk	1 sm (16 oz)	20	0	2	2	0
Iced Coffee w/ Skim Milk & Sugar	1 sm (16 oz)	80	0	21	19	0
Iced Coffee w/ Sugar	1 sm (16 oz)	70	0	19	17	0
Iced Latte	1 sm (16 oz)	120	6	10	10	0
Iced Latte Caramel Swirl	1 sm (16 oz)	220	6	35	34	0
Iced Latte Caramel Swirl w/ Skim Milk	1 sm (16 oz)	180	0	36	35	0
Iced Latte Lite	1 med (24 oz)	120	0	19	15	0
Iced Latte Mocha Swirl	1 sm (16 oz)	220	6	35	32	1
Iced Latte Mocha Swirl w/ Skim Milk	1 sm (16 oz)	180	0	36	32	1
Iced Latte w/ Skim Milk	1 sm (16 oz)	70	0	11	10	0
Iced Latte w/ Skim Milk & Sugar	1 sm (16 oz)	130	0	28	27	0
Iced Latte w/ Sugar	1 sm (16 oz)	170	7	27	27	0
Latte	1 sm (10 oz)	120	6	10	10	0
Latte Caramel Swirl	1 sm (10 oz)	220	6	35	34	0
Latte Lite	1 sm (10 oz)	80	0	13	10	0
Latte Lite Vanilla	1 sm (10 oz)	90	0	14	10	0
Latte Mocha Raspberry	1 med (16 oz)	340	9	54	48	2
Latte Mocha Spice	1 med (16 oz)	330	9	53	48	2
Latte Mocha Swirl	1 sm (10 oz)	220	6	35	32	1
Latte w/ Sugar	1 sm (10 oz)	170	6	27	27	0
Latte White Chocolate	1 med (16 oz)	320	9	50	43	0
Tea Regular or Decaffeinated	1 (10 oz)	0	0	0	0	0
Tea w/ Milk	1 (10 oz)	20	1	1	1	0
Tea w/ Milk & Sugar	1 (10 oz)	80	1	19	19	0
Tea w/ Skim Milk	1 (10 oz)	10	0	2	2	0

FOOD	PORTION	CAL	FAT	CARB	SUGAR	FIBER
Tea w/ Skim Milk & Sugar	1 (10 oz)	70	0	19	19	0
Tea w/ Sugar	1 (10 oz)	60	0	17	17	0
Turbo Shot	1 sm (1.75 oz)	0	0	0	0	0
CREAM CHEESE						
Blueberry Reduced Fat	1 serv (1.75 oz)	150	9	15	11	0
Onion & Chive Reduced Fat	1 serv (1.75 oz)	130	11	6	3	0
Plain	1 serv (1.75 oz)	150	15	3	3	0
Plain Reduced Fat	1 serv (1.75 oz)	100	8	5	2	0
Salmon Reduced Fat	1 serv (1.75 oz)	140	11	6	3	0
Strawberry Reduced Fat	1 serv (1.75 oz)	150	10	15	11	0
Veggie Reduced Fat	1 serv (1.75 oz)	120	10	6	2	0
SANDWICHES						
Bagel Bacon Egg Cheese	1	510	17	66	7	5
Bagel Egg Cheese	1	470	14	66	7	5
Bagel Ham Egg Cheese	1	510	16	67	7	5
Bagel Sausage Egg Cheese	1	640	29	67	7	5
Biscuit Egg Cheese	1	430	26	36	4	1
Biscuit Sausage Egg Cheese	1	610	40	36	4	1
Croissant Bacon Egg Cheese	1	510	31	39	6	2
Croissant Egg Cheese	1	470	28	39	6	2
Croissant Ham Egg Cheese	1	510	30	39	6	2

FOOD	PORTION	CAL	FAT	CARB	SUGAR	FIBER
Croissant Original Chicken	1	640	35	53	9	2
English Muffin Bacon Egg Cheese	1	360	16	34	3	2
English Muffin Egg Cheese	1	320	13	34	3	2
English Muffin Egg White & Cheese	1	270	5	34	3	.2
English Muffin Ham Egg Cheese	1	360	15	35	3	2
English Muffin Ham Egg White & Cheese	1	310	7	34	3	2
English Muffin Sausage Egg Cheese	1	490	28	35	3	2
English Muffin Wheat Egg White & Cheese	1	260	6	33	3	2
English Muffin Wheat Ham Egg White & Cheese	1	300	8	33	3	2
Flatbread Egg White Turkey	1	280	6	37	5	3
Flatbread Egg White Veggie	1	290	9	39	4	3
Flatbread Grilled Cheese	1	380	18	35	2	1
Flatbread Ham & Cheese	1	320	11	34	2	1
Flatbread Turkey Cheddar & Bacon	1	410	20	36	2	1
Pressed Cuban	1	680	33	50	6	2
SOUPS						
Broccoli Cheddar	1 serv (8 oz)	190	11	14	5	2
Chicken Noodle	1 serv (8 oz)	130	3	19	1	1

FOOD	PORTION	CAL	FAT	CARB	SUGAR	FIBER
EINSTEIN BROS BAGELS						
BAGELS AND BREADS						
Bagel Asiago Cheese	1 (4 oz)	310	5	56	5	2
Bagel Black Russian	1 (3.9 oz)	280	4	57	4	3
Bagel Blueberry	1 (3.8 oz)	300	1	65	11	3
Bagel Chocolate Chip	1 (3.8 oz)	290	3	58	10	3
Bagel Cinnamon Raisin	1 (3.8 oz)	290	1	63	13	3
Bagel Cinnamon Sugar	1 (3.9 oz)	290	3	63	12	2
Bagel Cranberry	1 (3.8 oz)	270	1	60	12	2
Bagel Croutons	1 serv (1 oz)	90	5	12	1	0
Bagel Egg	1 (3.5 oz)	300	5	54	6	2
Bagel Everything	1 (3.7 oz)	270	2	56	5	2
Bagel Garlic	1 (3.7 oz)	270	3	56	5	2
Bagel Green Chili	1 (5.4 oz)	350	8	58	6	2
Bagel Honey Whole Wheat	1 (3.6 oz)	260	1	57	8	3
Bagel Onion	1 (3.7 oz)	270	1	59	5	2
Bagel Plain	1 (3.5 oz)	260	1	56	5	2
Bagel Poppy	1 (3.7 oz)	280	3	56	5	2
Bagel Potato	1 (3.5 oz)	270	4	52	5	2
Bagel Power	1 (4 oz)	310	5	61	16	4
Bagel Pumpernickel	1 (3.5 oz)	240	2	53	4	3
Bagel Salt	1 (3.7 oz)	260	1	56	5	2
Bagel Sesame	1 (3.7 oz)	280	3	56	5	2
Bagel Six Cheese	1 (4.3 oz)	330	6	56	5	2
Bagel Spinach Florentine	1 (4.7 oz)	340	8	57	5	2
Bagel Poppers Cinnamon Sugar	1 (5 oz)	450	9	85	29	4
Bagel Poppers Pretzel w/ Nacho Cheese	1 (5 oz)	320	8	55	6	2
Bagel Poppers Sweet Cream Cheese	1 (6 oz)	440	7	85	30	3

FOOD	PORTION	CAL	FAT	CARB	SUGAR	FIBER
Bagel Thin Singles Everything	1 (2 oz)	150	2	25	2	1
Bagel Thin Singles Honey Whole Wheat	1 (2 oz)	140	2	27	4	4
Bagel Thin Singles Plain	1 (2 oz)	140	1	25	2	1
Bread Ciabatta	1 serv (4.25 oz)	300	4	58	1	2
Pizza Bagel Pepperoni	1 (6 oz)	450	15	59	7	3
Roll Challah	1 (2.75 oz)	210	3	39	5	1
BEVERAGES						
Americano	1 reg (12 oz)	0	0	0	0	0
Barq's Root Beer	1 reg (20 oz)	260	0	75	75	0
Cafe Latte Nonfat Milk	1 reg (12 oz)	100	0	15	15	0
Cafe Latte Reduced Fat Milk	1 reg (12 oz)	150	7	15	15	0
Cappuccino	1 reg (12 oz)	140	8	11	11	0
Cappuccino Nonfat Milk	1 reg (12 oz)	70	0	11	11	0
Cappuccino Reduced Fat Milk	1 reg (12 oz)	90	4	9	8	0
Chai Tea Latte	1 reg (12 oz)	230	3	47	45	0
Chai Tea Latte Nonfat Milk	1 reg (12 oz)	210	0	47	45	0
Chai Tea Latte Reduced Fat Milk	1 reg (12 oz)	220	2	47	45	0
Coca-Cola	1 reg (20 oz)	230	0	65	65	0
Coca-Cola Cherry	1 reg (20 oz)	250	0	70	70	0
Coffee Black All Sizes	1	0	0	0	0	0
Diet Coke	1 reg (20 oz)	0	0	0	0	0
Espresso Single	1 (2 oz)	0	0	0	0	0
Fanta Orange	1 (20 oz)	270	0	73	73	0
Frozen Blended Cafe Caramel	1 (18 oz)	520	9	100	66	0

FOOD	PORTION	CAL	FAT	CARB	SUGAR	FIBER
Frozen Blended Cafe Mocha	1 (18 oz)	510	8	102	64	0
Frozen Blended Strawberry	1 (18 oz)	450	19	75	64	3
Frozen Blended Wild Berry	1 (18 oz)	350	3	77	62	5
Half & Half	1 oz	40	3	1	1	0
Hi-C Fruit Punch	1 (20 oz)	270	0	74	74	0
Hot Chocolate	1 reg (12 oz)	270	8	37	36	1
Hot Chocolate Nonfat Milk	1 reg (12 oz)	220	2	37	36	1
Iced Americano	1 med	0	0	0	0	0
Iced Coffee	1 med	0	0	0	0	0
Iced Latte	1 med (12 oz)	110	6	9	9	0
Iced Latte Nonfat Milk	1 med (16 oz)	60	0	9	9	0
Iced Latte Reduced Fat Milk	1 med (16 oz)	90	4	9	9	0
Iced Mocha	1 med (16 oz)	220	6	37	32	0
Iced Mocha Nonfat Milk	1 med (16 oz)	180	0	39	33	0
Iced Mocha Reduced Fat Milk	1 med (16 oz)	200	4	39	33	0
Macchiato Caramel	1 reg (12 oz)	300	8	49	43	0
Macchiato Caramel Nonfat Milk	1 reg (12 oz)	260	0	55	50	0
Macchiato Caramel Reduced Fat Milk	1 reg (12 oz)	290	5	55	50	0
Minute Maid Lemonade Lite	1 reg (20 oz)	40	0	10	5	0
Mocha	1 reg (12 oz)	260	9	37	32	0
Mocha Nonfat Milk	1 reg (12 oz)	180	0	37	32	0
Mocha Reduced Fat Milk	1 reg (12 oz)	220	5	37	32	0
Nestea Iced Tea Unsweetened	1 reg (20 oz)	0	0	0	0	0
Pibb Xtra	1 reg (20 oz)	250	0	65	65	0

FOOD	PORTION	CAL	FAT	CARB	SUGAR	FIBER
Skim Milk	8 oz	80	0	15	13	0
Sprite	1 reg (20 oz)	230	0	63	63	0
Whole Milk	8 oz	150	8	11	11	0
DESSERTS						
Cinnamon Twist	1 (4 oz)	370	18	20	19	2
Coffee Cake Apple Cinnamon	1 serv (7 oz)	700	28	108	57	1
Coffee Cake Chocolate Chip	1 serv (6.4 oz)	800	36	114	62	3
Coffee Cake Mixed Berry	1 serv (7 oz)	710	29	110	59	2
Cookie Chocolate Chip	1 (2.75 oz)	360	18	48	29	2
Cookie Chocolate Mudslide	1 (2.8 oz)	320	17	46	38	1
Cookie Iced Sugar	1 (3.7 oz)	480	15	80	51	1
Cookie Oatmeal Raisin	1 (3 oz)	320	11	54	31	2
Marshmallow Crispy Treat	1 (4 oz)	410	7	86	37	0
Muffin Blueberry	1 (5 oz)	480	23	64	35	1
Muffin Double Chocolate	1 (5 oz)	440	24	54	32	2
Muffin Strawberry White Chocolate	1 (6 oz)	500	22	71	44	1
Strudel Cinnamon Walnut	1 piece (6 oz)	640	35	72	26	4
SALAD DRESSINGS						
Caesar	1 serving (3 oz)	410	44	3	3	0
Vinaigrette Chipotle	1 serv (3 oz)	290	26	13	11	1
Vinaigrette Raspberry	1 serv (3 oz)	410	44	3	3	0
SALADS						
Bros Bistro	1 (10.5 oz)	820	68	37	29	7
Bros Bistro Half	1 serv (5.3 oz)	410	34	19	15	3

FOOD	PORTION	CAL	FAT	CARB	SUGAR	FIBER
Bros Bistro w/ Chicken	1 (14.5 oz)	950	71	39	29	7
Bros Bistro w/ Chicken Half	1 serv (7.3 oz)	470	36	19	14	4
Caesar	1 (9.5 oz)	600	53	22	5	4
Caesar Half	1 serv (4.5 oz)	280	25	8	2	2
Caesar w/ Chicken	1 (14 oz)	730	56	23	5	4
Caesar w/ Chicken Half	1 (6.5 oz)	340	27	9	2	2
Chipotle	1 (11.7 oz)	590	37	52	14	11
Chipotle Half	1 serv (5.8 oz)	290	19	26	7	5
Chipotle w/ Chicken	1 (15.7 oz)	720	41	54	15	11
Chipotle w/ Chicken Half	1 serv (7.8 oz)	360	20	27	7	5
Fruit	1 (11 oz)	140	0	36	30	3
Fruit Cup	1 (5 oz)	60	0	16	14	2
Potato	1 serv (3 oz)	160	12	13	1	1
SANDWICHES						
Bagel Asiago Tasty Turkey	1 (13 oz)	540	18	66	9	4
Bagel Dogs Asiago	1 (7 oz)	550	28	56	5	2
Bagel Dogs Chicken Apple	1 (5 oz)	290	13	30	6	1
Bagel Dogs Original	1 (7 oz)	540	27	56	5	2
Bagel Thin Asparagus Mushroom & Swiss	1 (6 oz)	290	13	30	5	5
Bagel Thin BLT w/ Avocado	1 (7 oz)	400	25	35	7	7
Bagel Thin Panini Bacon & Cheese	1 (6 oz)	400	20	31	4	4
Bagel Thin Tuna	1 (8 oz)	320	16	32	7	5
Bagel Thin Turkey	1 (8 oz)	270	6	32	5	2

FOOD	PORTION	CAL	FAT	CARB	SUGAR	FIBER
Bagel Thin Turkey Sausage w/ Salsa	1 (6 oz)	240	6	30	6	4
Breakfast Wrap Sante Fe	1 (12 oz)	720	37	60	8	6
Breakfast Wrap Spicy Elmo	1 (11 oz)	720	40	56	6	6
Challah Club Mex	1 (11 oz)	740	48	44	8	2
Deli Albacore Tuna Salad	1 (9 oz)	390	12	50	7	4
Deli Chicken Salad	1 (10 oz)	480	17	56	12	6
Deli Ham	1 (11 oz)	610	31	56	9	4
Deli Open Face Melts Ham & Swiss	1 (9 oz)	480	15	60	8	3
Deli Open Face Melts Turkey & Cheddar	1 (9 oz)	490	15	58	6	3
Deli Turkey Breast	1 (11 oz)	590	29	53	7	4
Egg Bacon & Cheddar	1 (9 oz)	590	25	59	8	2
Egg Cheese Only	1 (8 oz)	510	20	58	7	2
Egg Ham & Swiss	1 (10 oz)	550	20	59	8	2
Egg Nova Lox & Bagel	1 (9 oz)	480	18	62	10	3
Egg Paninis Southwest Turkey Sausage	1 (12 oz)	680	29	64	5	4
Egg Paninis Spinach & Bacon	1 (12 oz)	830	47	65	4	5
Egg Spinach Mushroom & Swiss	1 (10 oz)	560	24	61	8	3
Egg Turkey Sausage & Cheddar	1 (10 oz)	580	24	59	8	2
Nova Lox & Bagel	1 (9 oz)	480	18	62	10	3
Panini Italian Chicken	1 (13 oz)	820	41	65	3	5
Panini Turkey Club	1 (13 oz)	790	41	66	5	6
Wrap California Chicken	1 (16 oz)	720	35	66	7	9
Wrap Chipotle Turkey	1 (13 oz)	750	38	71	12	9
Wrap Turkey Tornado	1 (7 oz)	270	4	33	4	5

FOOD	PORTION	CAL	FAT	CARB	SUGAR	FIBER
SOUPS						
Broccoli Cheese	1 cup (8.75 oz)	290	21	15	5	2
Chicken Noodle	1 cup (8.75 oz)	120	4	13	1	2
Turkey Chili	1 cup (8.75 oz)	170	5	17	5	5
SPREADS						
Butter Blend	1 serv (1 oz)	170	18	0	0	0
Cream Cheese Light Whipped Plain	1 serv (1.25 oz)	80	6	4	3	2
Cream Cheese Onion & Chive	1 serv (1.25 oz)	120	11	5	2	0
Cream Cheese Plain	1 serv (1.25 oz)	120	12	2	2	0
Cream Cheese Reduced Fat Blueberry	1 serv (1.25 oz)	120	9	11	9	0
Cream Cheese Reduced Fat Garden Vegetable	1 serv (1.25 oz)	110	9	5	2	0
Cream Cheese Reduced Fat Garlic Herb	1 serv (1.25 oz)	110	9	5	2	0
Cream Cheese Reduced Fat Honey Almond	1 serv (1.25 oz)	120	9	11	7	0
Cream Cheese Reduced Fat Jalapeno Salsa	1 serv (1.25 oz)	110	9	5	2	0
Cream Cheese Reduced Fat Plain	1 serv (1.25 oz)	110	9	4	2	0
Cream Cheese Reduced Fat Strawberry	1 serv (1.25 oz)	120	9	9	7	0
Cream Cheese Reduced Fat Sundried Tomato Basil	1 serv (1.25 oz)	110	9	4	2	0

FOOD	PORTION	CAL	FAT	CARB	SUGAR	FIBER
Cream Cheese Smoked Salmon	1 serv (1.25 oz)	110	11	4	2	0
Honey Butter	1 serv (1 oz)	140	12	8	7	0
Hummus	1 serv (1 oz)	70	3	6	0	4
Mayo Ancho	1 serv (1.5 oz)	310	33	1	1	0
Mustard Creamy	1 serv (1.5 oz)	270	29	2	1	0
Mustard Deli	1 tsp (5 g)	5	0	0	0	0
Mustard Yellow	1 tbsp (5 g)	0	0	0	0	0
Peanut Butter Creamy	1 serv (2 oz)	330	28	12	5	4
Salsa Ancho Lime	1 serv (1.5 oz)	20	1	3	2	0
Spicy Roasted Tomato	1 serv (1.5 oz)	210	22	4	1	1
ELEVATION BURGER						
DESSERTS						
Cone 1 Scoop Chocolate	1 (5 oz)	310	13	42	31	0
Cone 1 Scoop Coffee	1 (5 oz)	310	13	40	28	0
Cone 1 Scoop Vanilla	1 (5 oz)	310	15	38	22	0
Cookie	1 lg	380	22	43	23	4
Cookies	3 sm	270	15	33	18	3
MAIN MENU SELECTIONS						
Cheeseburger	1	420	21	29	4	1
Cheeseburger Wrapped In Lettuce	1	280	19	2	1	1
Elevation Salad w/o Dressing	1 (7.8 oz)	230	17	21	15	5
Fresh Fries	1 boat	520	26	64	3	5
Grilled Cheese	1	330	17	29	4	1
Half-The-Guilt Burger #1	1	480	19	50	4	4
Half-The-Guilt Burger #1 Wrapped In Lettuce	1	340	17	23	1	4
Half-The-Guilt Burger #2	1	500	22	50	6	5
Hamburger	1	330	14	29	4	1
Hamburger Wrapped In Lettuce	1	190	12	2	1	1

FOOD	PORTION	CAL	FAT	CARB	SUGAR	FIBER
Mandarin Oranges	1 serv (4 oz)	70	0	18	18	1
Side Salad w/o Dressing	1 (3.2 oz)	20	0	4	2	2
The Elevation Burger Double Meat	1	510	26	29	4	1
The Elevation Burger Double Meat Double Cheese	1	690	41	29	4	1
The Elevation Burger Double Meat Double Cheese Wrapped In Lettuce	1	550	39	2	1	0
The Elevation Burger Double Meat Wrapped In Lettuce	1	370	24	2	1	1
Veggie Burger #1	1	300	7	50	4	4
Veggie Burger #1 Wrapped In Lettuce	1	160	5	23	1	4
Veggie Burger #2	1	320	10	50	6	5
Veggie Burger #2 Wrapped In Lettuce	1	180	8	23	3	5
Vertigo Burger 3 Patties	1	690	38	29	4	1
Vertigo Burger Wrapped In Lettuce	1	550	36	2	1	1
SALAD DRESSINGS AND SAUCES						
Balsamic Mustard	1 serv (0.2 oz)	5	0	2	1	0
Dressing Blue Cheese	1 serv (1 oz)	130	14	1	0	0
Dressing Ranch	1 serv (1 oz)	160	17	1	1	0
Elevation Sauce	1 serv (0.2 oz)	5	0	2	1	0
Hot Pepper Relish	1 serv (0.7 oz)	0	0	0	0	0
SHAKES AND TOPPINGS						
Bananas	1 serv (1.4 oz)	35	0	9	5	1
Blueberries	1 serv (1.5 oz)	25	0	5	5	2
Malt Powder	1 serv (1 oz)	110	1	23	18	0

FOOD	PORTION	CAL	FAT	CARB	SUGAR	FIBER
Mangoes	1 serv (1.5 oz)	25	0	7	6	1
Oreo Cookies	1 serv (0.6 oz)	80	4	12	7	1
Organic Cheesecake Powder	1 tbsp	45	0	12	12	0
Shake Chocolate	1 (15.5 oz)	710	32	91	75	0
Shake Coffee	1 (15.5 oz)	710	32	86	70	0
Shake Vanilla	1 (15.5 oz)	710	37	81	55	0
Strawberries	1 serv (4.1 oz)	35	0	9	6	2
Syrup Black Cherry	1 serv (0.9 oz)	70	0	18	18	0
Syrup Chocolate	1 serv (3.6 oz)	260	0	63	52	3
Syrup Guava	1 serv (0.9 oz)	70	0	16	16	0
Syrup Key Lime Pie	1 serv (0.9 oz)	60	0	16	15	0
Syrup Mango	1 serv (0.9 oz)	90	0	22	21	0
Syrup Orange	1 serv (0.9 oz)	60	0	15	15	0
Syrup Pineapple	1 serv (0.9 oz)	70	0	16	15	0
FIVE GUYS BURGERS AND FRIES						
MAIN MENU SELECTIONS						
Bacon Burger	1 (9.8 oz)	780	50	39	8	2
Bacon Cheese Dog	1 (7 oz)	695	48	41	9	2
Bacon Dog	1 (6.4 oz)	625	42	40	8	2
Cheese Dog	1 (6.5 oz)	615	41	41	9	2
Cheeseburger	1 (10.6 oz)	840	55	40	9	2
Cheeseburger Bacon	1 (11 oz)	920	62	40	9	2
Fries	1 reg (8.6 oz)	620	30	78	2	6
Fries	1 lg (16 oz)	1464	71	184	5	14
Grilled Cheese	1 (4 oz)	430	26	41	10	3
Hamburger	1 (9.3 oz)	700	43	39	8	2
Hot Dog	1 (5.9 oz)	545	35	40	8	2
Little Burgers Bacon Burger	1 (6.5 oz)	560	33	39	8	2
Little Burgers Cheeseburger	1 (6.7 oz)	550	32	40	9	2

FOOD	PORTION	CAL	FAT	CARB	SUGAR	FIBER
Little Burgers Cheeseburger Bacon	1 (7.2 oz)	630	39	40	9	2
Little Burgers Hamburger	1 (6 oz)	480	26	39	8	2
Veggie Sandwich	1 (7.3 oz)	440	15	60	14	2
TOPPINGS						
A1 Steak Sauce	1 tbsp (0.6 oz)	15	0	3	2	0
Bacon	2 slices (0.5 oz)	80	7	0	0	0
BBQ Sauce	1 tbsp (0.6 oz)	60	8	16	10	0
Cheese	1 slice (0.7 oz)	70	6	tr	tr	0
Green Peppers	1 serv (0.8 oz)	5	0	2	tr	tr
Hot Sauce	1 tsp (5 g)	0	0	0	0	0
Jalapenos	1 serv (0.4 oz)	3	0	tr	0	0
Ketchup	1 tbsp (0.6 oz)	15	0	4	4	0
Lettuce	1 serv (1 oz)	4	0	1	tr	tr
Mayonnaise	1 serv (0.5 oz)	100	11	0	0	0
Mushrooms	1 serv (0.9 oz)	10	0	1	0	tr
Mustard	1 tbsp (0.6 oz)	0	0	0	0	0
Onions	1 serv (0.9 oz)	10	0	3	1	tr
Pickle Chips	6 (1 oz)	5	0	1	0	0
Relish	1 serv (0.5 oz)	15	0	4	3	0
Tomatoes	1 serv (1.8 oz)	9	0	2	2	tr

FRESHENS

FOOD	PORTION	CAL	FAT	CARB	SUGAR	FIBER
CREPES						
Breakfast Denver	1 serv	460	24	26	7	1
Breakfast Egg White Florentine	1 serv	270	8	24	5	2
Breakfast Steak & Egg	1 serv	480	26	25	6	1
Breakfast Wake Up	1 serv	420	22	23	5	1
Dessert Cheesecake Cherry	1 serv	590	19	93	23	2

FOOD	PORTION	CAL	FAT	CARB	SUGAR	FIBER
Dessert Cheesecake Supreme	1 serv	510	20	69	35	3
Dessert Nutella Supreme	1 serv	600	22	88	50	5
Dessert The Guilty Pleasure	1 serv	540	13	91	46	5
Honey Mustard Chicken	1 serv	470	14	52	16	3
Savory Buffalo Chicken	1 serv	480	14	48	12	5
Savory Caesar Salad	1 serv	500	19	50	14	5
Savory Fajita Chicken	1 serv	500	13	58	17	6
Savory Fajita Steak	1 serv	530	19	59	16	5
Savory Greek Salad	1 serv	370	9	52	15	5
Savory Harvest Salad	1 serv	520	12	73	29	6
Savory Havana Chicken	1 serv	470	15	46	11	3
Savory Pesto Chicken	1 serv	440	13	48	11	5
Savory Philly Cheese Chicken	1 serv	610	25	54	13	7
Savory Philly Cheese Steak	1 serv	650	30	55	12	6
Savory Pizza Cali	1 serv	270	30	48	12	5
Savory Southwest Chicken	1 serv	610	27	57	16	5
Savory Southwest Steak	1 serv	650	32	58	15	4
Savory Tomato Cheese & Basil	1 serv	460	18	49	11	5
SMOOTHIES						
Blended Fruit Berry Breeze	1	290	0	73	66	2
Blended Fruit Caribbean Craze	1	260	0	65	58	2
Blended Fruit Citrus Mango	1	390	7	83	67	1

FOOD	PORTION	CAL	FAT	CARB	SUGAR	FIBER
Blended Fruit Jamaican Jammer	1	290	0	63	56	2
Blended Fruit Orange Sunrise	1	260	3	57	44	2
Blended Fruit Peach Sunset	1	230	0	58	53	2
Blended Fruit Strawberry Kiwi	1	290	0	73	67	1
Blended Fruit Strawberry Shooter	1	250	0	64	59	1
Blended Fruit Strawberry Squeeze	1	250	0	54	48	1
Blended Fruit Tropical Pineapple	1	380	4	88	82	1
Fro-Yo Blasts Reese's Pieces & Peanut Butter	1	600	19	97	84	3
Fro-Yo Cookie Dough	1	490	6	103	82	1
Fro-Yo M&M's	1	490	10	93	83	2
Fro-Yo Oreo Overload	1	370	4	78	62	1
High Protein Peanut Butter	1	460	12	69	61	2
High Protein Strawberries 'N Cream	1	370	1	61	56	1
Indulgent Shake Chocolate	1	440	3	95	83	1
Indulgent Shake Oreo Cream	1	530	6	110	91	1
Indulgent Shake Strawberry	1	400	2	87	79	1
Indulgent Shake Vanilla	1	410	2	91	84	1
Low-Cal Mango Beach No Sugar Added	1	70	0	49	5	1

FOOD	PORTION	CAL	FAT	CARB	SUGAR	FIBER
Low-Cal Peach Breeze No Sugar Added	1	80	0	50	9	1
Low-Cal Strawberry Oasis No Sugar Added	1	70	0	50	9	1
Rainforest Energy Acai	1	280	3	62	57	3
Rainforest Energy Brazilian	1	290	3	67	59	3
Rainforest Energy Mangosteen	1	320	0	80	73	2
YOGURT						
Chocolate Cake Cone	1	150	0	35	26	1
Chocolate Cup	11 oz	280	1	66	56	2
Chocolate Waffle Cone	1	250	2	56	38	2
Granola Parfait w/ 2 Fruits	1 serv	400	8	76	45	6
Tart Cup	7 oz	190	0	40	35	0
Tart Cup	11 oz	300	0	63	55	0
Vanilla Cake Cone	1	160	0	35	28	0
Vanilla Cup	11 oz	290	0	66	60	1
Vanilla Cup	7 oz	180	0	42	38	0
Vanilla Waffle Cone	1	250	1	56	40	1

FRIENDLY'S

FOOD	PORTION	CAL	FAT	CARB	SUGAR	FIBER
BEVERAGES						
Milkshake Double Thick Vanilla	1	770	32	106	92	0
MAIN MENU SELECTIONS						
Apple Slices	1 serv	100	0	26	20	5
Applesauce	1 serv	110	0	27	25	1
Broccoli	1 serv	80	6	5	2	3
Burger All American	1	1190	68	103	12	8
Burger BBQ Fronion	1	1560	91	134	21	8
Burger Mushroom Swiss Bacon	1	1570	100	109	15	7

FOOD	PORTION	CAL	FAT	CARB	SUGAR	FIBER
Burger Soft Pretzel Bacon	1	1420	79	119	11	7
Burger The Vermonter	1	1420	87	102	4	7
Burger Ultimate Bacon Cheese	1	1400	86	103	11	7
BurgerMelt Deluxe Cheese Set-Up	1	1180	75	83	5	7
BurgerMelt Swiss Patty	1	1360	78	110	12	8
BurgerMelt Ultimate Grilled Cheese	1	1500	97	101	4	9
BurgerMelt Zesty Questo	1	1380	79	117	8	7
Carrot & Celery Sticks w/ Ranch Dressing	1 serv	100	7	6	3	2
Chicken Strips Basket w/o Dipping Sauce	5 pieces	1030	58	93	9	8
Chicken Strips Honey BBQ w/o Dipping Sauce	5 pieces	1560	74	188	88	0
Chicken Strips Kickin' Buffalo w/o Dipping Sauce	5 pieces	1530	109	97	10	8
Clamboat Basket	1 serv	1710	102	170	19	11
Coleslaw	1 serv	160	12	13	8	2
Corn	1 serv	160	7	20	9	4
Fishamajig	1	970	51	99	5	7
Friendly Frank	1	750	44	73	5	5
Friendly's BTL	1	990	57	99	7	7
Fronions Jumbo	1 serv	1430	90	140	31	7
Garlic Bread	1 serv	330	14	48	0	4
Grilled Cheese	1	790	37	96	4	6
Grilled Flounder	1 serv	980	48	100	10	7
Mandarin Oranges	1 serv	80	0	20	18	0

FOOD	PORTION	CAL	FAT	CARB	SUGAR	FIBER
Mashed Potatoes Homestyle	1 serv	240	12	29	4	2
Mini Mozzarella Cheese Sticks	1 serv	680	40	55	5	3
Mixed Vegetables	1 serv	110	6	13	6	4
New England Fish 'N Chips	1 serv	1150	70	106	15	9
Quesadillas Chicken	1 serv	1330	82	97	10	4
Quesadillas Chicken Fajita	1 serv	1540	91	106	13	7
Rice	1 serv	210	3	41	2	0
Shrimp Basket	1 serv	1090	60	110	17	9
Sirloin Steak Tips	1 serv	1140	51	92	28	13
Sliders Cheeseburger	1 serv	500	21	57	18	6
Sliders Chicken	1 serv	740	42	69	15	7
Spanish Rice	1 serv	330	15	41	2	0
SuperMelt Bruschetta Mozzarella	1	1140	54	105	6	7
SuperMelt Cheddar Jack Chicken	1	1070	49	98	5	6
SuperMelt Grilled Chicken Pesto	1	1360	82	98	7	6
SuperMelt Honey BBQ Chicken	1	1400	75	134	23	8
SuperMelt Kickin Buffalo Chicken	1	1430	86	118	7	7
SuperMelt Reuben	1	1130	56	105	10	6
SuperMelt Steak 'N Mushroom	1	1150	61	108	9	7
SuperMelt Tuna	1	1140	66	98	6	7
SuperMelt Turkey Club	1	990	46	102	9	7
Tuna Roll	1	920	57	73	5	6
Waffle Fries	1 serv	590	33	67	1	5

FOOD	PORTION	CAL	FAT	CARB	SUGAR	FIBER
Waffle Fries Loaded	1 serv	920	64	67	4	4
Wrap Buffalo Chicken	1	1510	94	123	6	9
Wrap Crispy Chicken	1	1140	54	132	14	10
Wrap Crispy Chicken Caesar	1	1500	94	123	7	9
Wrap Grilled Chicken Deluxe	1	1000	45	108	15	8
SALAD DRESSINGS AND TOPPINGS						
Dressing Bleu Cheese	1 serv	470	48	3	3	0
Dressing Honey Mustard	1 serv	360	30	24	18	0
Dressing Italian	1 serv	410	42	6	6	0
Dressing Italian Fat Free	1 serv	30	0	8	6	0
Dressing Peppercorn Parmesan Lite	1 serv	230	21	6	3	0
Dressing Ranch	1 serv	330	33	3	3	0
Dressing Salsa Ranch	1 serv	170	17	5	3	1
Dressing Sesame Oriental	1 serv	270	14	36	30	0
Dressing Thousand Island	1 serv	390	36	15	12	0
Dressing Vinegarette Dijon Low Fat	1 serv	110	3	21	21	0
Sauce BBQ	1 serv	90	0	20	11	0
Sauce Honey Mustard	1 serv	180	16	12	9	0
Vinegarette Balsamic	1 serv	180	15	9	9	0
SALADS						
Apple Walnut Chicken w/o Dressing	1 serv	390	18	22	9	5
Asian Chicken w/o Dressing	1 serv	490	20	41	21	6
Chicken Caesar	1 serv	1030	84	32	10	3
Chipotle Chicken w/o Dressing	1 serv	550	22	50	7	8

FOOD	PORTION	CAL	FAT	CARB	SUGAR	FIBER
Crispy Chicken w/o Dressing	1 serv	630	38	38	5	6
Kickin Buffalo Chicken w/o Dressing	1 serv	710	47	42	5	7
Side w/o Dressing	1 serv	60	1	10	2	2
Steak & Bleu Cheese w/o Dressing	1 serv	640	34	41	9	8
SOUPS						
Broccoli Cheddar	1 cup	200	13	14	3	1
Chili	1 cup	270	16	18	3	3
Chunky Chicken Noodle	1 cup	280	10	31	4	2
Homestyle Clam Chowder	1 cup	270	18	17	3	1
Minestrone	1 cup	90	1	15	2	2

FRUITFULL

FOOD	PORTION	CAL	FAT	CARB	SUGAR	FIBER
BREADS						
Almond Cherry	½ slice (2 oz)	226	11	29	17	1
Apple Spice	½ slice (2 oz)	186	7	29	18	1
Banana	½ slice (2 oz)	165	6	24	11	1
Cappuccino Chocolate Chip	½ slice (2 oz)	229	13	27	16	1
Carrot	½ slice (2 oz)	190	9	24	12	0
Chocolate	½ slice (2 oz)	120	0	26	16	2
Old Fashion Pound Cake	½ slice (2 oz)	227	13	25	14	0
Orange Cranberry	½ slice (2 oz)	130	0	28	12	0
Pumpkin	½ slice (2 oz)	130	0	30	19	1
Sweet Potato	½ slice (2 oz)	176	6	28	17	1
Zucchini	½ slice (2 oz)	190	9	24	13	1
FROZEN BARS						
Cream Banana	1 (4 oz)	110	3	18	13	0
Cream Coconut	1 (4 oz)	130	5	18	13	0
Cream Horchata	1 (4 oz)	240	14	23	21	tr
Cream Mango Cream	1 (4 oz)	170	7	26	20	tr

FOOD	PORTION	CAL	FAT	CARB	SUGAR	FIBER
Cream Peaches 'N' Cream	1 (4 oz)	150	5	24	21	2
Cream Pina Colada	1 (4 oz)	90	3	16	15	tr
Cream Raspberry Cream	1 (4 oz)	110	3	18	12	0
Cream Sapote Lucuma	1 (4 oz)	180	8	25	29	<2
Cream Strawberry Cream	1 (4 oz)	110	3	20	17	0
Juice Fuzzy Navel	1 (4 oz)	70	0	18	15	0
Juice Green Tea Melon	1 (4 oz)	90	0	21	16	–
Juice Guava	1 (4 oz)	70	0	17	11	–
Juice Lemon	1 (4 oz)	90	0	24	22	–
Juice Lime	1 (4 oz)	80	0	20	19	0
Juice Passionate Cherry	1 (4 oz)	80	0	20	16	–
Juice Pineapple	1 (4 oz)	80	0	20	10	0
Juice Raspberry	1 (4 oz)	70	0	18	18	0
Juice Strawberry	1 (4 oz)	70	0	18	13	0
Juice Tamarind	1 (4 oz)	90	0	21	21	–
Juice Tropical Splash	1 (4 oz)	80	0	19	17	0
Juice Watermelon	1 (4 oz)	60	0	13	13	–
Mamey Sapote Lucuma	1 (4 oz)	180	8	25	–	<2
SNACKS						
All About Almonds	1 pkg (1 oz)	170	15	5	0	4
Blueberry Thrill	1 pkg (1 oz)	150	8	14	9	3
Buzzworthy Banana	1 pkg (1.1 oz)	140	8	17	11	2
Calypso Cashews	1 pkg (1.1 oz)	170	13	7	2	1
Chocolate Covered Nuts	1 pkg (1.5 oz)	230	16	20	18	1
Chocolate Twisted Bliss	1 pkg (1.4 oz)	190	8	27	16	1
Cin-sational Apple Crunch	1 pkg (1 oz)	160	10	14	8	1
Dark Chocolate Covered Almonds	1 pkg (1.4 oz)	210	16	19	14	3
Dark Chocolate Covered Cashews	1 pkg (1.4 oz)	220	16	21	14	3

FOOD	PORTION	CAL	FAT	CARB	SUGAR	FIBER
Dark Chocolate Covered Cranberries	1 pkg (1.4 oz)	180	9	27	24	2
Debbie Loves Fruit	1 pkg (1 oz)	110	2	23	16	1
Eat Your Veggies	1 pkg (1.5 oz)	180	8	29	7	3
Got Nuts?	1 pkg (1.1 oz)	180	13	9	1	2
Hit The Road Jack	1 pkg (1.1 oz)	130	6	19	16	1
Honey I Ate The Peanuts	1 pkg (1 oz)	160	12	8	6	2
Just Peachy	1 pkg (1.4 oz)	140	0	35	22	0
Mammoth Malts	1 pkg (1 oz)	150	7	20	18	0
Nice Catch Swedish Fish	1 pkg (1.4 oz)	140	0	35	22	0
Off The Hook Gummy Worms	1 pkg (1.5 oz)	130	0	31	21	0
PB Pretzel Poppers	1 pkg (1 oz)	140	7	15	2	2
Power Pistachios	1 pkg (1.5 oz)	260	23	12	3	4
Pumpkin Seeds	1 pkg (1 oz)	180	15	3	0	1
Reggae Rice Crackers	1 pkg (1.1 oz)	110	0	26	1	0
Rockin' Raisins	1 pkg (1.4 oz)	170	7	28	19	1
Rocky Mountain Munch	1 pkg (1.1 oz)	120	4	22	14	1
Smokin' Nuts	1 pkg (1.3 oz)	170	15	6	2	3
Soft Twisters Green Apple	1 pkg (1 oz)	120	0	29	14	0
Soft Twisters Watermelon	1 pkg (1.3 oz)	120	0	29	14	0
Sour Wiggle Giggle	1 pkg (1.5 oz)	150	0	34	22	0
Strawberry Fields	1 pkg (1 oz)	140	7	18	9	1
Sunflower Seeds Tummy	1 pkg (1.1 oz)	190	14	8	1	2
Swinging Sesame Stix	1 pkg (1.1 oz)	180	13	12	0	2
Whassup Wasabi	1 pkg (1.1 oz)	150	7	17	1	2

HARDEE'S

BEVERAGES

Ice Cream Malt	1 (14.5 oz)	780	35	98	76	0
Ice Cream Shake	1 (14 oz)	710	33	86	68	0

FOOD	PORTION	CAL	FAT	CARB	SUGAR	FIBER
BREAKFAST SELECTIONS						
Big Country Breakfast Platter Bacon w/o Syrup Jam & Butter	1 (11.6 oz)	870	44	91	12	6
Biscuit Bacon Egg Cheese	1 (5.2 oz)	450	26	36	2	3
Biscuit Chicken Fillet	1 (6 oz)	550	32	47	3	4
Biscuit Cinnamon 'N' Raisin	1 (2.8 oz)	300	15	40	17	1
Biscuit Country Ham	1 (4.2 oz)	370	19	37	2	3
Biscuit Country Steak	1 (5 oz)	510	31	44	3	4
Biscuit Ham Egg Cheese	1 (6.1 oz)	440	24	37	2	3
Biscuit Jelly	1 (4 oz)	430	26	45	9	3
Biscuit Loaded Omelet	1 (6 oz)	520	33	37	2	3
Biscuit Made From Scratch	1 (3 oz)	300	15	36	2	3
Biscuit Monster	1 (8.3 oz)	720	49	38	3	3
Biscuit 'N' Gravy	1 (8 oz)	460	26	49	2	3
Biscuit Sausage	1 (4.4 oz)	490	33	37	3	3
Biscuit Sausage & Egg	1 (6 oz)	550	37	37	3	3
Breakfast Bowl Low Carb	1 (8.6 oz)	690	58	3	1	1
Breakfast Burrito Loaded	1 (8.9 oz)	710	45	40	1	2
Breakfast Sandwich Frisco	1 (6.8 oz)	440	19	43	5	2
Grits	1 serv (5 oz)	110	5	16	0	1
Hash Rounds	1 sm (3 oz)	260	17	26	1	3
Pancakes w/o Syrup Jam & Butter	3 (4.8 oz)	310	5	56	14	2
Sunrise Croissant w/ Ham	1 (5.7 oz)	440	27	28	4	1

FOOD	PORTION	CAL	FAT	CARB	SUGAR	FIBER
CHILDREN'S MENU SELECTIONS						
French Fries	1 serv (2.8 oz)	330	11	30	0	3
Kids Meal Cheeseburger	1 (7.1 oz)	540	26	61	6	4
Kids Meal Chicken Tenders	1 serv (5.7 oz)	400	19	37	0	4
Kids Meal Hamburger	1 (6.7 oz)	490	23	60	6	4
DESSERTS						
Apple Turnover w/o Cinnamon Sugar Topping	1 (3 oz)	270	13	35	11	1
Cookie Chocolate Chip	1 (2.4 oz)	290	11	44	26	0
Ice Cream Bowl Single Scoop	1 (4 oz)	240	13	27	22	0
Ice Cream Cone Single Scoop	1 (4.4 oz)	290	13	37	26	0
Peach Cobbler	1 sm (6.3 oz)	290	7	56	45	1
MAIN MENU SELECTIONS						
Burger Original Turkey	1 (8.2 oz)	390	17	32	7	3
Cheeseburger	1 sm (4.4 oz)	310	15	32	6	1
Cheeseburger Double	1 (5.8 oz)	410	21	34	7	2
Cheeseburger Little Thick	1 (5.8 oz)	420	23	34	8	3
Chicken Tenders Hand Breaded	3 (4.5 oz)	260	13	13	0	2
Cole Slaw	1 sm (4 oz)	170	10	20	16	2
Crispy Curls	1 sm (4 oz)	360	18	46	0	4
French Fries	1 sm (4 oz)	340	16	43	0	4
Fried Chicken Breast	1 (5.2 oz)	370	15	29	0	0
Fried Chicken Leg	1 (2.4 oz)	170	7	15	0	0
Fried Chicken Thigh	1 (4.2 oz)	330	15	30	0	0
Fried Chicken Wing	1 (2.3 oz)	200	8	23	0	0
Hamburger	1 sm (4 oz)	270	11	31	6	1

FOOD	PORTION	CAL	FAT	CARB	SUGAR	FIBER
Hot Ham 'N' Cheese	1 (4.6 oz)	280	11	29	4	1
Hot Ham 'N' Cheese Big	1 (8.4 oz)	480	19	48	6	3
Jumbo Chili Dog	1 (5 oz)	370	25	24	6	2
Mashed Potatoes	1 sm (5 oz)	90	2	17	1	0
Onion Rings Beer Battered	1 serv (4.3 oz)	410	24	45	5	3
Roast Beef Big	1 (7.2 oz)	460	20	46	5	4
Sandwich Charbroiled BBQ Chicken	1 (7.5 oz)	310	6	44	15	3
Sandwich Charbroiled Chicken Club	1 (8.6 oz)	540	31	38	10	3
Sandwich Fish Supreme	1 (7 oz)	530	34	37	9	3
Sandwich Hand Breaded Chicken Fillet	1 (10.9 oz)	680	38	56	7	4
Sandwich Low Carb Charbroiled Chicken Club	1 (8 oz)	340	22	13	8	1
Sandwich Roast Beef Regular	1 (4.5 oz)	290	14	28	4	2
Sandwich Spicy Chicken	1 (5.5 oz)	430	24	44	3	3
Side Salad w/o Dressing	1 (6.7 oz)	120	7	7	4	2
Thickburger ⅓ Lb Bacon Cheese	1 (11.7 oz)	850	56	51	7	4
Thickburger ⅓ Lb Cheeseburger	1 (8.8 oz)	630	33	53	10	3
Thickburger ⅓ Lb Frisco	1 (10.5 oz)	880	59	46	6	2
Thickburger ⅓ Lb Low Carb	1 (9.7 oz)	480	36	9	6	1
Thickburger ⅓ Lb Mushroom & Swiss	1 (9.2 oz)	670	38	50	5	3
Thickburger ⅓ Lb Original	1 (12.4 oz)	810	52	54	10	4

FOOD	PORTION	CAL	FAT	CARB	SUGAR	FIBER
Thickburger ⅔ Lb Double	1 (16.5 oz)	1160	78	55	10	4
Thickburger ⅔ Lb Monster	1 (13.4 oz)	1300	93	47	5	3
Thickburger Little	1 (8 oz)	570	39	35	7	3
Thickburger The Six Dollar	1 (14 oz)	940	63	60	16	4
IHOP						
Pancake Buttermilk	5	770	25	115	22	7
Pancake Buttermilk Short Stack	3	490	18	69	13	4
Pancake Chocolate Chip	4	720	24	112	32	8
Pancake Double Blueberry	4	800	17	144	57	11
Pancake Harvest Grain 'N Nut	4	920	49	95	22	10
Pancake New York Cheesecake	4	1100	44	152	53	8
Pancake Strawberry Banana	4	760	17	137	41	10
IVAR'S SEAFOOD BARS						
BEVERAGES						
Barq's Root Beer	1 (22 oz)	305	–	83	–	–
Cherry Coke	1 (22 oz)	288	–	77	–	–
Coca-Cola Classic	1 (22 oz)	267	–	75	–	–
Diet Coke	1 (22 oz)	3	–	0	–	–
Fanta Orange	1 (22 oz)	325	–	88	–	–
Hot Chocolate	1 (12 oz)	164	–	42	–	–
Minute Maid Lemonade	1 (22 oz)	308	–	77	–	–
Pibb Xtra	1 (22 oz)	267	–	72	–	–
Sprite	1 (22 oz)	271	–	69	–	–

FOOD	PORTION	CAL	FAT	CARB	SUGAR	FIBER
CHILDREN'S MENU SELECTIONS						
Kids Baby Prawns 'N Chips	1 serv (6 oz)	370	–	42	–	–
Kids Clams 'N Chips	1 serv (6 oz)	463	–	50	–	–
Kids Fish 'N Chips	1 serv (7 oz)	280	–	31	–	–
Little Chicken 'N Chips	1 serv (5.8 oz)	360	–	34	–	–
MAIN MENU SELECTIONS						
Baby Prawns 'N Chips	1 serv (10.6 oz)	640	–	74	–	–
Calamari 'N Chips	1 serv (13.4 oz)	680	–	83	–	–
Chicken 'N Chips	1 serv (12.7 oz)	790	–	75	–	–
Clams 'N Chips	1 serv (10 oz)	770	–	83	–	–
Coleslaw	1 serv (6 oz)	150	–	15	–	–
Corn Bread	1 serv (2.3 oz)	170	–	28	–	–
Crab Cocktail	1 (3.4 oz)	120	–	10	–	–
Dinner Grilled Chicken	1 (19 oz)	940	–	108	–	–
Dinner Grilled Halibut	1 (16 oz)	770	–	83	–	–
Dinner Grilled Mahi Mahi	1 (16 oz)	703	–	83	–	–
Dinner Grilled Salmon	1 (16 oz)	857	–	85	–	–
Fish 'N Chips	3 pieces (13 oz)	536	–	69	–	–
French Fries	1 side (10 oz)	430	–	70	–	–
Halibut 'N Chips	1 serv (15 oz)	660	–	74	–	–
Jumbo Prawns 'N Chips	1 serv (14 oz)	600	–	70	–	–
Oysters 'N Chips	1 serv (12.2 oz)	470	–	66	–	–
Salmon 'N Chips	1 serv (15 oz)	800	–	74	–	–

FOOD	PORTION	CAL	FAT	CARB	SUGAR	FIBER
Scallops 'N Chips	1 serv (12 oz)	611	–	68	–	–
Shrimp Cocktail	1 (3.4 oz)	120	–	10	–	–
Sole 'N Chips	3 pieces (15.5 oz)	610	–	69	–	–
SALAD DRESSINGS AND SAUCES						
Barbecue Sauce	1 serv (1.2 oz)	53	–	13	–	–
Caesar	1 serv (2 oz)	188	–	4	–	–
Caesar for Grilled Chicken	1 serv (2 oz)	144	–	5	–	–
Caesar for Crab Salmon or Shrimp	1 serv (2 oz)	188	–	4	–	–
Caesar Side	1 serv (0.8 oz)	71	–	2	–	–
Cocktail Sauce	1 serv (1.2 oz)	50	0	9	–	–
Ketchup	1 serv (1 oz)	29	–	0	–	–
Tartar Sauce	1 serv (2 oz)	164	–	2	–	–
SALADS						
Asian	1 (13.4 oz)	320	–	57	–	–
Caesar	1 (9.3 oz)	328	–	20	–	–
Caesar Crab	1 (12.3 oz)	410	–	21	–	–
Caesar Grilled Chicken	1 serv (13 oz)	630	–	39	–	–
Caesar Salmon	1 serv (15.3 oz)	639	–	21	–	–
Caesar Shrimp	1 serv (12.3 oz)	410	–	21	–	–
Caesar Side	1 (4.8 oz)	151	–	10	–	–
Side	1 (7.5 oz)	37	–	8	–	–
SOUPS						
Chowder Clamhattan	1 cup (8 oz)	80	–	12	–	–
Chowder Red Clam	1 cup (8 oz)	210	–	21	–	–
Chowder Smoked Salmon	1 cup (8 oz)	250	–	20	–	–
Chowder White Clam	1 cup (8 oz)	240	–	21	–	–

FOOD	PORTION	CAL	FAT	CARB	SUGAR	FIBER
Chowder White Clam Bread Bowl	1 serv (27 oz)	1150	–	171	–	–

JERSEY MIKE'S

SANDWICHES

FOOD	PORTION	CAL	FAT	CARB	SUGAR	FIBER
#05 Super Sub In A Tub	1 (11.9 oz)	290	14	13	5	2
#05 Super Sub Wheat	1 (16 oz)	80	19	67	11	5
#05 Super Sub White	1 (16 oz)	580	19	68	9	4
#06 Roast Beef & Provolone In A Tub	1 (12.2 oz)	430	20	9	5	2
#06 Roast Beef & Provolone Wheat	1 reg (16.2 oz)	720	25	64	11	5
#06 Roast Beef & Provolone White	1 reg (16.2 oz)	730	25	64	8	4
#07 Turkey Breast & Provolone In A Tub	1 (11.4 oz)	250	11	9	5	2
#07 Turkey Breast & Provolone Wheat	1 reg (15.4 oz)	540	16	64	11	5
#07 Turkey Breast & Provolone White	1 (15.4 oz)	550	15	64	8	4
#08 Club Sub w/ Mayonnaise In A Tub	1 (13.2 oz)	600	47	11	5	2
#08 Club Sub w/ Mayonnaise Wheat	1 (17.2 oz)	890	52	66	11	5
#08 Club Sub w/ Mayonnaise White	1 (17.2 oz)	890	52	67	9	4
#09 Club Sub Supreme w/ Mayonnaise In A Tub	1 (13.2 oz)	650	47	11	5	2
#09 Club Supreme w/ Mayonnaise Wheat	1 reg (17.2 oz)	940	52	66	11	5
#09 Club Supreme w/ Mayonnaise White	1 (17.2 oz)	940	52	66	9	4
#10 Albacore Tuna In A Tub	1 (12.2 oz)	620	55	12	5	3

FOOD	PORTION	CAL	FAT	CARB	SUGAR	FIBER
#10 Albacore Tuna Wheat	1 (16.2 oz)	910	59	66	11	6
#10 Albacore Tuna White	1 (16.2 oz)	910	59	67	9	4
#13 Original Italian In A Tub	1 (12.9 oz)	390	22	14	5	2
#13 Original Italian Wheat	1 reg (16.9 oz)	680	27	68	11	5
#13 Original Italian White	1 reg (16.9 oz)	680	27	69	9	4
#14 Veggie White	1 reg (15.7 oz)	750	36	69	10	5
American Classic In A Tub	1 (11.4 oz)	270	14	11	5	2
American Classic Wheat	1 reg (15.4 oz)	560	18	65	11	5
American Classic White	1 reg (15.4 oz)	560	18	66	8	4
BLT In A Tub	1 (8.2 oz)	280	21	8	5	2
BLT Wheat	1 reg (12.2 oz)	570	26	63	10	5
BLT White	1 reg (12.2 oz)	570	26	64	8	4
Hot Sub #15 Meatball & Cheese Wheat	1 reg (13.5 oz)	890	52	72	12	6
Hot Sub #15 Meatball & Cheese White	1 reg (13.5 oz)	890	51	72	10	5
Hot Sub #17 Chicken Philly Wheat	1 reg (13 oz)	630	25	65	12	4
Hot Sub BBQ Beef Wheat	1 reg (11.2 oz)	710	16	83	23	4
Hot Sub BBQ Beef White	1 reg (11.2 oz)	720	16	84	20	3

FOOD	PORTION	CAL	FAT	CARB	SUGAR	FIBER
Hot Sub Big Kahuna Chicken Wheat	1 reg (14.2 oz)	680	29	66	13	5
Hot Sub Big Kahuna Chicken White	1 reg (14.2 oz)	690	29	67	11	3
Hot Sub Big Kahuna Wheat	1 reg (14.2 oz)	670	28	65	12	5
Hot Sub Big Kahuna White	1 reg (14.2 oz)	680	28	66	10	3
Hot Sub Cheese Steak Buffalo Chicken Wheat	1 reg (20.2 oz)	940	55	73	17	5
Hot Sub Cheese Steak Buffalo Chicken White	1 reg (20.2 oz)	940	55	74	14	4
Hot Sub Cheese Steak California Chicken Wheat	1 reg (17.4 oz)	890	53	67	14	5
Hot Sub Cheese Steak California Chicken White	1 reg (17.4 oz)	890	52	67	12	4
Hot Sub Cheese Steak California Wheat	1 reg (17.4 oz)	870	51	65	12	5
Hot Sub Cheese Steak California White	1 reg (17.4 oz)	880	51	66	10	4
Hot Sub Cheese Steak Teriyaki Chicken Wheat	1 reg (14.9 oz)	680	25	74	20	4
Hot Sub Cheese Steak Teriyaki Chicken White	1 reg (14.9 oz)	680	25	75	18	3
Hot Sub Chicka Phila Roni Wheat	1 reg (12.5 oz)	620	19	62	7	3
Hot Sub Chicka Phila Roni White	1 reg (12.5 oz)	605	12	65	5	1
Hot Sub Chicken Parmesan Wheat	1 reg (11 oz)	650	22	77	7	5

FOOD	PORTION	CAL	FAT	CARB	SUGAR	FIBER
Hot Sub Chicken Philly White	1 reg (13 oz)	630	25	68	10	3
Hot Sub Chipotle Chicken Wheat	1 reg (14.4 oz)	910	56	68	12	4
Hot Sub Chipotle Chicken White	1 reg (14.4 oz)	920	56	68	10	3
Hot Sub Chipotle Steak Wheat	1 reg (14.4 oz)	900	55	66	11	4
Hot Sub Chipotle Steak White	1 reg (14.4 oz)	910	55	67	9	3
Hot Sub Chipotle Turkey Wheat	1 reg (17.4 oz)	865	50	67	10	6
Hot Sub Chipotle Turkey White	1 reg (17.4 oz)	870	50	67	8	4
Hot Sub Grilled Chicken Wheat	1 reg (12.7 oz)	670	33	60	8	4
Hot Sub Grilled Chicken White	1 reg (12.7 oz)	670	33	61	6	3
Hot Sub Pastrami & Swiss Wheat	1 reg (10.7 oz)	580	18	60	8	3
Hot Sub Pastrami & Swiss White	1 reg (10.7 oz)	590	17	61	6	2
Hot Sub Reuben Wheat	1 reg (12.2 oz)	700	27	72	14	5
Hot Sub Reuben White	1 reg (12.2 oz)	710	27	73	11	3
Hot Sub Sausage Wheat	1 reg (11.5 oz)	600	27	66	12	5
Hot Sub Sausage White	1 reg (11.4 oz)	600	26	66	10	4
Hot Sub Steak Philly Wheat	1 reg (13 oz)	620	24	64	11	4
Hot Sub Steak Philly White	1 reg (13 oz)	620	23	64	9	3

FOOD	PORTION	CAL	FAT	CARB	SUGAR	FIBER
Jersey Shore Favorite In A Tub	1 (11.4 oz)	270	14	12	5	2
Jersey Shore Favorite Wheat	1 reg (15.4 oz)	560	18	67	11	5
Jersey Shore Favorite White	1 reg (15.4 oz)	570	18	67	9	4
Veggie In A Tub	1 (11.7 oz)	460	32	14	7	3
Veggie Wheat	1 reg (15.72 oz)	720	33	65	11	6
Wrap Baja Chicken	1 (15.6 oz)	610	23	63	7	8
Wrap Buffalo Chicken	1 (14.6 oz)	740	37	62	6	6
Wrap Chicken Caesar	1 (12 oz)	580	23	58	4	6
Wrap Grilled Ham & Cheese	1 (14 oz)	740	41	63	11	5
Wrap Grilled Roast Beef & Cheese	1 (15 oz)	830	45	65	12	5
Wrap Grilled Veggie	1 (17 oz)	910	57	69	10	8
Wrap Turkey w/ Honey Mustard Sauce	1 (13 oz)	540	20	63	10	7
SOUPS						
Beef Steak & Black Bean	1 cup (8.7 oz)	140	2	21	3	9
Boston Clam Chowder	1 cup (8.5 oz)	130	6	15	0	0
Broccoli Cheese	1 cup (8.7 oz)	140	9	8	2	0
Cape Cod Clam Chowder	1 cup (8.7 oz)	140	6	17	1	0
Chicken & Dumplings	1 cup (8.7 oz)	250	18	16	4	0
Chicken Gumbo	1 cup (9 oz)	100	5	11	2	1
Chicken Noodle	1 cup (8.7 oz)	90	4	11	0	0
Chicken Pot Pie	1 cup (8.7 oz)	230	14	20	3	1
Chicken Tortilla	1 cup (8.7 oz)	140	3	22	2	5
Cream Of Broccoli	1 cup (8.7 oz)	90	6	9	3	1
Cream Of Potato	1 cup (8.7 oz)	180	8	17	0	1
Creamy Tomato Bisque	1 cup (8.5 oz)	90	4	11	5	1

FOOD	PORTION	CAL	FAT	CARB	SUGAR	FIBER
French Onion	1 cup (8.7 oz)	80	1	15	3	3
Italian Wedding	1 cup (8.5 oz)	120	5	13	1	1
Lumberjack Vegetable	1 cup (8.5 oz)	120	5	16	4	5
Maryland Crab	1 cup (8.7 oz)	70	1	12	4	2
Minestrone	1 cup (8.7 oz)	70	3	8	6	0
Potato w/ Bacon	1 cup (8.5 oz)	130	5	18	2	1
Spicy Chili w/ Beans	1 cup (9.6 oz)	240	8	25	5	7
Split Pea w/ Ham	1 cup (8.5 oz)	150	2	25	4	3
Timberline Chili w/ Beans	1 cup (8.7 oz)	280	9	31	9	7
Tomato Florentine	1 cup (8.7 oz)	90	1	17	6	1
Vegetable Beef & Barley	1 cup (8.7 oz)	90	3	11	1	2
Vegetarian Vegetable	1 cup (8.7 oz)	80	1	10	4	4
Wild & Brown Rice w/ Chicken	1 cup (8.7 oz)	310	15	17	1	1
Wisconsin Cheese	1 cup (8.5 oz)	220	16	16	8	0

JOE'S CRAB SHACK

DESSERTS

FOOD	PORTION	CAL	FAT	CARB	SUGAR	FIBER
Big Cheese Cheesecake	1 serv	980	64	85	70	3
Chocolate Shack Attack	1 serv	1530	63	225	155	10
Crabby Apple Crumble	1 serv	1400	51	227	161	4
Key Lime Wave	1 serv	1230	55	162	135	2
Sea Turtle Sundae	1	1240	57	167	125	6

MAIN MENU SELECTIONS

FOOD	PORTION	CAL	FAT	CARB	SUGAR	FIBER
Blackened Tilapia	1 serv	1190	64	44	4	6
Broccoli Flowers	1 serv	80	6	6	2	3
Bucket of Shrimp	12	190	3	9	5	1
Buckets of Crab Dungeness w/o Butter	1	480	3	69	6	7
Buckets of Crab King w/o Butter	1	430	3	68	6	7
Buckets Of Crab Snow w/o Butter	1	470	4	68	6	7

FOOD	PORTION	CAL	FAT	CARB	SUGAR	FIBER
Burger Surf 'N Turf	1	1260	85	67	8	4
Calamari Fried	1 serv	900	58	61	2	5
Cheeseburger Chipotle Bacon	1	1010	68	47	13	3
Cheesy New Potatoes	1 serv	250	15	19	1	2
Classic Sampler	1 serv	1460	103	90	5	8
Coleslaw	1 serv	110	7	13	10	2
Crab Cake Dinner	1	1470	109	82	14	9
Crab Daddy Feast w/o Butter	1	510	4	69	6	7
Crab Nachos	1 serv	2000	145	130	8	14
Crab Stuffed Mushrooms	1 serv	800	40	76	4	5
Crawfish Half & Half	1 serv	860	47	72	11	4
Crazy Good Crab Dip	1 serv	1270	87	92	4	7
Crunchy Catfish	1 serv	1440	94	123	10	10
Diablo Mussels	1 serv	1060	54	89	5	5
Dipping Butter	1 serv	400	44	0	0	0
Dirty Rice	1 serv	170	3	30	1	1
Double Dip	1 serv	1260	81	96	3	8
Ear Of Corn	1	60	1	14	2	2
Fish & Chips	1 serv	1430	92	99	12	10
Fish & Shrimp	1 serv	1540	92	111	18	7
French Fries	1 serv	370	19	47	0	5
Fried Oysters	1 serv	1060	64	104	1	9
Garlicky Mussels	1 serv	880	42	81	1	4
Get Stuffed Snapper	1 serv	830	43	48	6	4
Great Balls Of Fire	1 serv	970	66	75	4	8
Grilled Sunset Salmon	1 serv	890	45	66	25	8
Homestyle Chicken Tenders	1 serv	1450	81	93	15	6
Hush Puppies	1 serv	700	34	94	2	8
Joe's Steak Deal	1 serv	710	32	53	2	8

FOOD	PORTION	CAL	FAT	CARB	SUGAR	FIBER
Lobster Daddy Feast w/o Butter	1	580	4	69	6	7
Maui Mahi	1 serv	680	28	40	9	8
Mozzarella Sticks	1 serv	710	36	68	4	6
New England Clam Chowder	1 cup	250	13	22	1	2
Onion Strings	1 serv	470	23	61	4	6
Pan Fried Cheesy Chicken	1 serv	1590	100	110	8	7
Pasta-laya	1 serv	1820	94	161	10	12
Platter Caribbean Feast	1	1280	59	105	29	16
Platter East Coast	1	2110	144	143	9	13
Platter Fisherman's	1	1970	129	137	21	11
Platter Seaside	1	1540	92	117	19	8
Platter Shrimp	1	1490	84	144	33	18
Platter Shrimp Trio	1	1050	53	96	21	19
Platter The Big Hook	1	2750	168	220	27	26
Ribeye	1 serv	1150	82	26	4	5
Salmon Orleans	1 serv	1000	65	34	2	1
Sandwich Chicken Club Blackened	1	990	71	36	5	2
Sandwich Chicken Club Grilled	1	790	49	36	5	2
Sandwich Crab Cake	1	810	61	40	4	3
Sandwich Mahi Blackened	1	850	53	38	7	2
Seafood Fun-Do	1 serv	1310	69	127	2	7
Shrimp Coconut	1 serv	1230	72	127	24	25
Shrimp Crab Stuffed	1 serv	710	37	48	4	5
Shrimp Crispy	1 serv	1060	58	100	16	7
Shrimp Grilled Malibu	1 serv	540	19	55	9	5
Shrimp Pasta Alfredo	1 serv	1650	85	158	3	8
Shrimp Popcorn	1 serv	990	54	98	16	9

FOOD	PORTION	CAL	FAT	CARB	SUGAR	FIBER
Skillet Paella	1 serv	1990	84	196	17	12
Snapper Pontchartrain	1 serv	1090	74	44	5	6
Steak & Malibu Shrimp	1 serv	660	22	48	6	5
Steampots Bean Town	1	1470	78	73	6	7
Steampots Joe's Classic	1	1210	75	70	6	7
Steampots Old Bay	1	1200	74	72	6	7
Steampots Ragin' Cajun	1	1590	107	89	9	10
Steampots Samuel Adams	1	1180	74	72	6	7
Steampots Sunset Fire Grilled	1	1260	75	80	7	9
Steampots The Diablo	1	1420	84	96	11	9
Steampots The KJ	1	1330	85	77	7	7
Steampots The Orleans	1	1310	65	72	7	8
SALADS						
Aruba Chicken	1	780	49	37	22	7
Aruba Shrimp	1	860	61	60	23	15
Caesar	1	450	37	18	5	5
Caesar Chicken	1	670	46	18	5	5
Caesar Chicken Chipotle	1	760	46	42	9	10
Caesar Crab Cake Chipotle	1	970	72	52	11	11
Caesar Shrimp	1	530	38	19	5	5
Caesar Side	1	220	18	8	2	2
Classic Cobb Chicken	1	790	46	38	11	10
Classic Cobb Shrimp	1	650	39	39	11	10
Classic Cobb Snow	1	630	38	38	11	10
House Side w/o Dressing	1	120	7	10	3	2

LITTLE CAESARS

FOOD	PORTION	CAL	FAT	CARB	SUGAR	FIBER
DIPS AND SAUCES						
Crazy Sauce	1 serv (4 oz)	45	0	10	8	1
Dip Buffalo	1 serv (1.5 oz)	130	14	4	2	0

FOOD	PORTION	CAL	FAT	CARB	SUGAR	FIBER
Dip Buffalo Ranch	1 serv (1.5 oz)	220	24	3	2	0
Dip Buttery Garlic	1 serv (1.5 oz)	380	42	0	0	0
Dip Cheezy	1 serv (1.5 oz)	210	21	3	2	0
Dip Chipotle	1 serv (1.5 oz)	220	24	2	0	0
Dip Ranch	1 serv (1.5 oz)	250	26	3	2	0
MAIN MENU SELECTIONS						
Cheese Bread Italian	1 (1.6 oz)	130	7	13	1	0
Cheese Bread Pepperoni	1 (1.7 oz)	150	8	13	1	0
Crazy Bread	1 (1.3 oz)	100	3	15	1	1
Pizza 3 Meat Treat	⅛ pie (4.8 oz)	350	18	30	3	1
Pizza Baby Pan!Pan! Cheese & Pepperoni	1 pie (4.9 oz)	360	18	33	3	1
Pizza Baby Pan!Pan! Just Cheese	1 pie (4.7 oz)	320	15	33	3	1
Pizza Deep Dish Just Cheese	⅛ pie (4.8 oz)	320	13	38	3	1
Pizza Deep Dish Pepperoni	⅛ pie (5 oz)	360	16	38	4	1
Pizza Hot-N-Ready Just Cheese	⅛ pie (4 oz)	240	9	30	3	1
Pizza Hot-N-Ready Pepperoni	⅛ pie (4.2 oz)	280	11	30	3	1
Pizza Hulu Hawaiian Pineapple & Canadian Bacon	⅛ pie (5.2 oz)	280	9	34	6	1
Pizza Hulu Hawaiian Pineapple & Ham	⅛ pie (5.3 oz)	270	9	33	6	1

FOOD	PORTION	CAL	FAT	CARB	SUGAR	FIBER
Pizza Ultimate Supreme	⅛ pie (5.3 oz)	310	14	31	3	2
Pizza Ultimate Supreme Vegetarian	⅛ pie (5.4 oz)	270	10	32	4	2
Wings Barbecue	1 (1.2 oz)	70	4	3	2	0
Wings Hot	1 (1.2 oz)	60	5	1	0	0
Wings Mild	1 (1 oz)	60	4	1	0	0
Wings Oven Roasted	1 (0.9 oz)	50	4	0	0	0

LONG JOHN SILVER'S

BEVERAGES

FOOD	PORTION	CAL	FAT	CARB	SUGAR	FIBER
Diet Mountain Dew	1 med (32 oz)	0	0	0	0	0
Diet Pepsi	1 med (32 oz)	0	0	0	0	0
Dr Pepper	1 med (32 oz)	400	0	108	108	0
Iced Tea Unsweetened	1 med (32 oz)	0	0	0	0	0
Iceflow Lemonade	1 sm (16 oz)	190	0	47	40	0
Iceflow Strawberry Lemonade	1 sm (16 oz)	240	0	60	48	0
Lipton Raspberry Tea	1 med (32 oz)	320	0	84	84	0
Mountain Dew	1 med (32 oz)	440	0	116	116	0
Pepsi	1 med (32 oz)	400	0	112	108	0
Pepsi Wild Cherry	1 med (32 oz)	400	0	112	112	0
Sierra Mist	1 med (32 oz)	400	0	108	108	0
Tropicana Fruit Punch	1 med (32 oz)	440	0	120	120	0
Tropicana Lemonade	1 med (32 oz)	400	0	108	108	0

FOOD	PORTION	CAL	FAT	CARB	SUGAR	FIBER
DESSERTS						
Pie Chocolate Cream	1 slice (2.6 oz)	280	17	28	19	1
Pie Pineapple Cream	1 slice (3.1 oz)	300	17	35	25	0
MAIN MENU SELECTIONS						
Battered Alaskan Pollock	1 piece (3.2 oz)	140	16	17	0	0
Battered Shrimp	3 (1.5 oz)	130	9	8	0	0
Bites Broccoli Cheddar	5 (3.3 oz)	230	12	25	2	2
Bites Jalapeno Cheddar	5 (2.9 oz)	240	14	23	2	2
Breaded Clams Strips	1 box (3 oz)	320	19	29	1	2
Breaded Mozzarella Sticks	3 (1.8 oz)	150	9	13	0	1
Breadstick	1 (2 oz)	170	4	29	2	1
Buttered Langostino Lobster Bites	1 box (3.2 oz)	230	9	24	0	2
Chicken Strip	1 (1.8 oz)	140	8	9	0	0
Cole Slaw	1 serv (4 oz)	200	15	15	10	3
Corn Cobbette w/ Butter	1 (3.6 oz)	150	10	14	6	3
Corn Cobbette w/o Butter	1 (3.3 oz)	90	3	14	6	3
Crumblies	1 serv (1 oz)	170	12	14	0	1
Freshside Grille Salmon Entree	1 serv (10.7 oz)	280	7	27	5	3
Freshside Grille Shrimp Scampi Entree	1 serv (10.7 oz)	330	15	29	5	3
Freshside Grille Tilapia Entree	1 serv (10.2 oz)	250	5	27	4	3
Fries Basket Portion	1 serv (4 oz)	310	14	45	0	4
Fries Platter Portion	1 serv (3 oz)	230	10	34	0	3

FOOD	PORTION	CAL	FAT	CARB	SUGAR	FIBER
Grilled Pacific Salmon Filets	2 (4.5 oz)	150	5	2	1	0
Grilled Tilapia Filet	1 (4 oz)	110	3	1	1	0
Hushpuppy	1 (0.8 oz)	60	3	9	1	1
Jalapeno Peppers	1 (1.3 oz)	15	0	2	1	0
Longostino Lobster Stuffed Crab Cake	1 (2.2 oz)	170	9	16	0	1
Popcorn Shrimp	1 box (2.9 oz)	270	16	23	1	1
Rice	1 serv (5 oz)	180	1	37	1	2
Sandwich Alaskan Pollock	1 (6.6 oz)	470	23	49	4	3
Sandwich Chicken Strip	1 (6.6 oz)	440	30	47	2	4
Sandwich Ultimate Alaskan Pollock	1 (7.2 oz)	240	27	50	4	3
Sandwich Zesty Chicken Strip	1 (4.5 oz)	380	19	39	2	3
Shrimp Scampi	8 pieces (4.6 oz)	200	13	3	1	0
Soup Broccoli Cheese	1 bowl (7.4 oz)	220	18	8	2	1
Taco Baja Chicken Strip	1 (4.3 oz)	370	23	31	2	3
Taco Baja Fish	1 (4 oz)	360	23	30	2	3
Vegetable Medley	1 serv (4 oz)	50	2	8	3	3
SAUCES						
BBQ	1 serv (1 oz)	40	0	10	6	0
Cocktail	1 serv (1 oz)	25	0	6	5	0
Honey Mustard	1 serv (1 oz)	100	6	12	6	0
Ketchup	1 pkg (0.3 oz)	10	0	2	2	0
Lemon Juice	1 serv (4 g)	0	0	0	0	0
Louisiana Hot Sauce	1 tsp (5 g)	0	0	0	0	0
Malt Vinegar	1 serv (0.5 oz)	0	0	0	0	0
Marinara	1 serv (1 oz)	15	0	4	2	1
Ranch	1 serv (1 oz)	160	17	2	1	0

FOOD	PORTION	CAL	FAT	CARB	SUGAR	FIBER
Sweet & Sour	1 serv (1 oz)	45	0	12	7	0
Tartar	1 serv (1 oz)	100	9	4	3	0
MAGGIE MOO'S						
BEVERAGES						
Shake Caramel Cowpuccino	1 (15 oz)	740	43	79	70	0
Shake Cinnamoo Swirl	1 (16 oz)	780	44	87	73	1
Shake Cookies 'N' Cream	1 (15 oz)	740	44	77	65	0
Shake Moocha Cowpuccino	1 (15 oz)	710	41	78	69	0
Shake Peanut Butter S'Moo	1 (16 oz)	780	46	82	69	4
Shake Strawberries 'N' Cream	1 (15 oz)	620	37	66	58	1
Zoomer Caramel Coffee	1 (15 oz)	380	13	65	53	0
Zoomer Creamy Mango	1 (17 oz)	400	3	96	88	1
Zoomer Mocha Coffee	1 (17 oz)	460	11	90	74	0
Zoomer Raspberry Pomegranate	1 (17 oz)	460	0	141	104	3
Zoomer Strawberry Banana	1 (18 oz)	350	10	69	51	3
Zoomer Triple Berry Pomegranate	1 (17 oz)	460	1	115	106	3
CONES						
Dark Chocolate	1 (1.5 oz)	200	7	30	18	1
Dark Chocolate w/ Butterfinger	1 (2 oz)	260	10	41	24	1
Dark Chocolate w/ Heath Bar	1 (2 oz)	280	12	39	26	1
Dark Chocolate w/ Peanuts	1 (2 oz)	280	15	33	18	2
Plain	1 (1 oz)	120	3	22	10	0

FOOD	PORTION	CAL	FAT	CARB	SUGAR	FIBER
White Chocolate	1 (1.5 oz)	200	7	31	19	0
White Chocolate w/ Sprinkles	1 (2 oz)	210	7	34	22	0
ICE CREAM						
Amooretto Cream	1 serv (6 oz)	380	23	38	34	0
Apple Strudel	1 serv (6 oz)	380	21	44	39	0
Banana Pudding	1 serv (6 oz)	330	18	39	32	1
Black Cherry	1 serv (6 oz)	380	23	39	35	0
Blueberry Muffin	1 serv (6 oz)	390	20	48	37	1
Brownie Batter	1 serv (6 oz)	420	21	52	42	1
Butter Pecan	1 serv (6 oz)	380	21	44	40	0
Cake 6 inch Better Batter	1/8 cake (5.7 oz)	480	24	62	45	1
Cake 6 inch Chocolate Cream	1/8 cake (6.4 oz)	580	33	69	53	3
Cake 8 inch Caramel Drizzle	1/14 cake (6 oz)	530	33	55	45	11
Cake 8 inch Chocolate Espresso	1/14 cake (5.6 oz)	460	25	58	48	1
Cake 8 inch Chocolate Heaven	1/14 cake (5 oz)	400	22	45	38	2
Cake 8 inch Cookie Dreams	1/14 cake (5.3 oz)	440	22	57	41	1
Cake 8 inch Cookies 'N' Cream	1/14 cake (5.3 oz)	430	24	50	38	1
Cake 8 inch Cotton Candy Carnival	1/14 cake (5.9 oz)	490	25	65	50	1
Cake 8 inch Fudge Fantasy	1/14 cake (5.4 oz)	410	22	49	40	0
Cake 8 inch Maggie S'Mores	1/14 cake (7 oz)	610	23	94	61	2
Cake 8 inch Maggie's Mud	1/14 cake (5.3 oz)	440	25	49	41	2

FOOD	PORTION	CAL	FAT	CARB	SUGAR	FIBER
Cake 8 inch Pecan Perfection	1/14 cake (5.6 oz)	500	33	50	39	3
Cake 8 inch Sprinkle	1/14 cake (5.7 oz)	370	19	46	38	0
Cake 8 inch Strawberry Cheesecream	1/14 cake (6.3 oz)	530	23	74	46	1
Cake 8 inch Truffle Dream	1/14 cake (5.8 oz)	500	28	58	46	2
Cake 8 inch Turtle	1/14 cake (6.3 oz)	590	40	54	42	2
Cappuccino	1 serv (6 oz)	380	22	41	36	0
Caramel Apple	1 serv (6 oz)	400	21	47	41	0
Carrot Cake	1 serv (6 oz)	420	21	51	39	0
Cheesecake	1 serv (6 oz)	380	21	43	36	0
Choco Mallo	1 serv (6 oz)	360	19	43	36	1
Chocolate	1 serv (6 oz)	390	22	44	37	2
Chocolate Banana	1 serv (6 oz)	370	20	43	35	2
Chocolate Better Batter	1 serv (6 oz)	420	21	54	41	1
Chocolate Peanut Butter	1 serv (6 oz)	450	28	42	35	2
Chocolate Raspberry	1 serv (6 oz)	380	20	46	39	2
Cinnamoo	1 serv (6 oz)	380	23	39	33	0
Cinnamoo Bun	1 serv (6 oz)	530	23	74	40	1
Cocoa Amooretto	1 serv (6 oz)	390	23	42	36	1
Cool Mint	1 serv (6 oz)	380	23	38	34	0
Cotton Candy	1 serv (6 oz)	380	23	38	34	0
Creamy Coconut	1 serv (6 oz)	380	23	38	33	0
Cupcake Better Batter	1	430	21	58	45	1
Cupcake Caramel Pumpkin Pie	1	500	26	62	46	1
Cupcake Cherry Chocolate	1	280	13	39	22	1
Cupcake Chocolate	1	400	22	51	37	2

FOOD	PORTION	CAL	FAT	CARB	SUGAR	FIBER
Cupcake Chocolate Heaven	1	340	18	41	31	1
Cupcake Cool Swirl	1	370	19	47	36	0
Cupcake Cotton Candy Carnival	1	330	18	40	32	0
Cupcake Maggie O	1	360	18	45	29	1
Cupcake Pecan Pie	1	440	28	43	31	1
Cupcake Snowcap Blush	1	360	18	45	36	1
Cupcake Sprinkle	1	340	18	42	34	0
Dark Chocolate	1 serv	390	23	42	35	2
Egg Nog	1 serv (6 oz)	390	22	45	38	0
Espresso Bean	1 serv (6 oz)	380	22	41	36	0
French Vanilla	1 serv	390	22	43	38	0
Fresh Banana	1 serv (6 oz)	340	19	38	32	1
Key Lime	1 serv	380	18	54	48	0
Maggie's Fudge	1 serv	630	34	74	62	0
Mint Chocolate	1 serv (6 oz)	390	23	43	37	1
Mocha	1 serv (6 oz)	390	23	42	29	1
Peanut Butter	1 serv (6 oz)	480	33	38	31	1
Pina Cowlada	1 serv (6 oz)	360	21	37	33	0
Pink Bubblegum	1 serv (6 oz)	380	23	39	34	0
Pink Peppermint Stick	1 serv (6 oz)	420	21	51	47	0
Pistachio	1 serv (6 oz)	380	23	39	34	0
Pizza 10 inch Cheese	1/10 pie (5.4 oz)	340	18	40	31	0
Pizza Chocolate Lover's 10 inch	1/10 pie	390	20	48	35	1
Pizza Supreme 10 inch	1/10 pie (6.1 oz)	450	24	53	43	1
Pumpkin Pie	1 serv (6 oz)	370	21	41	36	0
Raspberry	1 serv (6 oz)	370	21	42	37	0
Red Velvet Cake	1 serv (6 oz)	420	21	54	41	1
Rum Raisin	1 serv (6 oz)	380	23	39	35	0

FOOD	PORTION	CAL	FAT	CARB	SUGAR	FIBER
Southern Peaches	1 serv (6 oz)	330	16	44	36	0
Strawberry	1 serv	350	21	37	33	0
Strawberry Banana No Sugar Added	1 serv (6 oz)	170	6	42	0	0
Udderly Cream	1 serv (6 oz)	380	23	38	34	0
Vanilla	1 serv (6 oz)	380	23	39	35	0
Vanilla Low Fat Lactose Free	1 serv (6 oz)	130	5	23	18	0
Very Yellow Marshmallow	1 serv (6 oz)	350	20	38	34	0
MANHATTAN BAGEL						
BAGELS AND BAKED GOODS						
Bagel Blueberry	1 (3.8 oz)	300	1	65	11	3
Bagel Blueberry Glaze	1 (4.5 oz)	360	0	83	25	3
Bagel Cheddar	1 (4 oz)	320	2	67	3	3
Bagel Chocolate Chip	1 (3.8 oz)	290	3	58	10	3
Bagel Cinnamon Raisin	1 (4 oz)	330	1	70	10	3
Bagel Egg	1 (4 oz)	320	2	67	3	3
Bagel Everything	1 (4.3 oz)	350	3	68	3	3
Bagel French Toast	1 (3.5 oz)	300	6	54	9	2
Bagel Garlic	1 (4.3 oz)	340	1	74	3	3
Bagel Honey Whole Wheat	1 (3.5 oz)	250	1	56	8	3
Bagel Honey Whole Wheat Everything	1 (3.8 oz)	280	3	59	8	3
Bagel Jalapeno Cheddar	1 (4 oz)	320	2	67	3	3
Bagel Onion	1 (4.3 oz)	340	1	74	3	3
Bagel Plain	1 (4 oz)	320	1	68	3	3
Bagel Poppy	1 (4.3 oz)	360	5	69	3	3
Bagel Pumpernickel	1 (3.5 oz)	240	2	53	4	3
Bagel Rye	1 (4 oz)	310	2	66	3	3
Bagel Salt	1 (4.3 oz)	320	1	68	3	3
Bagel Sesame Seed	1 (4.5 oz)	360	5	68	3	3

FOOD	PORTION	CAL	FAT	CARB	SUGAR	FIBER
Bagel Mini Plain	1 (1.8 oz)	130	1	28	1	1
Bagel Thin Honey Whole Wheat	1 (2 oz)	120	2	23	3	4
Bagel Thin Plain	1 (2 oz)	120	1	25	2	1

MARCO'S PIZZA

OTHER MENU SELECTIONS

FOOD	PORTION	CAL	FAT	CARB	SUGAR	FIBER
Cheezybread Bran	1 piece	80	2	11	1	0
Chicken Tumblers BBQ	1	67	2	7	3	0
Chicken Tumblers Hot & Spicy	1	57	2	5	0	0
Chicken Tumblers Naked	1	57	2	5	0	0
Chicken Wings BBQ	1	71	4	3	3	0
Chicken Wings Hot & Spicy	1	60	4	0	0	0
Chicken Wings Naked	1	60	4	0	0	0
Cinnasquares	1 piece	60	2	9	5	0
Salad Chicken Ranch	1 serv	240	13	10	2	3
Salad Italian	1 serv	230	17	11	3	3
Sub Chicken Club	½	385	16	34	2	2
Sub Ham & Cheese	½	400	21	33	2	1
Sub Italian	½	430	23	35	3	2
Sub Steak & Cheese	½	380	15	33	2	1
Sub Veggie	½	355	16	39	2	3

PIZZA

FOOD	PORTION	CAL	FAT	CARB	SUGAR	FIBER
Cheese Small	1 slice	200	6	23	2	1
Cheese Medium	1 slice	210	6	24	2	1
Cheese Large	1 slice	280	8	33	3	2
Chicken Fresco Small	1 slice	180	7	19	2	1
Chicken Fresco Medium	1 slice	260	10	26	3	1
Chicken Fresco Large	1 slice	350	13	35	4	2
Deep Pan Cheese	1 slice	290	8	36	3	2
Deep Pan Pepperoni	1 slice	330	12	36	3	2

FOOD	PORTION	CAL	FAT	CARB	SUGAR	FIBER
Deluxe Uno Small	1 slice	200	9	18	2	1
Deluxe Uno Medium	1 slice	280	12	26	2	1
Deluxe Uno Large	1 slice	380	16	35	3	2
Garden Small	1 slice	160	5	19	2	1
Garden Medium	1 slice	230	8	26	3	2
Garden Large	1 slice	310	10	36	4	2
Hawaiian Chicken Small	1 slice	180	6	18	2	1
Hawaiian Chicken Medium	1 slice	260	10	26	3	1
Hawaiian Chicken Large	1 slice	380	15	35	4	2
Meat Supremo Small	1 slice	210	10	18	2	1
Meat Supremo Medium	1 slice	300	15	25	2	1
Meat Supremo Large	1 slice	430	21	34	3	2
Pepperoni Small	1 slice	210	8	23	2	1
Pepperoni Medium	1 slice	230	9	24	2	1
Pepperoni Large	1 slice	310	11	33	3	2
White Cheezy Small	1 slice	170	7	17	1	1
White Cheezy Medium	1 slice	260	11	24	2	1
White Cheezy Large	1 slice	340	15	33	2	2

MCDONALD'S

BEVERAGES

FOOD	PORTION	CAL	FAT	CARB	SUGAR	FIBER
Apple Juice Minute Maid Juice Box	1 box (6.8 oz)	100	0	23	22	0
Coca-Cola Classic	1 sm (16 oz)	150	0	40	40	0
Coffee Black	1 sm (12 oz)	0	0	0	0	0
Coffee Cream	1 pkg (0.4 oz)	20	2	0	0	0
Diet Coke	1 sm (16 oz)	0	0	0	0	0
Dr Pepper	1 sm (16 oz)	150	0	39	39	0
Dr Pepper Diet	1 sm (16 oz)	0	0	0	0	0
Frappe Caramel	1 sm (12 oz)	450	20	62	56	0
Frappe Mocha	1 sm (12 oz)	450	20	62	56	1
Hi-C Orange Lavaburst	1 sm (16 oz)	160	0	44	44	0

FOOD	PORTION	CAL	FAT	CARB	SUGAR	FIBER
Hot Chocolate Peppermint w/ Nonfat Milk	1 (12 oz)	220	4	37	34	0
Iced Coffee Caramel	1 sm (16 oz)	130	5	21	20	1
Iced Coffee Hazelnut	1 sm (16 oz)	130	5	21	21	0
Iced Coffee Regular	1 sm (16 oz)	140	5	22	22	0
Iced Coffee Vanilla	1 sm (16 oz)	130	5	21	21	0
Iced Coffee w/ Sugar Free Vanilla Syrup	1 sm (16 oz)	60	5	8	1	0
Iced Mocha w/ Nonfat Milk	1 sm (12 oz)	230	7	35	29	0
Iced Tea	1 sm (16 oz)	0	0	0	0	0
McCafe Shake Chocolate	1 (12 oz)	570	17	91	76	1
McCafe Shake Strawberry	1 (12 oz)	560	18	89	79	0
McCafe Shake Vanilla	1 (12 oz)	530	17	84	63	0
Milk Lowfat 1%	1 jug (8.3 oz)	100	3	12	12	0
Orange Juice Minute Maid	1 sm (12 oz)	150	0	30	30	0
Peppermint Mocha w/ Nonfat Milk	1 sm (12 oz)	220	4	36	33	0
Powerade Mountain Blast	1 sm (16 oz)	100	0	27	21	0
Smoothie Strawberry Banana	1 (12 oz)	210	1	49	44	2
Smoothie Wild Berry	1 (12 oz)	210	1	48	4	3
Sprite	1 sm (16 oz)	150	0	39	39	0
Sweet Tea	1 sm (16 oz)	150	0	36	36	0
BREAKFAST SELECTIONS						
Big Breakfast Regular Biscuit	1 (9.5 oz)	740	48	51	3	3

FOOD	PORTION	CAL	FAT	CARB	SUGAR	FIBER
Big Breakfast w/ Hotcakes Regular Biscuit	1 (14.8 oz)	1090	56	111	17	6
Biscuit Regular Bacon Egg Cheese	1 (4.9 oz)	420	23	38	3	2
Biscuit Regular Sausage	1 (4.1 oz)	430	27	34	2	2
Biscuit Regular Sausage w/ Egg	1 (5.7 oz)	510	33	36	2	2
Chicken Biscuit Southern Style Regular	1 (5 oz)	410	20	41	3	2
Cinnamon Melts	1 serv (4 oz)	460	19	66	32	3
Fruit 'n Yogurt Parfait	1 (5.2 oz)	150	2	30	23	1
Hash Brown	1 (2 oz)	150	9	15	0	2
Hotcake Syrup	1 pkg (2 oz)	180	0	45	32	0
Hotcakes	1 serv (5.3 oz)	350	9	60	14	3
Hotcakes w/ Sausage	1 serv (6.8 oz)	520	24	61	14	3
McGriddles Bacon Egg Cheese	1 (5.8 oz)	410	18	48	15	2
McGriddles Sausage	1 serv (5 oz)	420	22	44	15	2
McGriddles Sausage Egg & Cheese	1 serv (7.1 oz)	550	31	48	15	2
McMuffin Egg	1 (4 oz)	300	12	30	3	2
McMuffin Sausage	1 (4 oz)	370	22	29	2	2
McMuffin Sausage w/ Egg	1 (5.8 oz)	450	27	30	2	2
Oatmeal Fruit & Maple	1 serv (9.2 oz)	290	5	57	32	5
Oatmeal Fruit & Maple w/o Brown Sugar	1 serv (9.2 oz)	260	5	48	18	5
DESSERTS						
Baked Hot Apple Pie	1 (2.7 oz)	250	13	32	13	4

FOOD	PORTION	CAL	FAT	CARB	SUGAR	FIBER
Cone Reduced Fat Vanilla	1 (3.7 oz)	170	5	27	20	0
Cookie Chocolate Chip	1 (1.2 oz)	160	8	21	15	1
Cookie Oatmeal Raisin	1 (1.1 oz)	150	6	22	13	1
Cookie Sugar	1 (1.1 oz)	160	7	21	11	0
McFlurry M&M's	1 (12 oz)	650	23	96	89	1
McFlurry Oreo Cookies	1 (12 oz)	510	17	80	64	1
Peanuts For Sundae	1 serv (0.3 oz)	45	4	2	0	1
Sundae Hot Caramel	1 (6.4 oz)	340	8	60	43	1
Sundae Hot Fudge	1 (6.3 oz)	330	9	53	48	1
Sundae Strawberry	1 (6.3 oz)	280	6	49	45	1
MAIN MENU SELECTIONS						
Angus Bacon & Cheese	1 (10.2 oz)	790	39	63	13	4
Angus Deluxe	1 (11.2 oz)	760	39	61	10	4
Angus Mushroom & Swiss	1 (10 oz)	770	40	59	8	4
Big Mac	1 (7.6 oz)	550	29	46	9	3
Cheeseburger	1 (4 oz)	300	12	33	7	2
Cheeseburger Double	1 (5.8 oz)	440	23	34	7	2
Chicken Breast Strips	3 (4.4 oz)	380	23	21	0	1
Chicken McNuggets	4 (2.3 oz)	190	12	12	0	1
Filet-O-Fish	1 (5 oz)	390	19	39	5	2
French Fries	1 sm (2.5 oz)	230	11	29	0	3
Grilled Onion Cheddar	1 (4.1 oz)	310	13	33	7	2
Hamburger	1 (3.5 oz)	250	9	31	6	2
McChicken	1 (5.1 oz)	360	16	40	5	2
McDouble	1 (5.3 oz)	390	19	33	7	2
McRib	1 (7.3 oz)	500	26	44	11	3
Quarter Pounder Double w/ Cheese	1 (10 oz)	750	43	42	10	3
Quarter Pounder w/ Cheese	1 (7.1 oz)	520	26	41	10	3

FOOD	PORTION	CAL	FAT	CARB	SUGAR	FIBER
Sandwich Classic Chicken Crispy	1 (7.5 oz)	510	22	55	10	3
Sandwich Classic Chicken Grilled	1 (7 oz)	350	9	42	8	3
Sandwich Club Chicken Crispy	1 (8.4 oz)	620	29	57	11	3
Sandwich Club Chicken Grilled	1 (7.9 oz)	460	16	43	9	3
Sandwich Ranch BLT Chicken Crispy	1 (7.6 oz)	540	23	56	11	3
Sandwich Ranch BLT Chicken Grilled	1 (7.1 oz)	380	10	42	9	3
Sandwich Southern Style Crispy Chicken	1 (5.6 oz)	420	19	43	7	2
Snack Wrap Angus Bacon & Cheese	1 (5 oz)	390	21	28	4	1
Snack Wrap Angus Deluxe	1 (5.9 oz)	410	25	27	3	2
Snack Wrap Angus Mushroom & Swiss	1 (5.7 oz)	430	25	27	2	2
Snack Wrap Chipotle BBQ Crispy	1 (4.1 oz)	330	15	34	4	1
Snack Wrap Chipotle BBQ Grilled	1 (4.1 oz)	250	8	27	5	1
Snack Wrap Honey Mustard Crispy	1 (4.1 oz)	320	15	33	2	1
Snack Wrap Honey Mustard Grilled	1 (4.1 oz)	250	8	27	2	1
Snack Wrap Ranch Crispy	1 (4.2 oz)	350	19	32	2	1
Snack Wrap Ranch Grilled	1 (4.2 oz)	270	12	25	2	1

FOOD	PORTION	CAL	FAT	CARB	SUGAR	FIBER
SALAD DRESSINGS AND SAUCES						
Dressing Newman's Own Creamy Caesar	1 pkg (2 oz)	190	18	4	2	0
Dressing Newman's Own Creamy Southwest	1 pkg (1.5 oz)	100	6	11	3	0
Dressing Newman's Own Low Fat Balsamic Vinaigrette	1 pkg (1.5 oz)	35	3	3	3	0
Dressing Newman's Own Low Fat Family Recipe Italian	1 pkg (1.5 oz)	50	3	7	2	0
Dressing Newman's Own Low Fat Sesame Ginger	1 pkg (1.5 oz)	90	3	15	9	1
Dressing Newman's Own Ranch	1 pkg (2 oz)	170	15	9	4	0
Honey	1 pkg (0.5 oz)	50	0	12	11	0
Ketchup	1 pkg (0.4 oz)	10	0	3	2	0
Sauce Chipotle Barbeque	1 pkg (1 oz)	50	0	11	10	0
Sauce Creamy Ranch	1 pkg (0.8 oz)	110	12	1	1	0
Sauce Honey Mustard	1 pkg (0.8 oz)	35	4	6	5	1
Sauce Hot Mustard	1 pkg (1 oz)	60	3	9	6	2
Sauce Spicy Buffalo	1 pkg (0.8 oz)	35	3	1	0	0
Sauce Sweet 'N Sour	1 pkg (1 oz)	50	0	12	10	0
Sauce Tangy Barbecue	1 pkg (1 oz)	50	0	12	10	0
Sauce Tartar	1 serv (1 oz)	140	15	0	0	0
SALADS						
Bacon Ranch w/ Crispy Chicken	1 (11.3 oz)	390	22	24	7	4
Bacon Ranch w/ Grilled Chicken	1 (10.8 oz)	230	9	10	5	4

FOOD	PORTION	CAL	FAT	CARB	SUGAR	FIBER
Bacon Ranch w/o Chicken	1 (7.9 oz)	140	7	10	4	3
Caesar w/ Crispy Chicken	1 (10.9 oz)	350	18	24	7	4
Caesar w/ Grilled Chicken	1 (10.4 oz)	190	5	10	5	4
Caesar w/o Chicken	1 (7.5 oz)	90	4	9	4	3
Croutons Butter Garlic	1 pkg (0.5 oz)	60	2	10	0	1
Fruit & Walnut Snack Size	1 pkg (5.7 oz)	210	8	31	25	2
Side Salad	1 (3.1 oz)	20	0	4	2	1
Southwest w/ Crispy Chicken	1 (12.3 oz)	450	21	42	13	7
Southwest w/ Grilled Chicken	1 (11.8 oz)	290	8	28	11	7
Southwest w/o Chicken	1 (8.1 oz)	140	5	20	6	6
MRS. FIELDS						
Bites Double Fudge	3 (1.6 oz)	200	10	27	21	1
Brownie Butterscotch Blondie	1 (2.1 oz)	260	10	38	28	0
Brownie Double Fudge	1 (2.1 oz)	260	13	34	27	1
Brownie Pecan Fudge	1 (2.1 oz)	270	15	32	25	2
Brownie Special Walnut Fudge & Blondie	1 (2.2 oz)	260	13	35	27	1
Brownie Toffee Fudge	1 (2.1 oz)	260	14	34	27	1
Brownie Walnut Fudge	1 (2.1 oz)	270	15	32	25	2
Cake Chocolate Chip	1 piece (2.9 oz)	350	17	45	27	tr
Coffee Cake Chocolate Chip	1 sm piece (2.2 oz)	240	11	30	16	1
Coffee Cake Chocolate Chip	1 lg (2.4 oz)	250	12	32	16	1
Cookie Butter	1 (1.5 oz)	200	8	29	15	tr

FOOD	PORTION	CAL	FAT	CARB	SUGAR	FIBER
Cookie Chocolate Covered Peanut Butter	1 (2.5 oz)	340	19	37	26	1
Cookie Chocolate Covered Semi-Sweet	1 (2.5 oz)	380	23	40	37	1
Cookie Chocolate Covered White Chunk Macadamia	1 (2.4 oz)	330	19	39	29	1
Cookie Cinnamon Sugar	1 (1.8 oz)	210	8	31	16	0
Cookie Cut Out	1 (2.4 oz)	280	11	44	28	0
Cookie Frosted Cinnamon Sugar	1 (2.1 oz)	270	11	39	25	0
Cookie Oatmeal Raisins & Walnuts	1 (1.7 oz)	200	9	27	16	1
Cookie Semi-Sweet Chocolate	1 (1.7 oz)	210	10	29	19	1
Cookie Semi-Sweet Chocolate w/ Walnuts	1 (1.7 oz)	220	11	28	17	1
Cookie Triple Chocolate	1 (1.7 oz)	210	10	28	19	1
Cookie White Chunk Macadamia	1 (1.7 oz)	230	12	28	19	0
Jelly Bellys	1 pkg (1.4 oz)	140	0	37	29	0
Mixed Nuts	1 pkg (2 oz)	350	32	13	2	3
Muffin Blueberry	1 (1.9 oz)	190	9	24	12	1
Muffin Chocolate Chip	1 (1.9 oz)	200	10	26	14	1
Nibbler Cinnamon Sugar	3 (1.4 oz)	180	8	25	12	0
Nibbler Debra's Special	3 (1.3 oz)	160	7	22	13	1
Nibbler Peanut Butter	3 (1.8 oz)	170	9	19	10	1
Nibbler Semi-Sweet Chocolate	3 (1.8 oz)	170	8	23	14	1
Nibbler Triple Chocolate	3 (1.8 oz)	160	8	22	15	1
Nibbler White Chunk Macadamia	3 (1.8 oz)	180	9	22	15	0
Taffy	1 pkg (2.4 oz)	160	2	38	23	0

FOOD	PORTION	CAL	FAT	CARB	SUGAR	FIBER
NAKED PIZZA						
10 Inch Pie Original Crust	1 slice	81	5	8	–	3
10 Inch Pie Thin Crust	1 slice	64	5	5	–	2
12 Inch Pie Original Crust	1 slice	132	6	16	–	6
12 Inch Pie Thin Crust	1 slice	91	5	10	–	3
14 Inch Pie Original Crust	1 slice	161	7	20	–	7
14 Inch Pie Thin Crust	1 slice	114	5	11	–	4
NATHAN'S						
Apple Pie	1 (3.49 oz)	314	19	33	9	0
Bacon Cheeseburger	1 (10.7 oz)	783	50	45	10	2
Cheese Dog	1 (5.05 oz)	390	25	30	5	1
Cheese Fries	1 reg (8 oz)	564	42	41	5	4
Cheesesteak	1 (12.31 oz)	849	45	70	1	2
Cheesesteak Supreme	1 (16.29 oz)	879	45	76	3	3
Cheesesteak Supreme Chicken	1 (13.81 oz)	601	19	70	3	3
Chicken Tender Pita	1 (11.94 oz)	823	52	66	15	5
Chicken Tender Platter	1 (17.69 oz)	1245	90	80	31	10
Chicken Tenders	3 (6.19 oz)	526	39	24	8	3
Chicken Wings	5 (6.65 oz)	400	27	12	0	0
Chili Dog	1 (5.05 oz)	400	23	33	5	2
Corn Dog On A Stick	1 (2.89 oz)	380	21	39	13	1
Corn On The Cob w/ Butter	1 (5.05 oz)	140	2	34	6	2
Double Burger w/ Cheese	1 (15.61 oz)	1178	84	45	10	2
Famous Hot Dog	1 (3.53 oz)	297	18	24	4	1
French Fries	1 reg (6.5 oz)	464	34	35	4	4
Funnel Cake	1 (4.21 oz)	580	29	73	43	1
Hot Dog Nuggets	6 (3.49 oz)	348	28	20	5	0

FOOD	PORTION	CAL	FAT	CARB	SUGAR	FIBER
Mozzarella Sticks + Sauce	3 (5.64 oz)	390	28	20	6	1
Onion Rings	1 sm (5.6 oz)	544	45	36	4	1
Platter Grilled Chicken	1 (15 oz)	504	56	58	24	7
Pretzel Dog	1 (4.02 oz)	390	16	49	7	1
Pretzel King Size	1 (2.28 oz)	180	1	38	1	1
Sandwich Chicken Tender	1 (9.65 oz)	706	43	58	12	5
Sandwich Grilled Chicken	1 (9.03 oz)	554	32	40	3	3
Wrap Grilled Chicken Caesar	1 (10.34 oz)	700	34	60	2	1
Wrap Krispy Southwest Chipotle	1 (11.71 oz)	750	39	62	3	1

OLD SPAGHETTI FACTORY

BEVERAGES

FOOD	PORTION	CAL	FAT	CARB	SUGAR	FIBER
Cherry Coke	1 (12 oz)	140	0	39	39	0
Coffee Black	1 (8 oz)	0	0	0	0	0
Coke	1 (12 oz)	130	0	37	37	0
Diet Coke	1 (12 oz)	0	0	0	0	0
Hot Tea	1 (8 oz)	0	0	0	0	0
Iced Tea Strawberry	1 (12 oz)	100	0	23	10	0
Italian Cream Soda	1 (7.5 oz)	140	3	25	24	0
Kid's Juice Bar	1 serv (2.4 oz)	60	0	15	14	0
Lemonade	1 (12 oz)	140	0	39	37	0
Lemonade Strawberry	1 (12 oz)	200	0	55	52	0
Masterpiece Shake	1 (8.5 oz)	700	39	81	63	1
Milk 2%	1 (13 oz)	180	7	17	17	0
Milk Skim	1 (13 oz)	130	1	18	18	0
Root Beer	1 (12 oz)	150	0	41	41	0
Sprite	1 (12 oz)	140	0	34	30	0

FOOD	PORTION	CAL	FAT	CARB	SUGAR	FIBER
CHILDREN'S MENU SELECTIONS						
Fettuccine Alfredo	1 serv (10.3 oz)	770	48	68	3	3
Macaroni & Cheese	1 serv (8 oz)	390	10	59	5	2
Ravioli	1 serv (10 oz)	420	14	55	9	5
Ravioli Spinach & Cheese	1 serv (6.6 oz)	310	12	38	5	4
Sandwich Grilled Cheese	1 (4.5 oz)	480	30	40	2	2
Spaghetti Marinara w/ Sicilian Meatballs	1 serv (13 oz)	570	16	75	8	5
Spaghetti w/ Brown Butter & Mizithra Cheese	1 serv (8.7 oz)	660	37	65	3	3
Spaghetti w/ Clam Sauce	1 serv (10 oz)	440	9	69	3	3
Spaghetti w/ Marinara Sauce	1 serv (15 oz)	560	5	108	11	7
Spaghetti w/ Meat Sauce	1 serv (10 oz)	410	6	70	6	4
Spinach Tortellini w/ Alfredo Sauce	1 serv (6.8 oz)	530	30	48	3	3
DESSERTS						
Cake Chocolate Truffle Mousse	1 serv (9 oz)	850	41	118	89	5
Ice Cream Spumoni	1 serv (3 oz)	180	9	21	17	0
Ice Cream Vanilla	1 serv (3 oz)	170	9	21	14	0
Mud Pie	1 serv (6 oz)	490	20	70	52	1
MAIN MENU SELECTIONS						
Angel Hair	1 serv (8 oz)	420	2	82	4	2
Appetizer Bay Shrimp Crostini	1 serv (9.3 oz)	720	41	54	3	3
Appetizer Garlic Fries	1 serv (18.4 oz)	1410	107	106	7	10

FOOD	PORTION	CAL	FAT	CARB	SUGAR	FIBER
Appetizer Portuguese Linguica	1 serv (17.5 oz)	1080	75	52	3	8
Baked Chicken	1 serv (18.3 oz)	1030	62	71	6	4
Baked Lasagna	1 serv (17.5 oz)	800	43	61	13	7
Bread Sicilian Garlic Cheese	4 serv (16 oz)	1310	76	110	10	6
Broccoli	1 sm (7.5 oz)	340	31	10	0	5
Burger Sliders	1 serv (23.6 oz)	1770	107	65	28	6
Cheese Manicotti w/ Marinara Sauce	1 serv (12 oz)	490	21	54	11	3
Chicken Marsala	1 serv (17.4 oz)	1050	57	75	7	3
Chicken Penne	1 serv (14.8 oz)	830	31	102	12	5
Dip Shrimp Spinach & Artichoke	4 serv (9.3 oz)	590	41	39	2	3
Factory Burger w/ Chips	1 serv (16.6 oz)	1370	84	71	12	4
Fettuccine Alfredo	1 serv (14.2 oz)	1080	70	91	5	4
Fettuccine or Penne	1 serv (8 oz)	420	2	85	3	4
Garlic Mizithra	1 serv (15 oz)	1240	77	103	7	4
Hearty Meal Clam Sauce	1 serv (25 oz)	1110	23	173	6	7
Hearty Meal Italian Sausage w/ Meat Sauce	1 serv (29 oz)	1350	42	177	14	12
Hearty Meal Marinara Sauce	1 serv (25 oz)	940	8	180	19	11

FOOD	PORTION	CAL	FAT	CARB	SUGAR	FIBER
Hearty Meal Meat Sauce	1 serv (25 oz)	1020	15	176	14	11
Hearty Meal Mizithra Cheese & Brown Butter	1 serv (22.4 oz)	1750	101	164	8	7
Hearty Meal Pot Pourri	1 serv (26 oz)	1280	43	176	13	9
Hearty Meal Sauteed Mushroom Sauce	1 serv (30 oz)	1120	26	184	22	12
Hearty Meal Sicilian Meatballs	1 serv (31 oz)	1350	36	186	19	13
Lasagna Vegetariano	1 serv (20.6 oz)	830	48	68	15	9
Meatloaf Italian	1 serv (18.5 oz)	1180	68	83	8	6
Olive Tapenade	4 serv (7.4 oz)	800	66	46	1	2
Panini Chicken Smoked Mozzarella w/ Chips	1 serv (14.4 oz)	1280	68	112	11	18
Parmigiana Chicken	1 serv (19.2 oz)	810	30	80	10	5
Pasta Gluten Free	1 serv (9 oz)	470	1	104	0	2
Pasta Whole Wheat	1 serv (8 oz)	390	2	85	4	14
Platter #1 Lasagna & Chicken Marsala	1 (27.5 oz)	1090	66	71	17	7
Platter #2 Ravioli & Spaghetti w/ Meat Sauce	1 (21 oz)	880	22	133	15	10
Platter #3 Spaghetti w/ Meat Sauce Sausage & Meatballs	1 (25 oz)	1360	64	114	9	9
Ravioli Crab	1 serv (11 oz)	810	45	73	3	5

FOOD	PORTION	CAL	FAT	CARB	SUGAR	FIBER
Ravioli Spinach & Cheese	1 serv (11 oz)	480	16	63	9	6
Ravioli Toasted Beef	4 serv (4 oz)	200	5	30	2	2
Ravioli Toasted Cheese	4 serv (4 oz)	210	6	30	3	2
Sandwich Sicilian Style Meatball w/ Chips	1 serv (16.4 oz)	1200	54	122	5	8
Sandwich Sicilian Style Sausage w/ Chips	1 serv (14.4 oz)	1140	55	117	4	9
Senior Meal Italian Sausage w/ Meat Sauce	1 serv (14 oz)	740	33	72	6	6
Senior Meal Pot Pourri	1 serv (10 oz)	520	19	69	5	4
Senior Meal Spaghetti Marinara	1 serv (10 oz)	370	4	72	8	5
Senior Meal Spaghetti Marinara w/ Sicilian Meatballs	1 serv (16 oz)	770	29	78	8	5
Senior Meal Spaghetti Mizithra & Brown Butter	1 serv (10 oz)	660	37	65	3	3
Senior Meal Spaghetti w/ Clam Sauce	1 serv (10 oz)	440	9	69	3	3
Senior Meal Spaghetti w/ Meat Sauce	1 serv (10 oz)	410	6	70	6	4
Senior Meal Spaghetti w/ Mushroom Sauce	1 serv (12 oz)	450	10	74	9	5
Side Alfredo Sauce	6 oz	640	67	7	0	0
Side Clam Sauce	6 oz	190	12	9	0	0
Side Marinara Sauce	6 oz	90	3	13	8	3
Side Marsala Sauce	6 oz	70	4	6	3	0
Side Meat Sauce	6 oz	140	7	10	5	2
Side Sausage	1 serv (4.5 oz)	340	27	3	0	2

FOOD	PORTION	CAL	FAT	CARB	SUGAR	FIBER
Side Sauteed Mushroom Sauce	9 oz	200	14	15	10	3
Side Sicilian Meatballs	2 (6 oz)	420	27	7	0	1
Spaghetti	1 serv (9 oz)	460	3	93	4	4
Spaghetti Vesuvius	1 serv (15 oz)	710	19	104	8	6
Spaghetti Squash	1 serv (20.7 oz)	540	36	45	13	8
Spaghetti w/ Clam Sauce	1 serv (15 oz)	660	14	104	4	4
Spaghetti w/ Italian Sausage w/ Meat Sauce	1 serv (19 oz)	940	36	107	8	8
Spaghetti w/ Meat Sauce	1 serv (15 oz)	610	9	105	8	7
Spaghetti w/ Mizithra Cheese & Brown Butter	1 serv (13.4 oz)	1040	59	99	5	4
Spaghetti w/ Pot Pourri	1 serv (16 oz)	780	26	106	8	6
Spaghetti w/ Sauteed Mushroom Sauce	1 serv (18 oz)	670	16	111	13	7
Spaghetti w/ Sicilian Meatballs	1 serv (21 oz)	960	31	114	12	7
Spinach Tortellini w/ Alfredo Sauce	1 serv (12 oz)	930	55	86	5	5
SALADS						
BLT	1 (15.4 oz)	1000	85	23	5	9
Caesar Upgrade	1 (7 oz)	440	37	14	2	3
Caesar Entree Chicken	1 (21.2 oz)	1130	90	29	5	6
Caesar Entree w/o Chicken	1 (14.5 oz)	820	72	25	5	6
House w/ 1000 Island	1 (5 oz)	230	17	16	5	1
House w/ Balsamic	1 (4.5 oz)	260	21	15	2	1
House w/ Blue Cheese	1 (5 oz)	280	24	13	2	1

FOOD	PORTION	CAL	FAT	CARB	SUGAR	FIBER
House w/ Caesar	1 (5 oz)	330	30	13	2	1
House w/ Creamy Pesto	1 (5 oz)	280	24	13	2	1
House w/ Fat Free Honey Mustard	1 (4.5 oz)	120	3	21	9	1
Senior Meal Caesar Chicken	1 serv (17 oz)	870	67	21	4	4
Senior Meal Caesar w/o Chicken	1 serv (10.2 oz)	560	48	17	4	4
SOUPS						
Chicken Mulligatawny	1 serv (9 oz)	260	19	20	6	1
Clam Chowder	1 serv (9 oz)	370	25	19	1	1
Cream Of Broccoli	1 serv (9 oz)	240	19	21	10	2
Minestrone	1 serv (9 oz)	60	2	10	2	2

ON THE BORDER

FOOD	PORTION	CAL	FAT	CARB	SUGAR	FIBER
CHILDREN'S MENU SELECTIONS						
Cheeseburger	1	530	42	17	–	0
Chicken Tenders	1 serv	450	32	29	–	2
Corn Dog	1	280	17	25	–	2
Hamburger	1	420	33	16	–	0
Mexican Plate Soft Taco Chicken	1 serv	270	11	23	–	1
Mexican Plate Taco Crispy Chicken	1 serv	260	12	18	–	3
Mexican Plate Taco Crispy Ground Beef	1 serv	320	20	19	–	4
Mexican Plate Taco Soft Ground Beef	1 serv	340	18	24	–	2
Nachos Bean & Cheese	1 serv	770	45	57	–	11
Nachos Cheese	1 serv	560	37	28	–	3
Sandwich Grilled Chicken	1	310	17	18	–	0

FOOD	PORTION	CAL	FAT	CARB	SUGAR	FIBER
DESSERTS						
Border Brownie Sundae w/ Vanilla Ice Cream	1	1360	72	162	–	7
Kahlua Ice Cream Pie	1 serv	950	50	111	–	6
Sizzling Apple Crisp	1 serv	1120	44	177	–	6
Sopapillas	5	1340	43	236	–	7
Sopapillas w/ Chocolate Sauce	2	540	18	92	–	4
Sopapillas w/ Honey	2	620	17	119	–	2
Sundae w/ Chocolate Syrup	1	370	18	51	–	1
Sundae w/ Strawberry Puree	1	330	17	41	–	1
MAIN MENU SELECTIONS						
Avocado Fries w/ Creamy Red Chile Sauce	1 serv	1120	83	89	–	11
Beans Black	1 side	180	3	29	–	10
Beans Refried	1 side	220	9	25	–	6
Big Bordurrito Chicken w/ Side Salad w/o Dressing w/ Rice	1 serv	1690	77	173	–	16
Big Bordurrito Steak w/ Side Salad w/o Dressing w/ Rice	1 serv	1750	89	171	–	17
Border Combo Baja	1 serv	1420	85	137	–	13
Border Combo New Mexico w/ Rice	1 serv	1090	68	90	–	8
Border Sampler	1 serv	2060	142	101	–	13
Burrito Classic Chicken w/o Sauce w/ Rice	1 serv	920	36	103	–	4
Burrito Classic Shredded Beef w/o Sauce w/ Rice	1 serv	1020	41	102	–	3

FOOD	PORTION	CAL	FAT	CARB	SUGAR	FIBER
Burrito Three Sauce Fajita Chicken w/ Rice	1 serv	1120	40	118	–	6
Burrito Three Sauce Fajita Steak w/ Rice	1 serv	1180	52	115	–	6
Carne Asada	1 serv	970	38	105	–	5
Chicken Queso	1 serv	1030	41	110	–	8
Chicken Salsa Fresca	1 serv	520	9	60	–	12
Chicken Tomatillo	1 serv	850	24	109	–	7
Chicken Flautas w/ Original Queso	1 serv	1250	87	65	–	9
Chile Con Queso	1 serv	80	6	3	–	0
Chile Relleno Cheese Stuffed w/ Ranchero Sauce	1 serv	570	49	26	–	7
Chips & Salsa	1 serv	430	22	52	–	5
Classic Chimichanga Chicken w/o Sauce w/ Rice	1 serv	1300	79	103	–	4
Classic Chimichanga Ground Beef w/o Sauce w/ Rice	1 serv	1420	90	105	–	6
Crispy Taco Chicken	1 serv	260	12	18	–	3
Crispy Taco Ground Beef	1 serv	320	20	19	–	4
Del Rio	1 serv	970	44	104	–	12
Empanadas Chicken w/ Original Queso	1 serv	1400	104	77	–	3
Empanadas Chicken w/ Chile Con Queso	1 serv	620	46	32	–	1
Empanadas Ground Beef w/ Chile Con Queso	1 serv	620	46	33	–	2
Empanadas Ground Beef w/ Original Queso	1 serv	1410	105	78	–	5

FOOD	PORTION	CAL	FAT	CARB	SUGAR	FIBER
Enchiladas Barbacoa w/ Rice	1 serv	1100	49	105	–	7
Enchiladas Cheese & Onion w/ Chile Con Carne	1 serv	310	21	18	–	2
Enchiladas Chicken w/ Sour Cream Sauce	1 serv	210	12	16	–	1
Enchiladas Green Chile Chicken w/ Rice	1 serv	850	34	103	–	5
Enchiladas Grilled Avocado w/ Red Chile Pesto & Rice	1 serv	1080	59	111	–	14
Enchiladas Grilled Pepper Jack Chicken w/ Rice	1 serv	1050	48	106	–	6
Enchiladas Grilled Smokey Beef Brisket w/ Rice	1 serv	980	46	100	–	5
Enchiladas Ground Beef w/ Chile Con Carne	1 serv	260	15	18	–	3
Enchiladas La Bandera	1 serv	940	40	102	–	6
Enchiladas Suizas w/ Rice	1 serv	1000	45	106	–	7
Fajita Monterey Ranch Chicken	1 serv	650	43	12	–	1
Fajita Grill Carnitas Pulled Pork	1 serv	920	83	3	–	3
Fajita Grill Grilled Vegetables w/ Portobello Mushrooms	1 serv	230	15	25	–	4
Fajita Grill Guajillo Steak Sauce	1 serv	45	3	6	–	0

FOOD	PORTION	CAL	FAT	CARB	SUGAR	FIBER
Fajita Grill Mesquite Chicken	1 serv	300	16	4	–	0
Fajita Grill Mesquite Steak	1 serv	390	28	1	–	0
Fajita Grill Salsa Red Chile Tomatillo	1 serv	10	0	2	–	1
Fajita Grill Seasoned Sauteed Shrimp	1 serv	390	33	2	–	0
Fajita Grill Veggies Baja Blend	1 serv	220	16	18	–	4
Fajita Grill Veggies Classic	1 serv	90	5	11	–	3
Fajita Grill Veggies El Diablo	1 serv	60	2	9	–	2
Fajitas The Ultimate	1 serv	1160	96	26	–	7
Firecracker Stuffed Jalapenos w/ Original Queso	1 serv	1910	135	124	–	5
Flautas Chicken w/ Chile Con Queso	1 serv	370	26	17	–	2
Grande Fajita Nachos Chicken	1 serv	1390	77	82	–	16
Grande Fajita Nachos Steak	1 serv	1450	89	79	–	16
Guacamole	1 side	50	5	3	–	3
Guacamole Live w/o Chips	1 serv	570	50	34	–	31
Mexican Rice	1 side	280	5	55	–	1
Mini Tacos Street Style Carnitas w/ Rice	1 serv	930	47	89	–	9
Mini Tacos Street Style Chicken w/ Rice	1 serv	890	40	88	–	8
Mini Tacos Street Style Steak w/ Rice	1 serv	980	51	85	–	8

FOOD	PORTION	CAL	FAT	CARB	SUGAR	FIBER
Original Queso Carne Style w/o Chips	1 bowl	510	36	17	–	2
Original Queso Carne Style w/o Chips	1 cup	350	24	11	–	2
Original Queso w/o Chips	1 cup	270	19	9	–	1
Original Queso w/o Chips	1 bowl	430	31	15	–	1
Quesadillas Fajita Chicken	1 serv	1180	82	55	–	5
Quesadillas Fajita Steak	1 serv	1210	88	54	–	6
Ranchiladas	1 serv	1260	66	96	–	6
Rice Cilantro Lime	1 side	390	3	83	–	1
Salmon Mexican Jalapeno BBQ	1 serv	590	21	45	–	24
Side Mixed Cheese	1 serv	110	9	0	0	0
Soft Taco Chicken	1 serv	270	11	23	–	1
Soft Taco Ground Beef	1 serv	340	18	24	–	2
Superior Dinner	1	1500	82	125	–	10
Tacos Achiote Chicken w/ Rice	1 serv	650	12	98	–	6
Tacos Al Carbon Especiales Chicken w/ Rice	1 serv	900	31	102	–	3
Tacos Al Carbon Especiales Steak w/ Rice	1 serv	960	41	101	–	3
Tacos Dos XX Fish w/ Creamy Red Chile Sauce	1 serv	550	39	34	–	1
Tacos Grilled Fish w/ Creamy Red Chile Sauce & Rice	1 serv	880	36	91	–	7
Tacos Pork Guajillo w/ Guajillo Sauce & Rice	1 serv	950	47	92	–	6

FOOD	PORTION	CAL	FAT	CARB	SUGAR	FIBER
Tacos Southwest Chicken w/ Creamy Red Chile Sauce & Rice	1 serv	1280	61	129	–	3
Tamale Pork w/ Enchilada Sauce	1 serv	310	19	21	–	4
Tortillas Homemade Flour	3	360	11	57	–	0
Tostadas Chicken	1 serv	130	5	12	–	2
Tostadas Ground Beef	1 serv	170	9	12	–	3
Tostadas Guacamole	1 serv	180	13	16	–	7
Tres Enchilada Dinner Cheese & Onion w/ Chile Con Carne & Rice	1 serv	1220	66	109	–	7
Tres Enchilada Dinner Chicken w/ Sour Cream Sauce & Rice	1 serv	920	39	102	–	5
Tres Enchilada Dinner Ground Beef w/ Chile Con Carne & Rice	1 serv	1060	48	109	–	10
SALAD DRESSINGS AND SAUCES						
Dressing Chipotle Honey Mustard	1 serv	320	31	12	–	0
Dressing Fat Free Mango Citrus Vinaigrette	1 serv	80	0	20	–	0
Dressing Smoked Jalapeno Vinaigrette	1 serv	250	24	8	–	0
Pico De Gallo	1 side	10	1	1	–	0
Queso	1 side	160	12	6	–	0
Sauce Green Chile	1 side	30	2	3	–	0
Sour Cream	1 side	60	5	2	–	0

FOOD	PORTION	CAL	FAT	CARB	SUGAR	FIBER
SALADS						
Citrus Chipotle Chicken w/ Mango Citrus Vinaigrette	1 serv	290	4	42	–	11
Grande Taco Chicken w/o Dressing	1 serv	1180	75	79	–	13
Grande Taco Ground Beef w/o Dressing	1 serv	1280	85	80	–	15
House Side w/o Dressing	1 serv	200	12	20	–	5
Sizzling Fajita Chicken w/o Dressing	1 serv	710	47	23	–	8
Sizzling Fajita Steak w/o Dressing	1 serv	780	57	21	–	8
SOUPS						
Chicken Tortilla	1 cup	300	16	24	–	3
Tortilla Soup	1 bowl	480	23	48	–	4
ORANGE JULIUS						
BEVERAGES						
Barq's	1 sm (17 oz)	180	0	48	48	0
Coca-Cola	1 sm (17 oz)	160	0	43	43	0
Coffee Black	1 (12 oz)	0	0	0	0	0
Diet Coca-Cola	1 sm (17 oz)	0	0	0	0	0
Diet Pepsi	1 sm (17 oz)	0	0	0	0	0
Dr Pepper	1 sm (17 oz)	160	0	43	43	0
Julius Bananarilla	1 sm (16 oz)	350	6	75	58	3
Julius Blackberry	1 sm (16 oz)	380	6	85	67	4
Julius Cool Cappuccino	1 sm (16 oz)	430	11	77	63	2
Julius Cool Mocha	1 sm (16 oz)	700	14	123	105	3
Julius Eggnog	1 sm (16 oz)	330	8	65	55	2
Julius Lemon	1 sm (16 oz)	280	0	77	76	0
Julius Mango	1 sm (16 oz)	250	0	67	64	1
Julius Orange	1 sm (16 oz)	230	0	61	59	0

FOOD	PORTION	CAL	FAT	CARB	SUGAR	FIBER
Julius Peach	1 sm (16 oz)	240	0	63	61	1
Julius Pina Colada	1 sm (16 oz)	330	5	74	64	2
Julius Pineapple	1 sm (16 oz)	230	0	61	59	1
Julius Pomegranate	1 sm (16 oz)	260	0	70	68	1
Julius Raspberry	1 sm (16 oz)	300	0	79	77	3
Julius Strawberry	1 sm (16 oz)	290	0	78	75	1
Julius Strawberry Banana	1 sm (16 oz)	380	6	83	69	3
Julius Tripleberry	1 sm (16 oz)	420	6	93	79	4
Julius Tropical	1 sm (16 oz)	370	6	80	63	3
Milk 2%	1 (8 oz)	110	5	11	11	0
Mountain Dew	1 sm (17 oz)	190	0	51	51	0
Mug	1 sm (17 oz)	160	0	47	47	0
Orange Juice	1 (12 oz)	170	0	41	36	0
Pepsi	1 sm (17 oz)	160	0	44	44	0
Sierra Mist	1 sm (17 oz)	170	0	43	43	0
Smoothie 3-Berry Blast	1 sm (12 oz)	310	1	74	61	4
Smoothie Banana Chill	1 sm (12 oz)	320	1	77	58	3
Smoothie Berry Banana Squeeze	1 sm (12 oz)	220	0	55	49	2
Smoothie Berry Lemon Lively	1 sm (12 oz)	290	1	70	56	3
Smoothie Blackberry Toner	1 sm (12 oz)	270	1	63	47	3
Smoothie Blackberry Storm	1 sm (12 oz)	360	4	82	64	3
Smoothie Cocoa Latte Swirl	1 sm (16 oz)	370	7	69	64	2
Smoothie Mango Passion	1 sm (12 oz)	230	0	54	46	1
Smoothie Orange Berry	1 sm (12 oz)	320	2	76	65	2
Smoothie Orange Swirl	1 sm (12 oz)	280	4	59	46	1

FOOD	PORTION	CAL	FAT	CARB	SUGAR	FIBER
Smoothie Peaches & Cream	1 sm (12 oz)	240	0	64	45	1
Smoothie Pomegranate & Berries	1 sm (12 oz)	250	0	57	49	2
Smoothie Raspberry Creme	1 sm (12 oz)	330	3	73	61	2
Smoothie Raspberry Crush	1 sm (12 oz)	160	0	41	32	4
Smoothie Strawberry Sensation	1 sm (12 oz)	280	0	65	57	2
Smoothie Strawberry Xtreme	1 sm (12 oz)	270	0	64	52	2
Smoothie Tropical Tango	1 (12 oz)	240	2	58	48	2
Smoothie Tropi-Colada	1 (12 oz)	330	3	73	61	1
Smoothie Light Berry Pom Twlight	1 (12 oz)	140	0	34	25	3
Smoothie Light Pineapple Daylight	1 (12 oz)	110	0	27	20	1
Smoothie Light Strawberry Delight	1 (12 oz)	110	0	27	20	2
Smoothie Light Tropical Sunlight	1 (12 oz)	130	0	33	26	2
Sprite	1 sm (17 oz)	150	0	42	42	0
FOOD						
Dog Bacon Cheese	1 (5.6 oz)	490	33	24	3	1
Dog Cheese	1 (5.4 oz)	460	31	24	3	1
Dog Chicago	1 (9.4 oz)	430	27	29	6	3
Dog Chili Melt	1 (5.8 oz)	470	33	25	3	1
Dog Chili Slaw	1 (6.5 oz)	480	33	27	3	2
Dog Classic	1 (5 oz)	390	27	22	4	1
Dog Pepperoni Cheese	1 (5.7 oz)	460	31	26	3	2
Dog Relish	1 (5.5 oz)	420	27	28	7	1
Dog Reuben	1 (6.9 oz)	520	36	24	3	2

FOOD	PORTION	CAL	FAT	CARB	SUGAR	FIBER
Dog Sauerkraut	1 (5.9 oz)	410	27	24	3	2
Dog Southwest Chili	1 (6.7 oz)	500	34	27	4	2
Dog Triple Cheese	1 (6.2 oz)	540	38	24	3	1
Pita Chicken Caesar	1 (6.6 oz)	450	22	45	2	6
Pita Chicken Fajita	1 (6.8 oz)	360	11	47	3	7
Pita Garden Veggie	1 (7.3 oz)	470	26	49	5	7
Pita Santa Fe Grilled Chicken	1 (6.8 oz)	450	21	47	2	7
Pita Steak Fajita	1 (8 oz)	410	14	51	3	7
Pita Turkey Club	1 (8 oz)	480	23	46	1	6
Sandwich Crispy Chicken	1 (7.4 oz)	600	30	59	8	7
Sandwich Grilled Chicken	1 (6.3 oz)	360	15	32	5	1
Sandwich Iron Grilled Classic Club	1 (9.4 oz)	600	24	55	4	3
Sandwich Iron Grilled Supreme BLT	1 (6 oz)	600	34	40	2	2
Sandwich Iron Grilled Turkey	1 (8.2 oz)	550	23	43	2	2

PANERA BREAD

BAKERY

FOOD	PORTION	CAL	FAT	CARB	SUGAR	FIBER
Asiago Cheese Loaf	1 slice (2 oz)	160	4	23	0	1
Bagel Asiago Cheese	1	330	6	55	3	2
Bagel Blueberry	1	330	2	68	10	2
Bagel Chocolate Chip	1	370	6	69	14	2
Bagel Cinnamon Crunch	1	430	8	80	29	2
Bagel Cinnamon Swirl & Raisin	1	320	3	64	11	3
Bagel Everything	1	300	3	59	4	2
Bagel French Toast	1	350	5	67	15	2
Bagel Jalapeno & Cheddar	1	310	3	56	3	2

FOOD	PORTION	CAL	FAT	CARB	SUGAR	FIBER
Bagel Plain	1	290	2	59	3	2
Bagel Sesame	1	310	3	59	3	2
Bagel Sweet Onion & Poppyseed	1	390	7	72	7	4
Bagel Whole Wheat	1	340	3	67	5	6
Baguette Whole Grain	1 slice (2 oz)	140	1	27	2	3
Bear Claw	1	550	28	67	32	3
Brownie Double Fudge w/ Icing	1	480	17	76	44	2
Cake Cinnamon Coffee Crumb	1 slice	470	25	54	30	1
Ciabatta	1 (6.25 oz)	460	6	84	3	3
Cinnamon Raisin	1 slice (2 oz)	180	3	34	11	1
Cinnamon Roll	1	620	24	89	33	3
Cobblestone	1	650	13	122	64	3
Cookie Candy	1	420	19	59	33	1
Cookie Chocolate Chipper	1	440	23	59	33	2
Cookie Chocolate Chipper	1 mini	110	6	15	8	1
Cookie Chocolate Duet w/ Walnuts	1	450	24	55	36	3
Cookie Easter Egg	1	480	22	67	38	1
Cookie Oatmeal Raisin	1	370	14	57	28	2
Cookie Shortbread	1	350	21	36	11	1
Cookie Toffee Nut	1	460	19	59	29	1
Country Loaf	1 slice (2 oz)	140	1	27	0	1
Croissant French	1	310	18	30	4	1
Focaccia	1 serv (2 oz)	180	1	28	1	1
Focaccia w/ Asiago Cheese	1 slice (2 oz)	160	5	23	1	1
French Baguette	1 slice (2 oz)	150	1	30	0	1
Honey Wheat Loaf	1 slice (2 oz)	170	3	30	4	2

FOOD	PORTION	CAL	FAT	CARB	SUGAR	FIBER
Hot Cross Bun	1	220	5	38	19	1
Muffie Chocolate Chip	1	320	14	46	27	2
Muffie Pumpkin	1	290	11	45	26	1
Muffin Apple Crunch	1	450	12	80	49	2
Muffin Carrot Walnut	1	500	21	72	37	3
Muffin Pumpkin	1	580	22	89	51	2
Muffin Wild Blueberry	1	440	17	66	39	2
Pastry Cheese	1	400	22	42	15	1
Pastry Cherry	1	500	18	77	45	2
Pastry Chocolate	1	410	24	46	18	2
Pastry Fresh Apple	1	380	17	44	17	1
Pastry Ring Apple Cherry Cheese	1 slice	230	11	30	16	1
Pecan Braid	1	470	26	52	23	2
Pecan Roll	1	730	39	87	48	5
Scone Cinnamon Chip	1	600	31	73	34	2
Scone Orange	1 mini	160	4	29	21	1
Scone Orange	1 lg	470	11	87	62	3
Scone Strawberries & Cream	1	420	19	57	27	1
Scone Strawberries & Cream	1 mini	140	6	19	9	0
Scone Wild Blueberry	1	440	18	63	25	2
Scone Wild Blueberry	1 mini	160	6	21	8	1
Sesame Semolina Loaf	1 slice (2 oz)	140	1	29	1	1
Sourdough Roll	1 (2.5 oz)	200	1	39	0	1
Sourdough Round Loaf	1 slice (2 oz)	140	1	28	0	1
Sourdough Soup Bowl	1 (8 oz)	590	3	118	1	4
Spring Petites	1 mini	230	12	27	12	0
Stone Milled Rye Loaf	1 slice (2 oz)	140	1	28	0	2
Three Cheese Loaf	1 slice (2 oz)	140	2	26	1	1
Tomato Basil XL Loaf	1 slice (2 oz)	140	1	27	1	1
White Whole Grain Loaf	1 slice (2 oz)	140	3	26	1	2
Whole Grain Loaf	1 slice (2 oz)	130	1	27	2	3

FOOD	PORTION	CAL	FAT	CARB	SUGAR	FIBER
BEVERAGES						
Apple Juice Organic	8 oz	120	0	29	29	0
Caffe Mocha	1 (11.5 oz)	380	16	50	42	2
Caramel Frozen	1 (16 oz)	600	33	97	82	0
Chocolate Milk Organic	8 oz	170	5	25	25	0
Hot Chocolate	1 (11 oz)	380	16	50	42	2
Iced Green Tea	1 (16 oz)	90	0	23	23	0
Iced Latte Chai Tea	1 (16 oz)	160	4	26	25	0
Latte Caffe	1 (8.5 oz)	120	5	11	11	0
Latte Caramel	1 (11.5 oz)	420	18	53	46	0
Latte Chai Tea	1 (10 oz)	200	5	32	32	0
Lemonade	1 (16 oz)	100	0	25	25	0
Mango Frozen	1 (16 oz)	330	10	61	56	2
Milk Organic	8 oz	120	5	12	12	0
Mocha Frozen	1 (16 oz)	570	20	94	78	2
Orange Juice	1 sm (8 oz)	110	0	26	26	1
Smoothie Black Cherry Low Fat	1 (16 oz)	290	2	63	53	2
Smoothie Mango Low Fat	1 (16 oz)	230	2	51	48	2
Smoothie Strawberry w/ Ginseng Low Fat	1 (16 oz)	260	2	59	53	2
Smoothie Wild Berry Low Fat	1 (16 oz)	290	2	67	65	1
CHILDREN'S MENU SELECTIONS						
Deli Sandwich Roast Beef	1	320	10	35	4	3
Deli Sandwich Smoked Ham	1	300	9	35	3	3
Deli Sandwich Smoked Turkey	1	290	8	35	3	3
Mac & Cheese	1 serv	490	30	37	7	1
Organic Yogurt All Flavors	1 tube	60	1	11	10	0

FOOD	PORTION	CAL	FAT	CARB	SUGAR	FIBER
Sandwich Grilled Cheese	1	360	13	46	4	4
Sandwich Peanut Butter & Jelly	1	410	18	56	21	4
CREAM CHEESE						
Chive & Onion	1 oz	70	6	2	1	0
Hazelnut Reduced Fat	1 oz	80	6	3	3	0
Honey Walnut Reduced Fat	1 oz	80	6	4	4	0
Plain	1 oz	100	6	1	1	0
Plain Reduced Fat	1 oz	70	6	1	1	0
Raspberry Reduced Fat	1 oz	70	5	4	3	1
Veggie Reduced Fat	1 oz	60	5	1	1	1
SALAD DRESSINGS						
BBQ Ranch	3 tbsp	140	12	8	7	0
Buttermilk Ranch Light	3 tbsp	80	4	9	3	1
Caesar	3 tbsp	150	16	2	1	0
Vinaigrette Asian Sesame Reduced Sugar	3 tbsp	90	8	6	4	0
Vinaigrette Balsamic Reduced Fat	3 tbsp	130	10	9	8	0
Vinaigrette Blue Cheese	3 tbsp	180	19	4	3	0
Vinaigrette Greek Herb	3 tbsp	220	24	1	0	0
Vinaigrette Thai Chili Low Fat	3 tbsp	60	2	10	7	0
Vinaigrette White Balsamic Apple	3 tbsp	150	12	11	10	0
SALADS						
Asian Sesame Chicken	1	410	20	31	6	3
BBQ Chopped Chicken	1	500	22	50	15	6
Caesar	1	390	27	25	2	3
Caesar Chicken	1	510	29	29	2	3
Chopped Chicken Cobb	1	500	36	11	2	3

FOOD	PORTION	CAL	FAT	CARB	SUGAR	FIBER
Chopped Steak & Blue Cheese	1	850	64	36	9	4
Classic Cafe	1	170	11	18	12	4
Fruit Cup	1	60	0	17	12	1
Fuji Apple w/ Chicken	1	520	31	35	21	6
Greek	1	380	34	14	4	5
Thai Chopped Chicken	1	390	15	36	13	5
SANDWICHES						
Asiago Roast Beef On Asiago Cheese	1	700	27	64	5	4
Bacon Turkey Bravo On XL Tomato Basil	1	800	29	83	6	4
Breakfast Asiago Cheese Bagel w/ Bacon	1	610	28	55	4	2
Breakfast Asiago Cheese Bagel w/ Egg & Cheese	1	480	18	54	3	2
Breakfast Asiago Cheese Bagel w/ Sausage	1	640	32	56	4	2
Breakfast Bacon Egg & Cheese On Ciabatta	1	510	24	44	2	2
Breakfast Egg & Cheese On Ciabatta	1	390	15	43	2	2
Breakfast French Toast Bagel w/ Sausage	1	670	31	69	15	2
Breakfast Jalapeno & Cheddar Bagel w/ Bacon	1	590	25	58	4	3
Breakfast Jalapeno & Cheddar Bagel w/ Egg & Cheese	1	470	16	57	3	3

FOOD	PORTION	CAL	FAT	CARB	SUGAR	FIBER
Breakfast Jalapeno & Cheddar Bagel w/ Sausage	1	630	29	59	4	3
Breakfast Power	1	340	14	31	2	4
Breakfast Sausage Egg & Cheese On Ciabatta	1	550	29	44	2	2
Breakfast Sweet Onion & Poppyseed Bagel w/ Steak	1	660	27	74	8	5
Chicken Caesar On Three Cheese	1	720	32	69	5	4
Italian Combo On Ciabatta	1	980	41	95	6	5
Jalapeno & Cheddar Bagel w/ Smoked Ham	1	500	16	58	3	3
Mediterranean Veggie On XL Tomato Basil	1	600	13	98	6	10
Napa Almond Chicken Salad On Sesame Semolina	1	690	26	90	12	5
Panini Chipotle Chicken On Artisan French	1	830	37	72	5	3
Panini Cuban Chicken	1	860	36	86	10	4
Panini Frontega Chicken On Focaccia	1	850	38	79	6	4
Panini Smokehouse Turkey On Three Cheese	1	690	25	64	4	4
Panini Steak & White Cheddar On French Baguette	1	950	35	112	3	5
Panini Tomato & Mozzarella On Ciabatta	1	770	10	96	10	6

FOOD	PORTION	CAL	FAT	CARB	SUGAR	FIBER
Panini Turkey Artichoke On Focaccia	1	740	26	86	8	5
Sierra Turkey w/ Asiago Cheese On Focaccia	1	920	49	79	5	4
Smoked Ham & Swiss On Stone Milled Rye	1	590	17	64	3	5
Smoked Turkey Breast On Country	1	420	3	66	3	3
Tuna Salad On Honey Wheat	1	470	16	65	12	5
SOUPS						
Baked Potato	1 serv (12 oz)	350	13	33	7	3
Broccoli Cheddar	1 serv (12 oz)	290	16	24	0	7
Chicken Noodle Low Fat	1 serv (12 oz)	140	3	23	9	0
Cream Of Chicken & Wild Rice	1 serv (12 oz)	310	17	29	4	3
Creamy Tomato	1 serv (12 oz)	380	23	36	9	5
French Onion	1 serv (12 oz)	250	11	30	6	3
Garden Vegetable w/ Pesto Low Fat	1 serv (12 oz)	160	4	28	8	6
New England Clam Chowder	1 serv (12 oz)	450	34	29	0	3
Vegetarian Black Bean Low Fat	1 serv (12 oz)	170	4	29	4	5

PAPA JOHNS

FOOD	PORTION	CAL	FAT	CARB	SUGAR	FIBER
DESSERTS						
Applepie	4 (6.7 oz)	480	10	90	43	2
Cinnamon Sweetsticks	4 (6.7 oz)	580	16	98	32	3
Cinnapie	4 (5.9 oz)	560	19	90	39	2
OTHER MENU SELECTIONS						
Breadsticks	2 (4 oz)	290	5	54	4	2
Breadsticks Garlic Parmesan	2 (4.4 oz)	340	10	54	5	2

FOOD	PORTION	CAL	FAT	CARB	SUGAR	FIBER
Cheesesticks	4 (4.8 oz)	370	16	41	4	2
Chickenstrips	2 (2.3 oz)	130	5	10	0	0
Wings BBQ	2 (2.8 oz)	190	12	6	2	0
Wings Buffalo	2 (2.8 oz)	170	13	3	1	0
Wings Honey Chipotle	2 (2.8 oz)	190	12	8	5	0
PIZZA						
BBQ Chicken & Bacon 8 inch	¼ pie (3.5 oz)	230	7	30	5	1
BBQ Chicken & Bacon 12 inch	⅛ pie (3.8 oz)	250	8	32	5	1
BBQ Chicken & Bacon 16 inch	⅒ pie (5.6 oz)	370	12	48	7	2
Cheese 12 inch	⅛ pie (3.2 oz)	210	8	26	3	1
Garden Fresh 8 inch	¼ pie (3.6 oz)	180	5	26	4	1
Garden Fresh 12 inch	⅛ pie (3.9 oz)	200	7	27	4	2
Garden Fresh 16 inch	⅒ pie (6 oz)	300	10	42	11	6
Hawaiian BBQ Chicken 12 inch	⅛ pie (4.1 oz)	250	8	33	6	1
Hawaiian BBQ Chicken 16 inch	⅒ pie (6 oz)	370	12	49	9	2
Original 16 inch	⅒ pie (4.6 oz)	300	10	40	5	2
Pepperoni 8 inch	¼ pie (3 oz)	210	9	25	3	1
Pepperoni 12 inch	⅛ pie (3.2 oz)	230	10	26	3	1
Pepperoni 16 inch	⅒ pie (4.8 oz)	340	14	40	5	2
Sausage 8 inch	¼ pie (3.1 oz)	220	9	25	3	1
Sausage 12 inch	⅛ pie (3.3 oz)	240	11	26	3	1
Sausage 16 inch	⅒ pie (4.9 oz)	350	15	40	5	2

FOOD	PORTION	CAL	FAT	CARB	SUGAR	FIBER
Spicy Italian 8 inch	¼ pie (3.4 oz)	240	12	25	3	1
Spicy Italian 12 inch	⅛ pie (3.6 oz)	270	13	27	3	1
Spicy Italian 16 inch	⅒ pie (5.5 oz)	400	20	41	5	2
Spinach Alfredo 8 inch	¼ pie (2.8 oz)	190	8	24	2	1
Spinach Alfredo 12 inch	⅛ pie (2.9 oz)	210	8	25	3	1
Spinach Alfredo 16 inch	⅒ pie (4.4 oz)	310	12	39	4	2
The Meats 8 inch	¼ pie (3.4 oz)	240	11	25	3	1
The Meats 12 inch	⅛ pie (3.6 oz)	250	12	26	3	1
The Meats 16 inch	⅒ pie (5.5 oz)	400	19	40	5	2
The Works 8 inch	¼ pie (3.6 oz)	210	9	26	3	1
The Works 12 inch	⅛ pie (3.9 oz)	230	9	27	3	1
The Works 16 inch	⅒ pie (5.9 oz)	350	14	42	5	2
Tuscan Six Cheese 8 inch	¼ pie (3 oz)	210	8	25	3	1
Tuscan Six Cheese 12 inch	⅛ pie (3.3 oz)	230	9	26	3	1
Tuscan Six Cheese 16 inch	⅒ pie (4.9 oz)	340	13	40	5	2
SAUCES AND SEASONINGS						
Crushed Red Pepper	1 pkg (1 g)	5	0	1	–	0
Parmesan Cheese	1 pkg (3.5 g)	15	1	0	–	0

FOOD	PORTION	CAL	FAT	CARB	SUGAR	FIBER
Sauce Barbeque	1 serv (1 oz)	45	0	11	10	0
Sauce Blue Cheese	1 serv (1 oz)	160	16	1	1	0
Sauce Buffalo	1 serv (1 oz)	15	1	2	2	0
Sauce Cheese	1 serv (1 oz)	40	4	1	1	0
Sauce Honey Mustard	1 serv (1 oz)	150	15	5	4	0
Sauce Pizza	1 serv (1 oz)	20	1	3	1	0
Sauce Ranch	1 serv (1 oz)	100	10	1	1	0
Sauce Special Garlic	1 serv (1 oz)	150	17	0	0	0
Special Seasoning	1 pkg (3 g)	5	0	1	0	0

PAPA MURPHY'S

PIZZA

FOOD	PORTION	CAL	FAT	CARB	SUGAR	FIBER
DeLite Thin Crust Large All Meat	1/10 pie	190	11	13	2	0
DeLite Thin Crust Large Cheese	1/10 pie	140	7	13	2	0
DeLite Thin Crust Large Hawaiian	1/10 pie	160	7	15	4	0
DeLite Thin Crust Large Pepperoni	1/10 pie	170	9	13	2	0
DeLite Thin Crust Large Veggie	1/10 pie	160	9	13	1	tr
Original Crust Family Size All Meat	1/12 pie	360	18	31	6	0
Original Crust Family Size Cheese	1/12 pie	270	11	30	6	0
Original Crust Family Size Cowboy	1/12 pie	350	18	32	6	tr
Original Crust Family Size Hawaiian	1/12 pie	290	11	33	9	tr
Original Crust Family Size Murphy's Combo	1/12 pie	360	18	33	6	tr
Original Crust Family Size Papa's Favorite	1/12 pie	360	18	33	6	tr

FOOD	PORTION	CAL	FAT	CARB	SUGAR	FIBER
Original Crust Family Size Pepperoni	1/12 pie	320	15	31	6	0
Original Crust Family Size Rancher	1/12 pie	330	16	31	6	tr
Original Crust Family Size Specialty Of The House	1/12 pie	320	15	32	6	tr
Original Crust Family Size Veggie Combo	1/12 pie	300	13	33	6	tr
Original Crust Family Size Veggie Mediterranean	1/12 pie	310	14	34	7	3
Original Crust Medium Cheese	1/8 pie	230	9	25	5	0
Stuffed Family Size 5 Meat	1/16 pie	370	16	39	7	0
Stuffed Family Size Big Murphy	1/16 pie	370	16	40	7	tr
Stuffed Family Size Chicago Style	1/16 pie	370	16	40	7	tr
Stuffed Family Size Chicken & Bacon	1/16 pie	370	15	39	6	0
Stuffed Large 5 Meat	1/12 pie	370	16	38	7	0
Stuffed Large Big Murphy	1/12 pie	360	15	39	7	tr
SALADS						
Club w/o Dressing & Croutons	1/2 serv (6.6 oz)	140	8	6	2	3
Garden w/o Dressing & Croutons	1 serv (7.2 oz)	100	6	8	2	3
Italian w/o Dressing & Croutons	1/2 serv (6.5 oz)	140	10	7	1	3

FOOD	PORTION	CAL	FAT	CARB	SUGAR	FIBER
P.F. CHANG'S CHINA BISTRO						
DESSERTS						
Banana Spring Rolls	¼ serv (4 oz)	240	10	36	–	0
Flourless Chocolate Dome	½ serv (4 oz)	270	16	41	–	2
Flourless Chocolate Dome Gluten Free	½ serv (4 oz)	270	16	41	–	2
Mini Apple Pie	1 serv	190	7	29	–	1
Mini Carrot Cake	1 serv	210	11	25	–	1
Mini Cheesecake	1 serv	210	13	22	–	1
Mini Great Wall	1 serv	160	7	22	–	1
Mini Red Velvet Cake	1 serv	220	11	28	–	1
Mini Tiramisu	1 serv	180	11	18	–	0
Mini Tres Leche Lemon Dream	1 serv	180	8	31	–	1
Mini Triple Chocolate Mousse	1 serv	300	22	25	–	1
Mini Triple Chocolate Mousse Gluten Free	1 serv	300	22	25	–	1
The Great Wall Of Chocolate	¼ serv (5 oz)	360	17	51	–	2
MAIN MENU SELECTIONS						
Almond & Cashew Chicken	⅓ serv (10 oz)	373	18	24	–	2
Asian Grilled Norwegian Salmon	½ serv (9 oz)	345	6	38	–	1
Asian Street Taco Mahi Mahi	½ serv (4 oz)	230	9	26	–	2
Asian Street Taco Red Cooked Pork	½ serv (3 oz)	140	5	19	–	1
Asian Street Taco Spicy Shrimp	½ serv (3 oz)	180	10	14	–	1

FOOD	PORTION	CAL	FAT	CARB	SUGAR	FIBER
Asian Street Taco Traditional Beef	½ serv (3 oz)	170	7	18	–	1
Beef A La Sichuan	⅓ serv (7 oz)	293	11	26	–	1
Beef w/ Broccoli	⅓ serv (7 oz)	290	12	21	–	2
Beef w/ Broccoli Gluten Free	⅓ serv (6 oz)	290	12	21	–	2
Buddha's Feast Steamed	½ serv (6 oz)	55	0	11	–	4
Buddha's Feast Steamed Gluten Free	½ serv (6 oz)	55	1	11	–	4
Buddha's Feast Stir Fried	½ serv (11 oz)	220	6	29	–	5
Buddha's Feast Stir Fried w/ White Rice	½ serv (11 oz)	310	5	54	–	3
Calamari Salt & Pepper	¼ serv (2 oz)	160	10	11	–	0
Chang's Spicy Chicken	⅓ serv (6 oz)	323	13	23	–	0
Chang's Spicy Chicken Gluten Free	⅓ serv (6 oz)	323	13	23	–	0
Chengdu Spiced Lamb	⅓ serv (5 oz)	237	12	11	–	1
Chicken w/ Black Bean Sauce	⅓ serv (7 oz)	300	16	14	–	0
Chopped Chicken w/ Ginger Dressing	1 (8 oz)	365	24	13	–	2
Coconut Curry Vegetables	½ serv (13 oz)	510	36	26	–	5
Crispy Green Beans w/o Sauce	¼ serv (4 oz)	260	18	21	–	2
Crispy Honey Chicken	⅓ serv (6 oz)	477	23	49	–	0
Crispy Honey Shrimp	½ serv (6 oz)	460	22	55	–	1
Crispy Wontons	2 (1 oz)	90	6	8	–	0
Double Pan Fried Noodles Combo	¼ serv (9 oz)	455	21	44	–	1
Double Pan Fried Noodles w/ Beef	¼ serv (8 oz)	395	17	44	–	2

FOOD	PORTION	CAL	FAT	CARB	SUGAR	FIBER
Double Pan Fried Noodles w/ Chicken	¼ serv (8 oz)	393	17	43	–	2
Double Pan Fried Noodles w/ Pork	¼ serv (8 oz)	413	21	42	–	2
Double Pan Fried Noodles w/ Shrimp	¼ serv (8 oz)	363	16	42	–	2
Double Pan Fried Noodles w/ Vegetable	¼ serv (8 oz)	190	5	30	–	2
Dumplings Pork Pan Fried	⅙ serv (1 oz)	70	4	6	–	0
Dumplings Pork Steamed	⅙ serv (1 oz)	60	2	6	–	0
Dumplings Shrimp Pan Fried	1 (1 oz)	60	2	6	–	0
Dumplings Shrimp Steamed	1 (1 oz)	45	0	6	–	0
Dumplings Steamed Edamame	⅓ serv (1 oz)	45	1	7	–	0
Dumplings Steamed Lemongrass Chicken	⅓ serv (1 oz)	40	1	5	–	0
Dumplings Steamed Pork & Leek	⅓ serv (1 oz)	50	2	5	–	1
Dumplings Steamed Shrimp & Pork	⅓ serv (1 oz)	40	1	5	–	1
Dumplings Vegetable Pan Fried	1 (1 oz)	60	2	8	–	0
Dumplings Vegetable Steamed	1 (1 oz)	45	0	8	–	0
Dynamite Shrimp	½ serv (4 oz)	290	12	6	–	0
Edamame w/ Kosher Salt	1 serv (3 oz)	130	4	11	–	5
Egg Rolls	1 (3 oz)	215	10	21	–	2
Eggplant Stir Fried	¼ serv (6 oz)	270	22	14	–	2

FOOD	PORTION	CAL	FAT	CARB	SUGAR	FIBER
Flaming Red Wontons	1/6 serv (2 oz)	80	5	5	–	0
Fried Rice Beef	1/4 serv (7 oz)	303	9	41	–	1
Fried Rice Beef Gluten Free	1/4 serv (7 oz)	293	9	41	–	1
Fried Rice Chicken	1/4 serv (7 oz)	303	9	39	–	1
Fried Rice Combo	1/4 serv (8 oz)	363	13	41	–	1
Fried Rice Pork	1/4 serv (7 oz)	320	13	39	–	1
Fried Rice Pork Gluten Free	1/4 serv (7 oz)	320	13	39	–	1
Fried Rice Shrimp	1/4 serv (7 oz)	273	8	39	–	1
Fried Rice Vegetable	1/4 serv (7 oz)	230	5	38	–	1
Garlic Noodles	1/4 serv (5 oz)	178	4	31	–	1
Garlic Snap Peas	1/3 lg serv (3 oz)	64	2	7	–	2
Garlic Snap Peas Gluten Free	1/3 lg serv (3 oz)	63	2	7	–	2
Ginger Chicken w/ Broccoli	1/3 serv (9 oz)	273	11	18	–	2
Ginger Chicken w/ Broccoli Gluten Free	1/3 serv (8 oz)	270	11	13	–	2
Hunan Hot Fish	1/3 serv (8 oz)	340	22	21	–	1
Kung Pao Chicken	1/3 serv (5 oz)	383	23	14	–	2
Kung Pao Scallops	1/3 serv (5 oz)	307	20	17	–	2
Kung Pao Shrimp	1/3 serv (5 oz)	208	17	12	–	2
Lettuce Wraps Chicken	1/4 serv (5 oz)	160	7	17	–	2
Lettuce Wraps Chicken Gluten Free	1/4 serv (5 oz)	158	7	15	–	2
Lettuce Wraps Vegetarian	1/4 serv (5 oz)	140	7	11	–	2
Lo Mein Beef	1 serv (7 oz)	270	9	33	–	2
Lo Mein Chicken	1 serv (7 oz)	267	9	30	–	2
Lo Mein Combo	1/3 serv (9 oz)	347	14	23	–	2
Lo Mein Pork	1 serv (7 oz)	290	13	30	–	2

FOOD	PORTION	CAL	FAT	CARB	SUGAR	FIBER
Lo Mein Shrimp	1 serv (7 oz)	227	6	30	–	2
Lo Mein Vegetable	⅓ serv (7 oz)	420	15	58	–	3
Lunch Bowl Buddha's Feast Steamed w/ Brown Rice	½ serv (9 oz)	210	2	39	–	5
Lunch Bowl Buddha's Feast Steamed w/ White Rice	½ serv (9 oz)	235	1	45	–	3
Ma Po Tofu	⅓ serv (10 oz)	350	23	17	–	2
Mahi Mahi	½ serv (10 oz)	420	17	42	–	2
Mandarin Chicken	½ serv (10 oz)	360	15	29	–	3
Mongolian Beef	⅓ serv (6 oz)	337	15	20	–	1
Mongolian Beef Gluten Free	⅓ serv (6 oz)	337	15	21	–	1
Moo Goo Gai Pan	⅓ serv (9 oz)	247	13	13	–	1
Mu Shu Chicken	½ serv (10 oz)	285	13	26	–	3
Mu Shu Pork	½ serv (10 oz)	320	19	16	–	3
Mu Shu Pork Pancake	1	90	2	14	–	0
Noodles Dan Dan	¼ serv (9 oz)	270	7	30	–	2
Norwegian Salmon Steamed w/ Ginger Gluten Free	½ serv (10 oz)	330	18	12	–	3
Norwegian Salmon w/ Ginger	½ serv (10 oz)	330	19	12	–	3
Oolong Marinated Sea Bass	½ serv (9 oz)	315	19	15	–	2
Orange Peel Beef	⅓ serv (5 oz)	283	13	21	–	1
Orange Peel Chicken	⅓ serv (5 oz)	333	15	20	–	1

FOOD	PORTION	CAL	FAT	CARB	SUGAR	FIBER
Orange Peel Shrimp	⅓ serv (5 oz)	187	14	14	–	1
Pepper Steak	⅓ serv (8 oz)	297	13	19	–	1
Pepper Steak Gluten Free	⅓ serv (8 oz)	300	13	19	–	1
Rice Brown Steamed	1 serv (6 oz)	190	2	40	–	3
Rice White Steamed	1 serv (6 oz)	220	0	49	–	1
Salt & Pepper Prawns	⅓ serv (6 oz)	197	11	8	–	2
Shanghai Cucumbers	⅓ lg serv (4 oz)	40	2	3	–	1
Shanghai Cucumbers Gluten Free	⅓ lg serv (4 oz)	40	2	3	–	1
Shanghai Shrimp w/ Garlic Sauce	½ serv (9 oz)	195	20	10	–	3
Shrimp w/ Candied Walnuts	⅓ serv (7 oz)	377	24	25	–	1
Shrimp w/ Lobster Sauce	½ serv (10 oz)	250	14	11	–	1
Shrimp w/ Lobster Sauce Gluten Free	½ serv (10 oz)	255	14	13	–	1
Sichuan Asparagus	⅓ lg serv (5 oz)	100	6	10	–	2
Sichuan Scallops	⅓ serv (7 oz)	295	15	26	–	1
Sichuan Shrimp	⅓ serv (5 oz)	173	7	10	–	0
Singapore Street Noodles	⅓ serv (6 oz)	300	6	42	–	3
Singapore Street Noodles Gluten Free	⅓ serv (7 oz)	300	7	41	–	3
Siu Mai Steamed Bacon & Egg	⅓ serv (1 oz)	70	3	8	–	0
Siu Mai Steamed Pork & Rice	⅓ serv (1 oz)	50	5	9	–	0
Spare Ribs Chang's	¼ serv (4 oz)	344	24	7	–	1

FOOD	PORTION	CAL	FAT	CARB	SUGAR	FIBER
Spare Ribs Northern Style	¼ serv (4 oz)	343	19	11	–	0
Spicy Green Beans	⅓ lg serv (5 oz)	110	6	13	–	4
Spinach Stir-Fried w/ Garlic	⅓ lg serv (5 oz)	53	3	5	–	3
Spinach Stir-Fried w/ Garlic Gluten Free	⅓ lg serv (3 oz)	53	3	5	–	3
Spring Roll	1 (1.5 oz)	156	8	17	–	2
Starters Seared Ahi Tuna	½ serv (4 oz)	160	11	7	–	1
Street Dumplings Shanghai	½ serv (2 oz)	140	5	19	–	1
Sweet & Sour Chicken	⅓ serv (5 oz)	370	19	38	–	0
Sweet & Sour Pork	½ serv (10 oz)	460	14	72	–	2
Tuna Tataki	⅓ serv (1 oz)	60	3	3	–	0
VIP Duck	½ serv (12 oz)	650	29	55	–	1
Wok Charred Beef	⅓ serv (8 oz)	317	17	16	–	1
Wok Seared Lamb	⅓ serv (7 oz)	283	16	9	–	1
Wontons Crab	2	163	10	13	–	0
SALAD DRESSINGS AND SAUCES						
Sauce Crispy Green Bean	1 serv (2 oz)	310	32	2	–	0
Sauce Plum	1 serv (2 oz)	200	0	50	–	0
Sauce Potsticker	1 serv (2 oz)	50	2	7	–	0
Sauce Shrimp Dumpling	1 serv (2 oz)	15	0	2	–	0
Sauce Sweet & Sour	1 serv (2 oz)	80	0	21	–	0
Sauce Sweet & Sour Mustard	1 serv (2 oz)	90	2	17	–	1
SOUPS						
Chicken Noodle	1 bowl (7 oz)	120	4	15	–	1

FOOD	PORTION	CAL	FAT	CARB	SUGAR	FIBER
Egg Drop	1 cup (7 oz)	60	3	8	–	0
Egg Drop Gluten Free	1 cup (7 oz)	60	3	8	–	0
Hot & Sour	1 bowl (7 oz)	80	3	9	–	0
Wonton	1 bowl (7 oz)	92	3	9	–	0
PIZZA HUT						
BEVERAGES						
Diet Pepsi	1 (16 oz)	0	0	0	0	0
Mountain Dew	1 (16 oz)	220	0	58	58	0
Pepsi	1 (16 oz)	200	0	56	54	0
Sierra Mist	1 (16 oz)	200	0	54	54	0
OTHER MENU SELECTIONS						
Breadstick	1 (1.5 oz)	140	5	19	2	1
Breadstick Cheese	1 (2 oz)	170	6	20	2	1
Dipping Sauce Marinara	1 serv (3 oz)	60	0	12	9	2
Dipping Sauce Ranch	1 serv (1.5 oz)	220	23	2	1	0
Dipping Sauce Wing Blue Cheese	1 serv (1.5 oz)	230	24	2	2	0
Dipping Sauce Wing Ranch	1 serv (1.5 oz)	220	23	2	1	0
Fried Cheese Sticks	4 (4.2 oz)	380	24	29	3	2
Tuscani Pasta Chicken Alfredo	1 serv (10 oz)	580	32	49	4	4
Tuscani Pasta Meaty Marinara	1 serv (9.5 oz)	450	20	44	8	5
Wedge Fries	1 serv (4.3 oz)	320	18	35	0	3
Wings Crispy Bone In All American	2 (1.9 oz)	200	14	8	0	1
Wings Crispy Bone In Buffalo Burnin Hot	2 (2.6 oz)	230	15	16	2	1
Wings Crispy Bone In Buffalo Medium	2 (2.6 oz)	230	15	16	2	2

FOOD	PORTION	CAL	FAT	CARB	SUGAR	FIBER
Wings Crispy Bone In Buffalo Mild	2 (2.6 oz)	230	15	16	2	1
Wings Crispy Bone In Garlic Parmesan	2 (2.5 oz)	300	25	9	1	1
Wings Crispy Bone In Honey BBQ	2 (2.9 oz)	260	14	24	12	1
Wings Crispy Bone In Lemon Pepper	2 (2.6 oz)	270	19	16	7	1
Wings Crispy Bone In Spicy BBQ	2 (2.9 oz)	240	14	19	11	1
Wings Crispy Bone In Spicy Asian	2 (2.9 oz)	250	15	21	13	1
Wings Traditional All American	2 (1.4 oz)	80	5	0	0	0
Wings Traditional Buffalo Medium	2 (2 oz)	110	6	8	2	1
Wings Traditional Buffalo Mild	2 (2 oz)	110	6	8	2	1
Wings Traditional Burnin Hot	2 (2 oz)	110	6	8	2	1
Wings Traditional Garlic Parmesan	2 (2 oz)	180	16	1	1	0
Wings Traditional Honey BBQ	2 (2.4 oz)	140	5	16	12	0
Wings Traditional Lemon Pepper	2 (2 oz)	150	10	8	7	0
Wings Traditional Spicy Asian	2 (2.3 oz)	130	5	13	13	0
Wings Traditional Spicy BBQ	2 (2.3 oz)	120	5	11	11	0
PIZZA						
Fit 'N Delicious 12 Inch Chicken Mushrooms & Jalapeno	1 slice (3.3 oz)	170	5	22	4	1

FOOD	PORTION	CAL	FAT	CARB	SUGAR	FIBER
Fit 'N Delicious 12 Inch Chicken Red Onion & Green Pepper	1 slice (3.3 oz)	180	5	23	5	1
Fit 'N Delicious 12 Inch Diced Red Tomato Mushroom & Jalapeno	1 slice (3.1 oz)	150	4	23	4	2
Fit 'N Delicious 12 Inch Green Pepper Red Onion & Diced Red Tomato	1 slice (3.1 oz)	150	4	24	5	2
Fit 'N Delicious 12 Inch Ham Pineapple & Diced Red Tomato	1 slice (2.9 oz)	160	5	24	6	1
Fit 'N Delicious 12 Inch Ham Red Onion & Mushrooms	1 slice (2.9 oz)	160	5	23	4	1
Hand Tossed 12 Inch Cheese Only	1 slice (2.9 oz)	220	8	26	4	1
Hand Tossed 12 Inch Cheese Only Garlic Parmesan	1 slice (3 oz)	220	8	26	4	1
Hand Tossed 12 Inch Dan's Original	1 slice (3.6 oz)	260	12	26	4	1
Hand Tossed 12 Inch Ham & Pineapple	1 slice (3.2 oz)	200	6	27	5	1
Hand Tossed 12 Inch Hawaiian Luau	1 slice (3.5 oz)	240	9	27	5	1
Hand Tossed 12 Inch Italian Sausage & Red Onion	1 slice (3.5 oz)	240	10	27	4	1
Hand Tossed 12 Inch Meat Lover's	1 slice (3.7 oz)	300	16	26	4	1
Hand Tossed 12 Inch Pepperoni	1 slice (2.9 oz)	230	9	25	3	1

FOOD	PORTION	CAL	FAT	CARB	SUGAR	FIBER
Hand Tossed 12 Inch Pepperoni Lover's	1 slice (3.3 oz)	270	13	26	4	1
Hand Tossed 12 Inch Pepperoni & Mushroom	1 slice (3.2 oz)	210	8	26	4	1
Hand Tossed 12 Inch Pepperoni Garlic Parmesan	1 slice (2.9 oz)	230	9	26	4	1
Hand Tossed 12 Inch Spicy Sicilian	1 slice (3.5 oz)	240	11	26	4	1
Hand Tossed 12 Inch Supreme	1 slice (3.7 oz)	260	12	26	4	1
Hand Tossed 12 Inch Triple Meat Italiano	1 slice (3.4 oz)	260	12	26	4	1
Hand Tossed 12 Inch Ultimate Cheese Lover's	1 slice (2.9 oz)	240	11	25	3	1
Hand Tossed 12 Inch Veggie Lover's	1 slice (3.6 oz)	200	6	27	4	2
Pan 12 Inch Cheese Only	1 slice (3.2 oz)	240	10	27	2	1
Pan 12 Inch Dan's Original	1 slice (3.9 oz)	280	14	27	2	1
Pan 12 Inch Ham & Pineapple	1 slice (3.4 oz)	230	9	28	3	1
Pan 12 Inch Hawaiian Luau	1 slice (3.6 oz)	260	12	28	3	1
Pan 12 Inch Italian Sausage & Red Onion	1 slice (3.7 oz)	270	13	28	3	1
Pan 12 Inch Meat Lover's	1 slice (4 oz)	330	19	27	2	1
Pan 12 Inch Pepperoni	1 slice (3.2 oz)	250	12	26	2	1

FOOD	PORTION	CAL	FAT	CARB	SUGAR	FIBER
Pan 12 Inch Pepperoni Lover's	1 slice (3.5 oz)	290	14	27	2	1
Pan 12 Inch Pepperoni & Mushroom	1 slice (3.4 oz)	240	10	27	2	1
Pan 12 Inch Spicy Sicilian	1 slice (3.7 oz)	270	13	27	2	2
Pan 12 Inch Supreme	1 slice (3.9 oz)	290	14	27	2	2
Pan 12 Inch Triple Meat Italiano	1 slice (3.6 oz)	290	15	27	2	1
Pan 12 Inch Ultimate Cheese Lover's	1 slice (3.2 oz)	270	13	26	2	1
Pan 12 Inch Veggie Lover's	1 slice (3.8 oz)	230	9	28	3	2
PANormous 9 Inch Cheese Only	1 pie (13.4 oz)	1100	45	124	10	6
PANormous 9 Inch Dan's Original	1 pie (15.9 oz)	1270	62	124	10	7
PANormous 9 Inch Ham & Pineapple	1 pie (14 oz)	1020	37	128	14	6
PANormous 9 Inch Hawaiian Luau	1 pie (14.8 oz)	1150	49	129	14	6
PANormous 9 Inch Italian Sausage & Red Onion	1 pie (15.4 oz)	1210	56	128	12	7
PANormous 9 Inch Meat Lover's	1 pie (16.3 oz)	1470	80	123	10	6
PANormous 9 Inch Pepperoni	1 pie (12.9 oz)	1100	48	121	9	6
PANormous 9 Inch Pepperoni Lover's	1 pie (16 oz)	1290	62	124	10	6
PANormous 9 Inch Pepperoni & Mushroom	1 pie (13.9 oz)	1050	42	123	10	7

FOOD	PORTION	CAL	FAT	CARB	SUGAR	FIBER
PANormous 9 Inch Spicy Sicilian	1 pie (15.4 oz)	1220	57	126	11	7
PANormous 9 Inch Supreme	1 pie (16.2 oz)	1270	62	125	11	7
PANormous 9 Inch Triple Meat Lover's	1 pie (14.9 oz)	1280	62	123	9	6
PANormous 9 Inch Veggie Lover's	1 pie (15.4 oz)	1010	38	127	12	8
Personal Pan 6 Inch Cheese Only	1 (7.2 oz)	590	24	69	7	3
Personal Pan 6 Inch Dan's Original	1 (8.8 oz)	720	36	69	7	4
Personal Pan 6 Inch Ham & Pineapple	1 (7.5 oz)	550	20	71	9	3
Personal Pan 6 Inch Hawaiian Luau	1 (8 oz)	620	25	71	9	3
Personal Pan 6 Inch Italian Sausage & Red Onion	1 (8.6 oz)	690	32	71	8	4
Personal Pan 6 Inch Meat Lover's	1 (9.2 oz)	830	46	68	7	3
Personal Pan 6 Inch Pepperoni	1 (7.1 oz)	610	26	67	6	3
Personal Pan 6 Inch Pepperoni Lover's	1 (8.1 oz)	720	34	69	7	3
Personal Pan 6 Inch Pepperoni & Mushroom	1 (7.5 oz)	570	23	68	7	4
Personal Pan 6 Inch Spicy Sicilian	1 (8.6 oz)	680	32	69	7	4
Personal Pan 6 Inch Supreme	1 (9 oz)	720	36	69	7	4
Personal Pan 6 Inch Triple Meat Italiano	1 (8.4 oz)	730	36	68	6	3

FOOD	PORTION	CAL	FAT	CARB	SUGAR	FIBER
Personal Pan 6 Inch Ultimate Cheese Lover's	1 (7.3 oz)	660	30	68	6	3
Personal Pan 6 Inch Veggie Lover's	1 (8.2 oz)	550	20	70	8	4
P'Zone Classic	½ serv (6.1 oz)	470	16	61	3	2
P'Zone Meaty	½ serv (6.6 oz)	550	23	61	2	2
P'Zone Pepperoni	½ serv (5.5 oz)	450	15	60	2	2
Stuffed Pizza Rollers	1 (2.7 oz)	220	10	24	3	1
Thin'N Crispy 12 Inch Cheese Only	1 slice (2.3 oz)	190	8	22	4	1
Thin'N Crispy 12 Inch Dan's Original	1 slice (3 oz)	240	12	22	4	1
Thin'N Crispy 12 Inch Ham & Pineapple	1 slice (2.6 oz)	180	6	23	5	1
Thin'N Crispy 12 Inch Hawaiian Luau	1 slice (2.8 oz)	220	10	24	5	1
Thin'N Crispy 12 Inch Italian Sausage & Red Onion	1 slice (2.8 oz)	220	10	23	4	1
Thin'N Crispy 12 Inch Meat Lover's	1 slice (3 oz)	280	16	22	4	1
Thin'N Crispy 12 Inch Pepperoni	1 slice (2.2 oz)	200	9	21	4	1
Thin'N Crispy 12 Inch Pepperoni Lover's	1 slice (2.6 oz)	250	13	22	4	1
Thin'N Crispy 12 Inch Pepperoni & Mushroom	1 slice (2.6 oz)	180	8	22	4	1
Thin'N Crispy 12 Inch Spicy Sicilian	1 slice (2.8 oz)	220	10	22	4	1

FOOD	PORTION	CAL	FAT	CARB	SUGAR	FIBER
Thin'N Crispy 12 Inch Supreme	1 slice (3.1 oz)	240	12	23	4	1
Thin'N Crispy 12 Inch Triple Meat Italiano	1 slice (2.7 oz)	240	12	22	4	1
Thin'N Crispy 12 Inch Ultimate Cheese Lover's	1 slice (2.3 oz)	220	11	21	4	1
Thin'N Crispy 12 Inch Veggie Lover's	1 slice (3 oz)	180	6	23	4	1

POPEYE'S

BEVERAGES

FOOD	PORTION	CAL	FAT	CARB	SUGAR	FIBER
Coffee Black	1 (16 oz)	0	0	0	0	0
Orange Juice	1 (10 oz)	140	0	33	30	0

BREAKFAST MENU SELECTIONS

FOOD	PORTION	CAL	FAT	CARB	SUGAR	FIBER
Biscuit Bacon	1 (5 oz)	400	25	37	2	3
Biscuit Chicken	1 (5.2 oz)	490	26	47	2	1
Biscuit Egg	1 (4.8 oz)	510	29	41	2	1
Biscuit Egg & Sausage	1 (6.5 oz)	690	45	43	2	1
Biscuit Sausage	1 (4.8 oz)	540	36	41	2	1
Biscuit Sausage & Gravy	1 (6.5 oz)	510	33	42	3	3
Grits	1 serv (5 oz)	370	5	80	0	7
Hashbrowns	1 serv (3.4 oz)	360	20	41	0	4

DESSERTS

FOOD	PORTION	CAL	FAT	CARB	SUGAR	FIBER
Apple Sauce	1 serv (4 oz)	50	0	12	8	2
Cheesecake Mardi Gras	1 serv (3 oz)	310	19	32	22	1
Pie Hot Sweet Potato	1 serv (3.5 oz)	350	19	41	10	2
Pie Mississippi Mud	1 serv (3 oz)	280	7	51	27	2
Pie Sliced Pecan	1 serv (3.3 oz)	410	21	52	22	1

MAIN MENU SELECTIONS

FOOD	PORTION	CAL	FAT	CARB	SUGAR	FIBER
Baguette	1 (1.3 oz)	90	2	18	1	1

FOOD	PORTION	CAL	FAT	CARB	SUGAR	FIBER
Biscuit	1 (2.1 oz)	260	15	26	1	2
Butterfly Shrimp	8 (3.5 oz)	290	17	21	0	3
Cajun Fries	1 reg (3 oz)	260	14	30	0	2
Cajun Rice	1 reg (4.3 oz)	170	5	25	4	1
Catfish Fillets	2 (5.2 oz)	460	29	27	0	1
Cheddar Cheese Tortilla	1 (1.6 oz)	140	5	21	0	1
Chicken Livers	10 (10 oz)	1190	80	65	3	6
Chicken Wrap Loaded	1 (4.6 oz)	310	13	33	0	3
Chicken Wrap Naked	1 (3.4 oz)	200	6	22	0	1
Coleslaw	1 reg (4.8 oz)	220	15	19	15	2
Corn On The Cob	1 (10 oz)	190	2	37	0	4
Green Beans	1 serv (3.5 oz)	40	2	6	1	2
Jalapeno	1 (6 g)	0	0	1	0	1
Jambalaya Chicken & Sausage	1 serv (5.3 oz)	220	11	20	0	1
Macaroni & Cheese	1 serv (5.5 oz)	200	7	26	3	1
Mashed Potatoes Gravy	1 serv (5 oz)	110	4	18	1	1
Mild Breast	1 (5.5 oz)	440	27	16	0	2
Mild Leg	1 (2.4 oz)	160	9	5	0	1
Mild Tenders	3 (4.4 oz)	340	14	26	0	1
Mild Thigh	1 (2.8 oz)	280	21	7	0	1
Mild Wing	1 (2.2 oz)	210	14	8	0	1
Naked Tenders	3 (4 oz)	170	2	2	0	0
Nuggets	4 (1.8 oz)	150	9	10	0	1
Onion Rings	6 (2.6 oz)	280	19	25	2	2
Po'Boy Catfish	1 (11.2 oz)	800	50	65	3	3
Po'Boy Chicken	1 (22.3 oz)	660	34	61	3	3
Po'Boy Naked BBQ Chicken	1 (7.4 oz)	340	7	49	11	2
Po'Boy Shrimp	1 (9.5 oz)	690	42	66	3	5
Popcorn Shrimp	1 serv (3.5 oz)	330	9	28	0	3

FOOD	PORTION	CAL	FAT	CARB	SUGAR	FIBER
Red Beans & Rice	1 reg (5.1 oz)	230	14	23	0	5
Spicy Breast	1 (5.5 oz)	420	27	13	0	3
Spicy Leg	1 (2.4 oz)	170	10	5	0	1
Spicy Thigh	1 (2.8 oz)	260	18	8	0	1
Spicy Wing	1 (2.2 oz)	210	14	8	0	1
Spicy Tenders	3 (4.4 oz)	310	15	16	0	2
SAUCES						
Cocktail	1 serv (1 oz)	30	0	6	6	0
Confetti Sauce	1 serv (1 oz)	65	0	16	10	0
Ranch	1 serv (1 oz)	150	15	3	1	0
Spicy BBQ	1 serv (1 oz)	45	0	10	8	0
Spicy Honey Mustard	1 serv (1 oz)	100	8	7	5	0
Tartar Sauce	1 serv (1 oz)	140	15	1	1	0

QUIZNOS

FOOD	PORTION	CAL	FAT	CARB	SUGAR	FIBER
SALAD DRESSINGS						
Acai Vinaigrette	1 reg	230	17	15	14	0
Balsamic Vinaigrette Fat Free	1 reg	130	0	29	20	0
Blue Cheese	1 reg	345	38	3	2	0
Honey Dijon	1 reg	450	44	14	13	0
Peppercorn Caesar	1 reg	480	50	5	3	0
Ranch	1 reg	350	36	5	3	0
Tzatziki	1 reg	450	46	3	2	0
SALADS						
Fresh Farmers Market Caprese Chicken w/o Dressing	1 reg	260	17	10	2	2
Fresh Farmers Market Chicken Caesar w/o Dressing	1 reg	130	5	6	3	2
Fresh Farmers Market Cobb w/o Dressing	1 reg	260	12	5	3	2

FOOD	PORTION	CAL	FAT	CARB	SUGAR	FIBER
Fresh Farmers Market Harvest Chicken w/o Dressing	1 reg	220	6	33	25	4
Fresh Farmers Market Mediterranean Chicken w/o Dressing	1 reg	180	7	13	3	4
SANDWICHES						
Classic Sub Classic Club	1 sm	570	34	41	8	3
Classic Sub Classic Italian	1 sm	520	29	43	8	4
Classic Sub Honey Bacon Club	1 sm	480	21	51	15	3
Classic Sub Honey Bourbon Chicken	1 sm	320	6	48	14	4
Classic Sub Pork Cuban	1 sm	450	22	39	5	3
Classic Sub The Traditional	1 sm	430	20	43	8	4
Classic Sub Tuna Melt	1 sm	690	47	40	6	3
Classic Sub Turkey Bacon Guacamole	1 sm	540	28	44	9	5
Classic Sub Turkey Ranch & Swiss	1 sm	420	18	44	8	4
Classic Sub Ultimate Turkey Club	1 sm	560	34	41	7	3
Classic Sub Veggie	1 sm	510	28	43	9	6
Flatbread Sammies Bistro Steak Melt	1	410	23	31	6	1
Flatbread Sammies Cantina Chicken	1	280	7	36	12	2
Flatbread Sammies Chicken Bacon Ranch	1	380	19	28	4	1
Flatbread Sammies Italiano	1	420	25	28	4	1

FOOD	PORTION	CAL	FAT	CARB	SUGAR	FIBER
Flatbread Sammies Roadhouse Steak	1	270	6	39	13	1
Flatbread Sammies Smoky Chipotle Turkey	1	390	23	29	4	1
Flatbread Sammies Veggie	1	340	20	29	5	3
Signature Sub Baja Chicken	1 sm	490	23	43	9	3
Signature Sub Black Angus On Rosemary Parmesan	1 sm	520	17	54	14	4
Signature Sub Buffalo Chicken	1 sm	470	22	45	7	3
Signature Sub Chicken Bacon Dipper	1 sm	630	38	43	8	3
Signature Sub Chicken Carbonara	1 sm	530	27	40	7	3
Signature Sub Chipotle Prime Rib	1 sm	600	34	42	7	3
Signature Sub Double Cheese Cheesesteak	1 sm	770	47	44	7	3
Signature Sub Harvest Chicken	1 sm	370	11	54	19	4
Signature Sub Honey Mustard Chicken	1 sm	520	26	44	10	3
Signature Sub Mesquite Chicken	1 sm	500	25	41	7	3
Signature Sub Peppercorn Steakhouse Dip	1 sm	630	37	44	7	3
Signature Sub Prime Rib & Blue	1 sm	570	29	42	7	3

FOOD	PORTION	CAL	FAT	CARB	SUGAR	FIBER
Signature Sub Prime Rib & Peppercorn	1 sm	620	36	43	7	3
Signature Sub Prime Rib Mushroom & Swiss	1 sm	600	34	42	6	3
Signature Sub Southern BBQ Pulled Pork	1 sm	520	22	46	12	3
Toasty Bullets Beef Bacon & Cheddar	1	450	18	48	8	2
Toasty Bullets Italian	1	500	25	47	8	3
Toasty Bullets Pesto Turkey	1	380	13	48	8	3
Toasty Bullets Tuna Melt	1	510	31	39	6	2
Toasty Bullets Turkey Club	1	460	21	48	8	3
Toasty Favorites Honey Cured Ham	1 sm	490	28	40	7	3
Toasty Favorites Meatball	1 sm	450	21	47	10	6
Toasty Favorites Oven Roasted Turkey	1 sm	500	28	42	7	3
Toasty Favorites Roast Beef	1 sm	500	28	42	8	3
Toasty Favorites Turkey & Ham	1 sm	500	29	41	7	3
Toasty Favorites Veggie Caprese	1 sm	400	21	41	7	4
Toasty Torpedoes Beef Bacon & Cheddar	1	800	31	93	16	5
Toasty Torpedoes Italian	1	860	40	93	16	5
Toasty Torpedoes Pesto Turkey	1	690	22	94	15	5

FOOD	PORTION	CAL	FAT	CARB	SUGAR	FIBER
Toasty Torpedoes Tuna Melt	1	980	56	88	12	4
Toasty Torpedoes Turkey Club	1	830	35	94	16	5
RAX						
BBQ Beef	1	399	20	43	–	–
BBQ Sandwich	1	716	51	37	–	–
Cheddar Melt	1	346	23	26	–	–
Deluxe	1	521	34	34	–	–
Grilled Chicken	1	526	33	32	–	–
Jr. Deluxe	1	367	25	25	–	–
Mushroom Melt	1	599	37	35	–	–
Philly Melt	1	537	32	35	–	–
Regular Rax	1	388	22	31	–	–
Turkey	1	484	32	32	–	–
Turkey Bacon Club	1	680	47	37	–	–
RED BURRITO						
Burrito Bean & Cheese	1 serv (7.4 oz)	430	16	54	2	6
Burrito Beef Bean & Cheese	1 serv (9.8 oz)	560	24	57	4	6
Burrito Grilled Chicken	1 serv (9 oz)	480	17	55	3	6
Burrito Grilled Steak	1 serv (9 oz)	520	20	56	3	6
Chips & Salsa	1 serv (7.4 oz)	300	22	60	3	1
Chips Side	1 serv (1.3 oz)	100	8	20	0	0
Fresh Salsa	1 serv (4 oz)	30	0	7	3	1
Hard Taco Beef	1 serv (3.3 oz)	170	12	13	1	1
Hard Taco Chicken	1 serv (4 oz)	160	9	12	0	1
Hard Taco Steak	1 serv (3.8 oz)	200	13	13	1	1

FOOD	PORTION	CAL	FAT	CARB	SUGAR	FIBER
Hot Sauce	1 serv (2 oz)	0	0	0	0	0
Jalapeno Coins	1 serv (1 oz)	5	0	1	0	1
Make It Wet	1 serv (3.6 oz)	140	10	5	1	1
Quesadilla	1 serv (5.7 oz)	560	33	40	1	2
Quesadilla Chicken	1 serv (8 oz)	720	45	42	1	2
Quesadilla Steak	1 serv (7.9 oz)	760	49	42	1	2
Queso	1 serv (3 oz)	110	8	5	2	0
Red Burrito Beef	1 serv (13.4 oz)	710	34	62	5	7
Red Burrito Chicken	1 serv (12.7 oz)	630	28	60	4	7
Red Burrito Steak	1 serv (12.6 oz)	660	31	60	4	7
Refried Bean In Tortilla Bowl	1 serv (4.8 oz)	360	18	38	1	7
Soft Taco Beef	1 serv (3.8 oz)	210	11	17	1	0
Soft Taco Chicken	1 serv (4.4 oz)	200	8	17	0	0
Soft Taco Southwest Chicken	1 serv (4 oz)	250	14	16	1	0
Soft Taco Steak	1 serv (4.3 oz)	240	12	18	1	0
Sour Cream	1 serv (1.4 oz)	50	4	3	3	0
Super Nachos	1 serv (10.7 oz)	690	29	90	5	5
Super Nachos Beef	1 serv (13 oz)	820	36	93	6	5
Super Nachos Chicken	1 serv (12.5 oz)	740	30	91	5	5
Super Nachos Steak	1 serv (12.4 oz)	740	38	106	6	14

FOOD	PORTION	CAL	FAT	CARB	SUGAR	FIBER
Taco Salad Beef	1 (20.3 oz)	1080	64	79	11	8
Taco Salad Chicken	1 (19 oz)	920	51	74	9	8
Taco Salad Steak	1 (18.7 oz)	1000	58	76	9	8

RED LOBSTER

BEVERAGES

FOOD	PORTION	CAL	FAT	CARB	SUGAR	FIBER
Boston Ice Tea	1 serv	50	0	12	–	–
Coke	1 serv	100	0	27	–	–
Diet Coke	1 serv	0	0	0	0	0
Dr Pepper	1 serv	150	0	27	–	–
Harbor Cafe Coffee	1 serv	0	0	0	0	0
Lemonade Light	1 serv	0	0	0	0	0
Lemonade Raspberry	1 serv	180	0	30	–	–
Tea Hot or Cold Unsweetened	1 serv	0	0	0	0	0
Wine Blush	1 glass	120	0	7	–	–
Wine Red	1 glass	120	0	7	–	–

MAIN MENU SELECTIONS

FOOD	PORTION	CAL	FAT	CARB	SUGAR	FIBER
Arctic Char Grilled Broiled or Blackened w/ Broccoli	1 half portion	340	15	13	–	–
Arctic Char Grilled Broiled or Blackened w/ Broccoli	1 full portion	630	29	21	–	–
Barramundi Grilled Broiled or Blackened w/ Broccoli	1 half portion	230	5	8	–	–
Barramundi Grilled Broiled or Blackened w/ Broccoli	1 full portion	420	10	11	–	–
Cobia Grilled Broiled or Blackened w/ Broccoli	1 full portion	760	54	8	–	–
Cobia Grilled Broiled or Blackened w/ Broccoli	1 half portion	400	26	6	–	–

FOOD	PORTION	CAL	FAT	CARB	SUGAR	FIBER
Cod Grilled Broiled or Blackened w/ Broccoli	1 half portion	170	2	8	–	–
Cod Grilled Broiled or Blackened w/ Broccoli	1 full portion	300	4	10	–	–
Corvina Grilled Broiled or Blackened w/ Broccoli	1 full portion	320	3	9	–	–
Corvina Grilled Broiled or Blackened w/ Broccoli	1 half portion	180	2	7	–	–
Flounder Grilled Broiled or Blackened w/ Broccoli	1 full portion	350	3	11	–	–
Flounder Grilled Broiled or Blackened w/ Broccoli	1 half portion	200	2	8	–	–
Grouper Grilled Broiled or Blackened w/ Broccoli	1 full portion	370	3	6	–	–
Grouper Grilled Broiled or Blackened w/ Broccoli	1 half portion	210	2	6	–	–
Haddock Grilled Broiled or Blackened w/ Broccoli	1 full portion	310	3	6	–	–
Haddock Grilled Broiled or Blackened w/ Broccoli	1 half portion	180	2	6	–	–
Lake Whitefish Grilled Broiled or Blackened w/ Broccoli	1 full portion	380	5	6	–	–
Lake Whitefish Grilled Broiled or Blackened w/ Broccoli	1 half portion	210	3	6	–	–

FOOD	PORTION	CAL	FAT	CARB	SUGAR	FIBER
Mahi Mahi Grilled Broiled or Blackened w/ Broccoli	1 full portion	360	2	7	–	–
Mahi Mahi Grilled Broiled or Blackened w/ Broccoli	1 half portion	200	2	6	–	–
Monchong Grilled Broiled or Blackened w/ Broccoli	1 full portion	340	3	9	–	–
Monchong Grilled Broiled or Blackened w/ Broccoli	1 half portion	190	2	7	–	–
Opah Grilled Broiled or Blackened w/ Broccoli	1 half portion	280	12	8	–	–
Opah Grilled Broiled or Blackened w/ Broccoli	1 full portion	510	24	11	–	–
Perch Grilled Broiled or Blackened w/ Broccoli	1 full portion	300	4	7	–	–
Perch Grilled Broiled or Blackened w/ Broccoli	1 half portion	170	2	6	–	–
Pompano Grilled Broiled or Blackened w/ Broccoli	1 full portion	430	16	7	–	–
Pompano Grilled Broiled or Blackened w/ Broccoli	1 half portion	240	8	6	–	–
Rainbow Trout Grilled Broiled or Blackened w/ Broccoli	1 half portion	220	10	6	–	–

FOOD	PORTION	CAL	FAT	CARB	SUGAR	FIBER
Red Rockfish Grilled Broiled or Blackened w/ Broccoli	1 full portion	300	4	10	–	–
Red Rockfish Grilled Broiled or Blackened w/ Broccoli	1 half portion	170	3	6	–	–
Salmon Grilled Broiled or Blackened w/ Broccoli	1 half portion	270	9	6	–	–
Salmon Grilled Broiled or Blackened w/ Broccoli	1 full portion	490	17	6	–	–
Seabass Grilled Broiled or Blackened w/ Broccoli	1 half portion	230	6	6	–	–
Snapper Grilled Broiled or Blackened w/ Broccoli	1 half portion	210	2	8	–	–
Sole Grilled Broiled or Blackened w/ Broccoli	1 half portion	140	2	6	–	–
Tilapia Grilled Broiled or Blackened w/ Broccoli	1 half portion	210	3	9	–	–
Tuna Grilled Broiled or Blackened w/ Broccoli	1 half portion	200	1	7	–	–
Wahoo Grilled Broiled or Blackened w/ Broccoli	1 half portion	220	3	8	–	–
Walleye Grilled Broiled or Blackened w/ Broccoli	1 half portion	170	2	7	–	–

FOOD	PORTION	CAL	FAT	CARB	SUGAR	FIBER
ROBEKS						
BAKED SELECTIONS						
Gourmet Pretzels Apple Cinnamon	1	470	25	78	38	3
Gourmet Pretzels Spinach Feta	1	430	9	70	7	3
Gourmet Pretzels Tomato Parmesan	1	420	10	67	7	3
Muffin Banana	1	310	11	43	20	5
Muffin Blueberry	1	300	10	42	18	5
Muffin Chocolate	1	320	11	45	17	5
Power Cookie Breakfast Bar	1	230	10	33	18	1
Power Cookie Chocolate Chip w/ Walnuts	1	404	12	60	31	5
Power Cookie Lemon Poppyseed	1	371	7	63	30	4
Power Cookie Oatmeal Raisin Walnut	1	375	7	64	33	6
Power Cookie Peanut Butter	1	426	14	59	25	3
BEVERAGES						
800 Lb Gorilla	1 (12 oz)	434	9	58	41	2
Freeze Lemon	1 (12 oz)	282	2	66	40	0
Freeze Orange	1 (12 oz)	290	1	63	47	0
Fresh Juice ABC	1 (12 oz)	150	0	33	19	2
Fresh Juice Apple	1 (12 oz)	180	0	45	45	0
Fresh Juice Carrot	1 (12 oz)	98	0	22	20	0
Fresh Juice Green-V	1 (12 oz)	96	1	19	11	2
Fresh Juice G-Snap	1 (12 oz)	120	1	24	14	3
Fresh Juice Lemonade Raspberry	1 (12 oz)	164	0	40	35	0

FOOD	PORTION	CAL	FAT	CARB	SUGAR	FIBER
Fresh Juice Monkey C	1 (12 oz)	186	1	44	32	2
Fresh Juice Orange	1 (12 oz)	168	1	39	31	1
Naturally Light Banana Mango	1	162	0	42	36	3
Naturally Light Pineapple Mango	1	172	0	44	40	3
Naturally Light Raspberry Banana	1	161	0	42	33	3
Naturally Light Strawberry Pineapple	1	131	0	33	29	3
Shake Bananasplit	1 (12 oz)	274	0	56	39	2
Shake P-Nut Power	1 (12 oz)	362	16	39	23	4
Smoothie Acai Energizer	1 (12 oz)	161	1	33	26	2
Smoothie Awesome Acai	1 (12 oz)	146	1	32	26	1
Smoothie Banzai Blueberry	1 (12 oz)	172	2	29	–	2
Smoothie Berry Brilliance	1 (12 oz)	192	1	45	38	2
Smoothie Big Wednesday	1 (12 oz)	201	1	49	42	2
Smoothie Cardio Cooler	1 (12 oz)	244	1	45	45	3
Smoothie Citrus Stinger	1 (12 oz)	198	1	44	24	2
Smoothie Cranberry Quest	1 (12 oz)	208	1	49	44	1
Smoothie Dr. Robeks	1 (12 oz)	186	1	42	31	2
Smoothie Green Tea Sensation	1 (12 oz)	199	2	37	27	0
Smoothie Guava Lava	1 (12 oz)	206	1	50	42	2
Smoothie Hummingbird	1 (12 oz)	211	1	50	43	2
Smoothie Infinite Orange	1 (12 oz)	182	1	42	31	2

FOOD	PORTION	CAL	FAT	CARB	SUGAR	FIBER
Smoothie Mahalo Mango	1 (12 oz)	201	1	50	45	2
Smoothie Malibu Peach	1 (12 oz)	181	0	44	38	1
Smoothie Outrageous Raspberry	1 (12 oz)	182	1	44	40	1
Smoothie Passionfruit Cove	1 (12 oz)	193	1	46	41	1
Smoothie Pina Koolada	1 (12 oz)	212	1	50	42	1
Smoothie Polar Pineapple	1 (12 oz)	183	1	45	40	1
Smoothie Pomegranate Passion	1 (12 oz)	190	0	46	40	1
Smoothie Pomegranate Power	1 (12 oz)	217	1	50	42	3
Smoothie Pro Arobek	1 (12 oz)	260	1	52	40	2
Smoothie Raspberry Romance	1 (12 oz)	209	0	50	41	2
Smoothie Robeks Rejuvenator	1 (12 oz)	221	1	51	42	2
Smoothie South Pacific Squeeze	1 (12 oz)	200	1	47	36	2
Smoothie Stawnana Berry	1 (12 oz)	188	0	44	37	1
Smoothie Venice Burner	1 (12 oz)	227	1	48	33	3
Smoothie Zen Berry	1 (12 oz)	217	1	51	29	4
SKIPPERS						
CHILDREN'S MENU SELECTIONS						
Kids Catch Chicken Tenderloin + Chips & Kids Side	1 serv	560	11	79	24	1
Kids Catch Fish Bites + Chips & Kids Side	1 serv	490	15	84	26	3

FOOD	PORTION	CAL	FAT	CARB	SUGAR	FIBER
Kids Catch Sandwich Grilled Cheese + Chips & Kids Side	1 serv	620	19	97	27	3
Kids Catch Shrimp + Chips & Kids Side	1 serv	520	11	91	25	2
MAIN MENU SELECTIONS						
Baked Potato Plain	1	210	0	48	3	5
Basket Chicken & Fish + Chips & Slaw	1 serv	620	27	59	5	1
Basket Chicken & Shrimp + Chips & Slaw	1 serv	760	25	84	5	1
Basket Chicken + Chips & Slaw	2 pieces	730	25	60	4	0
Basket Clam Strips + Chips & Slaw	1 serv	890	34	113	4	12
Basket Clams & Fish + Chips & Slaw	1 serv	740	32	91	5	8
Basket Original Recipe Shrimp + Chips & Slaw	1 serv	800	25	107	6	3
Basket Popcorn Shrimp + Chips & Slaw	1 serv	750	25	96	5	2
Basket Prawn & Fish + Chips & Slaw	1 serv	730	41	61	5	2
Basket Prawn Seafood + Chips & Slaw	1 serv	720	40	52	4	tr
Basket Shrimp & Fish + Chips & Slaw	1 serv	650	27	83	6	2
Basket Shrimp Trio + Chips & Slaw	1 serv	1040	38	123	7	4
Clam Chowder	1 cup	120	8	14	1	tr
Clam Strips	1 serv	270	6	39	0	6
Coleslaw	1 sm	170	16	7	4	0

FOOD	PORTION	CAL	FAT	CARB	SUGAR	FIBER
Fish Bites + Chips & Slaw	6 pieces	490	17	94	0	7
French Fries	1 reg	180	6	27	0	0
Grilled Veggies	1 serv	35	0	8	3	3
Halibut + Chips & Slaw	1 serv	580	30	51	4	0
Homestyle Chicken Tenderloin	1 piece	190	2	13	0	0
Hush Puppies	3 pieces	240	9	47	0	3
Original Fish Fillet	1 piece	80	4	12	1	1
Original Fish + Chips & Slaw	2 pieces	510	29	59	6	2
Original Shrimp	9 pieces	220	2	36	1	1
Sandwich Fish + Chips & Slaw	1 serv	800	34	105	14	4
Sandwich Fried Chicken + Chips & Slaw	1 serv	1260	49	117	12	3
Sandwich Grilled Chicken + Chips & Slaw	1 serv	1070	50	92	12	3
Skippers Platter + Chips & Slaw	1 serv	930	33	122	6	8
SALADS						
Caesar	1 sm	150	13	8	4	2
Caesar w/ Chicken	1 sm	340	17	8	4	2
Caesar w/ Salmon	1 sm	350	19	8	4	2
Green Salad w/o Dressing	1 sm	25	0	5	3	2

SMOOTHIE KING

FOOD	PORTION	CAL	FAT	CARB	SUGAR	FIBER
Acai Adventure	1 (20 oz)	435	5	92	74	4
Angel Food	1 (20 oz)	354	0	84	75	6
Banana Berry Treat	1 (20 oz)	364	0	86	75	5
Banana Boat	1 (20 oz)	524	12	97	77	6
Berry Punch	1 (20 oz)	360	0	91	84	4
Blackberry Dream	1 (20 oz)	365	1	88	68	2

FOOD	PORTION	CAL	FAT	CARB	SUGAR	FIBER
Blueberry Heaven	1 (20 oz)	325	1	73	64	2
Caribbean Way	1 (20 oz)	395	0	97	89	6
Celestial Cherry High	1 (20 oz)	257	0	64	55	3
Cherry Picket	1 (20 oz)	273	1	66	54	2
Coconut Surprise	1 (20 oz)	460	7	90	83	3
Coffee Smoothie Caramel	1 (20 oz)	340	1	66	56	0
Coffee Smoothie Mocha	1 (20 oz)	260	2	43	36	1
Coffee Smoothie Vanilla	1 (20 oz)	347	1	69	65	0
Cranberry Cooler	1 (20 oz)	496	0	120	89	3
Cranberry Supreme	1 (20 oz)	554	1	130	96	3
Fruit Fusion	1 (20 oz)	355	1	76	66	0
Go Goji	1 (20 oz)	433	0	104	104	0
Grape Expectations	1 (20 oz)	398	0	95	90	3
Grape Expectations II	1 (20 oz)	548	0	133	125	6
Green Tea Tango	1 (20 oz)	282	3	52	40	2
Hearty Apple	1 (20 oz)	405	1	86	75	2
High Protein Almond Mocha	1 (20 oz)	366	9	42	37	2
High Protein Banana	1 (20 oz)	322	9	32	23	4
High Protein Chocolate	1 (20 oz)	366	9	45	37	2
High Protein Lemon	1 (20 oz)	372	9	44	40	1
High Protein Pineapple	1 (20 oz)	320	9	29	23	2
Immune Builder	1 (20 oz)	380	1	89	77	6
Instant Vigor	1 (20 oz)	366	0	86	72	4
Island Impact	1 (20 oz)	311	0	73	65	1
Island Treat	1 (20 oz)	333	0	82	70	6
Kids' Kup Berry Interesting	1 (12 oz)	277	0	69	62	3
Kids' Kup Choc-A-Laka	1 (12 oz)	245	3	44	32	2
Kids' Kup CW Jr.	1 (12 oz)	270	0	68	59	5
Kids' Kup Gimmie-Grape	1 (12 oz)	265	0	64	60	2

FOOD	PORTION	CAL	FAT	CARB	SUGAR	FIBER
Kids' Kup Smarti Tarti	1 (12 oz)	200	0	49	46	0
Kiwi Island Treat	1 (20 oz)	498	1	116	96	0
Lemon Twist Banana	1 (20 oz)	358	0	87	82	3
Lemon Twist Strawberry	1 (20 oz)	438	0	107	104	3
Light & Fluffy	1 (20 oz)	395	0	99	89	6
Low Carb All Flavors	1 (20 oz)	268	9	7	3	1
Malts	1 (20 oz)	680	33	83	77	0
Mangofest	1 (20 oz)	285	0	72	69	1
Mangosteen Madness	1 (20 oz)	383	0	94	92	2
Mo'cuccino Caramel	1 (20 oz)	570	12	102	88	0
Mo'cuccino Mocha	1 (20 oz)	444	12	73	69	1
Mo'cuccino Vanilla	1 (20 oz)	525	12	92	85	0
Muscle Punch	1 (20 oz)	364	1	84	75	6
Muscle Punch Plus	1 (20 oz)	366	1	84	75	6
Orange Ka-Bam	1 (20 oz)	465	0	117	108	3
Organic Apple Acai	1 (20 oz)	353	5	74	58	4
Passion Passport	1 (20 oz)	395	0	96	93	2
Peach Slice	1 (20 oz)	314	0	72	55	1
Peach Slice Plus	1 (20 oz)	464	0	110	90	4
Peanut Power	1 (20 oz)	549	22	74	59	6
Peanut Power Plus Chocolate	1 (20 oz)	717	27	98	63	6
Peanut Power Plus Grape	1 (20 oz)	749	22	122	107	6
Peanut Power Plus Strawberry	1 (20 oz)	699	22	112	94	9
Pep Upper	1 (20 oz)	411	0	97	85	3
Pina Colada Island	1 (20 oz)	600	10	110	98	3
Pineapple Pleasure	1 (20 oz)	280	0	67	62	3
Pineapple Surf	1 (20 oz)	461	1	104	92	4
Pomegranate Punch	1 (20 oz)	464	0	110	108	1
Power Punch	1 (20 oz)	428	1	101	76	6
Power Punch Plus	1 (20 oz)	500	2	113	85	6

FOOD	PORTION	CAL	FAT	CARB	SUGAR	FIBER
Raspberry Collider	1 (20 oz)	338	0	86	74	4
Raspberry Sunrise	1 (20 oz)	392	0	95	73	2
Shakes	1 (20 oz)	670	33	81	76	0
Slim-N-Trim Chocolate	1 (20 oz)	297	2	57	48	3
Slim-N-Trim Orange Vanilla	1 (20 oz)	215	1	46	38	0
Slim-N-Trim Strawberry	1 (20 oz)	375	1	84	72	5
Slim-N-Trim Vanilla	1 (20 oz)	253	1	53	42	3
Strawberry Kiwi Breeze	1 (20 oz)	376	0	90	84	3
Strawberry X-treme	1 (20 oz)	366	0	92	70	6
Super Punch	1 (20 oz)	395	0	100	90	6
Super Punch Plus	1 (20 oz)	459	0	117	91	6
The Activator Chocolate	1 (20 oz)	404	1	83	56	5
The Activator Strawberry	1 (20 oz)	556	1	121	89	8
The Activator Vanilla	1 (20 oz)	406	1	83	54	5
The Hulk Chocolate	1 (20 oz)	876	31	124	90	6
The Hulk Strawberry	1 (20 oz)	1035	32	161	125	8
The Hulk Vanilla	1 (20 oz)	872	32	121	88	5
The Shredder Chocolate	1 (20 oz)	311	3	36	19	1
The Shredder Strawberry	1 (20 oz)	356	1	56	41	3
The Shredder Vanilla	1 (20 oz)	283	2	30	12	0
Yerba Mate Mango	1 (20 oz)	372	0	92	76	1
Yerba Mate Mixed Berry	1 (20 oz)	348	0	84	81	3
Yerba Mate Pomegranate	1 (20 oz)	372	0	91	73	2
Yogurt D-Lite	1 (20 oz)	333	4	59	47	0
Youth Fountain	1 (20 oz)	253	0	61	54	3

SONIC DRIVE-IN

ADD-ONS

Bacon	1 serv (0.5 oz)	70	5	0	0	0
Cheese	1 serv (0.7 oz)	60	5	2	1	0

FOOD	PORTION	CAL	FAT	CARB	SUGAR	FIBER
Chili	1 serv (1.2 oz)	50	4	2	1	1
Green Chilies	1 serv (1 oz)	5	0	1	0	0
Grilled Onions	1 serv (1 oz)	25	2	2	1	1
Jalapenos	1 serv (0.7 oz)	5	0	1	0	1
Slaw	1 serv (1 oz)	45	3	4	1	1
BEVERAGES						
Barq's Root Beer	1 sm (14 oz)	160	0	43	43	0
Coca-Cola	1 sm (14 oz)	140	0	39	39	0
Cream Pie Shake Banana	1 reg (14 oz)	590	19	98	83	1
Cream Pie Shake Chocolate	1 reg (14 oz)	660	19	114	96	0
Cream Pie Shake Coconut Cream	1 reg (14 oz)	580	20	93	82	0
CreamSlush Blue Coconut	1 reg (14 oz)	430	13	76	69	0
CreamSlush Cherry	1 reg (14 oz)	440	13	77	71	0
CreamSlush Grape	1 reg (14 oz)	430	13	76	70	0
CreamSlush Orange	1 reg (14 oz)	430	13	77	70	0
CreamSlush Strawberry	1 reg (14 oz)	450	12	84	72	1
CreamSlush Watermelon	1 reg (14 oz)	440	13	77	70	0
Diet Coke	1 sm (14 oz)	0	0	0	0	0
Dr Pepper	1 sm (14 oz)	130	0	37	37	0
Float Barq's Root Beer	1 reg (14 oz)	300	8	56	52	0
Float Coca-Cola	1 reg (14 oz)	290	8	54	50	0
Float Dr Pepper	1 reg (14 oz)	310	8	58	54	0
Limeade	1 sm (14 oz)	140	0	38	37	0
Limeade Cherry	1 sm (14 oz)	170	0	45	44	0
Limeade Strawberry	1 sm (14 oz)	170	0	45	41	0
Malt Banana	1 reg (14 oz)	490	17	78	65	1
Malt Caramel	1 reg (14 oz)	550	18	90	78	0
Malt Chocolate	1 reg (14 oz)	550	17	91	76	0

FOOD	PORTION	CAL	FAT	CARB	SUGAR	FIBER
Malt Hot Fudge	1 reg (14 oz)	580	22	87	73	1
Malt Peanut Butter	1 reg (14 oz)	870	36	78	65	0
Malt Peanut Butter Fudge	1 reg (14 oz)	620	29	83	69	1
Malt Pineapple	1 reg (14 oz)	510	17	82	68	0
Malt Strawberry	1 reg (14 oz)	520	17	85	71	1
Malt Vanilla	1 reg (14 oz)	480	18	72	64	0
Milk 1%	8.5 oz	110	3	13	12	0
Milk Chocolate 1%	8.5 oz	160	3	27	25	0
Shake Banana	1 reg (14 oz)	470	16	76	63	1
Shake Chocolate	1 reg (14 oz)	540	16	89	74	0
Shake Hot Fudge	1 reg (14 oz)	570	21	85	71	1
Shake Peanut Butter	1 reg (14 oz)	640	34	75	63	0
Shake Peanut Butter Fudge	1 reg (14 oz)	610	28	81	68	1
Shake Pineapple	1 reg (14 oz)	500	16	80	66	0
Shake Strawberry	1 reg (14 oz)	510	16	83	69	1
Shake Vanilla	1 reg (14 oz)	470	17	71	62	0
Sonic Blast Butterfinger	1 reg (14 oz)	580	22	88	72	0
Sonic Blast M&M's	1 reg (14 oz)	600	24	88	78	1
Sonic Blast Oreo	1 reg (14 oz)	540	21	80	67	1
Sonic Blast Reese's Peanut Butter Cup	1 reg (14 oz)	560	19	89	74	1
Sprite	1 sm (14 oz)	104	0	37	37	0
Sprite Zero	1 sm (14 oz)	5	0	0	0	0
BREAKFAST SELECTIONS						
Breakfast Burrito Jr.	1 (4.1 oz)	330	21	25	1	2
Breakfast Burrito Sausage Egg Cheese	1 (5.9 oz)	480	31	38	2	1
Breakfast Toaster Bacon Egg Cheese	1 (5.6 oz)	530	32	40	7	2
Breakfast Toaster Ham Egg Cheese	1 (6.5 oz)	490	26	40	6	2

FOOD	PORTION	CAL	FAT	CARB	SUGAR	FIBER
Breakfast Toaster Sausage Egg Cheese	1 (6.8 oz)	620	42	40	6	2
CroisSonic Bacon	1 (5.3 oz)	510	36	29	5	0
CroisSonic Sausage	1 (6.2 oz)	600	46	29	5	0
DESSERTS						
Apple Slices	1 serv (2.4 oz)	35	0	9	7	2
Apple Slices w/ Fat Free Caramel Dipping Sauce	1 serv (3.4 oz)	120	0	27	23	2
Banana Split	1 (10.8 oz)	420	9	80	57	2
Cone Vanilla	1 (4.7 oz)	180	6	30	22	0
Dish Vanilla	1 (6.5 oz)	240	9	36	32	0
Sundae Chocolate	1 (8.9 oz)	410	13	67	55	0
Sundae Hot Fudge	1 (8.9 oz)	440	18	63	52	1
Sundae Pineapple	1 (8.8 oz)	370	13	58	47	0
Sundae Strawberry	1 (8.8 oz)	380	13	61	49	1
MAIN MENU SELECTIONS						
California Cheeseburger	1 (9.3 oz)	690	39	57	13	5
Ched 'R' Bites	12 (3 oz)	280	15	22	0	1
Ched 'R' Peppers	4 (4.2 oz)	330	17	36	2	2
Chicken Strip Dinner	1 serv (13.5 oz)	930	43	100	7	7
Chicken Strips	2 (2.5 oz)	200	11	10	0	1
Chili Cheeseburger	1 (7.9 oz)	660	35	56	11	5
Coney Regular	1 (5.2 oz)	390	23	32	4	2
Corn Dog	1 (2.6 oz)	210	11	23	4	2
Crispy Chicken Bacon Ranch	1 serv (8.9 oz)	610	34	48	10	4
French Fries	1 sm (2.5 oz)	200	8	30	0	2
French Fries w/ Cheese	1 sm (3 oz)	270	13	32	1	2
French Fries w/ Chili & Cheese	1 sm (4.1 oz)	300	16	33	1	3

FOOD	PORTION	CAL	FAT	CARB	SUGAR	FIBER
Fritos Chili Pie	1 med (4.8 oz)	470	32	36	1	3
Green Chili Cheeseburger	1 (10 oz)	630	31	56	12	5
Grilled Chicken Bacon Ranch	1 serv (8.9 oz)	470	22	35	10	3
Hickory Cheeseburger	1 (8.3 oz)	640	31	61	17	5
Jalapeno Burger	1 (7.6 oz)	550	26	53	10	5
Jalapeno Cheeseburger	1 (8.3 oz)	620	31	54	11	5
Jr. Bacon Cheeseburger	1 (5 oz)	410	23	31	8	3
Jr. Burger	1 (4.1 oz)	310	15	30	7	3
Jr. Burger Deluxe	1 (4.7 oz)	350	20	28	4	3
Jr. Double Cheeseburger	1 (6.7 oz)	570	35	33	9	3
Jumbo Popcorn Chicken	1 sm (4 oz)	380	22	27	1	3
Mozzarella Sticks	1 serv (5 oz)	440	22	40	1	2
Onion Rings	1 med (5.5 oz)	440	21	55	14	3
Pickle-O's	1 serv (4 oz)	310	16	36	2	2
Sandwich Breaded Pork Fritter	1 (8.5 oz)	640	33	66	11	7
Sandwich Crispy Chicken	1 (7.9 oz)	550	32	46	8	4
Sandwich Fish	1 (8.6 oz)	650	31	71	12	7
Sandwich Grilled Cheese	1 (3.9 oz)	380	20	39	6	2
Sandwich Grilled Chicken	1 (7.8 oz)	400	19	32	8	3
Sonic Burger w/ Ketchup	1 (8.7 oz)	560	26	57	14	5
Sonic Burger w/ Mayonnaise	1 (8.7 oz)	650	37	55	11	5
Sonic Burger w/ Mustard	1 (8.5 oz)	560	26	54	11	5

FOOD	PORTION	CAL	FAT	CARB	SUGAR	FIBER
Sonic Cheeseburger w/ Ketchup	1 (9.3 oz)	630	31	59	15	5
Sonic Cheeseburger w/ Mayonnaise	1 (9.3 oz)	720	42	56	12	5
Sonic Cheeseburger w/ Mustard	1 (9.1 oz)	620	31	55	12	5
SuperSonic Cheeseburger w/ Ketchup	1 (12 oz)	900	53	60	16	5
SuperSonic Cheeseburger w/ Mayonnaise	1 (12 oz)	980	64	58	13	5
SuperSonic Cheeseburger w/ Mustard	1 (11.8 oz)	890	53	57	13	5
Thousand Island Burger	1 (8.7 oz)	610	32	56	13	5
Toaster Sandwich Bacon Cheeseburger	1 (8.5 oz)	670	39	52	13	3
Toaster Sandwich BLT	1 (5.2 oz)	500	29	45	7	2
Toaster Sandwich Chicken Club	1 (9 oz)	740	46	55	7	4
Toaster Sandwich Country Fried Steak	1 (8.5 oz)	670	37	71	6	4
Tots	1 sm (1.5 oz)	130	8	13	0	1
Tots w/ Cheese	1 sm (2.2 oz)	190	13	14	1	1
Tots w/ Chili & Cheese	1 sm (3.2 oz)	220	16	16	1	2
Wrap Crispy Chicken	1 (8.2 oz)	490	23	49	5	3
Wrap Fritos Chili Cheese	1 (8.5 oz)	670	39	66	3	4
Wrap Grilled Chicken	1 (8.8 oz)	390	14	39	5	2
SALAD DRESSINGS AND SAUCES						
Dressing Honey Mustard	1 serv (1.5 oz)	180	16	10	8	0

FOOD	PORTION	CAL	FAT	CARB	SUGAR	FIBER
Dressing Italian Fat Free	1 serv (1.5 oz)	40	0	10	3	0
Dressing Original Ranch	1 serv (1.5 oz)	190	20	2	1	0
Dressing Original Ranch Light	1 serv (1.5 oz)	110	5	14	3	0
Dressing Thousand Island	1 serv (1.5 oz)	190	19	7	5	0
Sauce BBQ	1 serv (1 oz)	45	0	11	7	0
Sauce Honey Mustard	1 serv (1 oz)	90	7	7	5	0
Sauce Marinara	1 serv (1 oz)	15	0	3	2	1
Sauce Ranch	1 serv (1 oz)	140	16	1	1	0
SALADS						
Crispy Chicken	1 serv (11.4 oz)	340	19	24	6	5
Grilled Chicken	1 serv (12 oz)	250	10	12	6	3

SOUPLANTATION

FOOD	PORTION	CAL	FAT	CARB	SUGAR	FIBER
BREADS AND MUFFINS						
Biscuit Buttermilk	1	190	8	25	2	0
Cornbread Buttermilk Low Fat	1 piece	140	2	27	4	2
Focaccia Bruschetta	1 piece	140	7	15	1	1
Focaccia Honey Wheat Crust BBQ Chicken	1 piece	200	8	23	4	2
Focaccia Honey Wheat Crust Buffalo Chicken	1 piece	170	7	20	2	2
Muffin Apple Cinnamon Bran 96% Fat Free	1	130	1	30	16	3
Muffin Apple Raisin	1	150	7	22	9	1
Muffin Banana Nut	1	150	7	22	9	1
Muffin Cappuccino Chip	1	190	6	31	15	1
Muffin Caribbean Key Lime	1	170	6	28	15	1
Muffin Carrot Pineapple w/ Oat Bran	1	150	6	23	13	2

FOOD	PORTION	CAL	FAT	CARB	SUGAR	FIBER
Muffin Cherry Nut	1	150	7	22	9	1
Muffin Chile Corn Low Fat	1	140	3	27	5	2
Muffin Chocolate Brownie	1	180	8	26	16	1
Muffin Chocolate Chip	1	170	8	22	10	1
Muffin Top Banana Crunch No Sugar Added	1	120	5	19	2	1
BREAKFAST MENU SELECTIONS						
Belgian Waffle	1	90	0	16	2	1
Biscuit Sweet Cinnamon w/ Frosting	1	270	13	37	14	0
Biscuit Sweet Maple Buttermilk	1	240	9	39	16	1
Biscuit Sweet Strawberry Buttermilk	1	250	9	40	19	1
Breakfast Burrito Country Ham & Egg	1	210	10	21	1	2
Breakfast Burrito Sweet Pepper Sausage Egg	1	210	11	20	1	2
Eggs Scrambled	½ cup	135	8	2	1	0
Focaccia Egg Scramble w/ Bacon	1 piece	180	8	20	1	1
French Toast	1 slice	150	4	25	4	1
Oatmeal Plain	¾ cup	110	2	19	0	3
Potatoes O'Brien	½ cup	140	6	19	3	2
Sticky Granola Clusters w/ Almonds	¼ cup	270	14	30	15	3
Sunrise Pasta Mediterranean	1 cup	210	12	19	3	2
DESSERTS						
Apple Medley Fat Free	½ cup	70	0	18	12	1
Banana Royale Fat Free	½ cup	80	0	20	12	1

FOOD	PORTION	CAL	FAT	CARB	SUGAR	FIBER
Cake Carrot & Cream Cheese Lava	1 piece	320	15	40	34	1
Cake Chocolate Lava	½ cup	330	8	62	47	0
Cobbler Apple	½ cup	360	10	67	10	1
Cobbler Caramel Apple	½ cup	390	12	68	50	2
Cobbler Cherry Apple	½ cup	330	10	57	29	2
Cookie Chocolate Chip	1 sm	75	3	10	6	0
Cookie Bar Chocolate Peanut Butter	1 piece	270	12	37	22	1
Frozen Yogurt Chocolate Nonfat	½ cup	110	0	22	17	1
Pudding Banana	½ cup	160	4	27	26	1
Pudding Butterscotch Low Fat	½ cup	140	3	24	24	0
Pudding Chocolate Low Fat	½ cup	150	3	25	24	0
Pudding Chocolate Low Fat No Sugar Added	½ cup	90	2	21	6	0
MAIN MENU SELECTIONS						
100% Whole Wheat Jalapeno & Salsa Pasta	1 cup	250	6	46	3	6
Alfredo 4 Cheese	1 cup	390	13	50	3	3
Alfredo Broccoli w/ Basil	1 cup	380	17	45	5	1
Alfredo Fettuccine	1 cup	390	18	41	4	2
Alfredo Fire Roasted Tomato Basil	1 cup	370	14	44	4	2
Arizona Marinara	1 cup	360	11	47	6	3
Baked Potato Topper Broccoli Cheese	1 cup	120	7	10	2	1
Beefy Meatball Stroganoff	1 cup	340	21	28	4	2
Bruschetta	1 cup	260	4	41	3	3
Bruschetta Creamy	1 cup	360	16	43	3	3

FOOD	PORTION	CAL	FAT	CARB	SUGAR	FIBER
Carbonara Pasta w/ Bacon	1 cup	290	10	43	3	2
Cheesy Scalloped Potatoes w/ Bacon	1 cup	240	17	15	2	1
Chicken Tetrazzini	1 cup	480	23	47	4	3
Creamy Cilantro Lime Pesto Hot Pasta	1 cup	360	20	37	3	1
Creamy Herb Chicken	1 cup	310	17	32	7	2
Curried Pineapple & Ginger	1 cup	200	2	40	9	2
Garden Vegetable w/ Italian Sausage	1 cup	300	10	42	2	3
Pesto Cilantro Lime	1 cup	370	21	36	3	2
SALAD DRESSINGS						
Avocado Ranch	2 tbsp	150	14	4	3	0
Bacon	2 tbsp	110	11	7	6	0
Blue Cheese	1 tbsp	130	13	3	1	0
Creamy Cucumber Reduced Calorie	2 tbsp	70	7	3	2	0
Creamy Italian	2 tbsp	120	13	0	0	0
Creamy Sesame Soy	2 tbsp	170	17	5	4	0
Green Chili Ranch	2 tbsp	150	14	4	3	0
Honey Mustard	2 tbsp	150	13	8	6	0
Honey Mustard Fat Free	2 tbsp	45	0	10	9	0
Italian Fat Free	2 tbsp	25	0	7	2	0
Vinaigrette Balsamic	2 tbsp	180	19	1	1	0
Vinaigrette Basil	2 tbsp	160	17	1	0	0
Vinaigrette Cranberry Orange Low Fat	2 tbsp	80	2	15	8	0
Vinaigrette Honey Lime Cilantro	2 tbsp	100	6	15	14	0
Vinaigrette Italian w/ Basil & Romano Cheese	2 tbsp	150	15	1	1	0

FOOD	PORTION	CAL	FAT	CARB	SUGAR	FIBER
SALADS						
100% Whole Wheat Arugula Citrus	½ cup	210	10	29	6	3
100% Whole Wheat Creamy Chipotle	½ cup	350	25	31	4	4
100% Whole Wheat Sicilian Penne w/ Feta & Pepperoni	½ cup	250	14	30	4	5
100% Whole Wheat Spicy Asian Peanut	½ cup	260	14	32	7	4
Ambrosia w/ Coconut	½ cup	190	9	30	23	2
Artichoke Rice	½ cup	190	12	19	2	1
Aunt Doris' Red Pepper Slaw Fat Free	½ cup	70	0	18	13	3
Azteca Taco w/ Turkey	1 cup	130	9	7	3	4
Baja Bean & Cilantro	½ cup	180	3	29	2	5
Bartlett Pear & Carmelized Walnut	1 cup	180	12	13	10	2
BBQ Smokehouse w/ Bacon & Peanuts	1 cup	290	17	25	5	2
Buffalo Chicken	1 cup	180	14	10	2	1
Caesar Asiago	1 cup	270	22	10	2	2
California Cobb w/ Bacon	1 cup	190	15	7	2	2
Cambay Curry w/ Almonds & Coconut	1 cup	220	17	17	11	4
Carrot Raisin	½ cup	90	3	17	15	2
Cherry Balsamic Blue Tossed	1 cup	220	16	16	9	1
Cherry Chipotle Spinach	1 cup	160	8	20	05	4
Chinese Krab	½ cup	160	8	19	4	3
Citrus Noodle w/ Snow Peas	½ cup	140	6	19	5	2
Classic Antipasto	1 cup	280	21	18	8	4

FOOD	PORTION	CAL	FAT	CARB	SUGAR	FIBER
Classic Greek	1 cup	120	9	4	2	2
Confetti Avocado Slaw	½ cup	140	9	12	4	3
Crunchy Island Pineapple	1 cup	160	8	20	12	2
Curried Rice w/ Mango Chutney	½ cup	170	2	36	9	1
Field Greens Citrus Vinaigrette	1 cup	150	12	10	4	2
Potato Bristo	½ cup	290	19	27	2	3
Potato Buffalo Blue	½ cup	190	13	16	3	2
SOUPS						
8 Vegetable Chicken Stew	1 cup	160	7	17	4	2
Albondigas Locas Meatball	1 cup	210	11	19	5	2
Asian Ginger Broth	1 cup	50	2	6	3	0
Basmati Lentil	1 cup	210	7	29	2	4
Beef & Barley Stew	1 cup	240	10	19	5	3
Better Than Mom's Beef Stew	1 cup	270	17	19	3	2
Big Chunk Chicken Noodle Low Fat	1 cup	170	3	19	3	1
Border Black Bean & Chorizo	1 cup	240	10	27	6	6
Broccoli Cheese	1 cup	270	19	17	7	1
Buffalo Chicken	1 cup	180	6	21	2	1
Canadian Cheese w/ Smoked Ham	1 cup	350	26	22	7	1
Cheese Stuffed Cappelletti	1 cup	250	11	31	9	2
Cheesy Corn Chowder w/ Bacon	1 cup	220	11	25	4	2

FOOD	PORTION	CAL	FAT	CARB	SUGAR	FIBER
Chesapeake Corn Chowder	1 cup	290	17	30	8	2
Chicken & Rice	1 cup	160	5	18	3	1
Chicken Dijon Reduced Sodium	1 cup	210	13	18	4	1
Chicken Divan	1 cup	240	15	18	4	1
Chicken Enchilada	1 cup	190	7	22	3	3
STEAK ESCAPE						
BEVERAGES						
Coca-Cola	16 oz	150	0	40	–	–
Diet Coke	16 oz	0	0	0	0	0
Lemonade	16 oz	167	0	44	–	–
Sprite	16 oz	150	0	39	–	–
SALADS						
Grilled Side	1 serv (5.9 oz)	40	1	8	–	–
Grilled w/ Chicken	1 serv (11.1 oz)	177	5	11	–	–
Grilled w/ Ham	1 serv (10.6 oz)	302	2	8	–	–
Grilled w/ Steak	1 serv (11.1 oz)	187	6	11	–	–
Grilled w/ Turkey	1 serv (10.6 oz)	132	2	8	–	–
SANDWICHES						
7 Inch Cajun Chicken	1 (8.6 oz)	408	5	58	–	–
7 Inch Capicola Portion	1 serv (1 oz)	31	1	tr	–	–
7 Inch Chicken Portion	1 serv (3.9 oz)	120	4	0	0	0
7 Inch Classic Italian Sub	1 (8.4 oz)	471	11	60	–	–
7 Inch Ham Portion	1 serv (3 oz)	75	1	3	–	–
7 Inch Salami Portion	1 serv (1 oz)	105	9	0	–	–
7 Inch Steak Portion	1 serv (3.9 oz)	130	5	0	0	0

FOOD	PORTION	CAL	FAT	CARB	SUGAR	FIBER
7 Inch Turkey Club	1 (7.9 oz)	380	2	62	–	–
7 Inch Turkey Portion	1 serv (2.9 oz)	75	1	3	–	–
7 Inch Vegetarian	1 (8.8 oz)	311	1	65	–	–
7 Inch Wild West BBQ	1 (9.6 oz)	455	6	60	–	–
Kids Chicken	1 (3.9 oz)	205	7	29	–	–
Kids Ham	1 (3.7 oz)	183	1	31	–	–
Kids Steak	1 (3.8 oz)	110	3	29	–	–
Kids Turkey	1 (3.7 oz)	183	1	31	–	–
SIDES						
Fries	1 serv (32 oz)	996	52	134	–	–
Fries	1 serv (12 oz)	498	26	67	–	–
Fries Kids	1 serv (2.9 oz)	249	13	34	–	–
Fries Loaded Bacon & Cheddar	1 serv (10.8 oz)	905	44	88	–	–
Fries Loaded Ranch & Bacon	1 serv (10.8 oz)	1044	71	84	–	–
Kids Chicken Tenders	2 (3.8 oz)	240	11	21	–	–
Smashed Potatoes Loaded Bacon & Cheddar	1 serv (16.7 oz)	636	26	91	–	–
Smashed Potatoes Loaded Ranch & Bacon	1 serv (16.7 oz)	692	34	87	–	–
Smashed Potatoes Plain	1 serv (13.8 oz)	246	0	53	–	–
Smashed Potatoes w/ Chicken	1 serv (19.9 oz)	383	4	56	–	–
Smashed Potatoes w/ Ham	1 serv (19.4 oz)	338	2	59	–	–
Smashed Potatoes w/ Steak	1 serv (19.9 oz)	393	5	56	–	–

FOOD	PORTION	CAL	FAT	CARB	SUGAR	FIBER
Smashed Potatoes w/ Turkey	1 serv (19.4 oz)	338	2	59	–	2
TOPPINGS						
BBQ Sauce	1 serv (1 oz)	40	0	9	–	–
Brown Mustard	1 serv (1 oz)	0	0	0	0	0
Cheddar	1 serv (1 oz)	116	8	1	–	–
Dressing Balsamic Vinaigrette	1 serv (1.5 oz)	90	9	3	–	–
Dressing Bleu Cheese	1 serv (1.5 oz)	184	18	3	–	–
Dressing Italian	1 serv (0.5 oz)	51	5	1	–	–
Dressing Ranch	1 serv (0.5 oz)	83	9	0	0	0
Lettuce	1 serv (1 oz)	2	0	0	0	0
Margarine	1 serv (1 oz)	203	23	0	0	0
Mayonnaise	1 serv (1 oz)	101	11	0	0	0
Parmesan	1 serv (1 oz)	30	2	tr	–	–
Peppers Mild	1 serv (1.5 oz)	11	0	4	–	–
Provolone	1 serv (0.75 oz)	80	6	0	0	0
Sour Cream	1 serv (1 oz)	61	6	1	–	–
Tomatoes	1 serv (2 oz)	24	0	2	–	–
White American	1 serv (1 oz)	101	9	3	–	–

TACO CABANA

FOOD	PORTION	CAL	FAT	CARB	SUGAR	FIBER
ADD-ONS						
Dressing Southwest Ranch	1 serv (1 oz)	112	11	2	0	0
Guacamole	1 serv (3 oz)	110	9	7	1	4
Pico De Gallo	1 serv (1 oz)	5	0	1	1	0
Queso	1 serv (3 oz)	200	15	5	5	0
Salsa Black Bean & Corn	1 serv (1 oz)	30	0	5	1	1
Salsa Fuego	1 serv (1 oz)	5	0	1	1	0
Salsa Pineapple	1 serv (1 oz)	20	0	5	5	0
Salsa Ranch	1 serv (1 oz)	35	4	1	1	0

FOOD	PORTION	CAL	FAT	CARB	SUGAR	FIBER
Salsa Roja	1 serv (1 oz)	5	0	1	1	0
Salsa Verde	1 serv (1 oz)	10	0	1	1	0
Shredded Cheese	1 serv (1 oz)	110	9	0	0	0
Sour Cream	1 serv (3 oz)	160	14	3	3	0
BREAKFAST MENU SELECTIONS						
Breakfast Burrito Bacon & Egg	1	410	18	41	2	2
Breakfast Burrito Barbacoa	1	510	25	40	2	2
Breakfast Burrito Chorizo & Egg	1	400	18	42	2	2
Breakfast Burrito Potato & Egg	1	440	21	48	2	2
Breakfast Taco Bacon & Egg	1	230	10	20	0	1
Breakfast Taco Barbacoa	1	250	12	19	0	1
Breakfast Taco Chorizo & Egg	1	200	9	20	0	1
Breakfast Taco Potato & Egg	1	210	10	23	0	1
Plates Huevos Rancheros	1 serv	770	38	67	1	9
Plates Steak Fajitas & Scrambled Eggs	1 serv	800	37	70	2	9
Platter Eggs Mexicana	1 serv	920	52	70	6	9
MAIN MENU SELECTIONS						
Black Beans	1 serv	80	0	14	2	2
Borracho Beans	1 serv	140	3	20	1	7
Burrito Bean & Cheese	1	730	35	77	3	11
Burrito Beef Ground	1	710	30	71	5	6
Burrito Beef Ultimo Ground	1	800	38	74	6	7
Burrito Black Bean	1	450	8	82	6	5

FOOD	PORTION	CAL	FAT	CARB	SUGAR	FIBER
Burrito Chicken Breast Fajita	1	630	24	65	5	3
Burrito Chicken Stewed	1	660	25	73	5	7
Burrito Chicken Ultimo Stewed	1	760	33	76	6	8
Burrito Steak Fajita	1	650	27	65	4	2
Chips	1 serv (2.5 oz)	180	16	37	1	5
Fajitas Chicken Personal	1 serv	740	20	98	8	13
Fajitas Chicken Platter	1 serv	1670	52	212	15	26
Fajitas Steak Personal	1 serv	760	24	98	7	12
Flautas Chicken	1	100	4	10	0	1
Refried Beans	1 serv	250	13	24	1	6
Taco Beef Ground	1	230	9	22	1	1
Taco Chicken Breast Fajita	1	190	4	21	0	1
Taco Steak Fajita	1	200	6	21	0	1
Taco Crispy Chicken Stewed	1	160	7	13	1	2
Taco Crispy Ground Beef	1	180	10	11	1	2
Taco Soft Bean & Cheese	1	300	14	32	0	4
Taco Soft Black Bean	1	200	4	34	2	2
Taco Soft Carne Guisada	1	190	6	21	0	1
Taco Soft Chicken Stewed	1	210	7	23	1	2
Tortilla Corn	1	70	1	15	0	2
Tortilla Flour	1	120	3	19	0	1

TACO JOHN'S

BREAKFAST SELECTIONS

FOOD	PORTION	CAL	FAT	CARB	SUGAR	FIBER
Breakfast Burrito Bacon	1 (7.6 oz)	550	25	56	5	7

FOOD	PORTION	CAL	FAT	CARB	SUGAR	FIBER
Breakfast Burrito Egg	1 (6.6 oz)	420	19	42	6	5
Breakfast Burrito Egg Bacon	1 (7 oz)	500	24	43	6	5
Breakfast Burrito Egg Sausage	1 (8.1 oz)	590	34	44	6	6
Breakfast Burrito Sausage	1 (8.6 oz)	640	35	56	5	7
Breakfast Taco Bacon	1 (3.7 oz)	270	13	25	1	2
Breakfast Taco Sausage	1 (4.2 oz)	310	18	25	1	2
Scrambler Burrito Bacon	1 (8.6 oz)	550	25	58	6	7
Scrambler Burrito Sausage	1 (9.6 oz)	640	32	58	7	7
Scrambler Potato Ole Bacon	1 sm (9.4 oz)	630	41	45	2	6
Scrambler Potato Ole Sausage	1 sm (10.5 oz)	720	50	45	5	6
DESSERTS						
Apple Grande	1 serv (3.4 oz)	270	12	39	15	2
Choco Taco	1 serv (4 oz)	390	20	48	32	1
Churro	1 serv (2 oz)	190	7	15	10	4
Cini-Sopapilla Bites	1 serv (2.6 oz)	210	5	37	7	4
Giant Goldfish Grahams	1 serv (0.5 oz)	70	2	11	4	1
MAIN MENU SELECTIONS						
Burrito Bean	1 (6.6 oz)	360	9	56	5	9
Burrito Beefy	1 (6.6 oz)	440	20	45	5	7
Burrito Chicken & Potato	1 (8.3 oz)	470	19	56	5	7
Burrito Chicken Grilled	1 (8.2 oz)	590	29	50	5	6
Burrito Combination	1 (6.6 oz)	400	14	50	5	8
Burrito Crunchy Chicken & Potato	1 (8.8 oz)	600	28	65	5	7

FOOD	PORTION	CAL	FAT	CARB	SUGAR	FIBER
Burrito Grilled Beef	1 (8.2 oz)	600	32	52	5	8
Burrito Meat & Potato	1 (8.3 oz)	500	23	58	5	8
Burrito Ranch Beef	1 (7.1 oz)	440	22	45	6	6
Burrito Ranch Chicken	1 (7 oz)	400	17	44	6	5
Burrito Smothered	1 (11.3 oz)	510	20	60	6	10
Burrito Super	1 (8.8 oz)	450	18	54	6	9
Chili w/o Crackers	1 serv (8 oz)	220	11	17	2	4
Chili w/o Crackers & Cheese	1 serv (7.5 oz)	160	6	17	2	4
Chilto	1 serv (4.6 oz)	360	15	40	5	5
Chips & Queso	1 serv (6.7 oz)	430	25	43	1	2
Crispy Taco	1 (3.2 oz)	180	10	13	1	2
Crunchy Chicken w/o Sauce	1 serv (5 oz)	450	27	24	0	0
Enchiliada Chili	1 serv (7.6 oz)	310	16	24	2	4
Mexi Rolls w/o Nachos	2 pieces (1.9 oz)	130	5	14	0	2
Mexican Rice	1 serv (6 oz)	250	6	45	2	0
Nachos	1 serv (5 oz)	380	23	38	0	1
Potato Oles	1 sm (5 oz)	430	26	45	1	6
Potato Oles Chili Cheese	1 serv (10.7 oz)	590	36	55	2	8
Potato Oles Super	1 serv (9.7 oz)	620	39	53	2	7
Quesadilla Melt Cheesey	1 (5.6 oz)	440	22	43	4	5
Quesadilla Melt Fajita Beef	1 serv (8.6 oz)	540	28	49	6	7
Quesadilla Melt Fajita Chicken	1 (8.6 oz)	510	23	47	6	6

FOOD	PORTION	CAL	FAT	CARB	SUGAR	FIBER
Refried Beans	1 serv (9.4 oz)	320	6	47	2	11
Refried Beans w/o Cheese	1 serv (8.9 oz)	260	2	47	2	11
Sierra Chicken Sandwich	1 (8.2 oz)	350	11	37	2	2
Softshell Taco	1 (4 oz)	220	11	21	1	2
Super Nachos	1 sm (6.9 oz)	450	27	38	1	3
Taco Bravo	1 (6.5 oz)	340	13	40	1	5
Taco Burger	1 (5 oz)	270	12	28	4	3
Taco Stuffed Grilled	1 (7.4 oz)	560	25	63	0	7
SALAD DRESSINGS AND TOPPINGS						
Bacon Ranch Dressing	1 serv (1.5 oz)	130	10	10	7	0
Creamy Italian Dressing	1 serv (1.5 oz)	130	15	3	1	0
Guacamole	1 serv (2 oz)	90	6	8	2	2
Hot Sauce	1 serv (1 oz)	10	0	1	0	0
House Dressing	1 serv (1.5 oz)	70	7	2	1	0
Mild Sauce	1 serv (1 oz)	10	0	1	0	0
Nacho Cheese	1 serv (3 oz)	120	9	5	0	0
Pico De Gallo	1 serv (1 oz)	10	0	1	0	0
Ranch Dressing	1 serv (1.5 oz)	140	16	3	1	0
Salsa	1 serv (2 oz)	20	0	4	2	1
Sour Cream	1 serv (2 oz)	120	12	2	0	0
Super Hot Sauce	1 serv (1 oz)	10	0	1	0	0
SALADS						
Softshell Taco Chicken	1 (4 oz)	190	6	19	0	1
Taco Crunchy Chicken w/o Dressing	1 serv (13.4 oz)	660	40	47	7	6
Taco w/o Dressing	1 serv (12.7 oz)	520	33	37	7	7

TASTI D-LITE

FOOD	PORTION	CAL	FAT	CARB	SUGAR	FIBER
Acai	4 oz	70	2	13	11	0
Banana	4 oz	70	1	13	11	0

FOOD	PORTION	CAL	FAT	CARB	SUGAR	FIBER
Banana 'N Peanut Butter	4 oz	90	3	13	11	0
Bananas Foster	4 oz	70	1	13	11	0
Burnt Sugar	4 oz	70	1	14	14	0
Buttercrunch	4 oz	80	3	13	11	0
Cappuccino	4 oz	70	2	13	10	0
Cherry Cake	4 oz	70	2	13	12	0
Chocoleche	4 oz	80	2	15	13	0
Cinnamon Crunch	4 oz	70	1	14	11	0
Coffee Liqueur	4 oz	70	2	12	10	0
Creme Brulee	4 oz	70	2	14	12	0
Egg Nog	4 oz	70	2	13	11	0
German Chocolate Cake	4 oz	80	2	14	13	0
Latte	4 oz	70	2	13	11	0
Mud Pie	4 oz	80	2	15	14	0
Nutella	4 oz	90	3	15	13	0
Peanut Butter Batter	4 oz	90	3	13	11	1
Peanut Cluster	4 oz	90	3	13	12	0
Pecan Praline	4 oz	70	2	14	12	0
Pina Colada	4 oz	80	2	14	12	0
Raspberry	4 oz	70	2	13	12	0
Rice Pudding	4 oz	80	1	15	12	0
Tapioca Pudding	4 oz	70	2	14	12	0
Tart 'N Tasti	4 oz	100	1	23	21	0
Tart 'N Tasti Acai	4 oz	100	2	20	18	0
Tart 'N Tasti Mango	4 oz	100	1	21	19	0
Tiramisu	4 oz	70	1	13	11	0
Toasted Almond Fudge	4 oz	80	1	14	14	0
Toffee Crunch	4 oz	90	3	14	14	0
WENDY'S						
BEVERAGES						
Barq's Root Beer	1 sm	180	0	50	50	0
Coca-Cola	1 sm	160	0	44	44	0

FOOD	PORTION	CAL	FAT	CARB	SUGAR	FIBER
Diet Coke	1 sm	0	0	0	0	0
Frosty Chocolate	1 sm	300	8	49	42	0
Frosty Vanilla	1 sm	280	7	47	40	0
Frosty Shake Caramel	1 sm	650	14	121	97	0
Frosty Shake Chocolate	1 sm	580	13	104	93	2
Frosty Shake Strawberry	1 sm	550	13	99	90	1
Frosty Shake Wild Berry	1 sm	520	13	90	79	1
Lemonade Light Minute Maid	1 sm	5	0	1	0	0
Sprite	1 sm	160	0	43	43	0
TruMoo Lowfat Chocolate Milk	1	140	3	22	20	0
TruMoo Lowfat Milk	1	100	3	12	11	0
Water Nestle Pure Life	1 serv	0	0	0	0	0
CHILDREN'S MENU SELECTIONS						
Kid's Meal Cheeseburger	1	290	13	25	5	1
Kid's Meal Chicken Nuggets	1 serv	180	11	11	1	1
Kid's Meal Hamburger	1	250	10	25	5	1
Sandwich Crispy Chicken	1	330	14	36	4	2
SALAD DRESSINGS AND TOPPINGS						
Buttery Best Spread	1 serv	50	5	0	0	0
Cheddar Cheese Shredded	1 serv	70	6	1	0	0
Croutons Gourmet	1 serv	80	3	12	0	0
Dipping Sauce Heartland Ranch	1 serv	120	12	3	2	0
Dressing Avocado Ranch	1 serv	100	10	2	1	0
Dressing Classic Ranch	1 serv	100	10	2	1	0

FOOD	PORTION	CAL	FAT	CARB	SUGAR	FIBER
Dressing Classic Ranch Light	1 serv	50	5	2	1	0
Dressing Creamy Red Jalapeno	1 serv	100	10	2	1	0
Dressing French Fat Free	1 serv	40	0	9	8	0
Dressing Italian Vinaigrette	1 serv	70	6	4	3	0
Dressing Lemon Garlic Caesar	1 serv	110	11	2	1	0
Dressing Thousand Island	1 serv	160	15	5	4	0
Dressing Vinaigrette Pomegranate	1 serv	60	3	8	7	0
Hot Chili Seasoning	1 pkg	5	0	1	1	0
Ketchup	1 pkg	10	0	3	2	0
Nugget Sauce Barbecue	1 serv	45	0	11	4	0
Nugget Sauce Honey Mustard	1 serv	80	6	7	3	0
Nugget Sauce Sweet & Sour	1 serv	50	0	12	11	0
Saltine Crackers	1 serv	25	1	4	0	0
Seasoned Tortilla Strips	1 serv	80	5	11	0	1
SALADS						
Apple Pecan Chicken	1 serv	340	11	28	20	5
Baja	1 serv	540	32	34	10	12
BLT Cobb w/o Dressing	1 serv	450	25	9	5	3
Caesar Side w/o Dressing & Croutons	1 serv	60	4	5	2	2
Garden Salad w/o Dressing & Croutons	1 serv	25	0	5	3	2
Spicy Chicken Caesar w/o Dressing & Croutons	1 serv	470	25	26	3	5

FOOD	PORTION	CAL	FAT	CARB	SUGAR	FIBER
SANDWICHES AND SIDES						
Bacon Deluxe Double	1	890	56	42	10	3
Bacon Deluxe Single	1	670	40	42	10	3
Baconator Double	1	970	63	40	10	2
Baconator Single	1	660	40	40	9	2
Baked Potato Plain	1 (10 oz)	270	0	61	3	7
Baked Potato w/ Sour Cream & Chives	1	320	4	63	4	7
Cheesy Cheddarburger	1	300	15	24	4	1
Chicken Nuggets	5	220	14	13	1	0
Chili	1 sm	210	6	21	6	6
Club Asiago Ranch w/ Homestyle Chicken	1	690	36	56	9	4
Club Asiago Ranch w/ Spicy Chicken	1	710	37	57	9	3
Club Asiago Ranch w/ Ultimate Chicken Grill	1	570	27	41	9	3
Double ½ Lb	1	800	48	42	10	3
Double Stack	1	400	21	26	5	1
Fries	1 med	420	21	55	0	6
Go Wrap Grilled Chicken	1	260	10	25	3	1
Go Wrap Homestyle Chicken	1	320	16	30	1	1
Go Wrap Spicy Chicken	1	340	16	31	1	1
Jr. Bacon Cheeseburger	1	400	24	25	5	2
Jr. Cheeseburger	1	290	13	26	5	1
Jr. Cheeseburger Deluxe	1	350	19	27	6	2
Jr. Hamburger	1	250	10	25	5	1
Sandwich Crispy Chicken	1	380	20	37	4	2

FOOD	PORTION	CAL	FAT	CARB	SUGAR	FIBER
Sandwich Homestyle Chicken Fillet	1	510	21	54	8	4
Sandwich Monterey Crispy Chicken	1	400	20	37	4	2
Sandwich Spicy Chicken Fillet	1	530	22	55	8	3
Sandwich Ultimate Chicken Grill	1	390	10	42	10	3
Single ¼ Lb	1	580	33	42	10	3
The "W"	1	580	33	40	9	3
Triple ¾ Lb	1	1060	67	42	10	3
Wrap Crispy Chicken Caesar	1	430	25	35	1	2

INDEX

(T) = Table